TEACHING PATIENTS WITH

ACUTE CONDITIONS

Springhouse Corporation
Springhouse, Pennsylvania

STAFF

Executive Director, Editorial
Stanley Loeb

Editorial Director
Matthew Cahill

Clinical Director
Barbara F. McVan, RN

Art Director
John Hubbard

Senior Editor
June Norris

Clinical Editor
Joan E. Mason, RN, EdM

Drug Information Editor
George J. Blake, RPh, MS

Editor
Edith McMahon

Copy Editors
Jane V. Cray (supervisor), Christina
Price

Designers
Stephanie Peters (associate art
director), Kristina Gabage, Donald
Knauss, Doug Miller (photographer)

Typography
David Kosten (director), Diane Paluba
(manager), Elizabeth Bergman, Joyce
Rossi Biletz, Phyllis Marron, Robin
Rantz, Valerie Rosenberger

Manufacturing
Deborah Meiris (manager), T.A. Landis

Production Coordination
Colleen M. Hayman

Editorial Assistants
Maree DeRosa, Beverly Lane, Mary
Madden

Library of Congress Cataloging-in-Publication Data

Teaching patients with acute conditions.
  p. cm.
  Includes bibliographical references and
index.
  1. Patient education—Study and teaching.
2. Nurse and patient.
I. Springhouse Corporation.
  [DNLM: 1. Acute Disease—nursing.
  2. Patient Education—methods—nurses' instruction. WY 100 T253]
RT90.T42 1992
615.5'07—dc20
DNLM/DLC
                                            92-2170
ISBN 0-87434-496-4   CIP

Contents

INTRODUCTION

As a nurse today, you face ever-increasing demands on your time and skills, especially with growing numbers of acutely ill patients. Whether these patients recover depends not only on the care they receive but also on their compliance with treatment and the teaching you provide. Unfortunately, with limited time available for care, let alone for teaching, your task may seem monumental. Fortunately, you can turn to *Teaching Patients with Acute Conditions* for help.

In this valuable book, you'll find virtually everything you need—from background information for you to reproducible instructional materials for your patients. The book's 11 chapters use the same easy-to-follow format. Organized primarily by body system, each chapter begins with a definition of the condition and points out difficulties to expect in teaching.

Following this introduction, you'll find a discussion of the condition's causes and pathophysiology. Then, you'll read about the complications that may occur—especially if the patient doesn't comply with prescribed treatment. Next, you'll find a discussion of the diagnostic workup that the patient may undergo, including what you must teach him about specific tests. In the section about treatments, you'll review activity, diet, drug, procedural, and surgical therapies.

At the end of each chapter, after a list of pertinent sources of information and support, you'll find reproducible patient-teaching aids. Printed in large, easy-to-read type and usually illustrated, these teaching aids can be photocopied and distributed to your patients. You'll save time because you'll no longer have to write out patient instructions or use incomplete forms. You'll have a wealth of teaching materials on such topics as avoiding infection, administering medications, preventing injury, using oxygen, preparing for diagnostic tests, and much more.

Besides patient-teaching aids, you'll find other features to help you teach quickly and effectively. These features include:
• sample teaching plans
• convenient and brief drug charts identifying adverse reactions and highlighting teaching points
• timesaving teaching tips
• answers to questions patients commonly ask.

With the help of all these features, you'll meet your goal of effectively teaching patients with acute conditions.

1

Cardiovascular Conditions

Contents

Myocardial infarction

Few disorders provoke as much fear and anxiety in a patient as does myocardial infarction (MI). Typically, the patient will worry not only about his immediate survival, but also about his quality of life after recovery. When severe, his anxiety can impair his ability to learn and cooperate. What's worse, it can increase his risk of complications. Obviously, then, helping to ease the patient's emotional distress ranks among your first nursing priorities. To achieve this and improve the patient's receptiveness to your teaching, you'll need to recognize anxiety, even when it's masked by denial and other coping mechanisms.

Shortly after the patient's hospitalized with an MI, you'll need to interpret for him the intensive care environment, with its bewildering array of equipment. You'll also need to explain immediate treatment measures to help ensure his compliance. For example, the doctor may schedule intracoronary or I.V. thrombolytic therapy or percutaneous transluminal coronary angioplasty (PTCA) to restore cardiac blood flow. Or the doctor may elect immediate open-heart surgery. Your teaching must be carefully timed and sensitive enough to see the patient through this acute period.

During recovery, you'll need to emphasize the importance of resuming activity gradually to give the heart time to heal. The patient may be anxious about beginning an exercise program, resuming sexual activity, or returning to work. Your teaching can help him understand that having an MI doesn't mean he should stop living; he must simply be careful not to overexert himself.

Because MI usually results from coronary artery disease (CAD), you'll find it helpful to refer to the previous chapter for additional teaching materials and ideas. There, you'll learn how to teach the patient to modify CAD risk factors—smoking, high serum cholesterol level, hypertension, obesity, sedentary life-style, and stress. By modifying them, the patient will reduce his risk of another MI.

Discuss the disorder

Tell the patient that an MI results from blocked coronary arterial flow, which reduces the oxygen supply to the affected area of the heart (see *When the blood supply stops,* page 4). This causes chest pain, ranging from a mild discomfort to a burning or crushing sensation that may radiate to the arm, jaw, neck, or shoulder blades. If blood flow isn't restored, the affected area of the heart becomes necrotic. Later, scar tissue forms but isn't able to contract. This reduces the heart's ability to pump blood, placing the

Richard K. Gibson, RN, MN, JD, CCRN, CS, wrote this chapter. He's a clinical nurse specialist in the surgical intensive care unit at Veterans Administration Hospital, San Diego.

CHECKLIST

Teaching topics in MI

□ How atherosclerosis, thromboembolism, or coronary artery spasm can occlude coronary blood flow
□ Area of infarction
□ Importance of following the prescribed treatment plan to aid recovery and forestall complications
□ Preparation for blood enzyme studies, serial ECGs, and other tests
□ Importance of bed rest
□ Exercise program and precautions
□ Dietary restrictions
□ Drug therapy for acute MI and for long-term care
□ Preparation for percutaneous transluminal coronary angioplasty, pulmonary artery catheterization, or other procedures
□ Preparation for coronary artery bypass surgery, if scheduled
□ Measures to reduce long-term complications, such as controlling weight, quitting smoking, and reducing stress
□ Support groups

patient at risk for another MI.

Discuss the causes of MI with the patient. By far the most common cause is atherosclerosis in one or more coronary arteries. This disorder is characterized by the buildup of fatty, fibrous plaques that narrow or occlude the arterial lumen. Thrombosis, or clot formation, often occurs in atherosclerotic arteries and is a contributing factor in many MIs.

Not all MIs result from atherosclerosis or thrombosis. Sudden smooth muscle contraction or spasm in a coronary artery can block blood flow to part of the heart as well. Coronary artery spasm can occur in both normal and atherosclerotic arteries, although its causes aren't well understood.

When the blood supply stops

Inform the patient that a myocardial infarction cuts off the blood supply to a portion of heart muscle, resulting in ischemia, injury, and infarction. Explain that the damaged heart produces changes in ECG waveforms. Note the characteristic changes explained below:
• *Ischemia* temporarily interrupts blood supply to myocardial tissue but generally doesn't cause cell death.

ECG changes: T wave inversion, resulting from altered tissue repolarization. (See waveform at top right.)
• *Injury* results from prolonged blood supply interruption, causing further cell injury.
ECG changes: elevated ST segment, resulting from altered depolarization. Consider an elevation greater than 1 mm significant. (See middle waveform.)

• *Infarction* ensues from complete lack of blood reaching the cell. This causes tissue necrosis.
ECG changes: pathologic Q wave (or Q-S segment), resulting from abnormal depolarization or from scar tissue that can't depolarize. Look for Q wave duration of 0.04 second or more or an amplitude measuring at least a third of the QRS complex.

CHANGES ON OPPOSITE SIDE

CHANGES ON DAMAGED SIDE

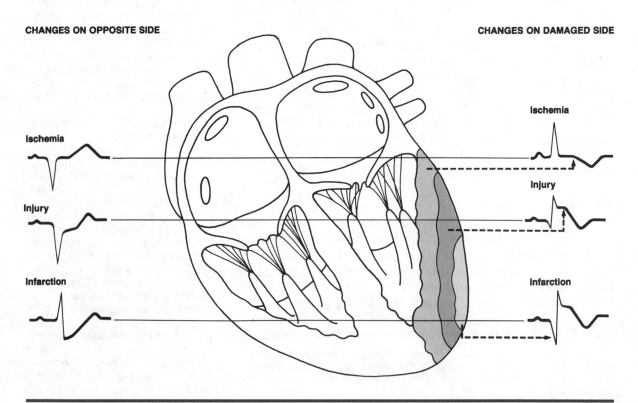

Ischemia

Injury

Infarction

Ischemia

Injury

Infarction

Complications
Stress to the patient that his compliance with prescribed treatment can significantly reduce the risk of another MI, congestive heart failure, or even death. Use discretion in deciding when and how to point out potential complications. Above all, you don't want to worsen the patient's anxiety.

Describe the diagnostic workup
Prepare the patient for tests to confirm an MI and determine the extent of damage to the heart. Later on, you'll need to teach about tests to detect the cause of chest pain, evaluate dysrhythmias, assess perfusion and scarring, and evaluate drug therapy.

Initial tests
Such tests include serial blood studies, electrocardiography (ECG), thallium and technetium scans, echocardiography, and cardiac catheterization.

Serial blood tests. Explain to the patient that blood samples will be collected regularly to detect fluctuations in cardiac enzyme level, reflecting evidence of MI.

ECG. Inform the patient that this 15-minute test evaluates the heart's function by graphically recording its electrical activity. It usually doesn't cause discomfort. The nurse will cleanse, dry, and possibly shave different sites on the patient's body, such as his chest and arms, and will apply a conductive jelly on them. Then she'll attach electrodes at these sites.

Explain that talking or limb movement will distort the ECG recordings and require additional testing time. The patient must lie still, relax, breathe normally, and remain quiet. Mention that this test will be repeated several times.

Resting thallium imaging. Inform the patient that this test assesses myocardial scarring and perfusion. It may be performed within the first few hours of onset of symptoms. Explain that he'll receive an injection of thallium, a radioisotope, and be placed in different positions while a scintillation camera scans multiple images of his heart. Reassure him that there is no known radiation danger from the thallium isotope.

Technetium scan. If the doctor orders a technetium scan, explain to the patient that the test detects damaged areas of heart muscle. The test takes about 45 minutes.

Tell the patient that the doctor will inject technetium pyrophosphate, a radioisotope, into an arm vein about 3 hours before the test. Reassure him that the injection causes only transient discomfort and that it involves negligible radiation exposure.

During the test, the patient will be placed in a supine position. A series of scans will be taken at different angles. Instruct him to remain still.

Echocardiography. Describe echocardiography as a safe and painless method of evaluating the size, shape, and motion of various cardiac structures. Mention that the procedure usually takes 15 to 30 minutes and that the patient may undergo other tests, such as an ECG or phonocardiography, simultaneously. Explain

6   Myocardial infarction

that before the test, conductive jelly will be applied to his chest. Tell the patient that he must remain still during the test because movement may distort results.

Inform the patient that during the test a technician will angle a transducer over the patient's chest to observe different parts of the heart, and may reposition him on his left side. While changes in heart function are recorded, the patient may be asked to breathe in and out slowly, to hold his breath, or to inhale a gas with a slightly sweet odor (amyl nitrite). Amyl nitrite may cause dizziness, flushing, and tachycardia. Reassure the patient that these effects quickly subside.

Cardiac catheterization. Inform the patient that cardiac catheterization evaluates the function of his heart and its vessels. The test reveals coronary artery stenosis or evaluates left ventricular function before coronary artery bypass surgery. It usually takes between 2 and 3 hours.

Inform the patient that after injecting a local anesthetic into the patient's groin, the doctor threads a catheter through an artery to the left side of the heart or through a vein to the right side of the heart and to the lungs. Next, the doctor will inject a contrast dye through the catheter. Instruct the patient to follow directions to cough or breathe deeply, and inform him that he may receive nitroglycerin during the test to dilate coronary vessels and to aid visualization.

Subsequent tests
After the patient's condition stabilizes, the doctor may order an exercise ECG (possibly with a thallium scan), an ambulatory ECG, or electrophysiologic studies.

Exercise ECG. Explain to the patient that an exercise ECG (also known as a stress test or a treadmill or graded exercise test) evaluates his heart's response to walking on a treadmill or pedaling a stationary bicycle. It usually takes about 30 minutes. Inform him that he mustn't eat or smoke cigarettes for 2 hours before the test. Explain that the test will make him perspire and that he should wear loose, lightweight clothing and snug-fitting shoes. Men usually don't wear a shirt during the test, and women usually wear a bra and a lightweight short-sleeved blouse or a patient gown with front closure.

Encourage the patient to express any fears about the test. Reassure him that a doctor will be present at all times. Emphasize that he can stop if he feels chest pain, leg discomfort, breathlessness, or severe fatigue. Tell the patient that before he begins, a technician will cleanse, shave (if necessary), and abrade sites on his chest and, possibly, his back. Then he'll attach electrodes at these sites.

If the patient's scheduled for a multistage treadmill test, tell him that the treadmill speed and incline increase at predetermined intervals and that he'll be told of each adjustment. If he's scheduled for a bicycle ergometer test, tell him that resistance to pedaling gradually increases as he tries to maintain a specific speed. Typically, he'll feel tired, out of breath, and sweaty during the test. Still, encourage him to report any of these sensations. Mention that his blood pressure and heart rate will be checked periodically.

Inform the patient that he may receive an injection of the radioisotope thallium during the test so the doctor can evaluate coronary blood flow. Reassure him that the injection involves negligible radiation exposure.

Tell the patient that after the test, his blood pressure and ECG will be monitored for 10 to 15 minutes. Explain that he should wait at least 1 hour before showering, and then he should use warm water. For more information, give him a copy of the patient-teaching aid *Learning about a stress test,* page 16.

Ambulatory ECG. Explain to the patient that this test records his heart's beat-by-beat response to normal activities over a prolonged period, usually 24 hours. (The test is also known as Holter monitoring or ambulatory monitoring.)

Inform the patient that a technician will cleanse, dry, and possibly shave different sites on the patient's body, such as his chest and arms, and will apply a conductive jelly on them. Then the technician will attach electrodes at these sites.

If the patient will be taking the test at home, tell him he'll wear a small, lightweight tape recorder with a belt or shoulder strap. Instruct him to record his activities and feelings in a diary. If applicable, teach him how to mark the tape at the onset of symptoms. Urge him not to tamper with the monitor or disconnect lead wires or electrodes.

Demonstrate how to check the recorder for proper function. Light flashes, for example, may indicate a loose electrode; the patient should test each one by depressing its center and should call the doctor if one comes off. Finally, provide the patient with a copy of the patient-teaching aid *Using your Holter monitor,* page 17.

Electrophysiologic studies. Explain to the patient that these tests evaluate his heart's electrical activity and may also monitor the effect of medication taken for an irregular heart rhythm. They take 2 to 5 hours.

Instruct him to avoid food, fluids, and nonprescription drugs for 6 hours before the test. Explain that a catheter insertion site on his groin will be shaved and cleansed.

Explain that after injection of a local anesthetic, a catheter will be inserted into the femoral vein and advanced into the right side of the heart. The patient will receive an I.V. sedative to help him relax. Tell him he may feel mild pressure at the groin site but that he should report any other discomfort. Explain that the doctor may try to induce extra heartbeats with the catheter.

Inform the patient that after the catheter is removed, pressure and then a heavy dressing are applied to the site to control bleeding. The nurse will check the site frequently for swelling. Tell the patient he may need to lie with his leg straight for a few hours after the test.

Teach about treatments
Initial treatment focuses on reducing pain and preventing further myocardial damage. If the doctor discovers a coronary artery

8 Myocardial infarction

Questions patients ask about activity after MI

When can I have sex again?
Usually, the doctor will give his okay for you to resume sex several weeks after your heart attack. Sex uses up about as much energy as climbing two flights of stairs or completing a session in week 3 or 4 of your walking program.

When can I start driving again?
Wait 3 to 4 weeks before driving and then start out with short trips. Driving increases stress and makes you tense your arm muscles—neither of which is good for your healing heart.

How will I know if I'm overdoing my exercise program?
You're overdoing it if you feel chest pain, dizziness, or extremely short of breath during exercise, or if you're tired for more than 45 minutes after exercise. To monitor your heart during exercise, take your pulse. If your pulse exceeds 110 beats/minute or if you notice a new irregularity, you're probably overdoing it. (If you're taking a beta blocker, though, your pulse rate may not rise this high during exercise.) If your pulse rate changes or you develop the symptoms above, just go back to a more comfortable exercise level.

thrombus, he may attempt to dissolve it with a thrombolytic drug, such as alteplase or streptokinase. Or, if thrombolytic therapy can't be instituted in time or isn't warranted, he may need to perform emergency surgery.

To help the patient recuperate, the doctor may recommend an exercise program and prescribe medications, as well as life-style changes. If these steps aren't sufficient to correct the patient's problem, the doctor may order coronary angioplasty or coronary artery bypass grafting (CABG).

Activity

Explain to the patient that 1 to 2 days of bed rest after an MI greatly reduces the demands on his heart and improves his chances for recovery. While he's in bed, encourage him to regularly wiggle his toes to reduce the risk of thromboembolism. However, caution against pressing his feet against the footboard, raising his legs off the bed, and performing any other activity that strains his heart.

Teach the patient about his prescribed activity program. Emphasize the need to resume activities gradually. For example, he'll progress from sponge baths in bed to unsupervised showers. Tell him to plan his daily activities so that he alternates light and heavy tasks and rests between them. Encourage him to share tasks with a family member, when necessary. Also encourage him to resume sexual activity after discharge. A satisfying sex life can help speed recovery. Before discharge, provide him with copies of the patient-teaching aids *Maintaining a safe level of activity,* pages 18 and 19, and *Resuming sex after a heart attack,* page 20.

Encourage the patient to initiate an exercise program, and give him a copy of the patient-teaching aid *Walking the road to recovery,* page 21. Warn against exercising in extreme heat or cold. Suggest walking in an enclosed shopping mall when the weather's inclement. Caution him to stop exercising immediately if he feels dizzy, faint, or short of breath or if he develops chest pain. Point out that exercise may bring on angina, which he may mistake for the chest pain of MI. Teach him how to treat angina.

Diet

Usually, the MI patient receives only clear fluids during the first days of hospitalization. Explain the reason for this: digesting solid foods places a greater strain on his heart. Tell the patient to avoid caffeine, which also stimulates his heart. (See *Caffeine warning.*)

Medication

If appropriate, explain to the patient that I.V. or intracoronary thrombolytic drug therapy helps to restore blood flow in the obstructed coronary arteries. (You may need to provide this explanation after therapy has been initiated.) Explain that these drugs need to be given within a few hours of the onset of MI to halt ischemia. Prepare him for frequent blood tests to monitor particles of dissolved clots. If the intracoronary route is chosen, prepare him for staying in bed with his leg straight.

Tell the patient about prescribed parenteral medications as you administer them. For instance, explain that I.V. nitroglycerin and morphine will help to relieve chest pain by increasing the oxygen supply to his heart; nitroprusside will lower his blood pressure, reducing the demand on his heart; lidocaine will control dysrhythmias; and dopamine or dobutamine will strengthen cardiac contractions.

After the patient's condition stabilizes, teach him about comfort-enhancing drugs that he may receive during hospitalization. These may include stool softeners to prevent straining during defecation, sedatives to decrease anxiety, and hypnotics to promote rest.

Long-term drug therapy may be prescribed to help control dysrhythmias, lower blood pressure, and strengthen cardiac contractions. See *Teaching patients about drugs for MI,* pages 10 to 13, for teaching points on antiarrhythmics, antihypertensives, cardiac glycosides, loop diuretics, and potassium-sparing diuretics.

Procedures
Before any procedure, give the patient a clear, simple explanation. Even if he fails to understand all the details, your concern and reassurance can improve his prospects for recovery. Mention that he'll receive supplemental oxygen through a nasal cannula for the first 24 to 48 hours and as needed thereafter to keep his heart and other tissues well oxygenated.

Percutaneous transluminal coronary angioplasty (PTCA). Inform the patient that although thrombolytic drugs dissolve the coronary artery clot, they do not expand arteries narrowed by CAD. Therefore, he may need to undergo PTCA to expand the affected arteries. Explain that PTCA involves threading a thin balloon-tipped catheter into the narrowed coronary artery. By injecting contrast dye through the catheter, the doctor can pinpoint the site of arterial narrowing under a fluoroscope. He then inflates the balloon catheter to expand and reopen the artery. Tell the patient that he'll receive a local anesthetic to numb the catheterization site, a sedative to promote relaxation, an anticoagulant to prevent embolism, and nitroglycerin to prevent coronary artery spasm. Warn the patient that he may feel flushed and experience brief chest pain as the contrast dye is infused.

Pulmonary artery catheterization. The doctor may order this procedure if the patient develops congestive heart failure, hypotension, hypertension, or oliguria. It may also be done to assess cardiac function or to monitor the effects of drug therapy. Explain

continued on page 14

Caffeine warning

Advise the MI patient to avoid caffeine. Explain that modifications in his diet are intended to help his heart rest and heal, whereas caffeine will stimulate his heart, causing it to beat harder and faster.

Large amounts of caffeine appear in coffee, cola, and tea. For instance, a 5-oz cup of coffee (brewed, drip method) contains 60 to 180 mg of caffeine. The same amount of imported brewed tea contains 25 to 110 mg of caffeine. A 12-oz glass of regular cola contains 30 to 46 mg of caffeine.

Suggest substituting decaffeinated coffee or tea, or other beverages. A 5-oz cup of brewed decaffeinated coffee, for example, contains only 2 to 5 mg of caffeine. A 12-oz glass of decaffeinated cola contains only trace amounts of caffeine. Also recommend substituting orange or lemon-lime soda, root beer, tonic water, ginger ale, or club soda for beverages that are high in caffeine.

10 Myocardial infarction

Teaching patients about drugs for MI

DRUG	ADVERSE REACTIONS	TEACHING POINTS
Antiarrhythmics		
amiodarone (Cordarone)	Be alert for diaphoresis, dyspnea, lethargy, tingling in the extremities, and weight loss or gain. Other: corneal microdeposits, photosensitivity, and bluish pigmentation.	• Tell the patient that if he misses a dose, he should take that dose as soon as possible, unless the next scheduled dose is less than 4 hours away. Tell him to never double-dose. • Demonstrate proper instillation of methylcellulose ophthalmic solution, if prescribed, which may reduce corneal microdeposits. Because corneal microdeposits usually don't interfere with vision, advise the patient that an eye examination is necessary only if vision changes occur. • Tell him that limiting sun exposure is the best way to prevent sunburn and that clothing provides more protection than a sunscreen. Also tell him to wear sunglasses if he experiences photosensitivity reactions.
disopyramide (Norpace)	Be alert for ankle edema, dizziness, drowsiness, excessive hunger, hypotension, impotence, irregular heart rate, rapid weight gain, shortness of breath, urinary retention, and weakness. Other: anorexia; constipation; and mouth, nose, and eye dryness.	• Because disopyramide may cause hypoglycemia, teach the patient these telltale symptoms: excessive hunger, weakness, drowsiness, and shakiness. If symptoms develop, he should eat sweets, such as candy, or drink a sugar-containing beverage, such as orange juice. Then he should call his doctor immediately. • Instruct him to rise slowly from a sitting or lying position to prevent dizziness or fainting from hypotension. • Tell him to avoid operating machinery until he has taken disopyramide for a while without experiencing adverse effects. • Suggest that he chew gum or ice chips to relieve mouth dryness and use artificial tears or saline eyewash for eye dryness. • Advise him to increase his dietary fiber and fluid intake and to use bulk laxatives if he experiences constipation. • Advise him to avoid alcohol, which can further reduce blood pressure. • Instruct him to take the drug on an empty stomach—1 hour before or 3 hours after a meal. • Tell him to take a missed dose as soon as possible, but warn him not to double-dose.
mexiletine (Mexitil)	Be alert for coordination difficulties, heartburn, dizziness, light-headedness, nausea, and nervousness. Other: tremors, confusion, drowsiness, headache, irregular heart rate, numbness, vomiting, sleep disturbance, and visual disturbances.	• Explain to the patient that he can reduce nausea by taking the drug with food. • Tell him to take a missed dose as soon as possible, but warn him not to double-dose.
procainamide (Procan SR, Pronestyl)	Be alert for hypotension and systemic lupus erythematosus-like syndrome (chills and fever, joint pain, malaise, and rash). Other: anorexia, bitter taste, diarrhea, dizziness, and GI upset.	• Instruct the patient to take procainamide on an empty stomach, if possible. • Advise him to reduce bothersome GI symptoms by taking procainamide with food. Caution him never to chew, break, or crush an extended-release tablet before swallowing it; this destroys the tablet's coating and releases the full drug dose all at once. • Tell him to take a missed dose as soon as possible, but warn him not to double-dose.

continued

Teaching patients about drugs for MI—*continued*

DRUG	ADVERSE REACTIONS	TEACHING POINTS
Antiarrhythmics—*continued*		
quinidine (Cardioquin, Cin-Quin, Duraquin)	Be alert for blurred vision, severe or prolonged diarrhea, hypotension, irregular heart rate, shortness of breath, syncope, and tinnitus. Other: anorexia, diarrhea, nausea, and vomiting.	• Advise the patient to take the drug with food to reduce GI upset. • Tell him to take a missed dose as soon as possible, but warn him not to double-dose. • Warn him to limit his use of antacids, which can raise blood levels of quinidine and exacerbate adverse effects.
tocainide (Tonocard)	Be alert for chest pain, chills, confusion, cough, dyspnea, easy bruising and bleeding, fever, hypotension, irregular heart rate, rash, sore throat, unsteadiness, sudden weight gain, and wheezing. Other: dizziness, fatigue, headache, nausea, numbness, sweating, and tremors.	• Explain to the patient that he can reduce nausea by taking the drug with food. • Tell him to weigh himself at least every other day and to report any sudden weight gain. • Tell him to take a missed dose as soon as possible, but warn him not to double-dose.
Antihypertensives		
captopril (Capoten) **enalapril maleate** (Vasotec) **lisinopril** (Prinivil, Zestril)	Be alert for chest pain, diaphoresis, severe diarrhea, dyspnea, fever, mouth sores, rapid heart rate, rash, sore throat, and severe vomiting. Other: altered taste, dizziness, fatigue, headache, and palpitations.	• Teach the patient to minimize postural hypotension by rising slowly from a sitting or lying position. • Tell him to drink 2 to 3 quarts of fluid a day, unless otherwise ordered. This will help prevent hypotension. • Instruct him to avoid foods with extremely high potassium levels (low-salt milk and salt substitutes) and to limit his intake of high-potassium foods, such as bananas and citrus fruits. • Advise him to check with his doctor or pharmacist before taking over-the-counter cold or allergy preparations. Many contain drugs that will increase blood pressure and counteract the effectiveness of this medication. • Tell him to take a missed dose as soon as possible, but warn him not to double-dose.
clonidine (Catapres)	Be alert for ankle edema, skin pallor, vivid dreams or nightmares, and persistent cough. Other: constipation, drowsiness, insomnia, dry mouth, and slow heart rate.	• Suggest to the patient that he take one of his scheduled daily doses just before bedtime to take advantage of the drug's tendency to cause drowsiness. • If he experiences constipation, instruct him to increase dietary fluids and fiber and to use bulk laxatives, as needed. • Tell him to chew gum, suck hard candy, or use mouth rinses to relieve dry mouth. • Instruct him to limit his alcohol intake and to avoid over-the-counter sympathomimetics, such as ephedrine-containing nasal sprays. • Tell him to take a missed dose within 6 hours, but warn him not to double-dose.
hydralazine (Apresoline)	Be alert for chest pain, numbness, palpitations, rapid heart rate, systemic lupus erythematosus-like syndrome (fever, joint pain, malaise, and rash), and tingling. Other: anorexia, diarrhea, headache, nasal congestion, and nausea.	• Instruct the patient to take the drug on an empty stomach—1 hour before or 3 hours after a meal. • Advise him to avoid over-the-counter sympathomimetics, such as ephedrine-containing nasal sprays. • If a four-doses-a-day schedule is prescribed, tell him to take a missed dose only up to 2 hours before his next scheduled dose; warn against double-dosing. Help him work out a regular medication schedule.

continued

Teaching patients about drugs for MI—*continued*

DRUG	ADVERSE REACTIONS	TEACHING POINTS
Antihypertensives—*continued*		
methyldopa (Aldomet)	Be alert for chest pain, depression, edema, fever, impotence, syncope, very slow heart rate, weakness, and weight gain. Other: decreased libido, diarrhea, dizziness, drowsiness, dry mouth, nausea, slightly slow heart rate, stuffy nose, and vomiting.	• Instruct the patient to take one of his daily doses at bedtime because the drug tends to cause drowsiness. • Reassure him that drowsiness is usually transient. Tell him to notify his doctor if it persists. • Tell him to rise slowly from a sitting or lying position to minimize postural hypertension. • Advise him to use chewing gum, hard candy, or mouth rinses to relieve dry mouth. • Advise him to limit his alcohol intake. • Advise him to check with his doctor or pharmacist before taking over-the-counter cold or allergy preparations. Many contain drugs that will increase blood pressure and counteract the effectiveness of this medication. • Tell him to take a missed dose as soon as possible, but warn him not to double-dose.
minoxidil (Loniten)	Be alert for distended neck veins, dyspnea, edema, rapid heart rate, and weight gain. Other: lengthening and darkening of fine body hair.	• Tell the patient to remove unwanted hair by shaving or using a depilatory. • If beta blockers are prescribed to control reflex tachycardia, explain that he must take both drugs on schedule to ensure their safety and effectiveness. Similarly, if diuretics are prescribed to control sodium and water retention, tell him he must also take them on schedule. • Tell him to weigh himself at least every other day and to report any sudden weight gain. • Advise him to avoid over-the-counter sympathomimetics, such as ephedrine-containing nasal sprays. • Tell him to take a missed daily dose within 8 hours of the scheduled time, but no later. Warn him not to double-dose.
prazosin (Minipress)	Be alert for chest pain, dyspnea, edema, rapid heart rate, and syncope. Other: drowsiness, gastric upset, headache, and dizziness.	• Advise the patient to take the initial dose at bedtime. Dizziness is most pronounced after this dose. • To reduce dizziness, tell him to take the drug with food. • Tell him to limit his alcohol intake to prevent dizziness. • Advise him to check with his doctor or pharmacist before taking over-the-counter cold or allergy preparations. Many contain drugs that will increase blood pressure and counteract the effectiveness of this medication. • Tell him to take a missed dose as soon as possible, but warn him not to double-dose.
Cardiac glycosides		
digoxin (Lanoxicaps, Lanoxin)	Be alert for abdominal pain, anorexia, visual disturbances, dizziness, drowsiness, fatigue, headache, irregular heart rate, loss of appetite, malaise, nausea, and vomiting. Other: breast enlargement.	• Teach the patient to take his pulse before taking digoxin and to report an unusually low pulse rate to his doctor. • Tell him to avoid antacids, kaolin and pectin mixtures, antidiarrheals, and laxatives, which decrease digoxin absorption. Also instruct him to limit his fiber intake, as dietary fiber can decrease digoxin absorption. • If he is also taking cholestyramine (Questran or Cholybar), advise him to wait at least 2 hours after taking digoxin before taking this medicine. • Tell him to establish a regular routine for taking digoxin each day. • Warn him not to take another person's tablets because different generic digoxin tablets are absorbed at different rates. • Instruct him to take a missed dose within 12 hours, but warn him not to double-dose.

continued

Teaching patients about drugs for MI—*continued*

DRUG	ADVERSE REACTIONS	TEACHING POINTS
Loop diuretics		
bumetanide (Bumex) **ethacrynic acid** (Edecrin) **furosemide** (Lasix)	Be alert for fever, hearing loss, increased thirst, jaundice, muscle cramps, nausea, tinnitus, unusual fatigue or weakness, urgent or burning urination, and vomiting. Other: anorexia, blurred vision, diarrhea, dizziness, muscle aches and cramps, and weight loss.	• If the patient takes the drug twice daily, tell him to take the second dose in late afternoon rather than at night, to prevent sleep interruption from nocturia. • Advise him to limit his alcohol intake to prevent dizziness. • Advise him to take the drug with meals to prevent GI distress. • Encourage intake of high-potassium foods (citrus fruits, tomatoes, bananas, dates, and apricots). Also remind him to take potassium supplements, if ordered. • Instruct him to record his weight daily to monitor fluid loss. To minimize postural hypotension, tell him to rise slowly from a lying or sitting position. • Advise him to check with his doctor or pharmacist before taking over-the-counter cold or allergy preparations. Many contain drugs that will increase blood pressure and counteract the effectiveness of this medication. • Instruct him to take a missed dose as soon as possible. Warn him not to double-dose.
Potassium-sparing diuretics		
amiloride (Midamor) **spironolactone** (Aldactone) **triamterene** (Dyrenium)	Be alert for confusion, irregular heart rate, muscle flaccidity, numbness, tingling in hands and feet, and weight changes. Other: decreased libido, diarrhea, headache, nausea, stomach cramps, vomiting, and weakness.	• Advise the patient to take the drug with food to relieve GI distress. • Tell him to weigh himself at least every other day and to report any unusual weight changes. • Advise him to check with his doctor or pharmacist before taking over-the-counter cold or allergy preparations. Many contain drugs that will increase blood pressure and counteract the effectiveness of this medication.
Thiazide and thiazide-like diuretics		
chlorothiazide (Diuril) **chlorthalidone** (Hygroton, Thalitone) **hydrochlorothiazide** (multiple brands) **metolazone** (Diulo, Zaroxolyn)	Be alert for excessive thirst, fever, irregular heart rate, lethargy, dry mouth, muscle cramps, rash, urgent or burning urination, weakness, and weak pulse. Other: anorexia, diarrhea, dizziness, GI distress, and restlessness.	• Instruct the patient not to take an evening dose just before bedtime, to prevent sleep interruption from nocturia. • Caution the diabetic patient that this drug may elevate his blood glucose level. • Instruct him to record his weight daily to monitor fluid loss. • Instruct him to avoid large doses of calcium supplements. • Advise him to check with his doctor or pharmacist before taking over-the-counter cold or allergy preparations. Many contain drugs that may increase his blood pressure and decrease the effectiveness of this medication. • Teach him to increase his intake of foods high in potassium, such as bananas and citrus fruits. • Tell him to take a missed daily dose within 8 hours. Otherwise, he should skip the missed dose. Warn him not to double-dose.

to the patient that a sheath will be inserted into the subclavian, jugular, or femoral vein under local anesthesia and then be sutured in place. Next, a thin balloon-tipped catheter will be introduced through the sheath. This balloon-tipped catheter will be carried by the circulation through the right atrium and right ventricle into the pulmonary artery. There, certain pressures will be measured until the patient's condition stabilizes.

Intra-aortic balloon pump (IABP) insertion. The doctor may insert an IABP to stabilize a patient with cardiogenic shock or uncontrollable chest pain or before performing CABG. The IABP also helps to maintain cardiac function during or just after surgery. It's typically used as an emergency procedure.

If appropriate, inform the patient or his family that the doctor will insert the balloon percutaneously through the femoral artery and into the descending aorta, slightly beyond the origin of the

Reversing ischemia with the intra-aortic balloon pump

Intra-aortic balloon catheter insertion is typically performed at the patient's bedside as an emergency procedure. If time permits, explain to the patient that the doctor will place a special catheter in the aorta to help his heart pump more easily. The intra-aortic balloon pump supports an ischemic heart in two ways: It improves myocardial perfusion, which increases the heart's oxygen supply, and it relieves the left ventricle's work load.

This illustration shows the balloon resting in the descending aorta, just below the left subclavian artery. Balloon inflation and deflation is closely coordinated with the patient's cardiac cycle.

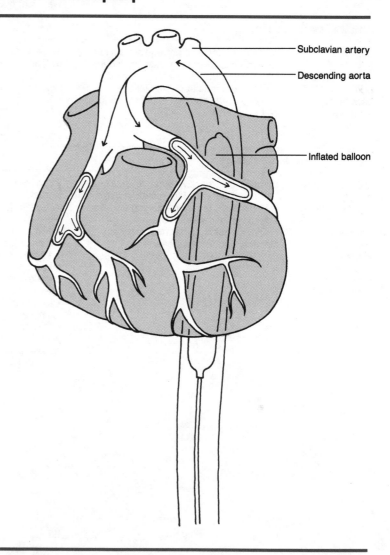

Subclavian artery

Descending aorta

Inflated balloon

left subclavian artery. Explain that the balloon inflates and deflates in synchrony with cardiac events, increasing the heart's oxygen supply and decreasing its oxygen demand.

Tell the patient or his family how the catheter is inserted and that it will be connected to a large console next to the patient's bed. Mention that the console has an alarm system, that any alarms will be answered promptly, and that the pumping sound of the console is normal. Explain that because of the catheter, he won't be able to sit up, bend his knee, or flex his hip more than 30 degrees. (See *Reversing ischemia with the intra-aortic balloon pump.*)

Surgery
If appropriate, prepare the patient for surgery. The doctor may perform CABG to treat acute MI or complications associated with cardiac catheterization or PTCA. He may also repair abnormalities, such as papillary muscle rupture or ventricular aneurysm, during open-heart surgery.

Other care measures
Educate the patient about the importance of correcting certain risk factors for MI, such as high blood pressure, high serum cholesterol level, and smoking. Also refer him to support and information groups.

Sources of information and support
American Cancer Society
90 Park Avenue, New York, N.Y. 10016
(212) 599-8200

American Heart Association
7320 Greenville Avenue, Dallas, Tex. 75231
(214) 750-5300

American Lung Association
1740 Broadway, New York, N.Y. 10019
(212) 315-8700

Further readings
American College of Cardiology/American Heart Association. "Guidelines for Exercise Testing," *Journal of the American College of Cardiology* 8(3):725-38, September 1986.
American Hospital Formulary Service. *AHFS Drug Information 89.* Bethesda, Md.: American Society of Hospital Pharmaceuticals, 1989.
Codini, M. "Management of Acute Myocardial Infarction," *Medical Clinics of North America* 70(4):769-90, July 1986.
Curran, C., and Mathewson, M. "Use of Cardiac Glycosides in the Critically Ill," *Critical Care Nurse* 7(6):31-42, November/December 1987.
Newton, K., and Killien, M. "Patient and Spouse Learning Needs During Recovery from Coronary Artery Bypass," *Progressive Cardiovascular Nursing* 3(2):62-9, April-June 1988.

Learning about a stress test

Dear Patient:

First of all, don't be intimidated by the name "stress test." The only stress involved is some carefully controlled physical exercise.

What the test does

A stress test tells your doctor how your heart functions while you're exercising. It may be combined with another test, called a thallium scan, to evaluate blood flow through your coronary arteries to the heart muscle itself.

What happens during the test

After not eating or drinking (except for normal medications) for at least 4 hours before the test, you'll go to the cardiology lab. There, the nurse will attach electrocardiogram (ECG) monitors to your chest and arms, along with a blood pressure cuff. Then, you'll either ride a stationary bike or walk on a treadmill at gradually increasing speeds and slopes. While you're exercising, you'll have your blood pressure taken frequently and an ECG will be run continuously. Be sure to report as soon as you feel tired, short of breath, or dizzy, or experience chest pain.

Thallium scan

If the test includes a thallium scan, the doctor will inject thallium into a vein in your arm while you're exercising (see illustration). Then, he'll ask you to continue exercising for several minutes.

Next, you'll be taken to the scanner room where the doctor will take pictures of your heart with a special scanner. These pictures will show how well your coronary arteries supply blood to your heart during exercise.

About 4 hours after you finish exercising, the doctor may take more pictures of your heart. They'll show him how well your coronary arteries supply blood to your heart after a rest period.

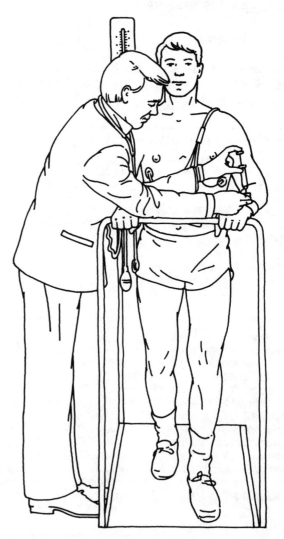

Using your Holter monitor

Dear Patient:

Your doctor has ordered a Holter monitor for you to wear for 24 hours. It works like a continuous electrocardiogram (ECG) by recording any irregular heartbeats you may have. The information from this recording will help your doctor judge how well your heart medication is working.

The monitor has various leads that the nurse will attach to your skin. She'll also show you how to wear the monitor on a belt or over your shoulder. If one of the leads becomes loose, secure it with a piece of tape.

While wearing the monitor, you can perform most of your usual activities. You'll even wear it to bed.

Practice these safety measures:
• Don't get the monitor wet—don't shower, bathe, or swim with it on.
• Avoid high-voltage areas, strong magnetic fields, and microwave ovens.

While you're wearing the monitor, the doctor wants you to write your activities and feelings. (You can use the diary below as an example.) Your diary will help your doctor establish a connection between your monitor tracing and your activities and feelings. Jot down the time of day when you perform any activity, such as taking medication, eating, drinking, moving your bowels, urinating, engaging in sexual activity, experiencing any strong emotions, exercising, or sleeping.

If your monitor has an event button, the nurse will show you how to press it should you experience anything unusual, such as a sudden, rapid heartbeat.

DAY	TIME	ACTIVITY	FEELINGS
Tuesday	10:30 am	Rode from hospital in car	Legs tired, some shortness of breath
	11:30 am	Watched TV in living room	Comfortable
	12:15 pm	Ate lunch, took Inderal	Indigestion
	1:30 pm	Walked next door to see neighbor	Shortness of breath
	2:45 pm	Walked home	Very tired, legs hurt
	3:00-4:00 pm	Urinated, took nap	Comfortable
	5:30 pm	Ate dinner, slowly	Comfortable
	7:20 pm	Had bowel movement	Shortness of breath
	9:00 pm	Watched TV-drank 1 beer	Heart beating fast for about one minute, no pain
	11:00 pm	Took Inderal, urinated, went to bed	Tired
Wednesday	8:15 am	Awoke, urinated, washed face and arms	Very tired, rapid heart beat for about 30 seconds
	10:30 am	Returned to hospital	Felt better

Maintaining a safe level of activity

Dear Patient:

Based on your condition and diagnostic test results, the doctor has determined the maximum level of activity that you can safely tolerate. This level is expressed as a MET (metabolic energy equivalent), which is a measure of energy and oxygen consumption. It predicts how much activity your cardiovascular system can safely support.

Find the column below corresponding to your MET level. You may engage in any of the activities listed, plus those under lower MET levels. Keep in mind that these are only general guidelines. Stop any activity that produces chest pain, prolonged shortness of breath, or excessive fatigue.

1 MET	1 to 2 METs	2 to 3 METs	3 to 4 METs	4 to 5 METs
Home activities				
• Bed rest • Sitting • Eating • Reading • Sewing • Watching television	• Dressing • Shaving • Brushing teeth • Washing at sink • Making bed • Desk work • Driving car • Playing cards • Knitting	• Tub bathing • Cooking • Waxing floor • Riding power lawn mower • Playing piano • Sexual intercourse	• General housework • Cleaning windows • Light gardening • Pushing light power mower	• Heavy housework • Heavy gardening • Home repairs, including painting and light carpentry • Raking leaves
Occupational activities				
• No activity allowed	• Typing (electric typewriter) • Operating a computer	• Driving small truck • Using hand tools • Typing (manual typewriter) • Repairing car	• Assembly-line work • Driving large truck • Bricklaying • Plastering	• Painting • Masonry • Paperhanging
Exercise or sports activities				
• No activity allowed	• Walking 1 mph (1.6 km/hr) on level ground	• Walking 2 mph (3.2 km/hr) on level ground • Bicycling 5 mph (8 km/hr) on level ground • Playing billiards • Fishing • Bowling • Golfing (with motor cart) • Operating motorboat • Riding horseback (at walk)	• Walking 3 mph (4.8 km/hr) • Bicycling 6 mph (9.7 km/hr) • Sailing • Golfing (pulling hand cart) • Pitching horseshoes • Archery • Badminton (doubles) • Horseback riding (at slow trot) • Fly-fishing	• Calisthenics • Table tennis • Golfing (carrying bag) • Tennis (doubles) • Dancing • Slow swimming

continued

Maintaining a safe level of activity—*continued*

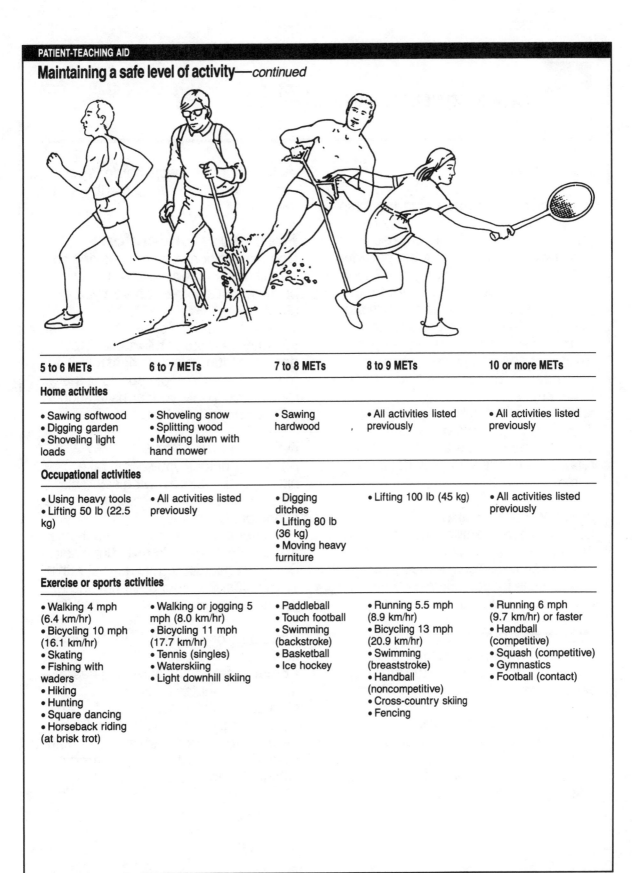

5 to 6 METs	6 to 7 METs	7 to 8 METs	8 to 9 METs	10 or more METs
Home activities				
• Sawing softwood • Digging garden • Shoveling light loads	• Shoveling snow • Splitting wood • Mowing lawn with hand mower	• Sawing hardwood	• All activities listed previously	• All activities listed previously
Occupational activities				
• Using heavy tools • Lifting 50 lb (22.5 kg)	• All activities listed previously	• Digging ditches • Lifting 80 lb (36 kg) • Moving heavy furniture	• Lifting 100 lb (45 kg)	• All activities listed previously
Exercise or sports activities				
• Walking 4 mph (6.4 km/hr) • Bicycling 10 mph (16.1 km/hr) • Skating • Fishing with waders • Hiking • Hunting • Square dancing • Horseback riding (at brisk trot)	• Walking or jogging 5 mph (8.0 km/hr) • Bicycling 11 mph (17.7 km/hr) • Tennis (singles) • Waterskiing • Light downhill skiing	• Paddleball • Touch football • Swimming (backstroke) • Basketball • Ice hockey	• Running 5.5 mph (8.9 km/hr) • Bicycling 13 mph (20.9 km/hr) • Swimming (breaststroke) • Handball (noncompetitive) • Cross-country skiing • Fencing	• Running 6 mph (9.7 km/hr) or faster • Handball (competitive) • Squash (competitive) • Gymnastics • Football (contact)

Resuming sex after a heart attack

Dear Patient:

After you're discharged from the hospital, you can expect to gradually resume most, if not all, of your usual activities, including sex. Most patients, in fact, can resume having sex 3 to 4 weeks after a heart attack. As far as physical demands, sex is a moderate form of exercise, no more stressful than a brisk walk. However, keep in mind that sex can place a strain on your heart if it's accompanied by emotional stress.

Read over the following guidelines. They can help you have a satisfying sex life. And be sure to discuss any related concerns with your doctor or nurse.

Setting significant

Choose a quiet, familiar setting for sex. A strange environment may cause stress.

Make sure the room temperature is comfortable for you. Excessive heat or cold makes your heart work harder.

When to have sex

Have sex when you're rested and relaxed. A good time is in the morning, after you've had a good night's sleep.

When not to have sex

Don't have sex when you're tired or upset. Also avoid having sex after drinking a lot of alcohol. Alcohol expands your blood vessels, which makes your heart work harder. And don't have sex after a big meal; wait a few hours.

Positioning for comfort

Choose positions that are relaxing and permit unrestricted breathing. Any position that's comfortable for you is okay.

Don't be afraid to experiment. At first, you may be more comfortable if your partner assumes a dominant role. You may also want to avoid positions that require you to use your arms to support yourself or your partner.

A few precautions

Ask your doctor if you should take nitroglycerin before having sex. This medication can prevent angina attacks during or after sex.

Remember, it's normal for your pulse and breathing rates to rise during sex. But they should return to normal within 15 minutes. Call your doctor at once if you have any of these symptoms after sex:
• sweating or palpitations for 15 minutes or longer
• breathlessness or increased heart rate for 15 minutes or longer
• chest pain that's not relieved by two or three nitroglycerin tablets (taken 5 minutes apart) or a rest period, or both
• sleeplessness after sex or extreme fatigue the next day.

PATIENT-TEACHING AID

Walking the road to recovery

Dear Patient:

This simple daily walking program can help to strengthen your heart and speed your recovery. Be sure to allow the full times for warm up and cool down.

To limber up your muscles, do stretching exercises, such as calf and shoulder stretches. For the calf stretch, place both hands on a wall, about shoulder height. Step with one foot toward the wall and lean against it, keeping your palms flat on the wall and your feet flat on the floor. Push against the wall until you feel a pull in your leg.

For the shoulder stretch, clasp your hands over your head and pull your shoulders backward.

WEEK	WARM UP	EXERCISE	COOL DOWN	TOTAL TIME
1	Stretch 2 min. Walk slowly 3 min.	Walk briskly 5 min.	Walk slowly 3 min. Stretch 2 min.	15 min
2	Stretch 2 min. Walk slowly 3 min.	Walk briskly 7 min.	Walk slowly 3 min. Stretch 2 min.	17 min
3	Stretch 2 min. Walk slowly 3 min.	Walk briskly 9 min.	Walk slowly 3 min. Stretch 2 min.	19 min
4	Stretch 2 min. Walk slowly 3 min.	Walk briskly 11 min.	Walk slowly 3 min. Stretch 2 min.	21 min
5	Stretch 2 min. Walk slowly 3 min.	Walk briskly 13 min.	Walk slowly 3 min. Stretch 2 min.	23 min
6	Stretch 2 min. Walk slowly 3 min.	Walk briskly 15 min.	Walk slowly 3 min. Stretch 2 min.	25 min
7	Stretch 2 min. Walk slowly 3 min.	Walk briskly 18 min.	Walk slowly 3 min. Stretch 2 min.	28 min
8	Stretch 2 min. Walk slowly 5 min.	Walk briskly 20 min.	Walk slowly 5 min. Stretch 2 min.	34 min
9	Stretch 2 min. Walk slowly 5 min.	Walk briskly 23 min.	Walk slowly 5 min. Stretch 2 min.	37 min
10	Stretch 2 min. Walk slowly 5 min.	Walk briskly 26 min.	Walk slowly 5 min. Stretch 2 min.	40 min
11	Stretch 2 min. Walk slowly 5 min.	Walk briskly 28 min.	Walk slowly 5 min. Stretch 2 min.	42 min
12 and after	Stretch 2 min. Walk slowly 5 min.	Walk briskly 30 min.	Walk slowly 5 min. Stretch 2 min.	44 min

PATIENT-TEACHING AID

Learning about digoxin

Dear Patient:

Your doctor has prescribed digoxin (the label may also read Lanoxin or Lanoxicaps) to strengthen your heart's ability to pump blood. This drug also slows down your pulse and regulates your heart rate.

Be sure to take your digoxin exactly as the label directs. Take it at the same time each day. That way, you'll be less likely to forget it.

However, if you do forget a dose, you can make it up within 12 hours of your scheduled administration time. Don't take two doses at the same time.

Check your pulse
Once a day, preferably in the morning *before* taking digoxin, check your pulse. If your pulse rate is less than 60 beats a minute or if your pulse rhythm isn't regular, call your doctor.

Report side effects
Because digoxin is one of the oldest drugs, a lot is known about its effects. Be sure to let your doctor know right away if you feel tired, drowsy, or dizzy or get a headache.

Also let your doctor know right away if you lose your appetite, throw up or feel like throwing up, or notice any changes in your vision, such as seeing halos.

Watch your diet
Some foods can change the way digoxin works. High-fiber foods, for instance, can reduce your body's absorption of digoxin. So, be sure to cut back on these foods. They include bran, raw and leafy vegetables, and most fruits.

Ask about other drugs
Before you take *any other drug,* talk to your pharmacist or doctor. That's because some drugs change the way digoxin works. You'll need to avoid antacids, antidiarrhea drugs (such as Kaopectate), and laxatives.

If your doctor has also prescribed cholestyramine (Questran or Cholybar) for you, you'll need to wait at least 2 hours after taking digoxin before taking this drug.

A few reminders
• Don't take another person's digoxin tablets.
• Don't change the brand of digoxin you've been taking. Another brand of digoxin may have a different effect on you.
• Don't let anyone else take your medication.
• Store your digoxin in a cool, dry area. Don't keep it in your bathroom medicine cabinet.
• Throw away any digoxin that is unused or several years old.

Inflammatory heart disease

Ordinarily, inflammation serves as a signal that the immune response is protecting the body from invading microorganisms. In the heart, however, inflammation damages more than it protects, leaving the patient vulnerable to cardiac disease for the rest of his life.

Clearly then, you'll focus on teaching the patient how inflammatory heart disease can impair cardiac function and how treatment and self-care measures help to preserve function and prevent recurrence. Of course, you'll also teach about diagnostic tests, surgery if needed, and other procedures. Keep in mind, though, that once the patient recovers and feels well, he may forget about his vulnerability to cardiac disease. That's why you'll need to carefully review complications, point out warning signs, and stress the need for ongoing monitoring.

Discuss the disorder

Explain to the patient which type of inflammatory heart disease he has—pericarditis (the most common), infective endocarditis, myocarditis, or rheumatic heart disease. All stem from infection and leave the heart vulnerable to recurrent inflammation (see *What causes inflammatory heart disease?* page 26). All, however, have different signs and symptoms, complications, treatments, and self-care requirements. And all affect the heart differently.

Pericarditis affects the pericardium—the thin, clear, fluid-containing sac that surrounds and protects the heart (see *How the pericardium protects the heart,* page 26). When inflammation starts, the pericardial sac loses fluid (see *Understanding pericarditis,* pages 24 and 25). This produces friction, as the heart muscle and pericardium rub together during normal contractions. Called friction rub, this hallmark of pericarditis can be detected on auscultation. Other symptoms include dyspnea and a dull or sharp chest pain that lasts from hours to days. The pain increases with breathing or turning, but usually subsides when the patient leans forward.

Infective endocarditis, an inflammation of the cardiac endothelium, may develop in patients with an acquired valvular or congenital cardiac lesion. It most commonly affects the mitral and aortic valves. In this disorder, circulating pathogens become trapped and form vegetative growths on inflamed areas. These growths may perforate the valve leaflets, obstruct the valve orifices, and spread to the chordae tendineae or to the papillary mus-

Linda S. Baas, RN, MSN, CCRN, who wrote this chapter, is a cardiovascular clinical nurse specialist at the University of Cincinnati Hospital. Ms. Baas is also engaged in doctoral studies at the University of Texas at Austin.

CHECKLIST

Teaching topics in inflammatory heart disease

☐ Explanation of the patient's type of inflammatory heart disease: pericarditis, infective endocarditis, myocarditis, or rheumatic heart disease
☐ Causes of inflammatory heart disease
☐ Complications and preventive measures
☐ Activity restrictions and dietary recommendations
☐ Drug therapy, including antibiotic and anti-inflammatory agents
☐ Possible surgical interventions, such as pericardiocentesis or parietal and visceral pericardiectomies
☐ Reportable signs, such as activity intolerance, shortness of breath, and weight gain.
☐ Sources of information and support

Understanding pericarditis

When discussing pericarditis with your patient, you'll want to describe how the body responds when a pathogen attacks the pericardium, the protective sac that encloses the heart. This sequence shows the course of bacterial inflammation in pericardial tissue, illustrating the body's defenses at work.

1. INFLAMMATION

Pericardial tissue damaged by bacteria or other substances releases chemical mediators of inflammation (such as prostaglandins, histamines, bradykinins, and serotonins) into the surrounding tissue, starting the inflammatory process. Friction occurs as the pericardial layers rub against each other.

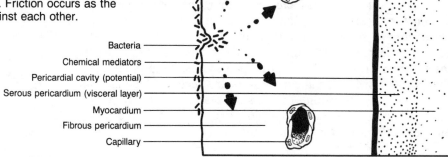

Bacteria
Chemical mediators
Pericardial cavity (potential)
Serous pericardium (visceral layer)
Myocardium
Fibrous pericardium
Capillary

2. VASODILATION AND CLOTTING

Histamines and other chemical mediators cause vasodilation and increased vessel permeability. Local blood flow to the area (hyperemia) increases. Vessel walls leak fluids and proteins (including fibrinogen) into tissues, causing extracellular edema. Clots of fibrinogen and tissue fluid form a wall, blocking tissue spaces and lymph vessels in the injured area. This wall impedes the spread of bacteria and toxins to adjoining healthy tissues.

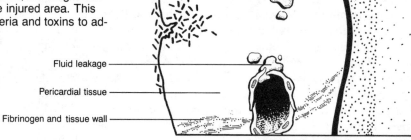

Fluid leakage

Pericardial tissue

Fibrinogen and tissue wall

3. PHAGOCYTOSIS: INITIAL RESPONSE

Macrophages already present in the tissues begin to phagocytize the invading bacteria, but usually fail to stop the infection.

Macrophage

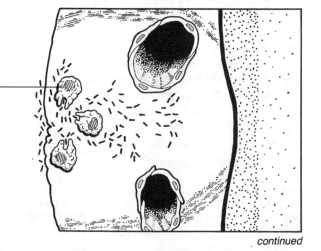

continued

Understanding pericarditis – *continued*

4. PHAGOCYTOSIS: ENHANCED RESPONSE

Substances released by the injured tissue stimulate neutrophil production in the bone marrow. Neutrophils then travel to the injury site through the bloodstream and join macrophages in destroying pathogens. Meanwhile, additional macrophages and monocytes migrate to the injured area and continue phagocytosis.

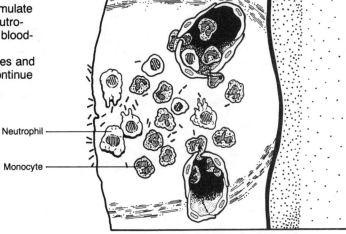

Neutrophil

Monocyte

5. EXUDATION

After several days, the infected area fills with an exudate composed of necrotic tissue and dead and dying bacteria, neutrophils, and macrophages. Thinner than pus, this exudate forms until all infection ceases, creating a cavity that remains until tissue destruction stops. The contents of the cavity autolyze and are gradually reabsorbed into healthy tissue.

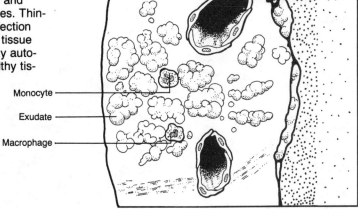

Monocyte

Exudate

Macrophage

6. FIBROSIS AND SCARRING

As the end products of the infection slowly disappear, fibrosis and scar tissue may form. Scarring, which can be extensive, may ultimately cause heart failure if it restricts movement.

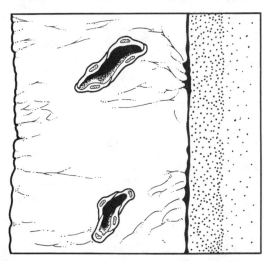

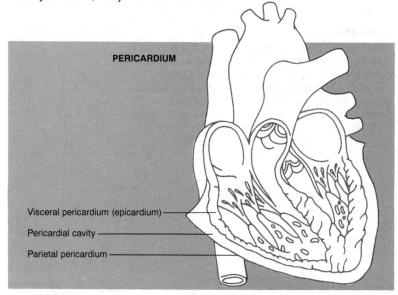

How the pericardium protects the heart

When teaching the pericarditis patient, show him an illustration of the pericardium. Seeing the pericardium and understanding its function may help him understand his condition and the need for treatment.

Point out that the pericardium, a double-walled, fluid-filled sac, surrounds the heart wall. Explain that the *visceral pericardium* (also called the epicardium) serves as the pericardium's inner wall and the heart wall's outer layer. The *parietal pericardium*, a smooth, translucent membrane, serves as the pericardium's outer wall. The cavity between the parietal and visceral pericardium contains 20 to 50 ml of lymphlike, lubricating fluid. Pressure in the *pericardial cavity,* normally negative, rises intermittently during ventricular filling, forcing excess fluid into the mediastinum's lymphatic channels.

Besides lubricating the beating heart and acting as a protective barrier between the heart and other organs, the pericardium also:
- holds the heart in a fixed position
- supports the great vessels, preventing them from kinking
- restrains ventricular dilation during exertion, preventing overstretching of the myocardium, a layer of the heart wall.

PERICARDIUM

Visceral pericardium (epicardium)
Pericardial cavity
Parietal pericardium

What causes inflammatory heart disease?

Use this list to help identify possible causes of the four most common types of inflammatory heart disease.

Pericarditis
- bacterial, fungal, or viral infection
- rheumatic fever
- cardiac injury (possibly from trauma or surgery)
- autoimmune diseases
- radiation

Infective endocarditis
- bacterial (streptococcal and staphylococcal) or fungal (*Candida, Aspergillus, Histoplasma*) infection
- I.V. drug abuse

Myocarditis
- bacterial, parasitic, or viral infection
- autoimmune disease
- chemotherapy or radiation therapy
- toxins

Rheumatic fever
- streptococcal infection that usually begins in the throat

cles, causing necrosis, dysfunction, and, rarely, rupture. As the vegetative growth continues, the patient develops vague, nonspecific symptoms of infection, such as fever, malaise, fatigue, headache, cough, anorexia, and weight loss.

Myocarditis, a focal or diffuse inflammation of the myocardium, produces more specific symptoms than infective endocarditis. Causing cellular changes that weaken the heart and reduce the force of contractions, myocarditis compromises cardiac output. Because the heart can't pump enough blood to meet activity demands, the patient may experience fatigue, dyspnea, palpitations, pericardial discomfort, or fever when he exerts himself. Typically, he may have no symptoms when he's at rest. (See *How myocarditis develops.*)

How myocarditis develops

When teaching about myocarditis, emphasize that prompt and effective treatment can lead to recovery, whereas delayed or inadequate treatment can lead to severe complications. To encourage compliance, explain to the patient how unchecked myocarditis develops into disabling heart disease.

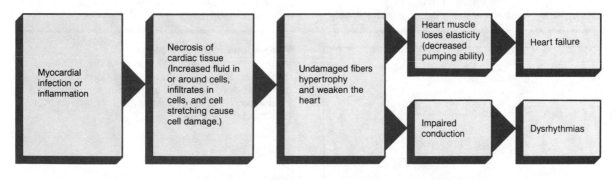

Rheumatic heart disease, which can affect one or more heart wall layers, is thought to reflect hypersensitivity to group A beta-hemolytic streptococcal infections of the throat or middle ear. Antibodies that combat these infections produce inflammatory lesions in other tissues, especially the joints and heart valves. Early stage valvular lesions injure the tissues and cause scar formation. Eventually, scarring distorts the valve and may lead to stenosis or regurgitation (see *How rheumatic fever affects heart valves,* page 28). The disease causes sudden sore throat, swollen and tender glands, pain on swallowing, a fever of 101° to 104° F. (38.3° to 40° C.), headache, and nausea. It also causes a lifelong heart murmur, which results from turbulence caused by blood flowing across heart valves that don't open sufficiently to allow smooth passage or don't close sufficiently to prevent backflow.

Complications

Inflammatory heart disease can have serious, even deadly, consequences. If the patient has pericarditis, explain that the disorder can progress to life-threatening cardiac tamponade if untreated. Signs of this complication include severe shortness of breath, sudden weight gain, edema, and an inability to carry out activities previously performed without difficulty. Other serious complications include chronic pericardial effusion, constrictive pericarditis, effusive-constrictive pericarditis, and adhesive pericarditis. Caution the patient to report jugular vein distention, shortness of breath, altered level of consciousness, and an erratic heart rate to the doctor promptly.

If the patient has infective endocarditis, point out possible complications: valvular stenosis, which restricts adequate opening, and valvular incompetence, which results in blood backflow. Other complications include heart failure, myocarditis, dysrhythmias, systemic emboli and infarctions (see *How infective endocarditis leads to embolism,* page 29). These complications can arise at any time, even weeks or months after treatment.

How rheumatic fever affects heart valves

Rheumatic fever causes gross changes in the mitral and aortic valves—edema, erosion of the valve leaflets along the closure line, and formation of beadlike vegetations along the inflamed leaflet edges. In many patients, the vegetations occur simultaneously on adjacent leaflets that scar and partially fuse as they heal.

These illustrations show a mitral valve in a possible progression from rheumatic inflammation to stenosis and regurgitation.

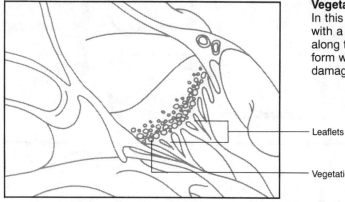

Vegetations form on leaflets
In this view, the mitral valve leaflets are inflamed, with a thin line of rheumatic vegetations formed along the delicate leaflet edges. These vegetations form when fibrin and platelets accumulate on the damaged valve surface.

— Leaflets

— Vegetations

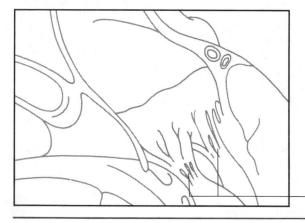

Stenosis reduces movement
In mitral stenosis, the most common valvular defect associated with recurrent rheumatic fever, inflammation causes shrinkage of the chordae tendineae as the leaflets fuse. This reduces valve movement. The left atrium attempts to force blood through the narrow valve opening into the left ventricle, eventually causing left atrial enlargement, pulmonary congestion, and right ventricular hypertrophy and failure. Unfortunately, symptoms of mitral stenosis don't usually appear until the valve opening narrows by about 50%.

— Chordae tendineae

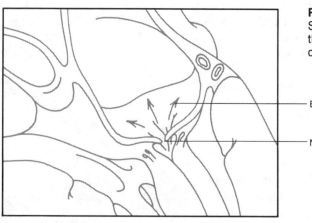

Regurgitation occurs
Some degree of regurgitation (backflow) of blood into the atrium may coexist with stenosis, because the dysfunctional valve cannot close tightly.

— Blood backflow

— Narrowed opening

How infective endocarditis leads to embolism

Besides impairing heart valves, infective endocarditis causes further complications when valve vegetations break away as emboli, travel through the bloodstream, and lodge in other organs, causing infarction. This flowchart shows the domino-like effect of infective endocarditis from infection to embolism.

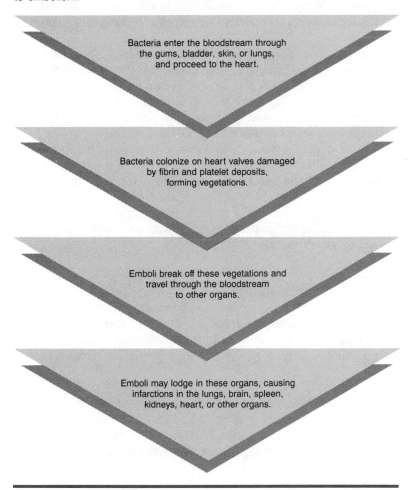

Bacteria enter the bloodstream through the gums, bladder, skin, or lungs, and proceed to the heart.

Bacteria colonize on heart valves damaged by fibrin and platelet deposits, forming vegetations.

Emboli break off these vegetations and travel through the bloodstream to other organs.

Emboli may lodge in these organs, causing infarctions in the lungs, brain, spleen, kidneys, heart, or other organs.

If the patient has myocarditis, explain that similar complications can result. These include congestive heart failure, dysrhythmias, heart block, and pulmonary or systemic emboli.

If the patient has rheumatic heart disease, mention that the most frequent complication is infective endocarditis. To help prevent this, the patient will need to take antibiotics before dental or other invasive procedures. Urge him to see his doctor immediately if he has a sore throat or other signs of streptococcal infection.

Describe the diagnostic workup

Inform the patient that he'll have blood tests, such as a white blood cell (WBC) count and erythrocyte sedimentation rate

What echocardiography tells about the heart

If the doctor orders echocardiography, tell your patient that this test assesses the size, shape, and motion of various heart structures and evaluates heart valve function.

What happens during the test
Explain that this ultrasonic procedure usually takes 15 to 30 minutes, unless the patient's having other tests, such as an ECG or phonocardiography, simultaneously. Mention that before the test, a technician will apply conductive jelly to the patient's chest before angling a microphone-like transducer over the area. Describe the mild pressure the patient may feel as this occurs. Advise him to remain still during the test because movement may distort results.

Add that the technician may direct him to lie on his left side and to breathe in and out slowly, hold his breath, or to inhale a gas with a slightly sweet odor (amyl nitrite). Amyl nitrite may cause dizziness, flushing and tachycardia. Reassure the patient that these effects subside quickly.

How the test works
Mention that the transducer transmits sound waves and receives the echoes that result from sound bouncing off the heart structures. Displayed on an oscilloscope screen, echo patterns represent various normal or abnormal structures.

(ESR), to detect infection. An elevated WBC count and increased ESR indicate inflammation. A blood culture may be performed to identify the causative microorganism. Additional tests may be performed depending on the suspected type of inflammatory heart disease.

If the doctor suspects pericarditis, the patient may undergo electrocardiography (ECG) to rule out myocardial infarction and angina and to detect other changes. He may also undergo echocardiography to detect fluid accumulation in the pericardium and, if the doctor suspects constrictive pericarditis, a computed tomography scan.

If the doctor suspects infective endocarditis, he'll order a blood culture to identify the infection (a positive result confirms the diagnosis) and echocardiography to evaluate valvular damage (see *What echocardiography tells about the heart*). He'll also order an ECG to detect dysrhythmias, and, possibly, cardiac catheterization to assess valvular damage.

If the doctor suspects myocarditis or rheumatic heart disease, teach the patient about any ordered tests. The only test that confirms myocarditis is endomyocardial biopsy (see *Preparing for endomyocardial biopsy*). In rheumatic heart disease, the patient's history and auscultation of a murmur confirm the diagnosis. However, echocardiography and cardiac catheterization may be performed to assess valvular damage, chamber size, and ventricular failure.

Teach about treatments
Regardless of the patient's type of inflammatory heart disease, you'll provide guidelines for activity, diet, and medication. If he has pericarditis, you may need to teach him about pericardiocentesis and possibly surgery.

Activity
Instruct the patient with acute pericarditis to rest in bed until his fever, pain, and malaise resolve. When he feels stronger, tell him to resume his normal activities. If he develops chronic pericarditis, however, advise him to limit strenuous activities, such as running or contact sports.

Tell the patient with acute infective endocarditis or rheumatic heart disease to limit his activities so he'll reduce the extent of valve dysfunction. As the infection is better controlled, instruct him to gradually increase his activities until he resumes his normal level. Tell him to monitor his activity tolerance so he'll know when he's overexerting himself. Give him a copy of the teaching aid *Recognizing warning signs in inflammatory heart disease*, page 33).

Explain to the acute myocarditis patient that he must reduce his activity to cut down on the heart's workload. Provide advice on how to save energy, such as by alternating light and heavy tasks and by resting frequently. If he develops heart failure symptoms, instruct him to rest in bed until he can tolerate activity.

When he's able to get around again, teach him how to monitor his activity tolerance, his breathing, and his weight, especially if symptoms of heart failure develop.

Diet
No matter what kind of inflammatory heart disease the patient has, instruct him to follow a low-fat, low-cholesterol diet as a precaution against coronary artery disease. If the patient develops heart failure symptoms, tell him to restrict fluids and sodium. If he has infective endocarditis, recommend a high-protein diet to help prevent the nutritional deficiencies that accompany this prolonged infection.

Medication
Inform the patient with pericarditis that nonsteroidal anti-inflammatory drugs (NSAIDs), such as indomethacin and aspirin, help relieve pain and reduce inflammation. If these drugs aren't effective, corticosteroids may be prescribed. Tell him he may also need antibiotics, if pericarditis is secondary to an infection.

Tell the patient with infective endocarditis that he'll receive antibiotics for 4 to 6 weeks to combat the infection. Drug therapy depends on the infecting microorganism. Urge him to notify the doctor if fever, anorexia, or other signs of relapse begin about 2 weeks after drug therapy ends. Make sure he understands the need for prophylactic antibiotics before, during, and after dental treatment and other invasive procedures. (Give him a copy of the patient-teaching aid *Preventing infection with antibiotics,* page 34). If heart failure occurs, advise him that he may need diuretics, inotropics, or vasodilators to improve heart function.

Teach the myocarditis patient that NSAIDs, such as ibuprofen (Motrin) and aspirin, relieve inflammation, whereas antibiotics combat the specific microorganism.

Instruct the patient with rheumatic heart disease that he'll receive a broad-spectrum antibiotic such as penicillin. Stress the importance of taking the full course of medication.

Procedures
If excessive fluid accumulates around the patient's heart, threatening cardiac function, the doctor may need to perform pericardiocentesis. See *What happens during pericardiocentesis,* page 32.

Surgery
Surgery is rarely needed to treat pericarditis complications. If the patient has persistent pericardial effusion (without constriction), however, the doctor may perform a parietal pericardiectomy. By removing part of the pericardium's parietal layer, this procedure allows excess pericardial fluid to drain. If constrictive pericarditis develops, the doctor may perform a visceral pericardiectomy by removing both the parietal and endocardial (visceral) layers, as necessary, to free the heart from constriction.

Preparing for endomyocardial biopsy

Explain to the patient that only endomyocardial biopsy can confirm myocarditis. Inform him that the procedure takes place in the cardiac catheterization laboratory or the operating room. Mention that many patients go home soon after the test.

Describe the procedure
Tell the patient that he'll be sedated but awake for the procedure so that he can report any unusual feelings or discomfort. Explain that his head and shoulders may be covered to provide a sterile area.

Then after the doctor numbs the patient's neck with a local anesthetic, he'll advance a catheter through the jugular vein and into the heart. Next, he threads a special device through the catheter to the right ventricle. After collecting a few heart cells, the doctor withdraws the catheter and applies light pressure to stop any bleeding at the site. Then he sends the cell samples for laboratory analysis to detect changes caused by myocardial inflammation. Advise the patient to rest a while before going home.

32   Inflammatory heart disease

What happens during pericardiocentesis

If your patient's having pericardiocentesis, explain that the procedure relieves the pressure and discomfort caused by fluid that collects in the pericardium and restricts heart function. To accomplish this, the doctor aspirates fluid through a needle positioned in the pericardial cavity.

Tell the patient that his chest will be cleaned and draped, to prevent infection, and numbed with anesthetic, to prevent pain. Reassure him that although he may feel some pressure, he won't feel pain. Then describe the monitors and devices, such as an ECG machine, that will monitor his heart's activity.

If the procedure will be performed in the operating room, tell the patient he may have a general anesthetic. Mention that the doctor may leave a flexible pericardial catheter in place temporarily so that excess fluid can be drained again, if necessary.

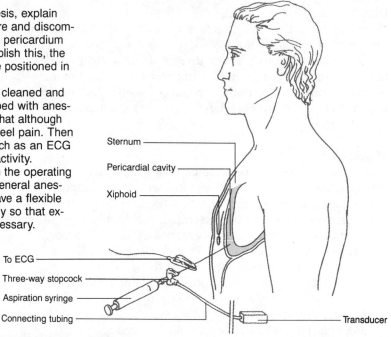

Sternum

Pericardial cavity

Xiphoid

To ECG

Three-way stopcock

Aspiration syringe

Connecting tubing

Transducer

Other care measures
Encourage the patient to comply with treatment and to see his doctor at once if he has a sore throat, flulike symptoms, or other indicators of recurrent disease. Point out that complications may still occur despite prompt treatment, but that slowing their progress will speed recovery.

Sources of information and support
American Heart Association
7320 Greenville Avenue, Dallas, Tex. 75231
(214) 373-6300

Coronary Club
9500 Euclid Avenue, Cleveland, Ohio 44106
(216) 444-3690

Further readings
Fraley, M.A. "Differential Diagnosis of Chest Pain," *Physician Assistant* 12(6):69, 73, 75, June, 1988.
"Infective Endocarditis: Basic Schema of Pathogenesis," *Hospital Medicine* 23(10):175-78, October 1987.
Kaplan, E.L. "A Comeback for Rheumatic Fever?" *Patient Care* 22(5):80-84, 87-88, 90, March 15, 1988.
Khan, A.H. "Pericarditis: Diagnosis and Treatment," *Hospital Medicine* 23(11):43, 46, 48-50, November 1987.
Trausch, P.A. "Infective Endocarditis: Nursing Care and Prevention," *Progress in Cardiovascular Nursing* 3(2):45-53, April-June 1988.

Recognizing warning signs in inflammatory heart disease

Dear Patient:

To prevent complications from inflammatory heart disease, you need to recognize the warning signs. They include chest pain, shortness of breath, unusual tiredness, sudden weight gain, and swollen hands or feet.

Don't be reluctant to tell your nurse or doctor about these warning signs, even though they may seem like nothing at first. The sooner you're treated, the better you'll feel.

Chest pain

If you have chest pain, tell your doctor right away. Describe where you feel the pain (for example, in the middle of your chest or on the left or right side) and how long the pain lasts. Then, describe its intensity (for example, sharp or dull or pressing or burning).

Think of what, if anything, seems to bring on the pain, such as breathing or turning. Also think of what, if anything, seems to relieve it, such as lying down or sitting forward.

Shortness of breath

Here's a way to tell if you're more short of breath than usual. Try talking while you go about a daily activity, such as folding the laundry or weeding the garden. If you find you can't talk without getting out of breath, slow down and check with your doctor.

Unusual fatigue

Rate your usual activities on a scale of 1 to 10. Give a score of 10 to the ones that take the most effort. Now, rate walking to the car, climbing the stairs, preparing dinner, and other activities.

If an activity is much harder to do than it used to be, or if yesterday's 5 becomes today's 10, check with your doctor.

Swelling and weight gain

Check your hands and feet for swelling. If they swell easily, tell your doctor.

Also check your weight each day at about the same time. Be sure to use the same scale and wear about the same amount of clothing. If you gain a lot of weight in a short time (say, 5 pounds in 1 week or 1 pound overnight), you could be retaining fluid. Tell your doctor.

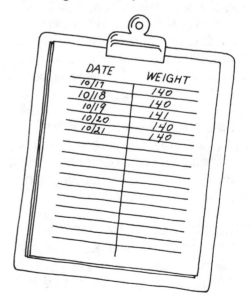

Preventing infection with antibiotics

Dear Patient:

If you're recovering from infective endocarditis or rheumatic fever, you need to avoid getting another infection, which could harm your heart valves. By taking an antibiotic drug, you can protect yourself from infection.

When to take an antibiotic
Take your antibiotic drug exactly as your doctor directs. This lets the drug do its job of fighting infection. If you've been exposed to an infection, an antibiotic helps your body defend itself by killing bacteria before they multiply and make you sick.

Your doctor may also tell you that you need to take antibiotics before you have dental work or any kind of surgery. Dental work, for instance, may allow germs to enter your bloodstream through your gums. Make sure you let your dentist or any other doctor know you have a heart valve disorder *before* any treatments.

If you forget your antibiotic
If you forget to finish or renew your prescription, let your doctor know right away. He can decide whether you need to continue your medicine.

When to call your doctor
Let your doctor know if you have any break in your skin or if you feel sick. That's because a cut, a puncture, a rash, or an abscess can introduce germs. A sore throat, fever, cold, or flu means that germs are already at work.

Be alert for signs and symptoms that your heart valves may be infected again. These include:
- shortness of breath
- fever
- fatigue
- weakness
- swollen ankles
- sudden weight gain, such as 5 pounds in a week or 1 pound overnight.

If you have any of these signs or symptoms, let your doctor know right away or go to the nearest emergency room.

An important reminder
Get a card from your local American Heart Association that tells dentists (and other health care providers) which antibiotics you need to prevent heart valve infection. Always carry the card with you. Each year, have the card checked to make sure you're carrying the latest advice.

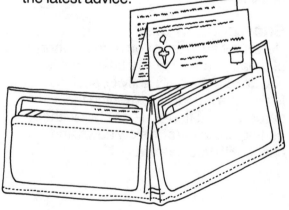

Deep vein thrombosis

You'll probably begin your teaching about deep vein thrombosis (DVT) by focusing on the acute phase. For instance, you'll instruct the patient about the need for immediate anticoagulant therapy—and possibly surgery—to prevent pain and potentially fatal complications, such as pulmonary embolism. You'll also explain the purpose of expected diagnostic tests, such as Doppler ultrasonography and impedance plethysmography.

As the patient recovers, you'll teach him about preventing or managing the long-term complications of the chronic venous insufficiencies that contribute to DVT: edema, varicose veins, and skin infection and ulceration. For example, he'll need to know how to apply antiembolism stockings and wear them, as directed. He'll need encouragement to elevate his legs periodically to improve venous return. He'll also need to learn about meticulous skin care and good nutrition to prevent skin ulcers and related infection. If he already has skin ulcers, he'll need to know how to care for them at home.

Discuss the disorder
Explain that DVT occurs when a blood clot, or thrombus, occludes a vein and blocks blood flow. (For more information, see *How a venous thrombus forms,* page 36.) Most thrombi develop in the deep veins of the leg, but they can also develop in the veins of the pelvis, kidneys, liver, right side of the heart, and arms. The disorder can lead to severe venous obstruction and injury, depending on thrombus size and collateral circulatory adequacy.

Tell the patient that DVT effects vary. Deep leg pain, swelling, and a faint blue-red skin discoloration constitute common signs and symptoms. Typically, the leg pain begins suddenly but diminishes when the patient elevates the leg. However, some patients have no symptoms, whereas others may have only a fever. The disorder most commonly occurs in hospitalized patients, especially those who've undergone surgery or who have heart disease. However, DVT can arise without warning in an otherwise healthy young adult.

Explain that DVT's exact cause remains unknown, but research links its development to three conditions: venous wall injury, venous stasis, and blood hypercoagulability (see *Managing DVT risk factors,* page 37).

Sally A. Boyle, RN, MSN, CEN, who wrote this chapter, is a critical care clinical nurse specialist at Temple University Hospital, Philadelphia.

CHECKLIST

Teaching topics in deep vein thrombosis

☐ How deep vein thrombosis (DVT) occurs
☐ Signs and symptoms of DVT
☐ Signs and symptoms of complications, such as pulmonary embolism and chronic venous insufficiency
☐ Preparation for tests, such as Doppler ultrasonography, impedance plethysmography, and blood studies
☐ Bed rest during the acute stage and daily exercise during rehabilitation
☐ Dietary guidelines to promote skin integrity and cardiovascular health
☐ Instructions for anticoagulant therapy
☐ Explanation of thrombectomy, if necessary
☐ Other care measures, such as use of antiembolism stockings, and ways to improve leg condition

How a venous thrombus forms

Before explaining deep vein thrombosis to the patient, review the sequence of pathophysiologic events that lead to thrombus formation.

Platelet aggregation
A venous thrombus begins forming when platelets adhere to the endothelium and then to each other. This platelet aggregate then becomes coated with a fibrin mesh, inducing further platelet aggregation.

Thrombus formation
Eventually, a macroscopic white thrombus forms, usually in a deep vein. This thrombus commonly obstructs the lumen and prevents blood flow between vein branches.

Stagnant blood then clots, forming a mesh of red blood cells, platelets, and fibrin. Called a red thrombus, this mass usually forms at a bifurcation. A red thrombus may retract and undergo lysis (decomposition), or it may completely occlude blood flow. With complete occlusion, blood backflow occurs unless sufficient collateral circulation develops.

Thrombus dissolution or breakup
What happens next involves two opposing processes. The thrombus dissolves in a few days (in most cases) from the normal fibrinolytic action of the thrombus, vein wall, and plasma. During this phase, large thrombus portions may break off and, as emboli, lodge in the pulmonary arterial tree. Meanwhile, a much slower process also takes place—inflammation in and around the vein wall, followed by fibroblastic thrombus organization. A thrombus that doesn't embolize may completely dissolve, leaving vein structure almost unimpaired. In some cases the thrombus may convert into fibrous tissue. Then, recanalization—usually with numerous small channels—may occur over several weeks.

The valves' role
Venous valves play a key part in venous thrombus formation. The initial platelet aggregate tends to develop in a valve pocket. If the thrombus organizes and recanalizes, it incorporates and then obliterates the valve cusps.

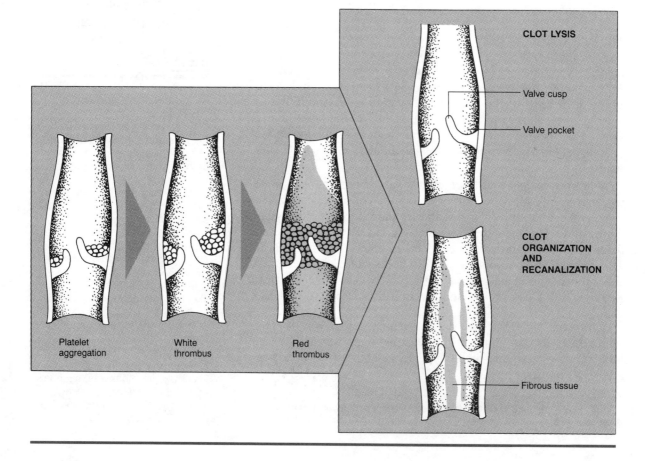

Platelet aggregation

White thrombus

Red thrombus

CLOT LYSIS

Valve cusp

Valve pocket

CLOT ORGANIZATION AND RECANALIZATION

Fibrous tissue

Managing DVT risk factors

Typically, educators point to Virchow's triad to explain deep vein thrombosis (DVT). This theory, though not conclusive, links DVT to three conditions: venous wall injury, venous stasis, and hypercoagulability.

As you teach your patient about DVT, suggest behaviors he can adopt to reduce DVT risk factors.

Prevent venous wall injury
Explain to the patient that he can prevent venous wall injuries by avoiding risky activities, such as rough sports, and by moving carefully to prevent falls or accidental collisions. Point out that venous wall injury can result from trauma, such as a fracture, dislocation, muscle injury, or venipuncture. Chemical agents (for example, X-ray contrast media), some antibiotic solutions, and irritation from an indwelling I.V. catheter can also injure the venous wall.

If the injury alters the vein's epithelial lining, the fibrinolytic activity that inhibits thrombus formation may be impaired. Without this activity, platelets collect at the injury site and become trapped by fibrin, red blood cells, and granular leukocytes. The aggregate thus formed begins the thrombus.

Reduce venous stasis
Advise the patient to help counteract venous stasis by elevating his legs when he rests, wearing antiembolism stockings, and giving up cigarette smoking.

Explain that venous stasis, which retards circulation and promotes thrombus formation, can develop from inactivity. Lacking an intrinsic force to propel blood, veins depend almost totally on voluntary muscle stimulation and competent one-way valves. Inactive voluntary muscles or incompetent valves contribute to venous stasis. Prolonged bed rest, congestive heart failure, obesity, pregnancy, and abdominal cancer, for example, represent conditions associated with venous stasis and DVT.

Control hypercoagulability
Advise the patient to follow his anticoagulant drug regimen exactly. That way, he may be able to prevent thrombus formation. Explain that hypercoagulability results when blood clots faster than normal. Hypercoagulability may result from anemia, cancer, polycythemia vera, liver disease, disseminated intravascular coagulation, trauma, or oral contraceptive use.

Complications
Inform the patient that without treatment, the thrombus may dislodge from the deep vein and be swept along in the bloodstream to the lungs, where it can cause a potentially lethal pulmonary embolism. Other possible complications include chronic venous insufficiency, skin ulceration, pain, and recurrent DVT.

Describe the diagnostic workup
Prepare the patient for routine coagulation studies and such tests as Doppler ultrasonography and impedance plethysmography to assess venous blood flow. If test findings are inconclusive, the doctor may order standard or radionuclide venography.

Doppler ultrasonography

Explain that this 10- to 20-minute test, which can detect DVT, evaluates how well blood circulates in the vessels. Tell the patient who will perform the test and where. Reassure him that the procedure doesn't involve risk or discomfort. Inform him that before the test he'll be asked to uncover his leg, arm, or neck and to loosen any restrictive clothing.

Tell the patient what to expect during the test: A small ultrasonic probe resembling a microphone will be touched to his skin at sites along blood vessels. Mention that he may be asked to hold his breath or perform Valsalva's maneuver during the test.

Impedance plethysmography

Inform the patient that this reliable, noninvasive test detects DVT in the leg. Tell him that it takes 30 to 45 minutes to examine both legs. Assure him that the test is safe and, in most cases, painless. Mention that he'll put on a hospital gown and lie on his back on an examination table or bed. The technician will cleanse, dry, and possibly shave sites on the lower legs and then attach electrodes smeared with conductive jelly. During the test the technician will wrap a pressure cuff around the patient's thigh. He'll inflate the cuff for 1 or 2 minutes and then quickly relieve the pressure. Usually the technician will repeat the test to confirm initial tracings. Emphasize that accurate test results require relaxed leg muscles and normal breathing. Reassure the patient that if he has any discomfort that interferes with leg relaxation, a mild analgesic may be given, as ordered.

Coagulation studies

If the patient's taking an anticoagulant, advise him to expect frequent blood studies to measure prothrombin time (pro time, or PT) and partial thromboplastin time (PTT). Tell him that these tests measure how fast his blood clots. They also help the doctor decide whether to adjust the patient's dosage. Tell the patient who will perform the venipuncture and when. Then mention that he may experience discomfort from the needle puncture and the tourniquet pressure. Reassure him that the actual procedure takes fewer than 3 minutes.

Explain that if the patient's PT or PTT values rise too high (indicating a risk for increased bleeding), the doctor may lower the anticoagulant dosage. If the values drop too low, the patient may be at risk for new clot formation, and his anticoagulant dosage may be increased.

Teach about treatments

If your patient has acute DVT, discuss the need for bed rest and immediate anticoagulant or thrombolytic therapy. As he begins to recover, shift your teaching focus to improving cardiovascular health. For example, encourage the patient to maintain a low-fat diet, to engage in regular exercise, and to wear antiembolism stockings to improve venous return. Prepare him for thrombectomy, if necessary. Teach him how to care for and prevent leg ulcers. Also review the warning signs of major complications, such as pulmonary embolism and chronic venous insufficiency.

Activity
During acute DVT, emphasize that bed rest helps to reduce oxygen and nutrient demands of the affected leg. Explain that immobilization can prevent the thrombus from breaking away and becoming an embolus. Add that the duration of bed rest depends on the patient's response to treatment. Instruct him to flex, extend, and rotate each foot several times an hour. Tell him that this can enhance venous return.

Later, once the acute stage subsides, advise the patient to resume his daily activities according to his doctor's instructions. Encourage him to start exercising regularly to help develop collateral circulation and improve venous return. Advise him to swim or participate in other water exercises—with his doctor's approval, of course. Caution him not to overdo any physical activity.

Diet
Inform the patient that by maintaining a healthful diet he can minimize complications—particularly skin ulcers—and improve his cardiovascular fitness. To minimize complications, instruct him to eat foods high in protein and rich in B complex and C vitamins. Tell him that vitamin C promotes healing and skin integrity, whereas the B complex vitamins help maintain blood vessel and smooth muscle tone. To help achieve cardiovascular fitness, help him investigate his eating habits. Then, review the basics of good nutrition with him, stressing general dietary restrictions, such as limiting salt and saturated fat intake.

If appropriate, encourage him to lose weight. Explain that excess weight compromises blood vessels and increases venous congestion. If he needs to diet, consult with a dietitian or nutritionist, or refer him to a self-help group, such as Weight Watchers or Overeaters Anonymous.

Medication
If the patient has acute DVT, he may receive parenteral anticoagulants or thrombolytics. Once his condition stabilizes, he'll be given an oral or self-injectable anticoagulant, such as warfarin or heparin. Explain that an anticoagulant decreases his blood's clotting ability. Instruct him to take his medication exactly as prescribed to keep an existing thrombus from expanding or new ones from forming. If appropriate, give him a copy of the patient-teaching aid *Learning about heparin*, page 42.

Before discharge, review the precautions the patient should take while using an anticoagulant. Instruct the patient to watch for adverse reactions, such as a bleeding nose or gums, chills, dark blue toes, discolored urine, fatigue, prolonged bleeding from cuts or bruises, red or tarry black stools, sore throat, excessive menstrual flow (in females), or coughing up blood. Tell him to contact his doctor if he experiences vomiting, diarrhea, or a fever that lasts longer than 24 hours. Remind him to keep all appointments for blood tests.

Advise the patient to wear a medical identification tag stating that he takes an anticoagulant. To reduce the risk of injury, suggest he shave with an electric razor, use a soft toothbrush, and install safety devices in the bathroom. If he notices a bruise, tell him to outline its margin with a felt-tipped marker and to call his doctor if the bruise extends outside the line. Instruct him to apply pressure on all cuts for 10 minutes. If he cuts an arm or leg, tell him to elevate it above his heart. If the bleeding doesn't stop, urge him to go at once to the nearest emergency department.

If the patient's receiving a thrombolytic drug, such as streptokinase or urokinase, explain that this drug breaks up or dissolves clots that occlude blood vessels. Administered in the hospital, thrombolytic drugs are given only when thrombi decrease circulation to major organs, such as the heart or lungs.

Advise the hospitalized patient to call the nurse immediately if he notices bleeding of any kind, fever, flushing, headache or muscle pain. He should also call her if he has a fast, slow, or irregular heartbeat; shortness of breath; tightness in his chest; wheezing, rash, itching, or hives; or swollen eyes, face, lips, or tongue. While he's receiving a thrombolytic, instruct him to stay in bed and to move around as little as possible.

Surgery

If necessary, prepare the patient for thrombectomy. Usually, the surgeon reserves thrombectomy for an acute thrombus in a large vein.

If anticoagulant or thrombolytic therapy fails or is contraindicated, the doctor may surgically place a tiny filter or "umbrella" in the inferior vena cava to intercept migrating thrombi and prevent pulmonary embolism. Discuss this surgery with the patient and review appropriate postoperative and self-care measures.

Other care measures

Teach the patient how to care for his feet and legs to prevent infection and skin ulcers. Instruct him to wash his feet daily in warm, soapy water and to blot them dry with a towel. Tell him to wear only leather shoes that fit properly. Point out that leather "breathes," allowing air to circulate to prevent conditions conducive to infection. Advise him to wear clean cotton socks daily.

Instruct the patient to check his feet for cuts, cracks, blisters, or red, swollen areas. Caution him against wearing tight-fitting garments or engaging in activities that can decrease leg circulation, such as sitting with crossed legs. Warn him not to pick at sores or apply adhesive tape to the skin of his feet. All of these actions may restrict blood flow or cause skin breaks that may admit infection. If the patient has leg ulcers, teach him how to change his dressings. Also give him a copy of the patient-teaching aid *Care and prevention of leg ulcers*, page 43.

To minimize venous stasis, instruct the patient to wear anti-embolism stockings whenever he's up and about. Give him a copy of the patient-teaching aid *How to apply antiembolism stockings*, page 80. Tell him what stocking size to buy and where to buy stockings. Tell him to wear them all day, every day. Remind him to check for and smooth out wrinkles throughout the day. Teach him how to maintain the elasticity of his stockings by using warm (not hot) wash water and soap (not detergent) and hanging the stockings to dry. Recommend purchasing two pairs of stockings, so he can wear one and wash the other. Mention that stockings should be difficult to put on; if they go on easily, they need to be replaced. If the patient has sharp or jagged fingernails, suggest he wear rubber gloves while applying stockings.

Review measures to improve venous circulation in the legs. Give him a copy of the patient-teaching aid *Taking steps toward healthier legs*, page 44.

Because life-threatening pulmonary embolism can develop suddenly, teach the patient to watch for and immediately report these warning signs: acute shortness of breath or severe chest pain, and a cough producing blood-tinged sputum. Also teach him to report early signs of chronic venous insufficiency, including leg pain, edema, skin changes (scaling, brown pigmentation), and dilated superficial veins.

Further readings

Fahey, V.A. "An In-depth Look at Deep Vein Thrombosis," *Nursing89* 19(1):86-93, January 1989.

Foley, W.T., et al. "When One Leg Swells," *Patient Care* 22(18):99-101, 104, 106+, November 15, 1988.

Hyers, T.M., et al. "Antithrombotic Therapy for Venous Thromboembolic Disease," *Chest* (Supplement) 95(2):37S-51S, February 1989.

McMahan, B.E. "Why Deep Vein Thrombosis Is So Dangerous," *Canadian Orthopaedic Nurses Association Journal* 10(2):9-11, June 1988.

Merli, G.J., et al. "Deep Vein Thrombosis: Prophylaxis in Acute Spinal Cord Injured Patients," *Archives of Physical Medicine and Rehabilitation* 69(9):661-64, September 1988.

"Steps to Take for Healthier Legs," *Patient Care* 22(18):155-56, November 15, 1988.

"The Risks of DVT in the Calf: Deep Vein Thrombosis," *Emergency Medicine* 21(6):59-60, March 30, 1989.

Learning about heparin

Dear Patient:

These directions will help you safely use heparin to control blood clotting. Review them at any time to refresh the instructions your nurse gave you when you learned to inject this drug.

Injecting heparin
Wash your hands and clean the injection site. Refer to the diagram below as you choose an area on your stomach between the iliac crests.

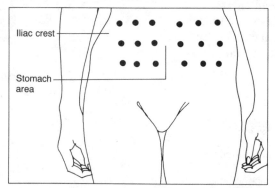

Now, pinch your skin gently and insert the needle deep into the underlying fat layer. Slowly inject the drug. Leave the needle in place for 10 seconds before you withdraw it. *Don't* massage or rub the area. Change your injection site each time you take this medicine.

Ensuring the right dose
Inject heparin exactly when your doctor directs. If you miss a dose, take it as soon as possible. If it's almost time for your next dose, though, forget the missed dose and don't double the next one. Instead, go back to your regular schedule.

Reporting side effects
Call your doctor at once if you cough up blood, have bleeding gums, nosebleeds, bruises, bloody (red-tinged) urine, black, tarry stools, or bloody or coffee ground–like vomit. If you're female, also call your doctor if you bleed unusually heavily during your period.

Also call your doctor if you have pain or swelling in your joints or stomach, unusual backaches, constipation, dizziness, or a severe or persistent headache.

Watching your diet
Eat cheese, eggs, liver, and leafy green vegetables in moderation. These foods may reduce heparin's effectiveness. Inform your doctor if you take vitamin C or E supplements. In large amounts, they may interfere with your medicine.

If you drink alcohol, limit yourself to one or two drinks a day.

Taking precautions with other drugs
Check with your doctor or pharmacist before taking other drugs, especially aspirin, which may cause bleeding.

Protecting yourself from injury
• Don't put toothpicks or sharp objects into your mouth. Don't walk barefoot. Avoid power tools and rough sports.
• Wear a medical tag that indicates you take an anticoagulant.
• Don't cut corns and calluses yourself. Consult a foot doctor.
• Tell your other doctors and your dentist that you're taking heparin.

Care and prevention of leg ulcers

Dear Patient:

You can help your leg ulcer heal and prevent new ulcers from forming by learning about your condition and its required care.

What is a leg ulcer?
It's an area of dying skin. Leg ulcers can form wherever an artery becomes blocked or constricted. When this happens, not enough blood gets to the skin and the tissue beneath it to nourish the area. Instead, blood tends to pool in your leg veins — sometimes from a condition called venous insufficiency.

Pressure then builds up in these congested leg vessels, and the blood supply to the tissues decreases. As the condition worsens, the skin becomes fragile, and an infection may develop from injury, pressure, and irritation. As a result, leg ulcers may develop.

Improving your circulation
To improve circulation in your legs, wear elastic support stockings. Called antiembolism stockings, these hose will help to return blood to your heart. They'll improve circulation to your existing ulcer and may help to keep new ones from forming.

Put your feet up. Rest and elevate your legs for as long and as often as your doctor directs. This will reduce your legs' needs for nutrients and oxygen and help to promote healing. Always raise your lower leg above heart level.

Promoting healing
Follow these measures to help your ulcer heal:
● Keep your ulcer clean to prevent infection. Always wash your hands before and after changing your dressing or touching the wound. This keeps the area germ-free.
● Follow your doctor's instructions exactly when changing your dressing and applying ointments or other medications.
● Be patient. Your ulcer may take 3 months to a year to heal.
● Check with your doctor if your ulcer grows larger, feels increasingly painful, or becomes foul-smelling.

Preventing ulcers
Follow these measures to prevent ulcers:
● Watch for signs of new ulcers. These signs include leg swelling, pain, and discolored skin that looks brownish or dark blue.
● Wear support stockings to help prevent ulcers, as well as to help heal an ulcer that's already developed.
● Be careful to avoid injury to your leg, which can lead to ulcer development. For example, avoid activities that involve rugged physical contact, such as roughhousing with children or dogs.
● Prevent falls by installing safety rails or a grab bar and placing a nonskid mat in your bathtub.
● Make sure to wear low, nonskid footwear whenever possible.

Taking steps toward healthier legs

Dear Patient:

Your doctor wants the circulation in your legs to improve. By developing healthier legs, you can help to promote healing and prevent complications, such as pain and swelling. Here's how you can have healthier legs.

Raise your legs
Rest your legs with your feet propped up higher than your heart. This helps gravity to move excess fluid out of your legs.

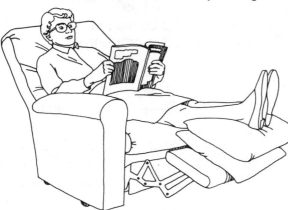

When you sit—at your desk, for example—prop up your feet with a footstool.

Watch your diet
Eat plenty of fresh fruits, vegetables, meats, and seafood. At the same time, avoid salty foods, which can increase swelling. Examples of salty foods include bacon, ham, corned beef, smoked fish, pickles, potato chips, and crackers.

When you shop, check package labels and choose products that are low in fat and salt.

Prevent infection
Wash your legs daily with soap and warm water to remove germs that could cause infection. Avoid using bath powders that could dry your skin.

Don't hesitate to call your doctor if you notice any signs of a leg infection, such as redness or swelling.

Exercise regularly
Get involved in swimming or other pool exercises, such as walking or jogging in water. Or ask your doctor if he can recommend other specific exercises for your legs.

Choose proper clothing
Avoid tight garments that could cut off circulation in your legs, such as garters, girdles, and knee-high hosiery. Wear tight elastic support stockings all day, every day.

Observe for warning signs
Make sure to inspect your legs every morning. Call your doctor if you notice these warning signs and symptoms of poor circulation:
• discolored skin (for example, brownish skin or bluish red areas)
• sores
• scales
• increasing leg pain or swelling.

Follow your treatment plan
Take your anticoagulant or other prescribed medication exactly as your doctor directs. And keep all appointments for follow-up visits with your doctor.

Dysrhythmias

Affecting a broad section of the population, dysrhythmias vary from mild, asymptomatic disturbances like sinus arrhythmia to life-threatening disturbances like ventricular fibrillation, which requires immediate intervention. This greatly complicates your teaching responsibilities. Not only are you teaching about diverse degrees of illness, but you're also teaching patients of diverse learning needs, ages, and health histories.

Regardless of your patient's status, your goal remains the same: to teach him about his specific dysrhythmia and its treatment. For some patients, treatment may mean implantation of a temporary or permanent pacemaker or an automatic implantable cardioverter defibrillator. If an implant is planned, you'll teach your patient not only about preoperative and postoperative care, but also about long-term follow-up.

Discuss the disorder

Tell the patient that a dysrhythmia is an abnormal change in his heart rate, rhythm, or both. Explain that normal conduction of the heart's electrical impulses can become disrupted for various reasons (both congenital and acquired). Briefly explain the normal conduction pathway: impulses usually originate in the sinoatrial node, then travel across the atria through the atrioventricular node to the bundle of His, and then disperse throughout the ventricles. Tell the patient that any disruption of this pathway can produce dysrhythmias.

As appropriate, discuss the characteristics and significance of the patient's dysrhythmia (see *Reviewing common dysrhythmias,* pages 46 and 47).

Complications

Reinforce the need to follow prescribed treatment by pointing out the possible consequences of untreated or improperly treated dysrhythmias. Without alarming the patient, explain that dysrhythmias alter cardiac output, which can lead to a wide range of complications—from palpitations, dizziness, and syncope to life-threatening thromboembolism or cardiac arrest.

Ann Aschoff, RN, BSN, and **Richard Gibson, RN, MN, JD, CCRN, CS,** contributed to this chapter. Ms. Aschoff is a nurse clinician I, cardiac electrophysiology, at the University of Iowa Hospitals and Clinics, Iowa City. Mr. Gibson is a clinical nurse specialist in the surgical intensive care unit at Veterans Administration Hospital, San Diego.

CHECKLIST

Teaching topics in dysrhythmias

☐ Explanation of normal cardiac conduction
☐ Explanation of the patient's specific dysrhythmia
☐ Preparation for diagnostic tests, such as an ECG, serum electrolyte studies, and electrophysiologic studies
☐ Activity instructions: regular exercise, appropriate warnings
☐ Dietary restrictions: moderate use of alcohol, caffeine, and tobacco; increased potassium intake, as ordered
☐ Antiarrhythmic drugs
☐ Prescribed treatments, such as carotid sinus massage, Valsalva's maneuver, temporary pacemaker implantation, electrocardioversion
☐ Preparation for implantation of permanent pacemaker or an automatic implantable cardioverter defibrillator (AICD), if necessary
☐ Guidelines for pacemaker or AICD use and maintenance, if necessary
☐ How to take pulse rate
☐ Sources of information and support

Reviewing common dysrhythmias

Study these descriptions to help you explain to your patient his type of dysrhythmia.

DYSRHYTHMIA	DESCRIPTION
Atrial fibrillation 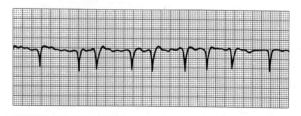	• Impulse forms in atrial ectopic areas. • Atrial rate exceeds 400 beats/minute. • Ventricular rate varies, and ventricular rhythm is grossly irregular. • Treatment depends on symptoms.
First-degree AV block 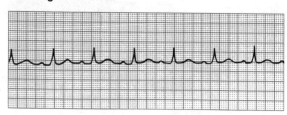	• Slowed AV node conduction with normal rate and rhythm. • Usually no treatment needed.
Second-degree AV block, Mobitz Type I (Wenckebach) 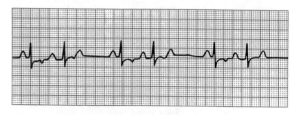	• PR interval gradually lengthens, after which an atrial impulse is fully blocked, creating a discrepancy between atrial and ventricular rates. • Ventricular rhythm is irregular; atrial rhythm, regular. • Second-degree heart block may progress to third-degree heart block. • Usually no treatment needed.
Second-degree AV block, Mobitz Type II 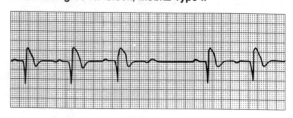	• Every second, third, or fourth atrial impulse is fully blocked, creating a discrepancy between atrial and ventricular rates. • Ventricular rhythm may be irregular with varying degrees of block. • Atrial rhythm is regular. PR interval is constant when conduction to the ventricles is present. • Second-degree heart block may progress to third-degree heart block. • Treatment depends on the patient's symptoms.
Third-degree AV block (complete heart block) 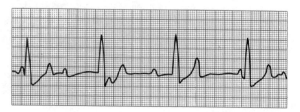	• Atrial impulses are blocked at AV node; atrial and ventricular impulses dissociated. • Atrial rhythm is regular; ventricular rhythm, slow and regular. • Onset may initiate pause before subsidiary pacemaker activates. During this pause, cardiac output decreases, causing syncope or ventricular standstill (asystole) characterized by convulsions (Stokes-Adams syndrome). • Patient may experience altered levels of awareness, syncope, or death if ventricular standstill occurs. • Treatment requires pacemaker insertion.

continued

Reviewing common dysrhythmias — *continued*

DYSRHYTHMIA	DESCRIPTION
Paroxysmal atrial tachycardia (PAT) 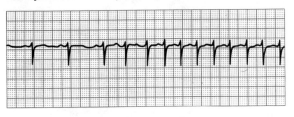	• Heart rate exceeds 140 beats/minute; rarely exceeds 250 beats/minute. • Sudden onset and termination of dysrhythmia. Tachycardia most often begins during sleep and awakens the patient. • PAT may cause palpitations, light-headedness, and exhaustion and may be aggravated by caffeine and stress. • When atrial rate is exactly twice the ventricular rate, patient is said to have PAT with 2:1 block (common in digitalis toxicity). • Treatment hinges on the patient's symptoms.
Premature ventricular contraction (PVC) Interpolated PVCs 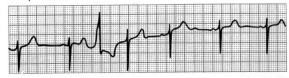 Multifocal PVCs 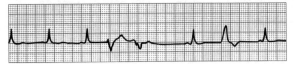 R-on-T phenomenon 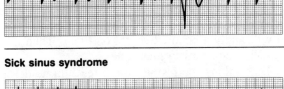	• Most common dysrhythmia. • PVC may be interpolated—falling exactly between two normal beats. • Focus can be unifocal (coming from one spot in ventricle) or multifocal (coming from more than one ventricular area). • PVCs are most ominous when clustered and multifocal, with R wave on T pattern (may precipitate ventricular tachycardia or fibrillation). • Beat occurs prematurely, usually followed by a complete compensatory pause after PVC; irregular pulse. • PVCs can occur singly, in pairs, or in threes, and can alternate with normal beats, as in ventricular bigeminy (one normal beat followed by PVC) or trigeminy (two normal beats followed by PVC). • Usually no treatment unless patient is symptomatic.
Sick sinus syndrome 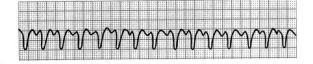	• Tachycardia and bradycardia may alternate and be interrupted by long sinus pauses, resulting in Stokes-Adams syndrome. • Permanent pacemaker may be necessary if patient has symptoms.
Ventricular tachycardia 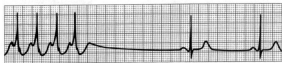	• Ventricular rate ranges from 100 to 300 beats/minute; rhythm is usually regular. • Because of dangerously low cardiac output, ventricular tachycardia can produce chest pain, anxiety, palpitations, dyspnea, syncope, shock, coma, and death. It can lead to ventricular fibrillation. • Electrophysiologic evaluation determines appropriate anti-arrhythmic therapy.

Describe the diagnostic workup

Prepare the patient for tests to identify his specific dysrhythmia and to monitor antiarrhythmic therapy. These may include blood tests, electrocardiography (ECG), ambulatory ECG, exercise ECG, and electrophysiologic studies.

Blood tests

Prepare the patient for venipuncture. The doctor may order blood tests to measure levels of serum electrolytes, such as potassium, or certain drugs, such as quinidine and propranolol. He may even order tests for illicit drugs, such as heroin, amphetamines, and cocaine, if he suspects them of being the underlying cause of dysrhythmia.

ECG

Inform the patient that this 15-minute test evaluates the heart's function by graphically recording its electrical activity. Reassure him that the ECG doesn't cause discomfort. The nurse will cleanse, dry, and possibly shave different body sites, such as the patient's chest and arms, and will apply a conductive gel on them. Then she'll attach electrodes to these sites.

Explain that talking or limb movement will distort the ECG recordings and require more testing time. The patient must lie still, relax, breathe normally, and remain quiet. Mention that this test will be repeated several times (see *Learning about an electrocardiogram,* page 56).

Ambulatory ECG

Explain to the patient that this test records his heart's beat-by-beat response to normal activities over a prolonged period, usually 24 hours. (The test is also known as Holter monitoring or ambulatory monitoring.)

Inform the patient that the technician will clean, dry, and possibly shave different sites on the patient's body, such as his chest and arms, and will apply a conductive gel on them. Then the technician will attach electrodes to these sites.

If the patient will be taking the test at home, tell him he'll wear a small, lightweight tape recorder with a belt or shoulder strap. Instruct him to record his activities and feelings in a diary.

If applicable, teach the patient how to mark the tape at the onset of symptoms. Urge him not to tamper with the monitor or disconnect lead wires or electrodes. Demonstrate how to check the recorder for proper function. Light flashes, for example, may indicate a loose electrode; the patient should test each one by depressing its center and should call the doctor if one comes off. Finally, provide the patient with a copy of the patient-teaching aid *Using your Holter monitor,* page 17.

Exercise ECG

Explain to the patient that an exercise ECG (also known as a stress test or a treadmill or graded exercise test) evaluates his heart's response to walking on a treadmill or pedaling a stationary bicycle. It usually takes about 30 minutes. Inform him that he mustn't eat food or smoke cigarettes for 2 hours before the test.

Explain that he should wear loose, lightweight clothing and snug-fitting shoes. Men usually don't wear a shirt during the test, and women usually wear a bra and a lightweight short-sleeved blouse or a patient gown with front closure.

Encourage the patient to express any fears about the test. Reassure him that a doctor will be present at all times. Emphasize that he can stop if he feels chest pain, leg discomfort, breathlessness, or severe fatigue. Tell the patient that before he begins, a technician will cleanse, shave, and abrade sites on the chest and, possibly, the back. Then he'll attach electrodes to these sites.

If the patient is scheduled for a multistage treadmill test, tell him that the treadmill speed and incline increase at predetermined intervals and that he'll be told of each adjustment. If he's scheduled for a bicycle ergometer test, explain that resistance to pedaling gradually increases as he tries to maintain a specific speed. Typically, he'll feel tired, out of breath, and sweaty during the test. Still, he should report any of these sensations. Mention that his blood pressure and heart rate will be checked periodically.

Inform the patient that he may receive an injection of thallium during the test so that the doctor can evaluate coronary blood flow. Reassure him that the injection involves negligible radiation exposure.

Tell the patient that after the test, his blood pressure and ECG will be monitored for 10 to 15 minutes. Explain that he should wait at least 1 hour before showering, and then he should use warm water. For more information, give him a copy of the patient-teaching aid *Learning about a stress test*, page 16.

Electrophysiologic studies
Explain to the patient that these tests evaluate his heart's electrical activity and may also monitor the effect of medication taken for an irregular heart rhythm. They take 2 to 5 hours.

Instruct him to avoid food, fluids, and nonprescription drugs for 6 hours before the test. Tell him that a catheter insertion site on his groin will be shaved and cleansed.

Explain that after injection of a local anesthetic, a catheter will be inserted into the femoral vein and advanced into the right side of the heart. The patient may receive an I.V. sedative to help him relax. Tell him that he may feel mild pressure at the groin site but that he should report any other discomfort. Explain that the doctor may try to induce extra heartbeats with the catheter.

Inform the patient that after the catheter is removed, pressure is applied to the site to prevent bleeding. The nurse will check the site frequently for swelling. Tell the patient he may need to lie with his leg straight for a few hours after the test.

Teach about treatments
Although teaching about physical activity and diet is important, your most crucial teaching will come in emphasizing compliance with the drug regimen, explaining conservative procedures for

managing dysrhythmias, and providing preoperative and postoperative teaching for a pacemaker implant or an AICD. Include family members in your discussions, specifying what they can do to help, such as learning cardiopulmonary resuscitation (CPR).

Activity
Tell the patient that most dysrhythmias, if managed properly, shouldn't interfere with normal activities. Encourage him to establish a regular exercise routine, under his doctor's supervision, to improve his overall cardiovascular fitness. Remind him to avoid overexertion, and warn him to stop exercising immediately if he experiences dizziness, light-headedness, dyspnea, or chest pain. Also warn against driving or operating heavy machinery if his dysrhythmia causes periodic dizziness or syncope.

Diet
Although dietary restrictions aren't usually required in managing many dysrhythmias, you can give your patient general guidelines to help prevent aggravating his condition. For example, caution him against overeating or consuming too much alcohol, and advise him to limit intake of caffeine and use of tobacco.

Explain the dangers of "holiday heart syndrome": the combination of increased food and alcohol consumption, smoking, and emotional excitement associated with holiday get-togethers can trigger or worsen his dysrhythmia. Because abnormal serum potassium levels can sometimes contribute to dysrhythmias, teach the patient to increase his intake of potassium-rich foods, as necessary. Such foods include bananas, citrus fruits, figs, leafy green vegetables, meats, and seafood.

Medication
Stress the importance of strict compliance with the prescribed drug regimen. Such a regimen usually consists of an antiarrhythmic, such as digitalis, verapamil, propranolol, quinidine, or procainamide, possibly given in combination with other drugs to treat an underlying cardiovascular disorder.

Point out that medications can only control, not cure, the patient's dysrhythmia. Tell him that he must continue taking antiarrhythmics and other prescribed drugs on schedule, even if he's free of symptoms. Advise the patient to call his doctor if he experiences adverse reactions. Tell him not to stop any medication until he contacts his doctor (see *Teaching patients about drugs for dysrhythmias*).

Procedures
Depending on the patient's type of dysrhythmia, teach about procedures to manage it. For example, teach the patient with paroxysmal atrial tachycardia how to quickly restore his heart's regular rhythm by performing carotid sinus massage or Valsalva's maneuver. Or teach the patient with sick sinus syndrome or recurrent conduction blocks about temporary pacemaker implantation. If the

Teaching patients about drugs for dysrhythmias

DRUG	ADVERSE REACTIONS	TEACHING POINTS
Antiarrhythmics		
amiodarone (Cordarone)	• Watch for diaphoresis, dyspnea, lethargy, tingling in the extremities, weight loss or gain, and yellow eyes or fingernails. • Other reactions include corneal microdeposits, hyperthyroidism or hypothyroidism, photophobia, and bluish pigmentation.	• Tell the patient to take a missed dose anytime in the same day or to skip it entirely. Warn him not to double the dose. • Advise having an eye examination if his vision changes. • Tell him that limiting sun exposure will prevent sunburn and skin discoloration. Suggest using a sunblocking agent with a skin protection factor of 15 when outdoors. • Stress the importance of keeping follow-up appointments to monitor thyroid and liver function.
disopyramide (Norpace)	• Watch for ankle edema, dizziness, drowsiness, excessive hunger, hypotension, impotence, irregular heart rate, rapid weight gain, shortness of breath, urine retention, and weakness. • Other reactions include anorexia, constipation, and mouth, nose, and eye dryness.	• Tell the patient who experiences excessive hunger, weakness, drowsiness, and shakiness to eat sweets or drink a sugar-containing beverage and then call his doctor at once. • Instruct him to rise slowly from a sitting or lying position to prevent dizziness or fainting from hypotension. • Tell him to avoid operating machinery until he no longer experiences adverse reactions to the drug. • Urge him to avoid alcohol, which can reduce blood pressure. • Instruct him to take the drug on an empty stomach—1 hour before or 3 hours after a meal for faster absorption. If stomach upset occurs, tell him to take the drug with meals. • Tell him to take a missed dose as soon as possible, but warn him not to double-dose.
encainide (Enkaid)	• Watch for blurred vision, dizziness, irregular heart rate, and tremors. • Other reactions include fatigue, headache, nausea, and palpitations.	• Instruct the patient to take a missed dose as soon as possible but not to double-dose. • Teach him how to take his pulse. Advise him to report an unusually low or high rate or a new irregularity. • Warn against driving or using machinery if dizziness occurs. • If the patient has a permanent pacemaker, explain that the device may need modification after encainide takes effect.
flecainide (Tambocor)	• Watch for ankle edema, chest pain, dizziness, irregular heart rate, shortness of breath, visual disturbances, and weight gain. • Other reactions include fatigue, headache, nausea, and palpitations.	• Tell him to take a missed dose as soon as possible, but warn him not to double-dose. • Teach him how to take his pulse. Advise him to report an unusually low or high rate or a new irregularity. • Warn against driving or using machinery if dizziness occurs. • Instruct the patient to weigh himself at least every other day and to report any sudden weight gain. • If the patient has a permanent pacemaker, explain that the device may need modification after flecainide takes effect.
mexiletine (Mexitil)	• Watch for ataxia, blurred vision, confusion, dizziness, headache, nystagmus, and tremors. • Other reactions include anorexia, constipation, and nausea.	• Tell the patient that he can help relieve nausea by taking the medicine with food or antacids. • Instruct him to take a missed dose as soon as possible, but warn him not to double-dose.
procainamide (Procan SR, Pronestyl)	• Watch for anorexia, nausea, and systemic lupus erythematosus–like syndrome (chills and fever, joint pain, malaise, and rash). • Other reactions include bitter taste, diarrhea, and dizziness.	• Advise the patient to reduce GI symptoms by taking procainamide with food. • Inform him that the tablet's shell may appear in the stool, but that the drug has been absorbed. • Tell him to take a missed dose as soon as possible, but warn him not to double-dose.
quinidine (Cardioquin, Cin-Quin, Duraquin)	• Watch for blurred vision, severe or prolonged diarrhea, hypotension, irregular heart rate, shortness of breath, syncope, and tinnitus. • Other reactions include anorexia, diarrhea, nausea, and vomiting.	• Advise the patient to take the drug with food to reduce GI upset, to take a missed dose as soon as possible, and never to double-dose. • Warn him to limit his use of antacids, which can alter urine pH. Such alteration increases quinidine reabsorption and elevates drug blood levels. • Small amounts of Alternagel may be taken 30 minutes after the dose to help bind stool if the patient is having diarrhea.

continued

52   Dysrhythmias

Teaching patients about drugs for dysrhythmias — *continued*

DRUG	ADVERSE REACTIONS	TEACHING POINTS
Antiarrhythmics — *continued*		
tocainide (Tonocard)	• Watch for chest pain, chills, confusion, cough, dyspnea, easy bruising and bleeding, fever, hypotension, irregular heart rate, rash, sore throat, unsteadiness, sudden weight gain, and wheezing. • Other reactions include dizziness, fatigue, headache, nausea, numbness, sweating, and tremors.	• Explain to the patient that he can reduce nausea by taking the drug with food. • Instruct him to weigh himself at least every other day and to report any sudden gain. • Tell him to take a missed dose as soon as possible, but warn him not to double-dose.
Beta-adrenergic blockers		
acebutolol (Sectral) **atenolol** (Tenormin) **labetalol** (Trandate) **metoprolol** (Lopressor) **nadolol** (Corgard) **pindolol** (Visken) **propranolol** (Inderal) **timolol** (Blocadren)	• Watch for bradycardia, depression, dizziness, dyspnea, rash, and wheezing. • Other reactions include diarrhea, fatigue, headache, impotence, insomnia, nasal stuffiness, nausea, vivid dreams and nightmares, and vomiting.	• Teach the patient to take his pulse before taking the drug and to notify his doctor if the rate falls below 50 beats/minute. • If the patient complains of insomnia, suggest that he take the drug no later than 2 hours before bedtime. • Instruct him to take labetalol, metoprolol, and propranolol with food to increase drug absorption. • If the patient takes one dose daily, instruct him to take a missed dose within 8 hours. If he takes two or more doses each day, instruct him to take a missed dose as soon as possible, but warn him not to double-dose. • Warn against suddenly discontinuing the drug. He must taper the dosage, as directed, to avoid serious complications.
Calcium channel blockers		
verapamil (Calan, Isoptin)	• Watch for ankle edema, bradycardia, chest pain, dyspnea, fainting, and tachycardia. • Other reactions include constipation, dizziness, flushing, headache, and nausea.	• To minimize dizziness, tell the patient to rise slowly from a sitting or lying position. • Explain that the drug won't relieve acute chest pain. He must continue to use sublingual nitroglycerin, if prescribed. • Reassure him that he can continue to eat and drink calcium-containing foods in reasonable amounts. • Teach him to prevent constipation by increasing his fluid and fiber intake and by using a bulk laxative, as necessary. • Advise him to limit alcohol intake to avoid dizziness. • Tell him to take a missed dose within 4 hours, but warn him not to double-dose.
Cardiac glycosides		
digoxin (Lanoxicaps, Lanoxin)	• Watch for abdominal pain, anorexia, blurred vision, color vision changes, diplopia, dizziness, drowsiness, fatigue, headache, irregular heart rate, malaise, and nausea.	• Teach the patient to take his pulse before taking digoxin and to report an unusually low, high, or irregular pulse rate. • Tell him to establish a daily routine for taking digoxin. • Instruct him to take a missed dose within 12 hours, but warn him not to double-dose. • Warn him not to take another person's tablets; different generic digoxin tablets are absorbed at different rates. • Tell the patient to not to take this drug with liquid antacids, kaolin-pectin mixtures (Kaopectate), or cholestyramine, since this may decrease absorption. Separating the administration times of these medications from that of digoxin by 2 hours probably will avoid this interaction.

patient experiences atrial fibrillation or certain other unstable dysrhythmias, teach him about electrocardioversion.

Carotid sinus massage. Show the patient how to locate the carotid sinus on both the right and left sides of his neck. Next, demonstrate how to *firmly* massage the right sinus for no more than 5 seconds. Then, depending on the doctor's orders, show him how to do the same for the left sinus. *Caution the patient never to massage both sinuses at once.* Have him perform the procedure in front of you to ensure that he's doing it correctly. Improper technique, such as using excessive pressure or massaging for too long, can block blood flow to the brain, possibly causing cerebrovascular accident. Or it can trigger new, more dangerous dysrhythmias.

Valsalva's maneuver. To teach the patient Valsalva's maneuver, simply tell him to inhale deeply, hold his breath, and strain hard for at least 10 seconds before exhaling. Explain that the resulting increase in intrathoracic pressure converts the dysrhythmia to a normal rhythm.

Temporary pacemaker implantation. If the patient is scheduled for temporary pacemaker implantation, prepare him for the procedure. Tell him that the doctor will insert a long, thin electrode lead wire into a peripheral vein and, guided by fluoroscopy, will advance it through the vena cava into the right atrium and into the right ventricle. Usually the subclavian or internal jugular vein is used; a brachial or femoral vein may also be used.

Explain that once the electrode lead is in place, the doctor will attach its other end to a battery-powered pacemaker pulse generator that will control the heart rate. Inform the patient that he may feel burning or stinging from the anesthetic used to numb the skin and transient pressure at the insertion site as the catheter is put in place.

Tell him that he may feel his heart flutter as the pacemaker is activated or adjusted, but reassure him that otherwise he'll feel no discomfort. Explain that the pacemaker will remain in place for up to several days until his dysrhythmia is controlled or until other measures, such as permanent pacemaker insertion or cardiac surgery, are taken. Tell him that he'll need to limit his activity. If a femoral vein is used, he'll have to remain in bed.

Electrocardioversion. Inform the patient that electrocardioversion uses an electric current to restore the normal heart rate and relieve symptoms. Instruct him to abstain from food and fluids for at least 8 hours before the procedure. If applicable, tell him that a blood sample will be taken to check his serum potassium level. Explain that he'll be given an I.V. sedative to induce sleep and that while he's asleep, an electric current will be delivered to his heart through paddles placed on his chest. Reassure him that he'll feel no pain or discomfort from the procedure and that he'll be able to eat and move about once the sedative wears off. Inform him that he may notice a reddened area of skin where the paddles were placed. The area may feel tender and itchy for a day or two.

Surgery
If the patient's dysrhythmia can't be controlled by medications or other conservative measures, the doctor may order surgery. The

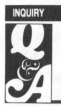

INQUIRY

Questions patients ask about AICDs

What activities can I safely pursue now that I have an AICD?

You may resume many of your previous activities. However, you have to keep in mind which ones may be dangerous if you have a dysrhythmia. For instance, you shouldn't drive a car or operate heavy machinery for at least a year after having the implant. You can exercise every day; just don't overdo it.

Must I take any other special precautions?

Avoid strong magnetic fields, including large radio transmitters and magnetic resonance imaging machines (used for diagnostic tests). Don't place any kind of magnet within 6 inches of the AICD battery. This may make it unresponsive.

Because your AICD may trigger an airport metal detector, tell airport authorities about your device before entering the metal detector. If you hear your AICD beeping, look around for a magnetic source, and try to move away from it. Call your doctor at once.

How will I know when the battery needs to be replaced?

The doctor will test the battery every 2 months for the first year and monthly after that. The test is painless and takes only a few minutes. Be sure to keep appointments to monitor battery function. This is essential to keep the AICD in proper working order.

What happens when my AICD discharges?

If you're awake, you'll feel a brief shock. If you're asleep, you may not sense the shock at all. Report AICD discharges at once to your doctor. If he's unavailable and you're having symptoms of arrhythmia, go to the nearest emergency department.

type of surgery selected depends on the patient's dysrhythmia and on possible underlying cardiovascular problems. It can involve complex open-heart surgery to correct structural defects, relatively uncomplicated permanent pacemaker implantation and, in recurrent life-threatening dysrhythmias, AICD insertion.

Pacemaker implantation. Inform the patient that a pacemaker triggers contraction of the heart muscle and controls the heart rate. Explain the implantation procedure, and make sure he understands preoperative and postoperative instructions. Tell him that he'll receive a sedative and local anesthetic before the procedure. Explain how the pacemaker pulse generator will be implanted under his skin in an unobtrusive area and how electrodes will be threaded through a vein into his heart's right chamber. Inform him that he may be on bed rest for the first 24 hours after implant surgery to allow the leads to seed, or attach well. Give the patient a copy of *Helping your pacemaker help you,* page 57, for detailed postoperative instructions.

If the patient had a temporary pacemaker implanted before permanent implantation, explain that it may be left in place for up to 24 hours after the permanent implantation, to serve as a backup. And, if thoracotomy was done during implantation to attach electrodes directly to the epicardium, teach him proper post-thoracotomy care. Mention that the doctor may provide instructions for testing the pacemaker. Give the patient a copy of the teaching aid *Checking your pacemaker by telephone,* page 58, for detailed instructions.

AICD implantation. If the patient is scheduled for AICD implantation, explain that the device provides an electrical shock to his heart to correct an abnormal heart rhythm. Explain the procedure and make sure he understands the preoperative and postoperative instructions.

Inform the patient that he'll receive a sedative and an anesthetic before surgery. Explain that after making an incision down the center of his chest or on the left side between his ribs, the surgeon will sew two small, rectangular patches onto the heart's surface. Attached to these patches are long, thin insulated wires that will be tunneled under the skin to a pocket made in the abdomen—where the AICD implant will be placed. Slightly larger than a deck of playing cards, the implant weighs about ½ lb (225 g). Inform the patient that he'll be hospitalized for about 1 week.

Instruct the patient to check both abdominal and chest incisions regularly for the first few weeks at home. Usually the patient can see the AICD under the skin and feel its edges. Inform him that fluid accumulation in the implant area is normal but that he should call the doctor immediately if he notices redness, swelling, or drainage, or if the area feels warm and painful. Advise him to wear loose clothing to avoid putting pressure on the area.

Explain to the family that touching the patient when the AICD discharges a shock will not harm them, although they may feel a slight buzz on the patient's skin. (For more information, see *Questions patients ask about AICDs.*)

Mention that after about 2 years, the patient will require hospitalization to replace the battery. Tell him to always carry his AICD information card and wear Medic-Alert identification.

Other care measures

Teach the patient—especially one with a pacemaker—how to take his pulse. Remind him to accurately record all daily pulse readings and to notify the doctor of any significant abnormalities—a rate 5 or more beats lower than his pacemaker's preset rate, a rate exceeding 100 beats/minute, or any unusually irregular rhythm. Teach the patient with atrial fibrillation how to take his carotid pulse rather than his radial pulse.

Teach the patient measures to reduce long-term complications of his dysrhythmia. Suggest that at least one family member learn CPR; this training could make the difference between life and death in a patient who develops sudden cardiac arrest or myocardial infarction.

Also make the patient aware of other cardiovascular disorders that can either contribute to or result from uncontrolled dysrhythmias. Discuss general risk factors for these disorders—stress, obesity, smoking, and sedentary life-style, among others. Refer the patient to a local chapter of the American Heart Association for more information.

Sources of information and support

American Heart Association
7320 Greenville Avenue, Dallas, Tex. 75231
(214) 750-5300

Coronary Club
9500 Euclid Avenue, Cleveland, Ohio 44106
(216) 444-3690

Heart Disease Research Foundation
50 Court Street, Brooklyn, N.Y. 11201
(718) 649-6210

Heartlife
P.O. Box 54305, Atlanta, Ga. 30308

Further readings

DeAngelis, R. "Rhythm: A Dysrhythmia Learning Program," *Critical Care Nurse* 8(7):77-78, October 1988.
Ducasse, R., et al. "Transtelephonic Cardiac Monitoring: A Comprehensive Review of Clinical Applications,"*Critical Care Nurse* 8(2):44, 46-51, March-April 1988.
Lazarus, M., et al. "Cardiac Arrhythmias: Diagnosis and Treatment," *Critical Care Nurse* 8(7):57-65, October 1988.
"Now and Then Arrhythmia," *Emergency Medicine* 20(8):179-80, 182, April 30, 1988.
Sargent, R.K. "Advances in the Treatment of Ventricular Dysrhythmias," *Emergency Care Quarterly* 3(2):18-26, August 1987.
Zorb, S. "Care of the Cardiac Patient: Assessment, Evaluation, and Nursing Implications. ECG Interpretation, Nursing Diagnosis, and Cardiac Medications, Part 1,"*Journal of Intravenous Nursing* 11(1):26-42, January-February 1988.

Learning about an electrocardiogram

Dear Patient:

The doctor has ordered an electrocardiogram for you. (The test is also called an ECG or EKG.) This test tells how well your heart works.

How your heart beats
Your heart is a pump that has its own built-in pacemaker. This pacemaker is actually a group of special cells in the upper right part of the heart.

About every second, this natural pacemaker releases an electrical impulse that travels down a path of muscle fibers and spreads throughout your heart.

This impulse makes your heart contract and pump blood through its chambers and into the rest of the body through the blood vessels.

How an ECG works
An ECG records the electrical impulses that travel through your heart. The ECG machine then converts these impulses to pencil-like "tracings" that print on long strips of graph paper. By looking at these tracings, the doctor can tell whether your heart is healthy or has a problem.

Before the test
The nurse will ask you to lie on your back, with the skin of your chest, arms, and legs exposed. Lie perfectly still and relax. (Don't even talk.) The test is painless and lasts about 15 minutes.

During the test
The nurse will attach a small metal plate called an electrode to each wrist and ankle using rubber tape and a sticky white jelly or a small, cold alcohol pad. Thin wires attached to the electrodes lead to the ECG machine.

Don't worry, you can't get a shock because the wires carry a tiny amount of electricity out of your heart. No electricity goes into your heart.

Next, the nurse will turn on the ECG machine to record the heart's electrical impulses picked up by the electrodes on your arms and legs. Then she'll attach six more electrodes (in the form of suction cups) to six dabs of sticky white jelly on your chest. Once again, the ECG machine will record your heart's electrical impulses.

After the test
When the test is over, the nurse will disconnect the electrodes. You'll be able to resume your usual activities. The doctor will probably tell you the results in a day or so.

Helping your pacemaker help you

Dear Patient:

Your doctor has inserted a pacemaker in your chest to produce the electrical impulses that help your heart beat correctly. Follow these guidelines to make sure your new pacemaker works correctly.

Check your pacemaker daily

To do so, count your pulse beats for 1 minute after you've been resting for at least 15 minutes—a good time to count is the first thing in the morning. Call the doctor if you detect an *unusually fast or slow* rate or if you have chest pain, dizziness, shortness of breath, prolonged hiccups, or muscle twitching.

Check the implantation site each day. Normally, the site bulges slightly. If it reddens, swells, drains, or becomes warm or painful, call the doctor. Remember to wear loose clothing to avoid putting pressure on the site.

Follow doctor's orders

Take your heart medication as prescribed to ensure a regular heart rhythm. Also follow the doctor's orders about diet and physical activity. Exercise every day, but *don't overdo it,* even if you think you have more energy than you did before getting your pacemaker. Avoid rough horseplay or lifting heavy objects. Be especially careful not to stress the muscles near the pacemaker.

Keep all scheduled doctor's appointments. Your pacemaker will need to be checked regularly at the doctor's office or over the telephone to make sure it's in good working order. Pacemaker batteries usually last about 10 years, and a brief hospitalization is necessary for replacement.

Take precautions

Always carry your pacemaker emergency card. The card lists your doctor, hospital, type of pacemaker, and date of implantation.

Don't get too close to gasoline engines, electric motors, or strong magnetic forces, such as those from a magnetic resonance imaging (MRI) machine used by hospitals for diagnostic testing. The MRI test uses a strong magnet and can permanently damage your pacemaker. Also, don't get too close to high-voltage fields created by overhead electric lines. (*Note:* Your microwave oven won't affect your pacemaker.)

If you need dental work or surgery, mention beforehand that you have a pacemaker. You may need an antibiotic to prevent infection.

Avoid driving for 1 month after implantation, and avoid long trips for at least 3 months. If you're traveling by plane, you must pass through an airport metal detector. Before doing so, let the airport authorities know you have a pacemaker.

If you have a nuclear pacemaker and plan to travel abroad, the Nuclear Regulatory Commission requires that you tell the pacemaker manufacturer of your travel itinerary, means of travel, and the name of your doctor.

Checking your pacemaker by telephone

Dear Patient:

Your doctor wants you to use a special device called a pacemaker transmitter so he can check your pacemaker by telephone. After the nurse explains how to operate the transmitter, use these directions as a guide when you go home.

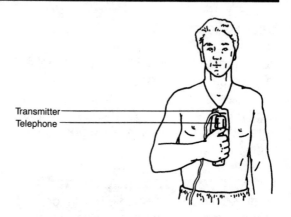

Transmitter
Telephone

Insert the battery
Before using your transmitter for the first time, remove the battery cover and insert the battery supplied by the manufacturer. You'll need to replace the battery every 2 or 3 months.

Position the transmitter
When you're ready to use the transmitter, put its chain around your neck. Then adjust the chain so the transmitter hangs comfortably at the middle of your chest. Open or take off your shirt (and undershirt, too) so the transmitter's chest electrodes rest against your bare skin.

Transmit the signal
Call your doctor. When his office is ready to receive your pacemaker's signal, set the transmitter's On/Off switch to the *On* position. Listen for a squealing sound. If you don't hear it, change the transmitter's battery before continuing.

Now place the telephone's mouthpiece against the transmitter's speaker. Hold the telephone steady, and try to remain still for about 30 seconds.

Follow instructions
After 30 seconds, hold the telephone to your ear, and listen for further instructions. For instance, the doctor may want you to repeat the procedure while you hold a *special magnet* over the pacemaker. If so, take care to hold the magnet flat and steady against your pacemaker. (Or ask someone to hold it for you.) Don't use the magnet unless the doctor asks you to do so.

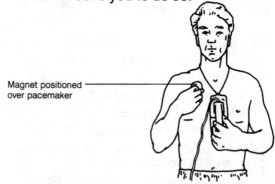

Magnet positioned
over pacemaker

If you receive no further directions, hang up the phone. Remove the transmitter from around your neck and turn off the switch. Keep it switched off whenever you're not using it.

Aneurysm

Without immediate intervention, a ruptured aneurysm can quickly progress to shock and death. To make matters worse, most patients with an aneurysm don't even know they're in danger because symptoms are uncommon. In fact, the diagnosis isn't made until the blood vessel ruptures or becomes apparent on an X-ray, or studies performed for another health problem detect it.

Whether your aneurysm patient requires immediate surgery or has time to consider treatment options, your foremost priority will be to help relieve his anxiety. Then, if time permits, you'll cover other topics, such as aneurysm sites, types, and causes; tests to detect the disorder; and treatments, including surgery, drug therapy, and self-care.

Discuss the disorder

Define an aneurysm as a localized, abnormal dilation in a blood vessel (like a bubble in wallpaper or an inner tube) or in the heart wall. Explain that most aneurysms affect the aorta, although they can occur anywhere in the cardiovascular system. If possible, pinpoint the patient's aneurysm on a diagram (see *Common aneurysm sites*, page 60).

To clarify how an arterial aneurysm impairs circulation, first review arterial anatomy. Explain that an artery has a hollow center and a tough, flexible surrounding wall. Tell the patient that the interior hollow *lumen* is the passageway for blood flow to various body parts. The delicate inner layer, or *tunica intima,* provides a smooth surface for blood flow. The strong and thick middle layer, or *tunica media,* consists of elastic fibers and a small amount of smooth muscle. The outer layer, called the *tunica externa* (adventitia), supports and protects the artery with elastic and collagenous fibers.

Inform the patient that arterial aneurysms are classified as fusiform, saccular, dissecting, or false. Focus your discussion on the kind that the patient has (see *Types of arterial aneurysms,* page 61).

Explain that two factors—mural and mechanical—influence an aneurysm's development. Mural factors refer to the strength and integrity of the vessel wall. For example, in an atherosclerotic aneurysm, fibrin deposits clog the artery, causing the arterial wall to lose its elasticity and to stiffen. Meanwhile, plaques accumulate and mural thrombi form on the wall, obstructing the lumen. Thrombi, which may break off and lodge in distal vessels, also

Lynne Patzek Miller, RN,C, who wrote this chapter, is a clinical systems manager at Doylestown Hospital, Doylestown, Pa.

CHECKLIST

Teaching topics in aneurysm

☐ Definition of aneurysm
☐ Common aneurysm sites
☐ Types of arterial aneurysms, including a berry aneurysm
☐ Causes of aneurysm, emphasizing mural and mechanical factors
☐ Signs and symptoms, such as pain, and complications, such as peripheral vascular insufficiency and increased intracranial pressure
☐ Tests to detect aneurysm, such as X-ray studies, abdominal ultrasonography, magnetic resonance imaging, computed tomography scan, angiography, echocardiography, and lumbar puncture
☐ Activity restrictions
☐ Medications to minimize aneurysm effects
☐ Surgical repair, such as resection and bypass
☐ Preoperative and postoperative care
☐ Other care measures, including blood pressure monitoring, proper skin care, and detection of warning signs and symptoms
☐ Source of information and support

Common aneurysm sites

After the doctor has located the patient's aneurysm, use a diagram like the one below to show the patient its location. (Note that the clusters of dots signify aneurysms.)

If the patient has a cerebral aneurysm, explain that this type commonly arises in the *cerebral artery* at the arterial junction in the circle of Willis, the loop of vessels near the brain's base.

If the patient's aneurysm lies in the *heart,* inform him that an aneurysm may form in the ventricles after a myocardial infarction.

Explain that an aortic aneurysm develops in the *aorta's abdominal section,* just below the renal arteries, or in the *descending aorta,* just below the subclavian artery to the diaphragm. Occasionally, aneurysms develop in the *ascending thoracic aorta* or in the *aortic arch.*

Tell the patient with a peripheral artery aneurysm that this type usually occurs in the *femoral or the popliteal artery* but that most peripheral artery aneurysms are named "false aneurysms" (they're actually pulsating hematomas). Peripheral atherosclerotic aneurysms, now rare, may become more common as the elderly population increases.

NONCEREBRAL ANEURYSM SITES

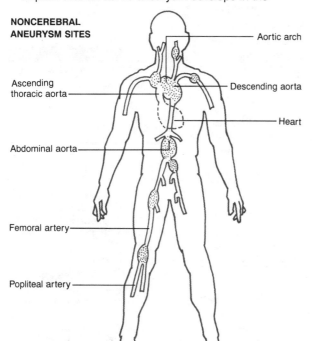

- Aortic arch
- Ascending thoracic aorta
- Descending aorta
- Heart
- Abdominal aorta
- Femoral artery
- Popliteal artery

CEREBRAL ANEURYSM SITES

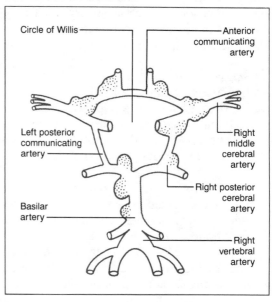

- Circle of Willis
- Anterior communicating artery
- Left posterior communicating artery
- Right middle cerebral artery
- Right posterior cerebral artery
- Basilar artery
- Right vertebral artery

narrow the lumen and critically impair blood flow. Over time, the artery weakens and bulges.

Mechanical factors, such as hypertension, trauma, infection, and congenital defects—even stress imposed on an artery by the pulse wave of each ventricular contraction—can also weaken vessel walls. Examples of mechanical factors that can stress the arterial wall are rising blood pressure and increasing blood volume, which normally occur in pregnancy. If the patient already has a risk factor, such as a congenital weakness in the vessel wall, an aneurysm may develop.

Finally, describe how signs and symptoms (if any) vary, depending on how quickly the aneurysm dilates and how it affects surrounding structures. Pain is the most common symptom. Its location and characteristics depend on the aneurysm's site. For example, a patient with a thoracic aortic aneurysm usually feels constant, boring chest pain when he lies supine. A patient with an abdominal aortic aneurysm may suffer low back pain or persistent or intermittent abdominal pain when lying down.

Explain that other symptoms stem from aneurysmal pressure on adjacent structures. For example, a thoracic aortic aneurysm may cause dyspnea from pressure on the trachea, main bronchus, or lung. Or it may produce dysphagia if the aneurysm presses on the esophagus. Individualize your teaching to the patient's symptoms and aneurysm site. For specific teaching points about a berry aneurysm, a leading cardiovascular disorder, see *Understanding a berry aneurysm,* page 62.

Complications
Many patients don't realize that they have an aneurysm until complications occur from rupture or until the blood supply to the tissues fed by the affected vessel decreases enough to cause health problems. For example, an *aortic aneurysm* or an aneurysm on a branch of the aorta may diminish the blood supply to abdominal organs and extremities, causing organ dysfunction or peripheral vascular insufficiency in the legs (or both): Severely impaired blood flow may cause tissue necrosis. If an aortic aneurysm ruptures and emergency intervention isn't undertaken, blood loss may cause shock and death.

A *cerebral aneurysm* typically produces no symptoms until the aneurysm ruptures, causing increased intracranial pressure, cerebral edema, paralysis, coma, and death.

An untreated *ventricular aneurysm* can lead to such complications as pulmonary edema, congestive heart failure, dysrhythmias, and cardiogenic shock. A rupture in this aneurysm typically causes death.

Describe the diagnostic workup
Several tests may help reveal an aneurysm, including routine X-ray studies, abdominal ultrasonography, magnetic resonance imaging (MRI), computed tomography (CT) scan, angiography, echocardiography, and lumbar puncture. Inform the patient that the tests he'll have depend on the suspected aneurysm's location.

Explain that some aneurysms are detected during a physical examination. For example, some abdominal aortic aneurysms are palpable. Frequently, abdominal bruits may be heard with a stethoscope.

X-ray studies
Prepare the patient for chest, abdominal, or skull X-ray studies to locate the aneurysm. Instruct him to put on a hospital gown and remove all jewelry from his neck and chest. Tell him that, depending on the area being studied, he'll need to assume various positions or hold his breath for a few seconds during the test until the technician records several images and views. Caution him to remain still while the X-ray films are taken to avoid distorting the images.

Types of arterial aneurysms

After diagnostic tests have identified the patient's aneurysm, describe its type: fusiform, saccular, dissecting, or false.

Fusiform aneurysm
The most common type of aneurysm, this spindle-shaped bulge encompasses the entire aorta like a spare tire.

Saccular aneurysm
The type most likely to rupture, this unilateral, pouchlike bulge has a narrow neck and resembles a bubble or a balloon.

Dissecting aneurysm
The most dangerous, painful type, this hemorrhagic separation or tear in the medial layer of the arterial wall creates a false compartment filled with blood.

False aneurysm
Commonly called a pulsating hematoma, this type usually results from penetrating trauma that causes a leak in the outer arterial wall, typically at an anastomosis, or graft, site. The lumen usually remains normal or nearly normal.

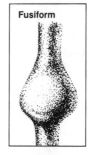

Fusiform

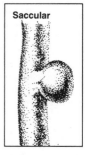

Saccular

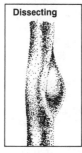

Dissecting

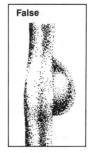

False

Understanding a berry aneurysm

Small, thin, blisterlike bulges that resemble a cluster of berries characterize a berry aneurysm. This saccular aneurysm commonly occurs at the bifurcations and branches of the circle of Willis.

Thought to be congenital, a berry aneurysm is also linked to hypertension, smoking, atherosclerosis, and age.

Signs and symptoms
Most patients experience no symptoms until the aneurysm ruptures, causing headache, loss of consciousness, and hemiplegia. Hemorrhagic effects range from mild to severe—from temporary paresis, confusion, and slurred speech to coma, seizures, and death.

Treatment
Surgical clipping is the treatment of choice. If the aneurysm ruptures before surgery, the patient should have complete bed rest in a darkened room to reduce bleeding and sensory stimulation (which may promote bleeding). Besides analgesics and sedatives, he may need antihypertensives, corticosteroids, anticonvulsants and, possibly, aminocaproic acid to destroy blood clots.

During recovery, the patient may require mechanical ventilation and intracranial pressure monitoring until his condition improves.

Interpreting the outcome
Prognosis hinges on cerebral damage, which correlates with symptoms and the aneurysm's grade:
• Grade I: asymptomatic or slight headache or stiff neck
• Grade II: moderate to severe headache and nuchal rigidity
• Grade III: drowsiness, confusion, and mild focal weakness
• Grade IV: vegetative state with decerebrate rigidity
• Grade V: deep coma with decerebrate rigidity.

Abdominal ultrasonography
Inform the patient that this painless, noninvasive test evaluates the major blood vessels in the abdomen for aneurysm formation. Explain that the equipment translates sound waves that bounce off anatomic structures into graphic images displayed or printed as a sonogram. Typically, the test takes about 30 minutes. During the test, the patient will lie on his back on an examining table while a technician applies conductive jelly to the patient's abdomen. Then the technician will use the transducer to scan the blood vessels, moving the instrument slowly over the abdominal area.

The patient may be asked to breathe deeply or to hold his breath briefly to obtain a clear image.

Magnetic resonance imaging
Tell the patient that this painless, noninvasive test relies on a powerful magnet, radio waves, and a computer to produce clear, cross-sectional images of the blood vessels. The test takes about 1 hour. Because no metal is allowed near the magnets in the MRI equipment area, instruct the patient to remove all jewelry and to inform his doctor or test examiner about any pacemaker, orthopedic pins or disks, shrapnel, or any other metal objects in his body.

Inform the patient that he'll be positioned on a table that slides into a cylinder housing the MRI magnets. Instruct him to lie still to avoid blurring the images. While the machine runs, he'll hear a loud knocking sound. If the noise bothers him, suggest that he ask for earplugs or earpads from the examiner, who can see and communicate with him from an adjoining room. After the test, the patient can resume his normal activities.

CT scan
Explain that a CT scan produces X-ray images of the cardiovascular system in 30 to 60 minutes. Reassure the patient that this noninvasive study causes no pain. If a contrast medium is ordered, instruct the patient not to eat or drink for 4 hours before the scan.

Describe what happens during the test. The patient will lie on a table, and the examiner will place a stabilizing strap across the body part to be scanned. Tell the patient that the table will slide into the scanner's circular opening. If the test calls for a contrast medium, it will be infused intravenously over about 5 minutes. Instruct him to report sensations of warmth, itching, or other discomfort immediately. (The examiner can see and communicate with him from an adjoining area.) Describe the noises that the scanner makes as it revolves around the patient.

Reassure the patient that he can resume his usual activities and diet after the test. However, if he received a contrast medium, he'll need to increase his fluid intake for the rest of the day to help expel the medium.

Angiography
Inform the patient that this procedure (also called arteriography) evaluates the arteries for abnormalities. Mention that the test may last from 30 minutes to 4 hours, depending on the arteries being examined.

Tell the patient that the skin over the artery to be examined may be shaved. Then the doctor will clean the shaved area, inject a local anesthetic, and insert and advance a catheter into the artery. He'll infuse a contrast medium through the catheter and take several X-rays to record the medium's passage. The patient may feel flushed or nauseated or have an unpleasant taste in his mouth. Reassure him that these feelings should pass quickly. Explain that he may be asked to turn on one side or to elevate an arm or leg but that he should stay perfectly still to avoid distorting the images when the doctor takes the films.

After the test, the doctor will remove the catheter and apply pressure to the catheter site for 15 to 30 minutes. He'll then apply a bulky dressing and add more pressure with a sandbag on the patient's arm or leg. Instruct the patient to keep his affected limb extended and immobile for as long as the doctor orders (usually 4 to 24 hours). During this time, the nurse will frequently check the pulse and circulation in the affected limb.

Echocardiography

Inform the patient that this painless test examines the chest (thoracic) area for an aneurysm by evaluating the size, shape, and motion of various cardiac structures. The process takes between 15 and 30 minutes.

Tell the patient that he'll lie on a table while a technician applies conductive jelly to the patient's chest and then angles a transducer over the same area. The technician may tell the patient to turn on his left side, to breathe in and out slowly, to hold his breath, or to inhale a gas (amyl nitrite) with a slightly sweet odor while the test equipment records changes in his heart function. Warn him that amyl nitrite may cause dizziness, flushing, and tachycardia but that these effects quickly subside. He should remain still during the test to keep from distorting the results.

Lumbar puncture

Explain that this test involves removing and analyzing spinal fluid to determine whether a cerebral aneurysm has ruptured. Mention that the procedure takes about 15 minutes and that the patient will feel some pressure when the doctor inserts the needle.

Describe how the patient will either sit with his head bent toward his knees or lie on the edge of a bed or table with his knees drawn up to his abdomen and his chin resting on his chest. After cleaning the lumbar area, the doctor will inject a local anesthetic and ask the patient to report any tingling or sharp pain. Next, the doctor will guide a hollow needle into the subarachnoid space surrounding the spinal cord. Tell the patient to remain still to avoid dislodging the needle. Inform him that he may be asked to breathe deeply or to straighten his legs and that he may feel the doctor apply pressure to the patient's jugular vein.

After the test, the doctor will remove the needle and apply an adhesive bandage. To prevent a headache, tell the patient to lie flat for as long as the doctor orders (usually 4 to 24 hours) and to keep his head at or below hip level. (He can still turn from side to side.) Advise him to increase his fluid intake for the rest of the

Teaching about nimodipine

If your patient has a cerebral aneurysm, the doctor may prescribe nimodipine (Nimotop), a calcium channel blocker. This drug affects calcium movement into blood vessel cells, thereby relaxing the blood vessel and minimizing or preventing bleeding. Nimodipine also spares neurologic function.

How to take the drug
Tell the patient to take nimodipine exactly as directed. If he forgets a dose, advise him to take it as soon as possible. If it's nearly time for his next dose, instruct him to skip the missed dose and take the next scheduled dose on time.

If the patient can't swallow, advise the caregiver to open the nimodipine capsule, mix the contents with fluid, and administer the medication through the patient's nasogastric tube.

Adverse effects
Fortunately, most patients experience few adverse effects from this drug. Urge the patient to seek medical advice at once, though, if he feels dizzy or lightheaded or if he develops a rapid heartbeat, a rash, or swelling in his ankles, feet, or lower legs.

Inform the patient that other adverse effects include a headache and nausea. Reassure him that these effects should subside as his body gets used to the drug.

day to help replenish lost cerebrospinal fluid and to prevent a headache.

Teach about treatments
Point out that surgery is the treatment of choice for aneurysm, although medications may reduce pressure, swelling, and pain. Treatment also involves activity restrictions, proper skin care, blood pressure monitoring, and staying alert for signs and symptoms of a ruptured aneurysm.

Activity
Tell the patient that his doctor will provide activity guidelines to follow until surgery. Warn him that overexertion can trigger a sudden rise in blood pressure. If this occurs, he may be ordered to bed to prevent complications.

Medication
Drug therapy typically aims to control blood pressure with antihypertensive agents and to reduce pulsatile blood flow and cardiac contractility with beta-adrenergic blockers, such as propranolol (Inderal). In a patient with a cerebral aneurysm, the doctor may order anticonvulsants to prevent seizures and corticosteroids to control edema.

Explain that sedatives or narcotics may be prescribed to reduce anxiety, stress, or pain. If so, these drugs will be monitored constantly because they can decrease consciousness and lower the respiratory rate. In turn, blood carbon dioxide levels increase, causing cerebral vessels to dilate, which leads to increasing cerebrospinal fluid pressure and a deteriorating condition.

If appropriate, tell the patient that nimodipine (Nimotop), a calcium channel blocker, may be prescribed in a ruptured cerebral aneurysm because it spares neurologic function (see *Teaching about nimodipine*).

Caution the patient to avoid aspirin, over-the-counter products containing aspirin, and foods and drugs with caffeine. Explain that caffeine, a stimulant, increases blood pressure. And aspirin hinders blood clot formation, which increases bleeding (should the aneurysm rupture).

Surgery
If the patient's having emergency surgery and time allows, briefly explain the procedure to him or to his family. If he isn't having surgery immediately, take the time to discuss the scheduled operation and possible complications. Make sure to cover preoperative and postoperative care and home care measures.

Types of aneurysm repair. Inform the patient that aneurysm repair may involve surgical resection, bypass and, occasionally, clipping or wrapping. Typically, the kind of surgery depends on the location, type, and size of the aneurysm; the patient's condition; and whether or not the aneurysm is intact.

Common sites for surgery include the thoracic aorta and the femoral-popliteal artery. The surgical procedures performed at these sites are a thoracic aortic bypass and a femoral-popliteal by-

Repairing an aortic aneurysm

If your patient has an aortic aneurysm—either ab-dominal or thoracic—and if he has time to learn about his impending operation, review the surgical procedure with him. If he's having emergency surgery, briefly describe aneurysmectomy to his family.

Inform them that the surgeon first resects the involved segment (below left). Next, he replaces the diseased section with biologically neutral graft material, such as Dacron or a derivative (below center). Then he cleans the diseased tissue of plaque or clotted blood and sutures this section around the graft (below right).

The section that once composed the aneurysm now covers the graft.

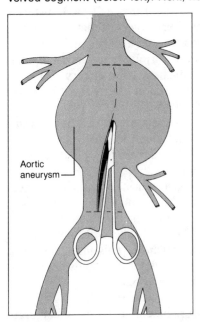

Aortic aneurysm

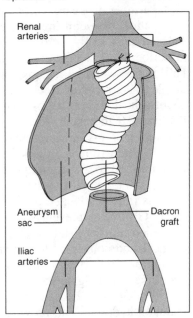

Renal arteries

Aneurysm sac

Iliac arteries

Dacron graft

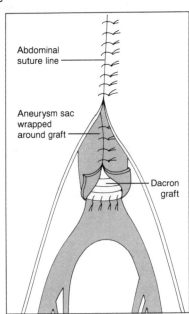

Abdominal suture line

Aneurysm sac wrapped around graft

Dacron graft

pass. Mention, though, that blood vessels may be repaired anywhere in the cardiovascular system.

If the patient's having bypass surgery, explain that the surgeon will graft an autologous or synthetic vessel above and below the aneurysm to divert blood flow around the diseased tissue.

If the patient's scheduled for a resection—for example, an aneurysmectomy—explain that the surgeon will remove the aneurysm and reconnect the ends of the blood vessel or heart muscle. Or he may remove the diseased portion and graft a replacement vessel to the healthy ends of the blood vessel (for more information, see *Repairing an aortic aneurysm*).

With a small aneurysm, the surgeon may clip or ligate the base of the aneurysm so that blood can't flow into it. If he decides to wrap the aneurysm, he'll support the arterial wall by wrapping it with a biologically neutral material, such as Dacron.

Preoperative care. Tell the patient that he'll bathe with a special antiseptic soap the day before surgery. Add that he may be shaved from his neck to his toes. If he has a cerebral aneurysm, his head will be shaved—at least partially. He won't be allowed to eat or drink after midnight before the surgery, although he may request a sleeping pill. He may also receive a sedative the morning of surgery to help him relax. If appropriate, tell him that peripheral pulses in his legs will be marked with an inklike substance. Caution him not to wash off the markings when he bathes with the antiseptic soap.

If the patient's scheduled for preoperative pulmonary artery catheterization or intracranial pressure monitoring, explain these procedures to him. Tell him that the catheter will remain in place during and after surgery, but reassure him that the catheter and arterial lines will cause little, if any, discomfort.

Postoperative care. Inform the patient that he'll be transferred to a critical care unit immediately after surgery. When he has recovered sufficiently, he'll be moved to a regular hospital room. Describe the type of dressing and the various tubes and equipment he'll notice when he regains consciousness after surgery. For example, if he receives mechanical ventilation briefly, he'll have an endotracheal (ET) tube inserted through his nose or mouth into his lungs. If the aneurysm was in his chest area, he'll have chest tubes to keep his lungs inflated properly and to allow blood and fluid to drain from the thoracic cavity. Explain that his tubes will be connected to a suction apparatus.

Tell the patient that he'll also have a urinary catheter to measure his fluid intake and output and that he may have a nasogastric (NG) tube to prevent vomiting, aspiration, and abdominal distention until peristalsis returns. The NG tube will be taped to his nose and connected to a suction machine. This may produce discomfort and dryness in the back of his throat. Advise him that the nurse will irrigate the tube every few hours.

Explain that the patient will receive I.V. fluid feedings to maintain hydration and provide nourishment. If he has a cerebral aneurysm, he'll be positioned on his side after surgery and the head of the bed will be raised 15 to 30 degrees to prevent increased intracranial pressure. If appropriate, inform him that the nurse will measure blood flow in his legs frequently with an ultrasonic instrument called a transducer.

Emphasize that the patient's priorities after surgery are resting and avoiding stress. Encourage him to request pain medicine as needed. Explain that he'll be able to sit up and swallow liquids when the ET and NG tubes are removed. Then he'll gradually start eating solid foods.

Urge the patient to practice coughing and deep-breathing exercises to avert pulmonary complications. Teach him how to splint his incision to minimize pain and how to use an incentive spirometer. Reassure him that coughing won't loosen or damage his graft or reopen his incision. However, caution the patient who's just had a cerebral artery repair not to cough too vigorously because bleeding may occur.

Show the patient how to perform active range-of-motion exercises with his legs to prevent clot formation. Tell him that his nurse will help him to walk as soon as possible. This will improve his circulation and help prevent complications. Also describe the antiembolism stockings that he'll wear to prevent complicatons.

Explain that his nurse will remove the stockings periodically to check his pulses and skin condition.

Home care. When the patient begins to feel stronger, review his prescribed activity program, stressing that he should increase activity gradually and set realistic goals for himself. If he's had surgery for a ruptured cerebral artery, he may have some neurologic impairment and need rehabilitation services. Encourage him and his family to use the services offered by the physical therapy and social service departments.

Make sure the patient understands which medications he'll be taking, how to take them, and which adverse reactions to watch for. In addition, teach him the warning signs of infection: redness, swelling, tenderness, or drainage at the incision site.

If he'll wear antiembolism stockings at home, teach him how to check his own pulses. Also advise him to check his skin for signs of infection or decreased circulation. He should know that cold, blue-tinged skin signals decreased circulation from thromboembolism in the artery, and that a fever or a color change or pain in the area fed by the affected artery can signal the development of an anastomotic aneurysm.

Other care measures

If your patient's at home awaiting surgery, discuss treatment measures with him and his family, and offer them the teaching aid *Living with an aneurysm,* page 68. Emphasize that controlling the patient's blood pressure will decrease the risk of the aneurysm's rupturing. Then teach him and his family how to take a blood pressure reading.

Also stress the importance of proper skin care. Explain that until the patient's aneurysm is surgically repaired, his circulation will be decreased, which heightens his risk of infection. Also, teach him and his family warning signs that call for medical attention. Finally, urge him to schedule and keep appointments for regular follow-up care.

Source of information and support

American Heart Association
7320 Greenville Ave., Dallas, Tex. 75231
(214) 373-6300

Further readings

Diamond, S. "Headaches that Herald Intracranial Emergencies," *Emergency Medicine* 20(2):20-24, 27, 31-32, January 30, 1988.
Downing, L.A., and Hill, M.N. "Action STAT! Aortic Dissection," *Nursing88* 18(6):58, June 1988.
MacDonald, E. "Aneurysmal Subarachnoid Hemorrhage," *Journal of Neuroscience Nursing* 21(5):313-21, October 1989.
Naftzger, M.E. "Recognition of Warning Signs in Intracranial Aneurysms," *Physician Assistant* 12(8):35-36, 43-45, 111-12, August 1988.
Smith, M.B., et al. "Traumatic Pseudoaneurysm," *Emergency Medicine* 21(13):147, 150, July 15, 1989.

Living with an aneurysm

Dear Patient:

Whether you're awaiting surgery or not, here are some tips to help you function safely and comfortably at home.

Slow down
Don't give up all activity, but do cut back enough to keep your blood pressure at a safe and steady level. For instance, taking a stroll around your neighborhood or in the park may be better for you than jogging.

Monitor your blood pressure
Learn to take your blood pressure regularly—as your nurse or doctor showed you. (Or ask someone else to take it for you.) Write down the results. Follow your doctor's guidelines for acceptable levels. Be sure to notify him if your blood pressure is higher or lower than those levels.

Eat sensibly
Keep your blood pressure on an even keel by eating sensibly. For example, restrict salt and follow a low-fat diet. Losing weight may help too.

Check your circulation
Examine your legs every day for changes in color and temperature and for numbness or tingling sensations, especially if you suspect that your aneurysm slows your circulation. Tell your doctor if you notice any changes.

Avoid infection
Protect yourself from complicatons caused by poor circulation in your legs, including infection and gangrene. Keep your skin clean, dry, and free of surface scratches that bacteria could enter.

Wash your feet in warm, soapy water every day. Then dry them thoroughly by blotting them with a towel. Be sure to dry between the toes. Check your feet daily for cuts, cracks, blisters, or red, swollen areas. Call your doctor if you cut your foot, even slightly.

Avoid wearing tight shoes or clothing that may further restrict your circulation. And don't wear elastic garters, sit with your knees crossed, or walk barefoot.

Take your medicine
Make sure you understand exactly how and when to take your medicine. And if you have questions about any medicine or possible side effects, call your nurse, doctor, or pharmacist. Also consult them before you take any nonprescription medicine—cold remedies, for example. Taken with prescription medicines, some nonprescription medicines may work against each other.

Recognize danger symptoms
Have someone call your doctor at once if you experience:
• a severe headache
• severe chest or abdominal pain
• cool, clammy skin
• disorientation or unusual sleepiness
• extreme restlessness or anxiety.

Respiratory Conditions

Contents

Pulmonary embolism

More than any other pulmonary disorder, pulmonary embolism is likely to complicate the recovery of hospitalized patients. As a result, you'll often encounter patients who'll need to learn about risk factors and symptoms of pulmonary embolism. (See *Classifying risks,* page 72.) But you'll also encounter patients admitted for an acute pulmonary embolism who require additional teaching about tests to confirm embolism and treatment to resolve it. Because acute pulmonary embolism typically causes dyspnea, you'll be teaching a patient who's understandably anxious about his condition, so he's willing to comply with therapy.

However, once the embolus resolves and the patient becomes asymptomatic, he may become less willing to comply with prolonged anticoagulant therapy to prevent recurrent emboli. Of course, you'll emphasize the need for such therapy. You'll also emphasize the need for periodic blood studies to monitor his anticoagulant drug level, especially during the first weeks of therapy, and close observation to watch for adverse drug effects. Similarly, you'll need to teach about symptoms of drug toxicity and safety measures to follow when taking the drug.

Discuss the disorder

Explain that pulmonary embolism is a blood clot that has traveled through the bloodstream and lodged in the artery of the lung. For more information, see *How a clot travels from the leg to the lung,* page 73. Tell the patient that the clot obstructs blood flow to a portion of the lung. As a result, this portion of the lung is ventilated, but not perfused. To compensate for this ventilation-perfusion mismatch, he must breathe faster and with more effort to avoid hypoxemia. He also may wheeze in response to distal airway constriction—the body's attempt to shunt ventilation from nonperfused to perfused areas of the lung.

Briefly discuss the probable cause of the pulmonary embolism: dislodged thrombi, usually originating in the deep veins of the leg. Thrombi form as the result of vascular wall damage, venous stasis, or hypercoagulability of the blood. The thrombi may have become dislodged during trauma, sudden muscular action, or a change in peripheral blood flow.

Complications

Emphasize that the patient can avoid or minimize atelectasis by strictly adhering to the treatment plan. Explain how atelectasis

Patricia L. Carroll, RN,C, MS, CEN, RRT, and **Sandra K. Crabtree Goodnough, BSN, MSN,** wrote this chapter. Ms. Carroll is a nurse consultant and owner of Educational Medical Consultants, Middletown, Conn. Ms. Goodnough is former director of research support services, Herman Hospital, Houston.

CHECKLIST

Teaching topics in pulmonary embolism

☐ An explanation of how emboli obstruct pulmonary blood flow
☐ Risks and causes of emboli
☐ Preparation for diagnostic tests, such as chest X-ray, perfusion and ventilation scans, ultrasonography, impedance plethysmography, and pulmonary angiography
☐ Preparation for clotting studies to monitor anticoagulant therapy
☐ Importance of exercise and proper positioning to prevent venous stasis
☐ Anticoagulant therapy
☐ How to use a sequential compression device and apply antiembolism stockings
☐ Signs and symptoms of recurrent pulmonary embolism and of complications, such as thrombophlebitis, ventricular failure, and dysrhythmias

72 Pulmonary embolism

Classifying risks

Which patients require special teaching about preventive measures for clot formation in the legs?

To help you decide, review the following predisposing factors that can put your patient at risk for pulmonary embolism.

Low risk (<6%)
A patient who has undergone minor surgery has a low risk of forming emboli if he is under age 40 and has no history of clots or other significant medical history (for example, chronic pulmonary disease or dysrhythmias).

Moderate risk (6 to 40%)
If the patient is over age 40 and has had abdominal, pelvic, or chest surgery or an uncomplicated myocardial infarction, his risk for pulmonary embolism is moderate.

High risk (>40%)
A patient over age 40 with a history of clots or cancer, who has had extensive major surgery, such as hip replacement, is at high risk for pulmonary embolism.

contributes to hypoxemia and may aggravate tachypnea and dyspnea. Note that the patient's at risk for atelectasis until the embolus resolves. Warn him that ultimately, pulmonary embolism can also cause pulmonary hypertension, reduced cardiac output, myocardial infarction, and heart failure. For an overview of pulmonary embolism pathology, see *Surveying potential damage from pulmonary embolism,* page 74.

Describe the diagnostic workup

Prepare the patient for diagnostic tests to detect pulmonary embolism and coagulation studies to evaluate his response to anticoagulant therapy.

To rule out other disorders, the doctor may order blood tests to determine white blood cell count, erythrocyte sedimentation rate, fibrin split products, and serum lactic dehydrogenase, aspartate aminotransferase, and bilirubin levels. He may also order a chest X-ray.

To help confirm a pulmonary embolism, the doctor may order a lung perfusion scan, a ventilation scan, arterial blood gas (ABG) measurements, pulmonary angiography, and an ECG. To detect peripheral venous thrombosis, he may schedule Doppler ultrasonography or impedance plethysmography.

Chest X-ray

Explain that a chest X-ray can rule out other pulmonary disorders and show areas of atelectasis. Mention that the test takes only minutes. However, additional time is required to check the quality of the X-ray film. Before the test, instruct the patient to remove his clothing above the waist, to take off all jewelry and metal objects from his neck and chest, and to put on a gown without snaps.

For an X-ray performed in the radiology department, inform the patient that he'll stand or sit in front of a machine. If the X-ray's done at bedside, someone will help him to a sitting position and place a cold, hard film plate behind his back. In either place, he'll be instructed to take a deep breath, hold it, and remain still for a few seconds while the film is taken. Reassure him that radiation exposure is minimal.

Lung perfusion scan

Inform the patient that this 30-minute test evaluates blood flow in the lungs. Tell him that he'll lie supine on a table while a radioactive protein substance is injected into an arm vein. This substance travels through the bloodstream to the lungs where it is detected by a large scanning camera. Pictures will be taken while the patient's supine, lying on his side, prone, and sitting. More dye will be injected when the patient's positioned on his stomach. Explain that these pictures measure the radioactivity in the lungs and can highlight areas not receiving adequate blood.

Reassure him that the amount of radioactivity in the dye is minimal. However, he may experience some discomfort from the venipuncture and from lying on a cold, hard table.

Ventilation scan

Tell the patient that this test, which takes about 30 minutes, evaluates lung ventilation during respiration. Instruct him to avoid eating a large meal, drinking a large volume of fluids, and smoking for 3 hours before the test. Unless directed otherwise, he may continue to take his medications. He should remove all jewelry and metal objects.

Explain that during the test the patient will be seated and instructed to breathe a radioactive gas through a mouthpiece or a tightly fitted face mask. He'll be instructed to breathe deeply, hold his breath, breathe out, and then breathe normally. He should remain still when he's asked to hold his breath. A nuclear scanner will monitor the gas distribution in the lungs. Assure him that the amount of radioactive gas is minimal and that it's mixed with air. Tell him to report any dyspnea or wheezing during the test.

ABG analysis

Prepare the patient for ABG analysis to evaluate how well the lungs are delivering oxygen to and eliminating carbon dioxide from the blood. Tell him which site will be used—the radial, brachial, or femoral artery. Instruct him to breathe normally during the test, and warn him that he may experience a brief cramping or throbbing pain at the puncture site.

Pulmonary angiography

Explain to the patient that this 1-hour test (also known as pulmonary arteriography) confirms pulmonary embolism. Pretest restrictions include fasting for 6 hours, or as ordered. He may continue his prescribed drugs unless the doctor orders otherwise. Instruct him to remove his clothing, except for socks, and to put on a gown that fastens in the front. He should void just before the test.

Inform him that during the test he'll remove the gown and lie supine on a table. He'll be covered with sheets and sterile drapes. The nurse will attach ECG electrodes to his arms and legs to monitor his heart during the test. She'll also apply a blood pressure cuff and start an I.V. line. After injecting a local anesthetic, the doctor will make a small incision or a percutaneous needle puncture in an antecubital, femoral, jugular, or subclavian vein. Warn the patient that he may feel pressure at the insertion site. Then the doctor will insert and advance a catheter through the vein to the right side of the heart and the pulmonary artery, where he'll measure pressures and withdraw blood samples.

Next, he'll inject a radiopaque dye into the catheter. Warn the patient that he may experience a flushed feeling, nausea, or a salty taste for a few minutes after the dye's injected. X-ray films will be taken as the dye circulates through the pulmonary vessels. When the test's over, the doctor will withdraw the catheter and apply a pressure dressing to the insertion site. Instruct the patient to tell the doctor if he experiences dyspnea, palpitations, chest pain, persistent nausea, paresthesias, or wheezing during the test.

Inform him that after the test his vital signs will be monitored during the first 1 or 2 hours, and the catheter insertion site

How a clot travels from the leg to the lung

Teach the patient that a blood clot may form in a leg vein if a blood vessel is torn, if blood accumulates in his legs, or if his blood clots more easily than normal.

Then if the clot breaks free, it will travel from the legs through progressively larger veins to the heart. Explain that the clot flows freely until it reaches the lungs where the blood vessels again become small. Here it can cause a blockage, stopping blood flow to the lungs.

Surveying potential damage from pulmonary embolism

In your patient teaching, stress the importance of complying with treatment to prevent recurrent emboli and potentially serious complications.

Discuss sources
Deep vein thrombosis represents the most common cause of pulmonary embolism. Besides the deep veins of the pelvis, thighs, and calves, other possible sources of thrombotic pulmonary emboli include the heart's right chambers, superficial veins, and central line catheters. Rare types include fat, air, amniotic fluid, and septic emboli.

Explain pathology
Thrombi may embolize spontaneously during clot dissolution or may be dislodged during trauma, sudden muscular action, or a change in peripheral blood flow. Rarely, emboli may result in pulmonary infarction, especially in patients with chronic cardiac or pulmonary disease.

   As the emboli form, platelets collect. This triggers the release of the vasoconstrictors serotonin and thromboxane A_2, causing pulmonary hypertension and impaired ventilation and perfusion. Unoxygenated blood is shunted into the arterial circulation, causing hypoxemia. To compensate, the patient's respiratory rate and effort will increase. This increases his oxygen consumption without improving oxygen levels.

   At first, excessive carbon dioxide diffuses out of the capillaries and is blown off by tachypnea, creating temporary respiratory alkalosis. Later, metabolic acidosis sets in as a result of anaerobic metabolism and the kidneys' failure to excrete enough hydrogen ions.

Emphasize outcomes
Eventually, pulmonary hypertension increases venous pressure, causing engorged neck veins, hepatomegaly, cerebral congestion, and myocardial dysfunction. It also reduces cardiac output. Together with hypoxemia, this causes ischemia of the major organs, producing confusion, disorientation, angina, dysrhythmias, hypotension, oliguria, and shock.

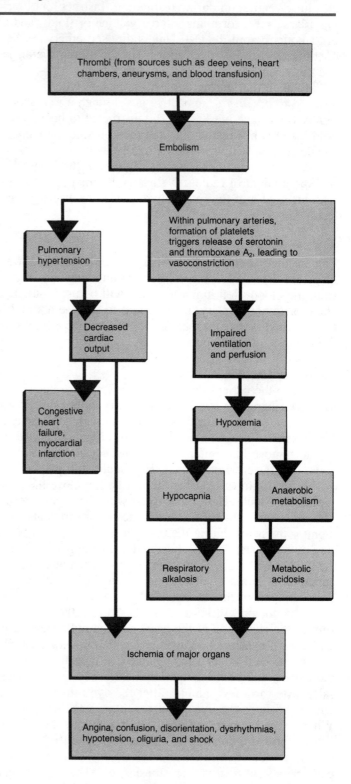

will be checked. If a femoral or antecubital vein was used, he may need to restrict activity in the affected limb for 4 to 6 hours. Instruct him to report wheezing, palpitations, chest pain, itching, nausea, vomiting, irritability, or euphoria after the test. Also tell him to report redness, swelling, or bleeding at the insertion site.

Electrocardiography

Inform the patient that this 15-minute test evaluates the heart's function by graphically recording its electrical activity. Pulmonary embolism doesn't cause specific ECG changes, but changes such as enlarged P waves, depressed ST segments, and inverted T waves may suggest pulmonary embolism.

Assure him that the test usually doesn't cause discomfort. Before the test, the technician will cleanse, dry, and possibly shave different sites on the patient's body, such as his chest and arms, and will apply a conductive jelly over them. Then he'll attach electrodes at these sites.

Point out that talking or moving his arms or legs will distort the ECG recordings and require additional testing time. He must lie still, relax, breathe normally, and remain quiet.

Doppler ultrasonography

Explain that this painless test, which takes 10 to 20 minutes, evaluates circulation in blood vessels. Inform the patient that he'll be asked to uncover his leg, arm, or neck and to loosen any restrictive clothing. Then a technician will pass a transducer coated with conductive jelly over the patient's skin, moving it along the vessels to be examined.

Impedance plethysmography

Inform the patient that this test helps detect blood clots in his leg veins. Tell him that the test takes 30 to 45 minutes to examine both legs. Assure him that it's painless and safe.

He'll put on a hospital gown and lie on his back on an examining table or bed. The technician will cleanse, dry, and possibly shave sites on his lower legs and then attach electrodes with conductive jelly.

Explain that during the test a pressure cuff will be wrapped around the patient's thigh and inflated for 1 or 2 minutes. Then it will be quickly released. Usually, the test is repeated to confirm initial tracings.

Coagulation tests

Teach the patient that in acute pulmonary embolism the doctor will monitor clotting time, thrombin time, or activated partial thromboplastin time to evaluate heparin therapy.

Once the patient begins oral anticoagulants, the doctor will monitor prothrombin time (PT) until the desired anticoagulant level is achieved. After discharge, when the patient's on anticoagulant therapy, remind him to return for periodic venipunctures to monitor PT. Usually, venipuncture will be performed once a week until PT stabilizes, then every 2 weeks and, eventually, once a month.

Questions patients ask about anti-coagulants

Why do I have to keep taking an anticoagulant now that I'm well enough to go home?
Even though you can breathe without any trouble now, you're still at risk for another pulmonary embolism. The doctor wants you to take an anticoagulant—probably for several months—to see you through this high-risk time. By taking this drug as he's prescribed, you can avoid another embolism—and a second stay in the hospital.

Why do I have to come in for blood tests while I'm taking this drug?
The drug makes your blood less likely to clot. Blood tests monitor how fast your blood clots while you're taking the medication. If it clots as quickly as normal, you'll need more medication. But if it takes too long to clot, you could experience bleeding, so you'll need less medication. Periodic blood tests allow the doctor to fine-tune your dosage to protect you from forming clots without risking bleeding.

Is there any way I can tell that the anticoagulant is working as it should?
No, not if it's working correctly. That's why you need the blood tests. You *will* know if the medication is too active: you'll note bleeding gums, nosebleeds, and dark stools or urine. These signs may indicate that your dosage needs to be adjusted.

Teach about treatments

Tell the patient that prevention of pulmonary embolism is just as important as treatment. Give him activity guidelines, including exercises for his legs. Explain how the anticoagulants should be taken, their adverse effects, and activity restrictions while taking them. If the patient is unable to take anticoagulants, teach him and his caregiver how to use a sequential compression device. Also outline how to use antiembolism stockings. Remember to teach about signs and symptoms of recurrent emboli and cardio-pulmonary complications.

Activity

Explain how prolonged standing, sitting, or inactivity can cause venous stasis, which sets the stage for peripheral venous thrombosis in the legs. Encourage the patient to exercise his legs frequently to promote blood flow. Show him exercises that he can easily do, such as rocking on his heels or toes.

If the patient's disabled or on bed rest, teach his family how to do passive leg exercises by flexing and extending the patient's feet at the ankles. Give them the teaching aid on passive range-of-motion exercises, pages 540 and 541.

Instruct the patient to elevate his legs 30 degrees or more whenever possible; for example, while he's watching television or working at a desk. He shouldn't bend his knees when he elevates his legs. This prevents blood from pooling in the legs. Tell him to avoid standing or sitting with his legs dangling or crossed.

Advise him to stop frequently for short walks on long car rides and to periodically stroll up and down the aisles on airplane trips.

Medication

Make sure the patient understands that the prescribed anticoagulants—warfarin or heparin—aim to prevent recurrent emboli. Discuss administration and adverse effects. Teach him to detect signs of drug toxicity, such as bleeding gums, epistaxis, bleeding hemorrhoids, red or purple skin spots, or excessive menstrual flow. (For more information on anticoagulant therapy, see *Teaching about drugs to prevent pulmonary embolism.*) Stress the importance of continuing anticoagulant therapy at home and returning for periodic blood tests (see *Questions patients ask about anti-coagulants*).

If the patient can't tolerate anticoagulants, the doctor may order aspirin or dipyridamole instead.

Procedures

Educate the patient about sequential compression—an alternative for patients who can't take anticoagulants. Explain that this procedure increases blood flow to the veins and decreases blood pooling to reduce the incidence of venous thrombosis during and after surgery. It's especially useful for patients on prolonged bed rest. Tell the patient that the sequential compression device (SCD)

Teaching about drugs to prevent pulmonary embolism

DRUG	ADVERSE REACTIONS	TEACHING POINTS
Anticoagulants		
heparin (Liquaemin, Lipo-Hepin)	• Watch for bleeding gums, signs of internal bleeding (bloody urine, tarry stools, hemoptysis, vomiting blood), unusually heavy bleeding from menses or cuts and wounds, easy bruising, and epistaxis. • Other reactions include chest pain; chills, fever; hives or rash; irritation, itching, or pain at injection site; leg pain; and numbness or tingling in hands and feet.	• Teach the patient how to administer an injection to prepare for self-care at home. • Caution the patient not to double-dose if he misses a dose; tell him to call the doctor instead. • Urge him to comply with regular checkups to monitor the drug's effectiveness. • Instruct him not to take aspirin and nonsteroidal anti-inflammatory drugs, such as ibuprofen (Advil), to avoid increased risk of bleeding. • Remind him to check with the doctor or pharmacist before taking other over-the-counter drugs. • Advise him not to play contact sports, such as football, to avoid injuries. Also, instruct him to brush his teeth with a soft toothbrush, shave with an electric razor (instead of a straight razor), use a nonslip mat in the bathtub, and always wear gloves for yard work. • Suggest that he wear a Medic Alert bracelet to identify himself as a heparin user.
warfarin (Coumadin, Panwarfin)	• Watch for bleeding gums, signs of internal bleeding (bloody urine, tarry stools, hemoptysis, vomiting blood), unusually heavy bleeding from menses or cuts and wounds, dark blue toes, easy bruising, chills, prolonged diarrhea, epistaxis, fatigue, fever, and sore throat. • Other reactions include diarrhea, ecchymoses, slight hair loss, and nausea.	• Instruct the patient to make up a missed dose within 8 hours. Warn him not to double-dose. • Inform him that he'll need frequent blood tests to monitor the drug's effects. • Teach him measures to reduce the risk of bleeding, such as placing a nonslip mat in the bathtub, shaving with an electric razor, using a soft toothbrush, and wearing gloves for yard work. Advise against contact sports. • Warn the female patient of childbearing age to avoid becoming pregnant. Warfarin can adversely affect fetal development and cause placental bleeding. • Instruct the patient to check with the doctor before taking any over-the-counter medications, including vitamins and pain killers or fever-reducing remedies, such as aspirin, acetaminophen (Tylenol), or Advil. Certain vitamins can reduce warfarin's effectiveness and aspirin-like drugs can increase warfarin's effect and cause bleeding. • Tell him to limit his alcohol consumption to one or two drinks daily. • Because vitamin K counteracts warfarin, emphasize the need to maintain a consistent intake of green, leafy vegetables that contain vitamin K and of fats, which enhance vitamin K absorption. Explain that following these guidelines is necessary to adjust his warfarin dosage precisely. Advise him not to drastically change his diet. For example, he shouldn't switch to a vegetarian or a weight-reduction diet without first consulting with the doctor. • Suggest that he wear a Medic Alert bracelet to identify himself as a warfarin user.

doesn't place him at increased risk for bleeding as anticoagulants do, yet it's as effective as a low heparin dose.

Assure the patient and his family that SCDs are convenient to use at home. Teach them how to use the device, and give them a copy of the teaching aid *Learning about sequential compression,* page 79. Mention that a community health nurse or therapist will follow up at home to help the patient use the device and answer any questions.

Other care measures

Stress the importance of coughing and deep-breathing exercises to prevent atelectasis. Then, teach the patient how to use antiembolism stockings to improve circulation in his legs (see *How to apply antiembolism stockings,* page 80). Emphasize that the stockings must fit properly and be applied smoothly. Explain the importance of avoiding compression in the popliteal space (the area behind the knee) from stockings or pillows used to elevate the legs. Remind him to avoid any clothing or positioning that puts pressure behind the knees or on the legs.

Advise the patient to remove throw rugs and small objects from floors to help prevent falls. If he does fall, tell him to notify his doctor. The doctor may want to examine him to rule out internal bleeding, especially in the joints.

Instruct the patient to immediately report calf pain and swelling, especially if pulling his toes back toward his head makes the calf hurt more (signs of thrombophlebitis) or lower leg and ankle swelling, hyperpigmentation, and ulceration (signs of postphlebitis syndrome). Show him how to measure his calves to detect nontender swelling (phlebothrombosis). Caution him to report symptoms of recurrent pulmonary embolism: dyspnea; tachypnea; chest pain (especially when trying to take a deep breath); hemoptysis; a dry, annoying cough; or apprehension or a feeling that "something isn't right."

Because pulmonary embolism increases pulmonary vascular resistance and taxes cardiac function, tell the patient with cardiopulmonary disease to immediately report signs of ventricular failure: fatigue, swelling of feet or ankles, unexplained steady weight gain, and chest tightness. And because pulmonary embolism can also precipitate dysrhythmias, such as atrial fibrillation or atrial flutter, tell the patient to report palpitations.

Further readings

Dickinson, S.P., and Bury, G.M. "Pulmonary Embolism-Anatomy of a Crisis," *Canadian Orthopaedic Nurses Association* 11(2):6-10, Summer 1989.

Gerdes, L. "Recognizing the Multisystemic Effects of Embolism," *Nursing87* 17(12):34-42, December 1987.

Hull, R.D., et al. "Preventing Pulmonary Embolism," *Patient Care* 23(4):63-66, 71-72, 75-76+, February 28, 1989.

Sandin, K.J., and Smith, B.S. "Above-knee Amputation with Insidious Pulmonary Embolism and Hypercoagulability Secondary to Protein C Deficiency," *Archives of Physical Medicine and Rehabilitation* 70(9):699-701, September 1989.

Schiff, M.J. "Finding and Fighting Pulmonary Embolism," *Emergency Medicine* 21(7):47-48, 50-51, April 15, 1989.

"Silent Pulmonary Embolism in the Office," *Emergency Medicine* 21(13):151, 154, July 15, 1989.

Vermilya, S.K. "Future Indications for Thrombolytic Therapy with Tissue Plasminogen Activator," *Journal of Emergency Nursing* (Supplement) 15(2):204-07, March-April 1989.

Young, H.L. "Peripheral Vascular Disease: Venous Disorders of the Lower Limb," part 2, *British Journal of Occupational Therapy* 52(4):130-32, April 1989.

Learning about sequential compression

Dear Caregiver:

The sequential compression device ordered by the doctor for the patient in your care will discourage clots from forming in leg veins. The device increases blood flow and prevents blood from pooling in the legs.

How the device works
This device has plastic sleeves that fit around the patient's legs and a controller that attaches to the sleeves with tubing.

Turned on, the controller automatically inflates and deflates the sleeves, beginning at the ankles and moving up the legs. This wavelike milking action, called "sequential compression," increases blood flow. After a few minutes, the patient probably won't be aware of the changes.

How to apply the sleeves
1 First, have the patient lie down on his back.

2 Spread the sleeve flat with the tubing connector near the patient's foot. Place his leg on top of the sleeve. The sleeve's opening should be at the side of his knee. The sleeve's solid part should lie under his knee.

Tubing connector
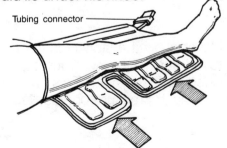

3 Once the sleeve is in position, fold the section that has Velcro strips *on the outer surface* over the patient's leg. Remember to remove all wrinkles.

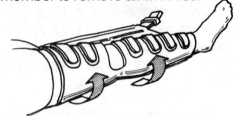

4 Now fold the outer section of the sleeve with Velcro *on the underside* over the inner section, and fasten the strips. The sleeve should be snug around the leg, but with enough room so that you can fit two fingers into the open space at the front of the knee.

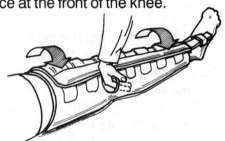

5 Follow the same steps to apply the second sleeve on the other leg. Then attach the tubing connectors on both sleeves to the controller. Be sure to align the arrows on both the controller and the sleeve tubing for a proper connection. Now turn the controller on for the recommended time.

When to call the doctor
Tell the patient to notify the doctor if he experiences tightness, numbness, or tingling in the legs or toes or any increase in pain.

PATIENT-TEACHING AID

How to apply antiembolism stockings

Dear Patient:

To improve circulation in your lower legs, the doctor wants you to apply antiembolism stockings in the morning before getting out of bed and to remove them at night once you're in bed. Follow these steps to apply the stockings.

1 Lightly dust your ankle with powder to ease stocking application.

2 Insert your hand into the stocking from the top, and grab the heel pocket from the inside. Turn the stocking inside out so that the foot section is inside the stocking leg.

3 Hook the index and middle fingers of both your hands into the foot section. Ease the stocking over your toes, stretching it sideways as you move it up your foot. Point your toes to help ease on the stocking.

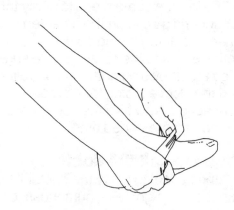

4 Center your heel in the heel pocket. Then, gather the loose material at your ankle, and slide the rest of the stocking up over your heel with short pulls, alternating front and back.

5 Insert your index and middle fingers into the gathered stocking at your ankle, and ease the stocking up your leg to the knee.

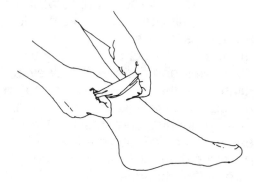

Stretch the stocking toward the knee, front and back, to distribute the material evenly. The stocking should fit snugly, with no wrinkles.

6 Make sure the top of the stocking is below the crease at the back of your knee. If the top of the stocking sits in the crease, it can put pressure on the vein and decrease circulation to your legs.

7 Never allow the stockings to be rolled part way down your leg or bunched up in any way. This can create too much pressure on your leg veins.

Pneumonia

Despite the availability of vaccines and anti-infective drugs, pneumonia remains a leading cause of death and disability, especially among already debilitated patients. For this reason, your teaching will underscore the need for complying with prescribed treatment. However, if dyspnea, tachypnea, fever, coughing, and fatigue interfere with the patient's ability to learn, you'll need to modify your plan. You'll give simple test explanations, concise directions for taking medications, and brief instructions about relieving symptoms and clearing lung secretions with such procedures as deep breathing and pursed-lip breathing, therapeutic coughing, and oxygen administration.

As the patient's condition improves, you'll cover pneumonia's causes, its development, and its symptoms. Keep in mind, though, that the patient may lose his motivation to comply with treatment as he starts to feel better. Bearing this in mind, you'll caution him about risk factors for recurrent pneumonia. To prevent a relapse, you'll urge him to take all prescribed medications as directed and stress the importance of adequate rest. Finally, you'll teach him how to prevent passing the infection to others and discuss immunization. (For more information, refer to *Teaching the pneumonia patient,* page 82.)

Discuss the disorder

Inform the patient that pneumonia is a lung infection that interferes with oxygen and carbon dioxide exchange. Explain that it develops when pathogens overwhelm the body's respiratory defenses. Normally, the upper and lower airways stop most pathogens from reaching the alveoli. If these mechanisms are inadequate, the immune system releases phagocytes and macrophages to digest the pathogens. However, pneumonia can develop if all natural defenses fail. (See *How the body fights respiratory infection,* page 83.)

Indicate that subsequent fluid accumulation and tissue changes impair gas exchange, which can cause consolidation, especially in weak or debilitated patients. This occurs when a partial lobe, an entire lobe, or most of the lung fills with mucus, pus, and other liquid material.

Point out the cardinal signs and symptoms of pneumonia: fever, pleuritic chest pain, shaking chills, dyspnea, tachypnea, and coughing. Explain that sputum color may vary, depending on the causative organism: Colorless sputum implies a noninfectious process; creamy yellow sputum suggests staphylococcal pneumonia; green sputum denotes pneumonia caused by *Pseudomonas* organisms; and sputum that looks like currant jelly indicates pneumonia

Marci Majors, RN, MSN, who wrote this chapter, is the director of cardiopulmonary rehabilitation for the Franciscan Health System of Cincinnati.

CHECKLIST

Teaching topics in pneumonia

☐ Respiratory defense mechanisms and how pneumonia develops
☐ Signs and symptoms
☐ Pneumonia classifications: by cause, location, and type
☐ Risk factors, including chronic health conditions and smoking
☐ Treatment, such as activity restrictions, drug therapy, breathing and coughing exercises, chest physiotherapy, hydration, and oxygen therapy
☐ Preventive measures, including pneumococcal and influenza vaccinations for high-risk patients and methods to prevent spreading infection, such as proper hand washing and tissue disposal
☐ Sources of information and support

Teaching the pneumonia patient

A standard plan can help you organize strategies for teaching pneumonia patients. But once you've assessed a particular patient's learning needs, you need to adapt the plan accordingly. Here's how.

Assess first
Suppose Martha Browning, a 59-year-old widow, was recently admitted to the unit. Mrs. Browning lives with her divorced daughter and cares for her 4-year-old grandson, Robbie, while her daughter works.

From Mrs. Browning's chart, you see she has a 3-year history of chronic obstructive pulmonary disease (COPD). Last week, however, her usually mild dyspnea grew severe. She began coughing up large amounts of thick, "rusty" sputum. Three days ago, she was hospitalized with pneumonia. Yesterday, sputum culture results confirmed pneumococcal pneumonia.

You also see that she's receiving continuous oxygen by nasal cannula at 2 liters/minute, chest physiotherapy, and oral antibiotics.

While you take Mrs. Browning's pulse, she asks you to help her to the bathroom. As you do, you notice that she tires easily and her dyspnea worsens even with assisted walking. She pauses to catch her breath and anxiously grips your arm, breathing rapidly. When at last she gets back to bed, she gasps, "How can I ever take care of my grandson again? I can hardly breathe. My daughter's got to go to work. Please help me."

Identify Mrs. Browning's learning needs
Obviously, Mrs. Browning is motivated to learn. But how best can she benefit from your teaching? Compare what she already knows about pneumonia with the content of a standard teaching plan. Then include or modify teaching points as needed. A standard teaching plan for a pneumonia patient covers:
• respiratory defense mechanisms and how pneumonia develops
• causes (bacteria, viruses, or other organisms) and risk factors
• signs and symptoms
• diagnostic studies, such as chest X-ray and sputum culture
• treatment, including drug therapy, therapeutic breathing and coughing techniques, chest physiotherapy, and hydration and oxygen therapies
• prevention, including ways to avoid spreading infection and immunization.

After talking with Mrs. Browning, you know that she's well aware of what happens in COPD, but she needs to know more about how pneumonia has aggravated her breathing problems. She also needs an explanation of her treatment regimen, including why

and how to comply with therapy. She should have reassurance that she can recover with time. What's more, she needs to review breathing and coughing exercises (to expel excess sputum) and infection prevention measures (to avoid repeated bouts of pneumonia).

Set learning outcomes
Now use the standard teaching plan to help you and Mrs. Browning set learning outcomes. Specifically, Mrs. Browning should be able to:

```
-list the predisposing factors for pneumonia (such as
exposure to infectious organisms, smoking, and pre-
existing health conditions) and express ways to avoid or
eliminate them at home
-name the signs and symptoms of pneumonia
-explain the rationale for complying with prescribed
antibiotic therapy
-discuss strategy to alternate rest and activity to promote
full recovery
-perform breathing and coughing exercises daily
-demonstrate ways to prevent spreading infection--for
example, by proper tissue disposal and hand washing methods.
```

Select teaching tools and techniques
Because Mrs. Browning tires easily, leaving her with little energy for learning, plan brief *demonstrations* of proper breathing and coughing techniques. Consider also using *audiocassette tapes* to explain relaxation techniques to relieve anxiety.

Then employ *booklets, posters,* and *lung models* to illustrate pneumonia pathophysiology. Informally, for instance, while you're giving routine care, plan to stress bits of information, such as proper tissue disposal and hand washing. Affirm Mrs. Browning's efforts to learn about self-care. And encourage her to ask questions and express her concerns about her condition.

Evaluate your teaching
Appropriate evaluation methods include *direct observation* and *discussion*. For example, does Mrs. Browning appear alert as you talk? Or does she yawn? Does she ask and answer questions related to her condition? Or does she try to change the subject— for instance, to her grandson?

Can she perform accurate *return demonstrations?* When you ask what she'll do in a *simulated situation* (for instance, how she will alternate rest and activity when she goes home), can she give an acceptable plan? The answers to these questions will help you modify your teaching to meet new learning needs as they arise.

How the body fights respiratory infection

As you explain the pathophysiology of pneumonia to your patient, point out how his upper airway structures form a front-line defense against infection. Add that lower airway structures stand ready to expel pathogens that escape upper airway defenses. Finally, explain how the immune system backs up failed airway defenses by destroying any remaining pathogens.

Upper airway defenses
Explain that nasal hairs trap inhaled dust and grit. Mucus then traps finer particles, such as bacteria, which the cilia move to the oropharynx (mouth area).

At the same time, turbinates—bony structures that project into the nasal cavity—humidify and warm the air, which keeps secretions warm and moist.

In the pharynx, the soft palate and epiglottis separate air and food, preventing choking. Add that gag and cough reflexes also prevent choking, and the cough reflex clears secretions that might harbor bacteria.

Lower airway defenses
Tell the patient that his lower airways—containing the larynx, trachea, bronchi, and lungs—form a second line of defense against infection. Entering the trachea, particles small enough to pass through the upper airway defenses fall into a blanket of cilia and mucus that carries these invaders away from the lungs—a process known as the mucociliary escalator. In this process, continuously undulating cilia move contaminated mucus to the pharynx (where it's swallowed), to the larynx (where coughing expectorates it), or to the nose (where sneezing and blowing expel it).

Macrophages: Last line of defense
Inform the patient that specialized reticuloendothelial cells called macrophages greet any bacteria and foreign particles that escape airway defenses and reach the pulmonary alveoli. Explain that macrophages carry out phagocytosis. First, bacteria attach to the cell surfaces, initiating opsonization—an antibody coating that enables phagocytosis. Then the macrophages surround the bacteria by forming pseudopods—footlike extensions. Phagosomes digest the bacteria and merge with lysosomes to form phagolysosomes, which help destroy the bacteria. Finally, the macrophages release digestive debris and continue to fight infection.

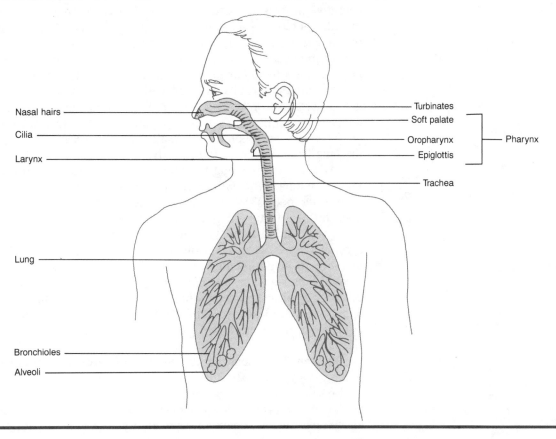

Questions patients ask about pneumonia

I can't seem to stop coughing. Should I be taking cough medicine?
No, right now you need to cough. Coughing rids your lungs of excess mucus produced by your infection. Without coughing, these secretions will remain in your lungs, allowing your infection to multiply and spread. If your cough keeps you awake at night or exhausts you, though, consult your doctor before your next appointment.

The doctor says I have "walking pneumonia." Does this mean I'm not very sick?
No. The term simply describes pneumonia with mild symptoms. Even though your sickness hasn't forced you to bed, your infection is serious and can

spread—both in you and to others. That's why you should follow your treatment plan and also take every precaution to avoid passing your infection to anyone else.

How long does pneumonia last? I've felt sick for what seems forever.
Complete recovery from pneumonia may take several weeks (especially if you're elderly, have another illness, or if the infection has spread). Your body uses a lot of energy fighting pneumonia. And like a runner after a marathon, your body needs time and rest to get back to normal. Don't sabotage your recovery by asking your body to do more than it has energy for. Follow your doctor's instructions to rest regularly.

---

caused by *Klebsiella*. (For more information, see *Questions patients ask about pneumonia*.)

Inform the patient that pneumonia may be classified by its causative organism, location, or type. Causative organisms may include bacteria, viruses, fungi, and protozoa. (See *Classifying pneumonia*.) Pneumonia may be located in the distal airways and alveoli (bronchopneumonia), part of a lobe (lobular pneumonia), or an entire lobe (lobar pneumonia). Finally, of the two types, primary pneumonia results from inhalation or aspiration of a pathogen, whereas secondary pneumonia may follow initial lung damage from a noxious chemical or other insult (superinfection). Or secondary pneumonia may result from the spread of bacteria to the lung from elsewhere in the body.

Discuss predisposing factors that influence the patient's risk for pneumonia. *Viral infections,* such as a cold or influenza, may weaken the body's defenses against pneumonia-causing viruses. *Age,* too, is a factor. Individuals under age 1 or over age 65 have the fewest natural immune factors. With aging, too, chronic disease and less efficient lung function are more likely, predisposing the body to lung infection. *Smoking* also is associated with decreased lung function, and *alcohol consumption* impairs the lung's defenses against infection. What's more, intoxication suppresses upper airway reflexes for gagging and coughing, placing the patient at risk for aspiration of gastric contents, especially while he's sleeping.

Inform the patient that *chronic lung disease,* such as emphysema, asthma, or cystic fibrosis, heightens the risk for pneumonia (and results in more serious disease than in otherwise healthy patients). A *depressed immune system* associated with cancer (particularly lung cancer), chemotherapy, an organ or bone marrow transplant, splenectomy, leukemia, or acquired immunodeficiency

Classifying pneumonia

Explain to the patient that pneumonia's origin can be classified as bacterial, viral, fungal, or protozoal. Then review the clinical features of his form of pneumonia with him.

Bacterial pneumonia
This form of pneumonia results from such organisms as *Streptococcus pneumoniae, Klebsiella pneumoniae, Staphylococcus aureus, Haemophilus influenzae, Legionella pneumophila,* and *Mycoplasma pneumoniae* ("atypical pneumonia").

Streptococcus pneumoniae. Usually preceded by an upper respiratory tract infection, this pneumonia starts suddenly with a single, shaking chill. Typified by pleuritic chest pain, rusty sputum, and a sustained fever between 102° and 104° F. (39° and 40° C.), it most commonly affects patients with chronic heart and lung disease.

Klebsiella pneumoniae. Clinical features of this pneumonia include fever, recurrent chills, and a cough that produces rusty, bloody, sticky sputum. The patient's breathing may be shallow and labored, and his lips and nail beds may appear dusky from impaired gas exchange. This type of pneumonia typically strikes patients with chronic alcoholism, lung disease, or diabetes.

Staphylococcus aureus. A fever between 102° and 104° F., recurrent, shaking chills, bloody sputum, and rapid, labored breathing characterize staphylococcal pneumonia. This bacteria commonly affects patients compromised by cystic fibrosis or by a viral illness, such as influenza.

Haemophilus influenzae. Typically colonizing the lower respiratory tract of patients with chronic bronchitis, this organism causes pneumonia that is characterized by coryza and pleural effusions.

Legionella pneumophila. Inhabiting air and water treatment systems, this organism causes legionnaires' disease. This form of pneumonia typically begins gradually and may include fever, cough, chills, muscle pain, headache, mucoid sputum, nausea, vomiting, and diarrhea.

Mycoplasma pneumoniae. Pneumonia from this organism begins gradually. Symptoms include malaise, fever, headache, sore throat, dry cough, skin rash, and enlarged lymph nodes in the neck.

Aspiration pneumonia. Various organisms are responsible for *aspiration pneumonia,* although bacterial infection of the lower airways is the most common form of this disorder. It may result from organisms aspirated from gastric or oropharyngeal contents (for example, during vomiting, coughing, or choking) or introduced during intubation. Arising from damage in the respiratory tract lining, this disorder causes breathing difficulty, low blood pressure, rapid heart rate, and dusky lips and nail beds from a lack of oxygen. A cavity or an abscess may form in the lung if a foreign body is present.

Viral pneumonia
This is the most common pneumonia—causative viruses include the influenza virus, adenovirus, respiratory syncytial virus (RSV), and measles, chicken pox, and cytomegalovirus (CMV).

Influenza. In pneumonia caused by influenza, an initially unproductive cough progresses to a productive cough with purulent sputum. The patient experiences breathing difficulty, marked duskiness from decreased oxygen, a high fever, chills, pain behind the breastbone, a frontal headache, and muscle pain.

Adenovirus. Pneumonia caused by this virus begins insidiously and most commonly affects young adults. Symptoms include a sore throat, fever, a cough with small amounts of mucoid sputum, chills, malaise, and pain behind the breastbone. The patient also may have little or no appetite, inflamed nasal passages, and enlarged lymph nodes.

Respiratory syncytial virus. Symptoms of pneumonia associated with this virus include listlessness; irritability; rapid, labored breathing; fever; severe malaise; and, possibly, cough or croup with slight sputum production. RSV affects mostly infants and children.

Rubeola (measles). Pneumonia from the measles virus produces fever, breathing difficulty, a cough with little sputum, inflamed nasal passages, a rash, and enlarged lymph nodes in the neck.

Varicella (chicken pox). The varicella virus causes pneumonia in about 30% of adults who contract chicken pox. This disease features rapid, labored breathing, dusky lips and nail beds, pleuritic chest pain, and a cough that may produce blood.

Cytomegalovirus. Difficult to distinguish from other nonbacterial pneumonias, pneumonia from CMV causes a fever, cough, shaking chills, breathing difficulty, dusky lips and nail beds, and weakness. In neonates, this form of pneumonia may be devastating, affecting multiple systems. In adults, the disease resembles mononucleosis; in immunocompromised patients, symptoms range from clinically unapparent to life-threatening illness.

Fungal pneumonia
The fungus *Aspergillus fumigatus* produces pneumonia characterized by rapid, labored breathing, a persistent fever, a cough, and pleuritic chest pain. This type of pneumonia occurs most commonly in immunocompromised patients.

Protozoal pneumonia
Caused by *Pneumocystis carinii,* protozoal pneumonia has an abrupt onset and produces rapid, labored breathing, fever, a dry cough, crackles, and dusky lips and nail beds. This form of pneumonia commonly strikes patients with acquired immunodeficiency syndrome (AIDS).

syndrome, increases susceptibility to pneumonia. Conditions associated with *impaired breathing or chest expansion* also increase the chance. Such conditions include prolonged bed rest, use of general anesthetics or narcotics, chest or abdominal surgery, abdominal distention (including pregnancy), and neuromuscular diseases (such as Guillain-Barré syndrome). *Other risk factors* include chronic illnesses, such as sickle cell anemia, diabetes, and cardiac and renal disorders, and exposure to contaminated air or water.

Complications

Emphasize that untreated or inadequately treated pneumonia can lead to life-threatening complications, such as septic shock, hypoxemia, and respiratory failure. And with inadequate treatment, the infection can spread within the patient's lung, causing empyema or lung abscess. It also may spread by the bloodstream or by cross-contamination to other parts of the body, causing bacteremia, endocarditis, pericarditis, or meningitis.

Describe the diagnostic workup

Prepare the patient for tests to diagnose pneumonia and evaluate his condition. Standard tests include a chest X-ray, sputum analysis, and blood studies.

Chest X-ray

Inform the patient that a chest X-ray can detect and monitor the progress of pneumonia. Tell him that the test will take only minutes and that he'll wear a gown without metal snaps but may keep his pants, socks, and shoes on. Instruct him to remove all jewelry from his neck and chest.

If the test is performed in the radiology department, inform the patient that he'll stand or sit in front of a large, camera-like machine. If the test is done at his bedside, someone will help him to a sitting position and place a cold, hard film plate behind his back. Then he'll be asked to take a deep breath, hold it, and remain still for a few seconds while the X-ray film is taken. Reassure him that radiation exposure is minimal.

Sputum analysis and blood studies

Explain that a sputum analysis, including a Gram stain and culture and sensitivity studies, can guide the selection of antimicrobial therapy.

To obtain a sputum sample, instruct the patient to cough deeply and expectorate into the provided sterile container. Tell him to notify you as soon as he produces the sample so that you can send it to the laboratory for analysis.

If the patient is seriously ill, blood cultures may also be ordered. Inform the patient why a blood sample is necessary and discuss when and how it will be drawn.

If the sputum analysis and blood culture results don't identify the causative organism and the patient remains ill despite conventional therapy, the doctor may order more invasive studies, such as bronchoscopy, transtracheal aspiration, and needle or open-lung biopsy. Provide instructions for these tests as necessary.

Teach about treatments

Explain that treatment includes rest, medication, and procedures to remove excess secretions, such as deep-breathing exercises, therapeutic coughing, hydration therapy, and chest physiotherapy. If the patient had healthy lungs and adequate defenses before getting ill, reassure him about his prospects for complete recovery.

Activity

Urge the patient to obtain adequate rest to promote full recovery and prevent a relapse. Tell him that the doctor will advise him when he can resume his usual activities and return to work. Explain that convalescent time depends on his age, health history, and the severity of his pneumonia. For example, a young, usually healthy patient can resume his typical activities within a week of recovery. However, a middle-aged or chronically ill patient may need several weeks before regaining his usual strength, vigor, and feeling of well-being. Accordingly, caution the patient that he may tire easily, and encourage him to alternate activity with rest to conserve his energy.

Medication

Inform the patient that the doctor usually prescribes a broad-spectrum antibiotic, such as penicillin or erythromycin, based on results of the Gram stain of the sputum. Once culture and sensitivity tests identify pneumonia's cause, the doctor may prescribe an antibiotic that is specific to the infecting organism. Discuss the patient's medication and give directions for taking it. For more specific teaching points, refer to *Teaching about drugs for pneumonia,* pages 88 to 90.

Explain that early antibiotic treatment usually cures bacterial pneumonia, particularly in young, previously healthy patients. Athough the patient's condition may improve dramatically after only a few days of treatment, emphasize that he'll need to complete the entire prescription (7 to 10 days) to prevent a relapse. Stress that recurrent pneumonia can be far more serious than the initial illness.

If necessary, discuss medications, such as gentamicin, for hospital-acquired pneumonia or pneumonia associated with immunosuppression, which can be caused by a vast range of organisms.

Procedures

Teach the patient procedures to clear lung secretions, such as breathing and coughing exercises, hydration therapy, chest physiotherapy, and home oxygen administration.

Breathing and coughing exercises. Show the patient how to perform deep breathing and pursed-lip breathing. Begin by demonstrating the proper position for maximum effectiveness. Instruct him to sit upright, placing both feet on the floor. If he must remain in bed, have him assume a high Fowler's position. Then demonstrate prolonged deep inspiration through the nose and slow exhalation through pursed lips.

Tell the patient that effective coughing can help him expel lung secretions. Suggest he use the position he used for deep

continued on page 90

Teaching about drugs for pneumonia

DRUG	ADVERSE REACTIONS	TEACHING POINTS
Antibacterials		
Aminopenicillins		
amoxicillin (Amoxil) **amoxicillin/ clavulanate potassium** (Augmentin) **ampicillin** (Omnipen, Polycillin) **bacampicillin** (Spectrobid)	• Watch for abdominal cramps, severe diarrhea, signs of hypersensitivity (such as hives, itching, rash, wheezing), and unusual thirst or weight loss. • Other reactions include mild diarrhea, nausea, sore mouth or tongue, and vomiting.	• If the patient is taking ampicillin or bacampicillin, tell him to take the drug 1 hour before meals or 2 hours after meals (on an empty stomach). If he's taking amoxicillin or amoxicillin/clavulanate potassium, advise him to take the drug without regard to mealtimes. However, if amoxicillin or amoxicillin/clavulanate potassium causes GI upset, suggest he take the drug with meals. • Instruct him to complete the prescribed therapeutic course. Remind him to take every dose. • If he's taking the suspension form of the drug, remind him to check the label for storage directions. • Tell the female patient taking ampicillin to avoid using oral contraceptives. Suggest another method of birth control.
Cephalosporins		
cefaclor (Ceclor) **cephalexin** (Keflex) **cephradine** (Anspor, Velosef)	• Watch for abdominal pain and distention; diarrhea (severe, watery, perhaps bloody); fever; hives; itching; nausea; rash; unusual fatigue, thirst, weakness, or weight loss; vomiting; and wheezing. • Other reactions include mild diarrhea, mild GI upset, and a sore mouth or tongue.	• Instruct the patient to complete the prescribed therapeutic course. Remind him to take every dose. • Suggest taking the drug with food or milk to decrease GI upset. • Tell him to store the reconstituted suspension form in the refrigerator and to shake the bottle well before pouring a dose. Inform him that the suspension form remains stable for 14 days if refrigerated. • If diarrhea develops after taking this drug, advise him to consult the doctor before taking an antidiarrheal medication.
Natural penicillins		
penicillin G potassium (Pentids) **penicillin V potassium** (PenVee K, V-Cillin K)	• Watch for signs of hypersensitivity (such as hives, itching, rash, and wheezing). • Other reactions include a darkened or discolored tongue, mild diarrhea, nausea, and vomiting.	• Tell the patient to take this drug 1 hour before meals or 2 hours after meals (on an empty stomach). Also instruct him to avoid fruit juices while taking penicillin G. • Urge him to complete the therapeutic course, even if he feels well. Remind him to take every dose and to take a missed dose within 8 hours. • Identify the signs and symptoms of hypersensitivity, and tell the patient to report any of them immediately.
Penicillinase-resistant penicillins		
cloxacillin (Tegopen) **dicloxacillin** (Dynapen) **nafcillin** (Nafcil, Unipen) **oxacillin** (Prostaphlin)	• Watch for signs of hypersensitivity (such as hives, itching, rash, or wheezing). • Other reactions include mild diarrhea, nausea, and vomiting.	• Tell the patient to take this drug 1 hour before meals or 2 hours after meals (on an empty stomach). • Instruct him to complete the therapeutic course, even if he feels well before the end. Remind him to take every dose and to take a missed dose within 8 hours. • Identify the signs and symptoms of hypersensitivity. Instruct him to notify his doctor immediately if any of them occur.
Sulfonamides		
co-trimoxazole (Bactrim, Septra)	• Watch for aching joints or muscles; fever; itching; pallor; skin blistering, peeling, rash, or redness; sore throat; unusual bleeding, bruising, fatigue, or weakness; and yellowing of the eyes or skin. • Other reactions include anorexia, diarrhea, dizziness, headache, nausea, photosensitivity, and vomiting.	• Instruct the patient to take this drug 1 hour before meals or 2 hours after meals (on an empty stomach). • Tell him to complete the prescribed therapeutic course. Remind him to take every dose and to take a missed dose within 8 hours. After 8 hours, advise him to skip that dose. • Warn him to avoid direct sunlight and ultraviolet light to prevent a photosensitivity reaction. • Point out that the initials "DS" on a co-trimoxazole drug label mean "double strength."

continued

Teaching about drugs for pneumonia — *continued*

DRUG	ADVERSE REACTIONS	TEACHING POINTS
Antibacterials – *continued*		
Miscellaneous antibiotics **clindamycin** (Cleocin)	• Watch for abdominal cramps or pain; nausea; severe abdominal distention; severe diarrhea (possibly bloody); unusual thirst, fatigue, weakness, or weight loss; and vomiting. • Other reactions include itching, mild diarrhea, and rash.	• Instruct the patient not to take antidiarrheals, especially those containing kaolin and pectin, while taking this drug. These substances may decrease absorption of clindamycin. Tell the patient to report diarrhea to the doctor *immediately.* • Instruct him to complete the prescribed therapeutic course. Remind him to take every dose. If he misses a dose, instruct him to take the missed dose within 8 hours. • Advise him not to refrigerate the reconstituted solution because it will thicken. Mention that the drug remains stable at room temperature for 2 weeks. • Tell him to take the capsule form of this drug with a full glass of water.
erythromycin base (E-Mycin, Erythrocin) **erythromycin estolate** (Ilosone) **erythromycin ethylsuccinate** (EryPed, Pediamycin) **erythromycin stearate** (Erypar, Erythrocin)	• Watch for amber or darkly colored urine, fever, pale stools, severe abdominal pain, unusual fatigue or weakness, yellowing of eyes or skin (more common with Ilosone). • Other reactions include abdominal cramps, diarrhea, nausea, sore mouth or tongue, and vomiting.	• Tell the patient who has received the base or stearate form of the drug to take it 1 hour before or 2 hours after meals (on an empty stomach). If he has received the estolate or ethylsuccinate form, tell him that he can take the drug without regard to meals and that food may actually enhance absorption. • Instruct him to complete the prescribed therapeutic course. Remind him to take every dose and to take any missed doses within 8 hours. • Advise him to take the drug with a full glass of water. Tell him *not* to take the drug with fruit juice. • Caution him not to swallow chewable tablets whole.
Antifungal		
flucytosine (Ancobon)	• Watch for bruising, confusion, dizziness, drowsiness, fatigue, fever, rash, sore throat, and unusual bleeding or weakness. • Other reactions include diarrhea, headache, nausea, and vomiting.	• Instruct the patient to complete the prescribed therapeutic course. Inform him that therapy may take weeks or months. • Tell him to take capsules over a 15-minute period to reduce nausea and vomiting.
Antiprotozoal		
pentamidine (Nebu-Pent)	• Watch for bronchospasm or cough (with inhalational form of drug) and delayed reaction (up to several months) after I.V. drug, including anxiety; chills; cold sweats; cool, pale skin or flushed and dry skin; drowsiness; hunger or loss of appetite; increased bruising or bleeding; nausea; rapid or irregular pulse rate; rash; shakiness; and unusual tiredness or weakness. • Other reactions (to I.V. pentamidine) include blurred vision, confusion, dizziness, fainting or light-headedness, fever, hallucinations, headache, and sore throat.	• Discuss proper home inhalational use of this drug. Tell the patient how to minimize bronchospasm and coughing by using an inhalational bronchodilator, as prescribed, 5 minutes before dosing. • Warn the patient *never* to reconstitute the drug with saline solution or to mix it with other drugs. • Explain that the drug should be administered only with an approved nebulizer (Respigard II), as directed by the doctor. • Review directions for proper pressure and flow rate with nebulizer use. Instruct the patient to continue inhalational therapy until the drug chamber empties (30 to 45 minutes).

continued

90 Pneumonia

Teaching about drugs for pneumonia — *continued*

DRUG	ADVERSE REACTIONS	TEACHING POINTS
Antiviral		
amantadine (Symmetrel)	• Watch for confusion, difficulty with urinating, fainting, hallucinations, and mood or other mental changes. • Other reactions include anorexia, anxiety, difficulty with concentrating, dizziness, insomnia, irritability, light-headedness, nausea, nightmares, oral or nasal dryness, and skin blotches.	• Instruct the patient to complete the prescribed therapeutic course. Remind him to take every dose. • Tell him to take the drug after meals to ensure optimum absorption. • Advise him to use caution when driving or operating machinery. Tell him not to drink alcohol, which can worsen central nervous system symptoms. • Warn him that sudden sitting up or standing may cause dizziness. Advise him to change positions slowly. • If the patient has a dry mouth, nose, or throat, advise him to chew sugarless gum or to dissolve ice chips in his mouth. • Reassure the patient with skin blotches that these usually disappear within 2 to 12 weeks of stopping the drug. • If the patient has insomnia, tell him to take the dose several hours before bedtime.

breathing. Show him how to flex his body at the waist if he's sitting or to bend his knees if he's in a high Fowler's position. If he must lie flat, direct him to lie on his side and bend his knees.

Instruct the patient to breathe deeply through his nose, hold his breath for a few seconds, and cough twice to bring up any sputum. Next, instruct him to inhale by sniffing gently and then to expectorate into a strong tissue. (Swallowed mucus can upset his stomach.) Tell him to inspect his secretions for changes and to report any unusual color, amount, or consistency.

Hydration therapy. Urge the patient to drink 2 to 3 quarts of fluid a day. This promotes adequate hydration and keeps mucus secretions thin and fluid for easier removal. Without adequate hydration, infected secretions become thick and tenacious. Fever and tachypnea also increase mucoid thickening, thereby providing an excellent medium for growth of the infecting organism.

If the patient has a cardiovascular or renal disorder that prohibits increased fluid intake, suggest he try inhaling steam from hot shower water or from a pan of boiling water. (To prevent scalding himself, he should avoid close contact with the steam.)

Chest physiotherapy. Include the patient's family when you discuss chest physiotherapy. Explain that postural drainage, percussion, and vibration help to mobilize and remove mucus from the lungs. Show your patient how to position himself for gravity drainage of the affected segment or lobe. Ambulatory and upright positions naturally drain the upper lobes. The lower lobes (with the exception of the superior segments) are best drained with the patient in the prone Trendelenburg position.

Have a family member demonstrate percussion to ensure correct technique. Along with percussion, provide instructions for deep breathing with vibration during exhalation.

Oxygen therapy. If the patient will be receiving oxygen at home, give him a copy of the teaching aid *Using oxygen safely and effectively,* page 92.

Other care measures

Urge the patient to avoid irritants that stimulate secretions, such as cigarette smoke, dust, and significant environmental pollution. Refer him to community programs or agencies that can help him stop smoking.

Discuss ways to avoid spreading infection to others. Remind the patient to sneeze and cough into tissues and to dispose of the tissues in a waxed or plastic bag. Advise him to wash his hands thoroughly after handling contaminated tissues. Give him a copy of the teaching aid *Tips for proper hand washing,* page 114.

Because pneumonia caused by influenza usually carries a poor prognosis—even with treatment—encourage the patient to obtain yearly flu immunization, unless he has a demonstrated allergy to eggs or to a previous flu vaccine.

Encourage the high-risk patient (over age 65, with chronic heart, renal, or lung disease, sickle cell anemia, or diabetes) to ask the doctor about the pneumococcal pneumonia (Pneumovax) vaccination, which he would receive only once.

Refer the patient to the local chapter of the American Lung Association for more information about pneumonia.

Sources of information and support

American Lung Association
1740 Broadway, New York, N.Y. 10019
(212) 315-8700

Coalition on Smoking or Health
1607 New Hampshire Avenue, NW, Washington, D.C. 20009
(202) 234-9375

Further readings

Bentley, D.W. "Bacterial Pneumonia in the Elderly," *Hospital Practice* 23(12):99-104, 107-09, 114-16, December 15, 1988.
Bryan, C.S. "Serious Infections in the Elderly: Preventing Pneumonia and Influenza Deaths in 1989-1990," *Consultant* 29(11):25-28, November 1989.
Caruthers, D.D. "Infectious Pneumonia in the Elderly," *American Journal of Nursing* 90(2):56-60, February 1990.
Everett, D. "For a Child With Pneumonia, There's No Place Like Home," *RN* 53(3):85-88, March 1990.
Fein, A.M., et al. "Nonresolving Pneumonia," *Emergency Medicine* 20(17):127-28, 130-33, October 15, 1988.
Mack, D.L., et al. "Foreign-Body Aspiration Presenting as Recurrent Pneumonia: A Case Report," *Respiratory Care* 33(11):1027-29, November 1988.
Mason, C.M., et al. "Prevention of Nosocomial Pneumonia," *Emergency Medicine* 22(5):31-32, 34, 37, March 15, 1990.
Niederman, M.S. "Pneumonia: The Ongoing Challenge," *Emergency Medicine* 21(7):77-79, 82-85, 88, April 15, 1989.

PATIENT-TEACHING AID

Using oxygen safely and effectively

Dear Patient:

To help you breathe easier, the doctor wants you to receive extra oxygen. You'll use an oxygen concentrator, a liquid oxygen unit, or an oxygen tank. Your prescribed oxygen flow rate is _____ liters a minute for _____ hours a day.

Obtaining equipment
When you obtain your home oxygen system from your medical equipment supplier, you'll learn how to set it up, check for problems, and clean it.

Your system will include a humidifier to warm and add moisture to the prescribed oxygen and a nasal cannula or a face mask through which you'll breathe the oxygen. Keep the supplier's phone number handy in case of problems.

Also get a backup system suitable to use in an emergency.

General guidelines
When using an oxygen tank, an oxygen concentrator, or liquid oxygen, be sure to follow these important guidelines:
• Check the water level in the humidifier bottle often. If it's near or below the refill line, pour out any remaining water and refill it with sterile or distilled water.
• If your nose dries up, use a water-soluble lubricant like K-Y Jelly.
• If you'll need a new supply of oxygen, order it 2 or 3 days in advance or when the register reads ¼ full.
• Maintain the oxygen flow at the prescribed rate. If you're not sure whether oxygen is flowing, check the tubing for

kinks, blockages, or disconnection. Then, make sure the system's on. If you're still unsure, invert the nasal cannula in a glass of water. If bubbles appear, oxygen is flowing through the system. Shake off extra water before reinserting the cannula.

Safety tips
• Oxygen is highly combustible. Alert your local fire department that oxygen is in the house, and keep an all-purpose fire extinguisher on hand.
• If a fire does occur, turn off the oxygen immediately and leave the house.
• Don't smoke — and don't allow others to smoke — near the oxygen system. Keep the system away from heat and open flames, such as a gas stove.
• Don't run oxygen tubing under clothing, bed covers, furniture, or carpets.
• Keep the oxygen system upright.
• Make sure the oxygen's turned off when it's not in use.

When to call the doctor
You may not be getting enough oxygen if you have these signs: difficult, irregular breathing, restlessness, anxiety, tiredness or drowsiness, blue fingernail beds or lips, confusion, or distractibility.

You may be getting too much oxygen if you notice these signs: headaches, slurred speech, sleepiness or difficulty waking up, or shallow, slow breathing.

If any of these signs develops, call your doctor immediately. And — above all — *never change the oxygen flow rate* without checking with the doctor first.

Pleural disorders

When pleural effusion, empyema, or pleurisy causes sharp, stabbing chest pain and impairs breathing, your patient will certainly feel apprehensive. And when diagnostic tests (such as pleural biopsy) and treatments (such as thoracentesis) are ordered, he's likely to feel increasingly frightened. Clearly, one of your major teaching goals will be to relieve his anxiety by helping him understand his disorder.

Begin by discussing how the pleural system functions. If the patient understands normal lung function, he'll better comprehend why his disorder causes his symptoms. Then he can apply the information he's learned as you teach him about tests, treatments, and self-care.

Discuss the disorder

Tell the patient that a pleural disorder refers to a lung problem. Then describe how normal pleural function promotes smooth and efficient respiration (for more information, see *Looking at the pleura,* page 94).

Review the causes of the patient's disorder. If the patient has *pleural effusion,* explain that excess fluid in the pleural space causes his signs and symptoms. Add that the causes may be classified as transudative or exudative (for more information, see *Pleural effusion: Transudative or exudative?* page 94).

Now describe the signs and symptoms of pleural effusion, including a dry cough, shortness of breath, chest pain that intensifies with coughing and deep breathing, tachycardia, and tachypnea. Other signs include a dull sound on percussion, a pleural friction rub, and decreased chest motion and breath sounds.

If the patient has *empyema,* explain that pus or necrotic tissue is found in the pleural space. The infection is typically associated with pneumonitis, cancer, esophageal perforation or rupture, tuberculosis, chest trauma, or chest surgery. Signs and symptoms include chest pain, cough, fever, malaise, night sweats, and weight loss. Other signs include absent or distant breath sounds and decreased respiratory excursion on the affected side.

If the patient has *pleurisy,* explain that this disorder is characterized by inflammation of the pleural linings (the parietal pleura and the visceral pleura). Pleurisy may complicate such disorders as cancer, chest trauma, Dressler's syndrome, pneumonia, pulmonary infarction, rheumatoid arthritis, systemic lupus erythematosus, tuberculosis, uremia, or viral illness. Signs and symptoms include dyspnea; sharp, stabbing pain that increases with respiration; and a pleural friction rub.

Heidi Volpe, RN,C, BSN, who wrote this chapter, is a research coordinator at Albert Einstein Medical Center, Philadelphia.

CHECKLIST

Teaching topics in pleural disorders

☐ How the pleural system functions
☐ An explanation of pleural effusion, empyema, pleurisy, and chylothorax, including causes and signs and symptoms
☐ Possible complications of pleural disorders
☐ Diagnostic workup, such as a health history, physical examination, chest X-rays, computed tomography, pleural biopsy, and thoracentesis
☐ Importance of balancing rest and activity
☐ Dietary guidelines
☐ Drug therapy, including antibiotic and anticancer drugs via chest tube, antibiotics given I.V. or I.M., and oral drugs for symptomatic relief
☐ Oxygen therapy to relieve dyspnea and thoracentesis to remove fluid
☐ Comfort measures, such as the orthopneic position to ease breathing and chest binding for support and pain relief
☐ Sources of information and support

Pleural effusion: Transudative or exudative?

Don't let a diagnosis such as *transudative pleural effusion* or *exudative pleural effusion* leave your patient puzzled over the nature of his disorder. Use the information below to answer questions about the causes of pleural effusion.

Transudative effusion
Associated with disorders or procedures that increase intra-vascular fluid, such as:
• congestive heart failure (most common cause)
• ascites
• cirrhosis
• hepatic hydrothorax
• hypoalbuminemia
• misplaced subclavian or internal jugular vein catheter
• nephrotic syndrome
• peritoneal dialysis
• pulmonary edema
• pulmonary embolism
• renal failure with fluid overload
• urinary tract obstruction.

Exudative effusion
Associated with underlying lung infections, such as:
• tuberculosis (most common cause)
• cancer
• collagen vascular disease
• fungal disease
• pulmonary infarction.

Looking at the pleura

Help your patient visualize the pleura as it relates to lung function and respiration. Point out that the pleural layers protect the lungs. The outer *parietal pleura* lines the inside of the thoracic cage. The inner *visceral pleura* envelops the lung itself. Between the parietal pleura and the visceral pleura, the *pleural space* (only a potential space) contains a thin film (10 to 20 ml) of fluid. This lubricates the pleural surfaces and prevents friction between the pleural layers when they expand with inhalation.

Now explain that breathing occurs through hollow tubes in the lungs. Beginning at the patient's mouth, the largest tube, called the *trachea* (or the windpipe) leads to hollow tubes called *bronchi,* which resemble tree branches, gradually becoming smaller. Each bronchus eventually branches into *bronchioles* and finally terminates in clusters of air sacs. In these tiny air sacs, called *alveoli,* the exchange of oxygen and carbon dioxide takes place. Tell the patient that any disorder of the pleura interferes with smooth and efficient gas exchange, thus hindering respiration.

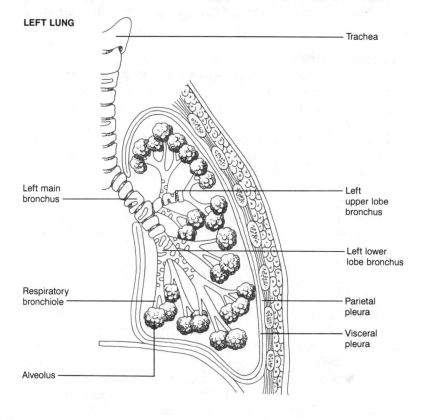

LEFT LUNG

Trachea

Left main bronchus

Left upper lobe bronchus

Left lower lobe bronchus

Respiratory bronchiole

Parietal pleura

Visceral pleura

Alveolus

If the patient has *chylothorax,* explain that this rare disorder results when chyle accumulates in the pleural space (for more information, see *Teaching about chylothorax*).

Complications
Tell the patient that untreated or poorly treated pleural effusion or pleurisy may lead to respiratory failure and systemic sepsis.

Teaching about chylothorax

Inform the patient that chylothorax is a rare pleural disorder, resulting from the accumulation of chyle in the pleural space. A milky fluid produced during digestion, chyle consists of triglyceride fats and lymph. This substance passes from the lymphatic circulation to the venous circulation at the thoracic duct. Dyspnea and chest tightness result as large amounts of chyle fill the pleural space. Be prepared to answer the patient's questions about this disorder.

What causes chylothorax?
Although chylothorax may have a congenital source, most commonly it stems from lymphoma, traumatic injury, thoracic surgery, or thoracic duct injury. Rare causes include tuberculosis, aortic aneurysm, mediastinal fibrosis, left subclavian thrombosis, pancreatitis, filariasis, and Noonan's syndrome.

How is chylothorax diagnosed?
Diagnostic tests to confirm chylothorax include a chest X-ray (which typically shows mediastinal widening), thoracic-abdominal computed tomography, lymphangiography, and thoracentesis with pleural fluid analysis.

How is chylothorax treated?
Treatment commonly depends on the disorder's cause. Usually, therapy begins with conservative measures, such as repetitive thoracentesis, chest tube thoracostomy with tetracycline pleurodesis, or chest tube drainage. (If chylothorax results from traumatic injury, reassure the patient that the disorder tends to resolve with conservative treatment in 10 to 14 days.)

Nutritional therapy aims to rest and heal the GI tract with a medium-chain triglyceride (MCT) diet supplement, such as MCT Oil, or total parenteral nutrition.

If these measures fail, the doctor may recommend surgical ligation of the thoracic duct or, if the disorder is associated with cancer, radiation therapy to the mediastinum.

Describe the diagnostic workup
Review the tests that confirm a pleural disorder. The workup may include a health history, physical examination, chest X-rays, computed tomography (CT) scan, pleural biopsy, and a pleural fluid aspiration (thoracentesis) and analysis.

Health history
Tell the patient that he'll answer questions about his medical history, in search of predisposing factors, and about the onset and duration of symptoms. Mention that cigarette smoking is commonly linked to pleural disease. Then ask about the patient's smoking history.

Physical examination
Inform the patient that pleural disorders may produce varied and widespread symptoms that reflect the underlying disorder. As a result, the determination of the cause of a pleural disorder may require examination of all body systems. However, examination of the respiratory system commonly reveals significant findings.

Chest X-rays
Tell the patient with suspected pleural effusion, empyema, or chylothorax that chest X-rays can detect pleural disorders and monitor treatment. Mention that the test takes only a few minutes.

Inform the patient that before the test he must undress from the waist up, remove all jewelry from his neck and chest, and put on a hospital gown. If the test takes place in the radiology department, he'll stand or sit in front of an X-ray machine. If the test takes place at the patient's bedside, he'll sit up while the X-ray technician places a cold, hard film plate behind the patient's back. In either case, he'll need to take a deep breath and hold it for a few seconds while the X-ray machine takes the films. Reassure him that the amount of radiation exposure is minimal.

CT scan

Explain that a CT scan helps to diagnose or evaluate pleural effusion and empyema. The scan will take about 90 minutes. If a contrast medium will be used to enhance the cross-sectional chest images, instruct the patient to fast for 4 hours before the test. Just before the CT scan, he'll be asked to remove all jewelry or metal objects that could interfere with a clear image.

During the test, the patient will lie on his back on an X-ray table that moves into the center of a large, noisy, tunnel-shaped machine. Ask him if he suffers from claustrophobia; if so, the doctor may prescribe a mild sedative. When the patient receives the contrast medium through his arm vein, advise him that he may experience a transient feeling of warmth. Instruct him to report any nausea, vomiting, dizziness, headache, or urticaria at once. Reassure him that such reactions are rare. Also tell him to relax and breathe normally during the test and not to move— movement may blur the images and prolong the test. Reassure him that the radiation exposure is minimal.

Pleural biopsy

If the patient is having a biopsy for pleural effusion, tell him that the biopsy takes 30 to 45 minutes. First he'll have his vital signs checked. Then he'll assume a special position: He may sit on the edge of the bed and lean forward on the overbed table with his arms resting on a pillow and his feet resting on a stool; he may straddle a chair; or he may sit in bed in semi-Fowler's position. Just before the biopsy, the doctor will clean the biopsy site with an antiseptic solution. Then he'll inject a local anesthetic to numb the site.

Explain that the doctor will probably use an ultrasound device to guide a needle (an Abrams' or a Cope's needle) through the chest wall to obtain a sample of pleural tissue. The patient may feel some pressure as the needle enters the chest cavity. Caution him not to move, breathe deeply, or cough while the needle's in place. Instruct him to let the doctor know if he feels short of breath, dizzy, weak, or sweaty, or as if his heart is racing.

Inform the patient that afterward the doctor will apply pressure and a bandage to the site. The patient will have a chest X-ray to check for complications, and his vital signs will be monitored frequently for a few hours. Instruct the patient to tell the doctor if he feels faint or experiences increased breathing difficulty, chest pain, or uncontrollable coughing.

Tell the patient that the biopsy sample will be sent to the laboratory for analysis to identify the cause of his disorder.

If the doctor decides to make a chest incision to obtain a tissue sample, the biopsy will be done in the operating room. Be sure to describe basic preoperative and postoperative procedures.

What pleural fluid findings mean

Be prepared if your patient asks you to clarify what his test results mean, especially if he's having pleural fluid studies. Use this chart to help you interpret test findings.

TEST	SIGNIFICANCE OF RESULTS
Gram stain and culture and sensitivity studies	Positive results identifying gram-positive or gram-negative organisms suggest bacterial infection at an early stage. In the later stages, the fluid may look grossly purulent with a positive Gram stain; yet cultures may be negative from antibiotic therapy.
Acid-fast stain and culture	Positive results suggest tuberculosis.
Red blood cell (RBC) count	An RBC count around 10,000/mm³ in pink or light red pleural fluid suggests tissue damage. A count over 100,000/mm³ in grossly bloody pleural fluid suggests intrapleural cancer, pulmonary infarction, tuberculosis, or closed chest trauma. (If the patient has a hemothorax, the pleural fluid's hematocrit value will be similar to that of capillary blood.)
Leukocyte count	Fewer than 1,000/mm³ suggests a transudate. More than 1,000/mm³ may indicate an exudate.
Lymphocyte count	A value over 50% suggests tuberculosis, lymphoma, or other cancer.
Blood clots	These formations in pleural fluid may reflect neoplasm, tuberculosis, or other infection.
Specific gravity	A value exceeding 1.016 points to neoplasm, tuberculosis, or other infection; a value under 1.014 may indicate congestive heart failure (CHF).
Total protein	A protein level below 3 g/dl suggests CHF or another transudative process; a protein level above 3 g/dl suggests neoplasm, tuberculosis, or other infection.
Lactate dehydrogenase	Levels rise above normal in cancer and other conditions associated with exudates; levels fall below normal in heart failure and other conditions associated with transudates.
Glucose	Pleural fluid levels below the serum glucose level may suggest cancer, bacterial infection, or nonseptic inflammation.
pH	A pH value under 7.30 suggests empyema or other inflammation.
Sediment	Sediment detected in pleural fluid may represent malignant cells, cellular debris, or cholesterol crystals.

Thoracentesis
Inform the patient that thoracentesis (also called pleural aspiration) may determine the cause of pleural effusion once it's been confirmed by physical examination and chest X-ray. Explain that the doctor will send the pleural fluid sample to the laboratory for analysis (for more information, see *What pleural fluid findings mean*). Describe the procedure, and give the patient a copy of the teaching aid *Learning about thoracentesis,* pages 101 and 102.

Teach about treatments
Depending on the patient's disorder, treatments include medication, thoracentesis, oxygen therapy, coughing and deep-breathing, adequate rest and nutrition and, as a last resort, surgery.

Using the orthopneic position

Is your patient losing sleep because he can't breathe comfortably when he lies down? Show him how to assume the orthopneic position.

The illustration shows how pillows can be propped behind the patient's back to keep him upright and positioned on the overbed table. This will help to support and cushion the weight of his arms, shoulders, and head.

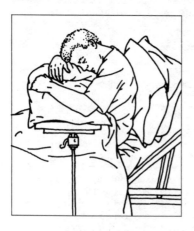

Activity
Most patients with pleural disorders experience fatigue and breathlessness. Explain that the patient's disorder deprives his body of adequate oxygen. The lower his oxygen level, the greater his fatigue. Emphasize that he'll need to find the right balance between rest (for healing) and activity (to prevent complications, such as pneumonia). Encourage him to take short naps (long ones may interfere with a good night's sleep), to alternate exercise and rest periods, and to schedule treatments and take medication when they won't interrupt rest periods. If he has trouble breathing when lying down, recommend the orthopneic position (see *Using the orthopneic position*).

Diet
Nutrition problems are common in patients with pleural disorders. Your patient may complain of impaired taste and smell (from nasal congestion), coughing attacks that make eating difficult, and a bad taste in his mouth (from sputum and accompanying nausea). Encourage him to brush and floss his teeth and rinse with mouthwash frequently. Also suggest that he eat small, protein-rich meals or snacks to conserve energy and ease digestion. Urge him to drink plenty of fluids, unless the doctor directs otherwise (for example, in pleural effusion from congestive heart failure, additional fluids may be harmful).

Medication
Tell the patient that medications are the primary treatment for pleural disorders. Discuss the drugs prescribed for the patient's particular disorder, explaining that they may be discontinued after the disorder is controlled. Pleurodesis, accomplished by using tetracycline or bleomycin, may be ordered in pleural effusion. Antibiotics may be used for empyema, and symptomatic drug therapy, including antitussives, nonsteroidal anti-inflammatory drugs (NSAIDs) and, possibly, narcotic analgesics, may be used for pleurisy.

Pleurodesis. If the patient has pleural effusion, explain that he may receive a solution of tetracycline hydrochloride (Achromycin) or bleomycin sulfate (Blenoxane) through a chest tube to produce inflammation and adhesions. Called pleurodesis, this condition may deter pleural fluid from reaccumulating. Explain that the inflammation and adhesions in the pleural space eliminate areas for further effusion. After the instillation, direct the patient to change his position frequently to help distribute the drug. Reassure him that adverse effects are usually mild because the instillation method confines the drug to the pleural space until the drug is withdrawn.

If the patient's effusion aspirate contains malignant cells, tell him that an anticancer agent, such as nitrogen mustard (Mustargen), may be instilled through the chest tube.

Antibiotic therapy. If the patient has empyema, inform him that high doses of antibiotic drugs may destroy the organism causing the infection. Typically, he'll receive the antibiotic via a chest tube or parenterally (I.V. or I.M.). Before starting the therapy, the patient will undergo culture and sensitivity tests.

Symptomatic therapy. Tell the patient with pleurisy that drug treatment aims to relieve his symptoms. If the doctor recommends *antitussive therapy* to help control the patient's cough, tell the patient that he can obtain some antitussives, such as the combination of dextromethorphan and guaifenesin (Robitussin-DM), without a prescription. Caution him about adverse effects, including insomnia, irritability, nervousness, and unusual excitement. The drug may also cause dizziness, drowsiness, and gastric upset.

Warn the patient to avoid alcohol when taking this drug because alcohol may increase central nervous system (CNS) depression. Caution him to avoid activities that require alertness if the medication makes him feel drowsy.

If an *NSAID,* such as ibuprofen (Motrin), is prescribed, inform the patient that this drug reduces inflammation. Clarify the dosage, and caution him that this drug may cause behavioral changes, confusion, diarrhea, dizziness, drowsiness, edema, fainting, GI upset, headache, insomnia, loss of appetite, nausea, rashes, vertigo, vomiting, and weight gain. Reassure him, however, that adverse effects are usually mild with short-term therapy. Tell him that taking the drug with food can reduce GI upset, the most common adverse effect.

If the patient needs a *narcotic analgesic* for severe pleuritic pain, the doctor may prescribe morphine (Duramorph), codeine, or meperidine (Demerol). Mention that most narcotic analgesics have antitussive properties. One such drug, codeine sulfate, helps to suppress coughing at the same time that it relieves pain. Point out the adverse effects of these controlled substances, including possible breathing difficulties, confusion, constipation, dizziness, drowsiness, dry mouth, euphoria, nausea, urine retention, and vomiting.

Advise the patient to avoid alcohol when taking a narcotic analgesic because alcohol may increase CNS depression. Instruct him to avoid activities requiring alertness if the drug makes him feel drowsy or clumsy. Finally, caution him that prolonged use can lead to physical and psychological dependence and tolerance.

Procedures

Inform the patient that oxygen therapy is usually necessary for pleural effusion or empyema. Explain that the flow rate, type of delivery system, and duration of therapy will vary, depending on the patient's disorder and the severity of his dyspnea. Tailor your teaching to the patient's disorder.

Tell the patient with pleural effusion, empyema, or pleurisy with pleural effusion that thoracentesis may be performed to drain the pleural space and relieve breathing difficulties. Add that thoracentesis may be followed by insertion of a chest tube (to remove fluid or air) and closed drainage. Describe the chest tube insertion and drainage procedure to the patient, as appropriate.

Surgery

If the patient has severe empyema, explain that decortication (removal of the visceral pleura) may be performed. Rib resection may also be necessary to allow for open drainage and lung expansion. Describe these operations and provide preoperative and postoperative guidelines as needed.

Other care measures

Teach the patient how to do coughing and deep-breathing exercises.

If the doctor recommends chest support for the patient with pleurisy, show the patient how to tape his chest to provide support and firm pressure at the pain site. Even without chest binding, he can apply pressure to relieve discomfort, especially during coughing and deep breathing. Demonstrate how to use a folded blanket or pillow as a splinting device.

Finally, urge the patient to ensure continuing recovery by scheduling and keeping appointments for follow-up examinations and tests.

Sources of information and support

American Lung Association
1740 Broadway, New York, N.Y. 10019
(212) 315-8700

National Jewish Center for Immunology and Respiratory Medicine
1400 Jackson Street, Denver, Colo. 80206
(303) 388-4461

Respiratory Health Association
55 Paramus Road, Paramus, N.J. 07652
(201) 843-4111

Further readings

Bunch, D. "Air Pollution and Respiratory Health," *American Association of Respiratory Care* 13(12):26-28, 30, December 1989.

Chilman, A.M., and Thomas, M., eds. *Understanding Nursing Care,* 3rd ed. New York: Churchill Livingstone, 1987.

Connor, P., et al. "Two Stages of Care for Pleural Effusion," *RN* 52(2):30-34, February 1989.

Davis, N.B. "Danger Signs: Pleural Friction Rub," *Nursing88* 18(1):70-71, January 1988.

Feinsilver, S.H., et al. "Effusions: Fast-track Management," *Patient Care* 22(19):30-54, November 30, 1988.

Glatt, A.E. "Acute Pleurisy in an Intravenous Drug Abuser," *Hospital Practice* 25(2):155, 158, 160+, February 15, 1990.

Heath, G.G., et al. "Chylothorax: An Overview," *Choices in Respiratory Management* 19(1):18-19, January 1989.

Kronenberg, R.S. "Asbestos Inhalation and Cigarette Smoking Make a Lethal Combination," *Occupational Health Safety* 58(3):50-53, 55-56, 68, March 1989.

Olson, E. "The Hazards of Immobility," *American Journal of Nursing* 90(3):43-44, 46-48, March 1990.

Smyrnios, N.A., et al. "Pleural Effusion in an Asymptomatic Patient," *Chest* 97(1):192-96, January 1990.

Learning about thoracentesis

Dear Patient:

Your doctor wants you to have thoracentesis. In this procedure, the doctor uses a needle to remove extra fluid from the area around your lung called the pleural space. He'll send a sample of this fluid to the laboratory where it will be studied to find out what's causing your disorder.

The procedure is usually done in your hospital room, and it takes about 10 or 15 minutes.

Getting ready

The nurse will ask you to put on a hospital gown that opens down the back so the doctor can easily reach the right location for the procedure.

Then the nurse will take your vital signs. She'll take your temperature and pulse rate. She'll also check your breathing rate and your blood pressure.

Next, the doctor will examine your back and chest and choose an area for inserting the needle. Then that area will be shaved and cleaned.

Just before the procedure, the nurse will help you to assume a special position. If the doctor decides to perform thoracentesis from your back, you may sit on the edge of the bed and lean forward on your overbed table. The nurse will help you rest your arms on a pillow and your feet on a stool (as shown above right).

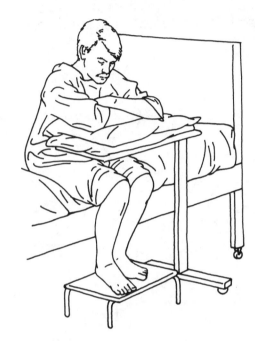

Or she may ask you to straddle a chair (as shown below).

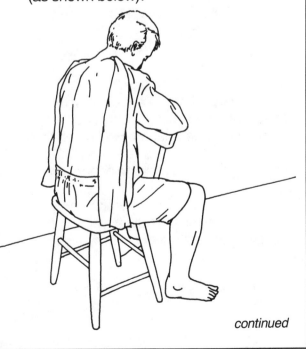

continued

Learning about thoracentesis — *continued*

If the doctor decides to perform thoracentesis by obtaining a fluid sample from your chest, the nurse will help you sit up in bed with the head of your bed raised. This is called the semi-Fowler's position.

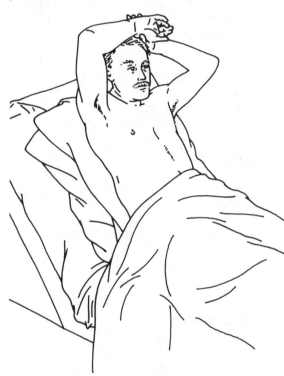

During the procedure
Immediately before thoracentesis, the doctor will clean your chest or back with a cold antiseptic solution. He'll numb the area by injecting a local anesthetic. This may cause a slight stinging or burning sensation.

Then he'll perform thoracentesis by inserting a special needle between your ribs and into your chest cavity where the fluid lies.

You shouldn't feel much discomfort, but you may feel some pressure when the needle's inserted.

Don't move, and don't breathe deeply or cough when the needle's in place because this could damage your lung.

Be sure to let the doctor or nurse know if you feel short of breath, dizzy, weak, or sweaty, or if your heart is racing.

Now, the doctor will use the needle and a syringe to withdraw excess pleural fluid. If you have lots of fluid, he may also use a suction device. Usually, he'll take out 1 to 2 quarts of fluid. If your lung holds more, you may need thoracentesis again later.

After the procedure
When the doctor removes the needle, you may feel the urge to cough. (Go ahead. It's safe to do so.) Then he'll apply pressure and a snug bandage to the wound.

Immediately after thoracentesis, you'll have an X-ray to monitor your progress and check for complications. Your nurse will check your vital signs frequently for the next few hours.

If the doctor withdrew a lot of fluid, you may notice that you're breathing more easily.

What to watch for
If you feel faint, tell the doctor. He may give you some oxygen. And be sure to report any other discomfort, such as difficult breathing, chest pain, or uncontrollable coughing—these can signal complications.

Acute bronchitis

Because acute bronchitis occurs commonly, you're likely to teach about it often. Typically, you'll begin by describing the disorder and how bronchial inflammation affects the respiratory tract.

You'll explain that acute bronchitis is usually mild and self-limiting, unless the patient has an underlying disorder, such as a respiratory or cardiac one. Your teaching will usually focus on helping him take an active role in managing his symptoms. You'll emphasize the need for rest, a balanced diet, and increased fluid intake. You may also discuss therapeutic devices, such as home humidifiers, used to help mobilize lung secretions. And you'll show the patient how to breathe effectively and do controlled coughing exercises to prevent airway obstruction and unnecessary fatigue.

Because upper respiratory tract infections represent the major cause of acute bronchitis, you'll teach how proper hand washing and other infection-control measures can help prevent recurrence.

Discuss the disorder

Tell the patient that acute bronchitis may follow a cold or another respiratory tract infection. It usually results from viruses, such as rhinoviruses, adenoviruses, and *Mycoplasma pneumoniae*. If the patient's resistance to infection diminishes, normal flora colonize, which may lead to a secondary bacterial infection. Acute bronchitis can also result from bacteria, such as *Haemophilus influenzae* and *Streptococcus pneumoniae*. What's more, it can result from inhalation of industrial pollutants or chemicals or from aspiration of food or other foreign objects.

Explain that acute bronchitis is an inflammation of the bronchial tubes, which lead from the trachea to the lungs (see *What happens in acute bronchitis,* page 104). Describe how this disorder affects both the upper (nose, mouth, oropharynx, and larynx) and lower (trachea, bronchi, and bronchioles) respiratory tracts.

Inform the patient that early symptoms mimic those of the common cold or flu: chills, chest discomfort, sore throat, slight fever, and dry cough. As the illness progresses, breathing becomes more difficult. The cough becomes irritating and productive, producing thick, mucopurulent, and, possibly, blood-tinged sputum. Typically, cold symptoms subside in a few days, but the cough persists for 2 to 3 weeks. For more information, see *Reviewing the cough mechanism,* page 105.

Karen K. McDowell, RN, who wrote this chapter, is a staff nurse at Wilson Memorial Hospital in Johnson City, N.Y.

CHECKLIST

Teaching topics in acute bronchitis

☐ How acute bronchitis develops
☐ Major symptoms of acute bronchitis
☐ Review of the coughing mechanism
☐ Possible complications: pneumonia and chronic obstructive pulmonary disease
☐ Diagnosis by physical examination
☐ Importance of bed rest, a balanced diet, and increased fluid intake
☐ Role of drug therapy
☐ Over-the-counter remedies to avoid
☐ Breathing and coughing exercises
☐ How to take a temperature
☐ Measures to prevent recurrent infections, such as proper hand washing and annual influenza vaccine
☐ Source of information and support

What happens in acute bronchitis

In acute bronchitis, viral pathogens or inhaled irritants produce widespread inflammation in the tracheobronchial tree. This leads to increased mucus production and a narrowed or blocked airway.

As inflammation progresses, the mucus-producing goblet cells undergo hypertrophy, as do the ciliated epithelial cells that line the respiratory tract. Hypersecretion from the goblet cells blocks free movement of the cilia, which normally propel dust, irritants, and mucus from the airways.

As a result, the airway remains blocked, and mucus and debris accumulate in the respiratory tract.

CROSS SECTION OF NORMAL BRONCHIAL TUBE

NARROWED BRONCHIAL TUBE IN ACUTE BRONCHITIS

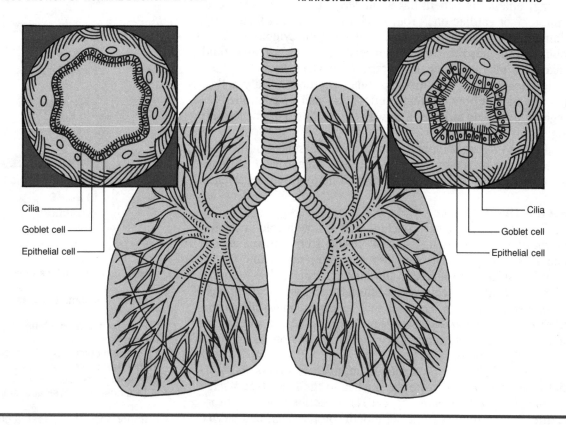

Cilia
Goblet cell
Epithelial cell

Cilia
Goblet cell
Epithelial cell

Complications
Warn the patient that acute bronchitis can lead to pneumonia. Infants and elderly patients are most susceptible to complications because their immune systems are less able to fend off infections. Point out that persistent fever may signal developing pneumonia. Urge the patient to call his doctor if symptoms are severe or persist beyond a week. Instruct him to take his temperature daily. Give him a copy of the teaching aid *How to take a temperature correctly,* pages 112 and 113.

If appropriate, explain that frequent episodes of acute bronchitis may progress to chronic obstructive pulmonary disease (COPD). That's why it's so important to avoid upper respiratory tract infections. COPD is characterized by chronic airway obstruction and breathing difficulty, increased sputum production, dyspnea on exertion, and a persistent, productive cough that causes fatigue.

Describe the diagnostic workup

Inform the patient that the key to diagnosing acute bronchitis is a thorough physical examination. Explain that you or the doctor will listen to his lungs for crackles (which sound like firecrackers) and rhonchi (which sound like bubbling). Ask if he has experienced fever, midsternal chest pain, malaise, and sore throat. If his sputum is thick with mucus and pus, he may need to provide a specimen for bacterial analysis. If so, show him how to expectorate from deep within his lungs to produce a pure sputum sample.

Advise him that the doctor may order a chest X-ray if he suspects other diseases or complications.

Teach about treatments

Explain that treatment aims to relieve symptoms until the bronchi heal. Outline the role of rest, fluids, and, possibly, medications. Teach the patient to wash his hands properly and to follow other recommendations to prevent recurrent infection.

Reviewing the cough mechanism

When you teach patients with acute bronchitis, emphasize the positive effects of coughing in clearing sputum from the airway passages.

Explain that sensory nerve endings, or cough receptors, detect an irritant or obstruction. These cough receptors are thought to be located in the nose, sinuses, auditory canals, nasopharynx, larynx, trachea, bronchi, pleurae, diaphragm, and, possibly, the pericardium and GI tract.

Once a cough receptor is stimulated, the sensory signals travel by way of the vagus and glossopharyngeal nerves to the "cough center" in the medulla. There, the decision is made to cough—a three-step process.

Step 1
The cough decision is relayed to the abdominal and intercostal muscles. Then, a deep inspiration occurs.

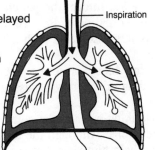

Inspiration

Step 2
This triggers closure of the epiglottis, which seals off lung air.

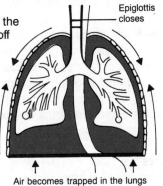

Epiglottis closes

Air becomes trapped in the lungs

Step 3
Next, the diaphragm relaxes, and the intercostal and abdominal muscles contract, causing air pressure to build in the lungs. The building air pressure forces the epiglottis open, releasing a pressurized burst of air. This sudden, forceful, and noisy expiration—the cough—propels the irritant or obstruction upward and out of the airway.

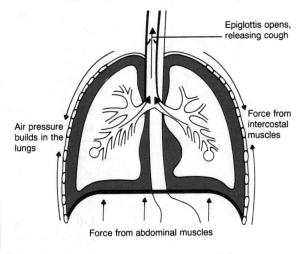

Epiglottis opens, releasing cough

Air pressure builds in the lungs

Force from intercostal muscles

Force from abdominal muscles

Activity

Advise the patient to limit daily activities and to rest frequently. Explain that bed rest minimizes irritation of the inflamed bronchi and promotes healing.

Diet

Encourage the patient to eat a well-balanced diet to maintain his strength. Advise him to drink 10 to 12 glasses of fluid daily to help eliminate secretions. If he must limit his fluid intake because of a cardiac or renal disorder, suggest that he use a humidifier to help liquefy his secretions. Caution him to avoid alcoholic beverages because they suppress upper airway reflexes and increase the risk of superinfection.

Medication

Explain that drug therapy varies according to the patient's condition and may include antibiotics, antipyretic analgesics, or other drugs. (For more information, see *Teaching about drugs for acute bronchitis.*)

Antibiotics. If the patient has no underlying disorder, antibiotic therapy usually isn't necessary. However, if his sputum contains pus, a sign of bacterial infection, his doctor may prescribe a broad-spectrum antibiotic. Other indications for antibiotic therapy include persistent fever, lingering cold symptoms, and prolonged sputum production.

Instruct the patient to take an antibiotic with a full glass of water to promote complete absorption and to prevent the pill from lodging in his esophagus. If the patient has ever had a hypersensitivity reaction to an antibiotic, tell him to let the doctor know before he prescribes any medication.

Antipyretic analgesics. Inform the patient that aspirin or acetaminophen reduces fever and pain. Be sure to discuss the risks of GI and bleeding disorders associated with aspirin use in children and in older patients.

Other drugs. If the doctor prescribes a bronchodilator, tell the patient that this drug opens airway passages to make breathing easier.

If the patient is taking an over-the-counter cough suppressant, explain its limitations. Although the drug may reduce his coughing spasms and help him sleep better, it won't relieve acute bronchitis. Remind him to practice productive coughing to help clear his airways.

Caution the patient about using an over-the-counter cold remedy for this condition. Advise him to avoid medications that contain antihistamines, which dry out, rather than liquefy, respiratory tract secretions. Warn against cough expectorants because they haven't proved effective and against decongestants because they aren't recommended for acute bronchitis and may raise his blood pressure.

Other care measures

Specify techniques for effective breathing and coughing, and measures to prevent further infections.

continued on page 110

Teaching about drugs for acute bronchitis

DRUG	ADVERSE REACTIONS	TEACHING POINTS
Antibiotics		
amoxicillin/clavulanate potassium (Augmentin) **amoxicillin trihydrate** (Amoxil)	• Watch for abdominal cramps, severe diarrhea, signs of hypersensitivity (hives, pruritus, rash, wheezing), unusual thirst, and weight loss. • Other reactions include mild diarrhea, nausea, sore mouth or tongue, and vomiting.	• Advise the patient to chew tablets thoroughly or crush before swallowing and to wash them down with liquid to ensure adequate drug absorption. The capsule may be emptied and contents swallowed with water. • Tell him to report diarrhea promptly. • Instruct him to complete the prescribed course of therapy. Remind him to take every dose, even if he feels better after taking the drug for a while. • If the drug causes GI upset, advise the patient to take it with meals.
cefaclor (Ceclor)	• Watch for abdominal pain and distention, diarrhea (severe, watery, perhaps bloody), fever, hives, nausea, pruritus, rash, unusual fatigue, thirst, weakness, weight loss, vomiting, and wheezing. • Other reactions include mild diarrhea or GI upset and sore mouth or tongue.	• Instruct the patient to complete the prescribed course of therapy. Remind him to take every dose, even if he feels better after taking the drug for a while. • Suggest taking the drug with food or milk to decrease GI upset. • Tell the patient to store the reconstituted suspension form in the refrigerator and to shake it well before using. Inform him that the suspension remains stable for about 14 days when refrigerated. • If he develops diarrhea, tell him to consult the doctor before taking an antidiarrheal drug. • Inform the diabetic patient that this drug may cause false-positive results on some urine glucose tests. Advise him to check with the doctor before changing his diet or medication dosage.
co-trimoxazole (trimethoprim-sulfamethoxazole) (Bactrim, Septra)	• Watch for aching joints or muscles; fever; pallor; pruritus; skin blistering, peeling, rash, or redness; sore throat; unusual bleeding, bruising, fatigue or weakness; and yellowing of eyes or skin. • Other reactions include anorexia, diarrhea, dizziness, headache, nausea, photosensitivity, and vomiting.	• Tell the patient to take this drug on an empty stomach 1 hour before or 2 hours after meals. • Instruct him to complete the prescribed course of therapy. Remind him to take every dose, even if he feels better after taking the drug for a while. • Tell him to drink a full glass of water with each dose and extra water throughout the day to prevent formation of urine crystals. • Warn him to avoid direct sunlight and ultraviolet light to prevent photosensitivity reaction. • Advise him to notify his doctor before undergoing surgery requiring general anesthesia. • Explain that "DS" on the drug container label means "double strength."
erythromycin (E-Mycin, Erythrocin, Ilosone, Pediamycin)	• Watch for amber or dark urine, fever, pale stools, severe abdominal pain, unusual fatigue or weakness, and yellowing of eyes or skin (more common with Ilosone). • Other reactions include anorexia, diarrhea, dizziness, headache, nausea, photosensitivity, rash, and vomiting.	• Instruct the patient to complete the prescribed course of therapy. Remind him to take every dose, even if he feels better after taking the drug for a while. • Tell him not to swallow chewable tablets whole. • Advise him to take this drug on an empty stomach 1 hour before or 2 hours after meals with a full glass of water. If prescribed, he can take enteric-coated estolate, or ethylsuccinate forms without regard to meals.

continued

Teaching about drugs for acute bronchitis — *continued*

DRUG	ADVERSE REACTIONS	TEACHING POINTS
Antibiotics — *continued*		
tetracycline (Achromycin, Tetracyn)	• Watch for diarrhea; increased pigmentation of skin or mucous membranes; unusual fatigue, thirst, or weakness; and urinary frequency or increased volume. • Other reactions include abdominal cramps or burning, discolored tongue, dizziness, genital or rectal itching, light-headedness, nausea, photosensitivity, sore mouth or tongue, and vomiting.	• Instruct the patient to complete the prescribed course of therapy. Remind him to take every dose, even if he feels better after taking the drug for a while. • Advise him to take this drug on an empty stomach 1 hour before or 2 hours after meals. Tell him not to take it with milk. • Caution him to take the drug at least 1 hour before bedtime to prevent esophageal irritation. • Instruct him to store reconstituted solutions in the refrigerator. They're stable for 48 hours. • Warn the pregnant patient or the parent of the patient under age 8 that this drug may permanently discolor teeth, cause enamel defects, and retard bone growth. • Teach the patient good oral hygiene. Show him how to inspect his tongue for signs of candidal infection. If signs indicating superinfection occur, instruct him to stop taking the drug and to notify the doctor. • Warn him to avoid exposure to direct sunlight and ultraviolet light. Instruct him to use a sunscreen if exposure is unavoidable, and tell him that photosensitivity may continue after he stops the drug. • Advise him not to use medication that has changed color, taste, or appearance.
Antipyretic analgesics		
acetaminophen (Tylenol)	• Watch for possible liver damage with prolonged use. • Other reactions include hives and rash.	• Advise the patient to notify the doctor if his fever rises above 103° F. (39.5° C.) or if it persists for more than 3 days. • Suggest the liquid drug form for patients who have difficulty swallowing tablets.
aspirin (Bayer, Ecotrin, Measurin)	• Watch for bleeding gums, dyspnea, easy bruising, hearing loss, tarry stools, tinnitus, and vomiting blood. • Other reactions include gastric upset and heartburn.	• Advise parents not to give this drug to children with flulike symptoms because of its link to Reye's syndrome. • Tell the patient to avoid antacids, which can reduce the drug's effectiveness. • Warn him to avoid taking the drug with alcohol to prevent GI bleeding. • Instruct the patient who has difficulty swallowing tablets that this drug can be crushed and mixed with soft food or dissolved in liquid.
Bronchodilators		
terbutaline (Brethine)	• Watch for chest pain, diaphoresis, dizziness, dyspnea, flushing, headache, pallor, pounding heartbeat, and vomiting. • Other reactions include anxiety, fear, heartburn, insomnia, nausea, and palpitations.	• Tell the patient to notify his doctor if he gets minimal or no relief from the prescribed dosage. • Warn him that increasing the dosage can cause serious complications, such as severe wheezing, stroke, myocardial infarction, and, possibly, death. Also advise against taking the prescribed dosage more frequently than ordered. Excessive use can cause respiratory distress or reduce the drug's effectiveness. Tell him to stop using the drug and notify the doctor if he develops any signs of serious complications. • Tell him not to take over-the-counter drugs containing central nervous system (CNS) stimulants, such as ephedrine and epinephrine, to avoid worsened adverse reactions and toxicity. • Teach him how to use an inhaler. • Suggest that the patient gargle or rinse his mouth with water after using an oral inhaler to minimize any bitter aftertaste.

continued

Teaching about drugs for acute bronchitis — *continued*

DRUG	ADVERSE REACTIONS	TEACHING POINTS
Bronchodilators — *continued*		
theophylline (Bronkodyl, Elixophyllin, Theo-Dur, Theolair, Theospan-SR, Theostat)	• Watch for anorexia, diarrhea, dizziness, flushing, headache, insomnia, irritability, light-headedness, nausea, palpitations, pulse rate or rhythm changes, restlessness, seizures, tachypnea, tremulousness, and vomiting. • Other reactions include mild dyspepsia and bitter taste.	• Tell the patient not to take over-the-counter drugs containing CNS stimulants, such as ephedrine or epinephrine, to avoid increased CNS stimulation. • Advise him that beverages containing xanthines, such as coffee and tea, can magnify the drug's effects. • Because cigarette smoking increases drug metabolism, tell him not to stop smoking abruptly during therapy to avoid drug toxicity. • Instruct him that taking this drug on an empty stomach about 1 hour before or 3 hours after meals will result in best absorption. • Advise him to notify the doctor if he experiences new flulike symptoms or develops a high fever, which may influence the drug's effectiveness.
Cough suppressants		
codeine (Phenergan VC with codeine)	• Watch for confusion, dizziness, respiratory difficulty, and sedation. • Other reactions include constipation, drowsiness, dry mouth, and nausea.	• Explain that this drug should help control his nonproductive cough. Advise him to consult his doctor if his cough becomes productive. • Warn him that prolonged use can lead to physical and psychological dependence and tolerance. • Advise against taking this drug with alcohol to avoid increased CNS depression. • Because this drug can impair mental and physical function, advise him to cautiously use a motor vehicle, heavy machinery, or tools. • Suggest that he use sugarless chewing gum or hard candy or ice chips to relieve mouth and throat dryness.
hydrocodone bitartrate (Hycodan Syrup, Hydrocodone Syrup, Hydropane Syrup, Mycodone Syrup)	• Watch for sedation and drowsiness. • Other reactions include nausea and vomiting, which occur most frequently in ambulatory patients.	• Explain that this drug should help control his nonproductive cough. Advise him to consult his doctor if his cough becomes productive. • Caution the ambulatory patient to avoid activities that require alertness, such as driving a car, operating heavy machinery, or using power tools. • Mention that this syrup contains a small amount of homatropine methylbromide to deter potential abuse. • Inform the patient that prolonged use of this drug can lead to physical and psychological dependence and tolerance.
dextromethorphan (Benylin DM, Comtrex, Coricidin Cough Syrup, DM Cough, Novahistine DMX, NyQuil, Robitussin-DM, Triaminicol, Tussi-Organidin-DM, Vicks Children's Cough Syrup)	• Watch for insomnia, irritability, nervousness, and unusual excitement. • Other reactions include dizziness, drowsiness, and gastric upset.	• Explain that this drug should help control coughing. Because dextromethorphan is usually given with antihistamines, sympathomimetics, or other drugs, advise the patient to consult his doctor or pharmacist before taking any other cough or cold formulas. • Advise against taking this drug with alcohol to avoid increased CNS depression. • Instruct him not to drive a car, operate heavy machinery, or use tools if the drug makes him drowsy. • Suggest that he use sugarless chewing gum or hard candy or ice chips to relieve mouth and throat dryness.

Practicing breathing and coughing exercises. Show the patient how to perform deep-breathing exercises to keep his airways open and mobilize secretions. Tell him to inhale deeply through his nose, then exhale through pursed lips. Instruct him to breathe by using his diaphragm and abdominal muscles, not just his chest muscles. Advise him to breathe slowly and not through his mouth, which will dry secretions. Explain that nose breathing filters and humidifies air.

Teach the patient how to do coughing exercises to help remove sputum from his airway. Give him a copy of the teaching aid *How to do controlled coughing exercises.* Suggest that he humidify his home to help him expectorate more easily. Also, advise him to use a cool-mist humidifier to add moisture to dry room air and to frequently breathe the steam mist from a hot shower. Alternatively, suggest that he place pans of water around the house—for example, near a hot radiator or heat register. Explain that evaporating water adds moisture to the room air.

Preventing recurrent infection. To prevent recurrent episodes of acute bronchitis, discuss ways to avoid infection. Give the patient a copy of the teaching aid *Tips for proper hand washing,* page 114. Remind him to wash his hands after contact with an infected person or after handling objects that have been touched by an infected person. Tell him to refrain from breathing through his mouth, which increases the likelihood of infection. And he shouldn't rub his eyes, which may transmit infection from his fingers through his tear ducts. Remind children to avoid putting their fingers in their mouths or noses.

If the patient smokes, encourage him to join a smoking cessation program. Explain that smoke paralyzes the ciliated epithelia that normally remove debris and infectious microbes from the respiratory tract. Also advise him to avoid dust and occupational irritants or pollutants. Encourage elderly and asthmatic patients to have an influenza vaccine annually, unless they have previously had a reaction to it or are allergic to eggs.

Source of information and support

American Lung Association
1740 Broadway, New York, N.Y. 10019
212-315-8700

Further readings

Biller, P.L. "Diagnosis and Management of Acute Bronchitis and Pneumonia in the Ambulatory Setting," *Nurse Practitioner* 12(10):12-28, October 1987.
Dunlay, J., et al. "A Placebo-controlled, Double-blind Trial of Erythromycin in Adults with Acute Bronchitis," *Journal of Family Practice* 25(2):137-41, August 1987.
Ellner, J. "Management of Acute and Chronic Respiratory Tract Infections," *American Journal of Medicine* 85(3A):2-5, September 16, 1988.
Hanley, M.V. "Ineffective Airway Clearance Related to Airway Infection," *Nursing Clinics of North America* 22(1):135-49, March 1987.
Marcoux, J.P., et al. "COPD: Controlling Bronchitis Flare-ups," *Patient Care* 21(9):99-104, May 15, 1987.

PATIENT-TEACHING AID

How to do controlled coughing exercises

Dear Patient:

Learning how to do coughing exercises will help you save energy and remove mucus from your airways. Here's what to do.

1 Sit on the edge of your chair or bed. Rest your feet flat on the floor, or use a stool if your feet don't touch the floor. Lean slightly forward.

2 To help stimulate your cough reflex, slowly take a deep breath. Place your hands on your stomach. Breathe in through your nose, letting your stomach expand as far as it can.

3 Next, purse your lips and slowly breathe out through your mouth, as

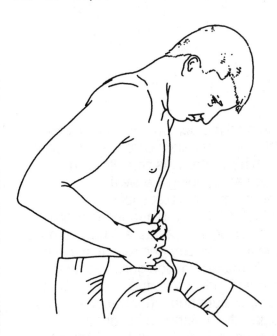

shown. Concentrate on pulling your stomach inward. Try to exhale twice as long as you inhaled.

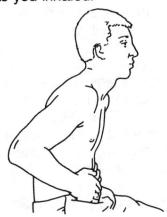

4 Cough *twice* with your mouth slightly open. Once isn't enough: The first cough loosens mucus; the second cough helps remove it.

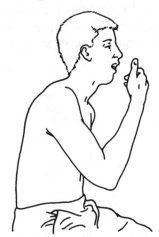

5 Pause for a moment. Then breathe in through your nose by sniffing gently. Don't breathe deeply. If you do, the mucus you brought up may slide back into your lungs.

How to take a temperature correctly

Dear Patient:

A fever usually means that your body is fighting an infection or some other illness. To find out if you or a family member has a fever, you'll probably use a mercury or digital thermometer. You can take a temperature orally, rectally, or under the arm. A normal oral temperature is 97° to 99.5° F. (36.1° to 37.5° C.). Normal rectal temperature is about 1 degree higher and underarm temperature, 1 to 2 degrees lower.

Using a mercury thermometer
Before using a mercury thermometer, wipe it with an alcohol-soaked gauze pad and rinse it off.

1 With your thumb and forefinger, grasp the thermometer at the end opposite the bulb. Then quickly snap your wrist to shake down the mercury.

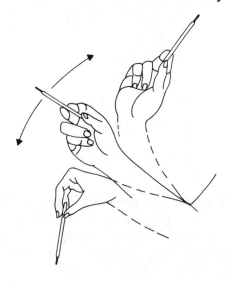

2 Next, hold the thermometer at eye level in good light and rotate it slowly until you see the mercury line clearly. Look for a reading of 95° F. (35° C.) or lower. Now you're ready to take a temperature.

3 *To take an oral temperature,* place the bulb of the thermometer under the tongue, as far back as possible.

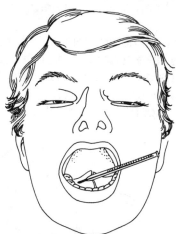

Remind the person not to bite on the thermometer and not to keep it in place with his teeth. This can affect an accurate reading. Leave the thermometer in place for 4 to 5 minutes—the time needed to register the correct temperature. Then, remove the thermometer and read it at eye level.

To make sure you get an accurate reading, never take the person's oral temperature right after he's smoked a cigarette or sipped a hot or cold beverage. Instead, wait for 20 to 30 minutes.

continued

How to take a temperature correctly — *continued*

● *To take another person's rectal temperature,* first dip the bulb end of the *rectal* thermometer in petrolatum (Vaseline). Then, position the person on his side with his top leg bent. Position an infant on his stomach, as shown here.

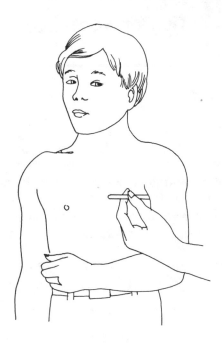

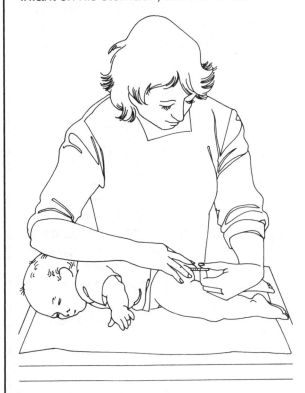

Gently insert the thermometer into the rectum—about ½ inch for a baby, 1 inch for a child, and 1½ inches for an adult.

Hold the thermometer in place for 3 minutes. Next, carefully remove it and wipe it with a tissue. Read the thermometer at eye level.

● *To take an underarm temperature,* put the thermometer's bulb in one armpit, and fold that arm across the chest. (This secures the thermometer.) Remove the thermometer after 10 minutes, and read it at eye level.

Using a digital thermometer

If you wish, you can use a digital thermometer instead of a mercury one to take an oral temperature reading. Here's how.

1 Remove the thermometer from its protective case.

2 Next, position the thermometer tip under the tongue, as far back as possible. Leave the thermometer in place for at least 45 seconds.

3 Remove the thermometer and read the numbers on display. This is the temperature. Clean the thermometer as the manufacturer instructs, and return it to the protective case.

PATIENT-TEACHING AID

Tips for proper hand washing

Dear Patient:

Everyday activities, such as petting your dog or sorting money, leave unwanted germs on your hands. These germs may enter your body and cause an infection. To prevent this, wash your hands several times daily—and always before meals. Here's how.

1 Wet your hands under lots of running water. This carries away contaminants.

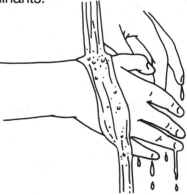

2 Lather your hands and wrists with soap. Although soap and water don't actually kill germs, they do loosen the skin oils and deposits that harbor germs. While you're washing, give your fingernails a good scrub, too.

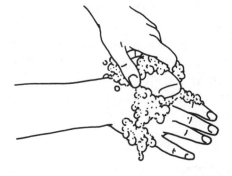

3 Now, thoroughly rinse your hands in running water. Make sure your fingers point downward. That way runoff water won't travel up your arms to bring new germs down to your hands.

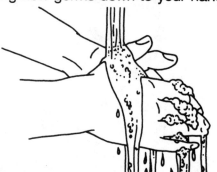

4 If you're at home, dry your hands with a clean cloth or paper towel. Don't dry off with a used towel, which may put germs right back on your hands. If you're in a public place, a hot-air hand dryer is best, but clean paper towels will do.

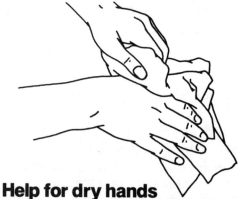

Help for dry hands
If your hands become dry or scratchy from frequent hand washing, soothe them with a hand lotion. And don't use strong soaps. They aren't needed for good hygiene, and they may cause drying or even allergic reactions.

Influenza

Highly contagious, influenza strikes millions of people each year, keeping them home from work and school and sending some to the hospital with complications. For these reasons, your teaching will include how to avoid getting "the flu," how to relieve symptoms if a flu infection does occur, and how to recognize serious, possibly life-threatening complications. It will also include measures to prevent contagion.

Discuss the disorder

Inform the patient that the flu, an acute upper respiratory tract infection, is caused by a myxovirus—type A, type B, or type C. Type A, the most prevalent, and type B occur every year. Type C is endemic and occurs sporadically (for more information, see *Avoiding the flu,* page 116). Mention that types A and B change their genetic makeup slightly each year, which explains the ineffectiveness of previously developed vaccines and previously developed natural immunity.

Tell the patient that influenza infects all age-groups, but its incidence is highest in children between ages 5 and 14. Its effects are severest—even life-threatening—in elderly adults, very young children, and persons with chronic disorders.

Explain that the virus can survive for up to 72 hours outside the body. It's transmitted by air or by person-to-person contact, making objects handled by a flu victim a potential source of infection. Add that the incubation period for the virus lasts from 18 to 36 hours, with a 3-day period of communicability that begins before the patient is symptomatic.

Inform the patient that the primary infection site is the ciliated respiratory epithelium. The mucous membranes of the upper airways and the tracheobronchial tree become inflamed, swollen, and congested. The process impairs the patient's respiratory defenses, leaving him vulnerable to a secondary infection (see *How flu viruses multiply,* page 116).

Describe the typically abrupt onset of illness. Fever may begin near 102° F. (38.9° C.) and rise as high as 106° F. (41.1° C.) in severe infections. Respiratory symptoms—sore throat, dry cough, runny nose, and sneezing—typically accompany red, watery eyes; muscle aches in the lower back and legs; and a frontal headache. Point out that the severity of flu symptoms varies greatly and that symptoms should subside in 3 to 4 days. Forewarn the patient that he may continue to feel tired and weak for days or even weeks.

Eileen VanParys, RN, MSN, EdD, who wrote this chapter, is assistant chairman of the Abington Memorial Hospital School of Nursing, Abington, Pa.

CHECKLIST

Teaching topics in influenza

☐ Explanation of influenza, emphasizing how it spreads, who's at risk, and how to avoid it
☐ Complications requiring medical attention
☐ Diagnosing the flu by evaluating symptoms
☐ Treating symptoms with rest, fluids, aspirin, and other drugs
☐ Flu prevention with vaccines and antiviral agents
☐ How Reye's syndrome relates to the flu and aspirin
☐ The difference between *Haemophilus influenzae* type B infection and the flu
☐ Self-care measures, including humidification and infection prevention
☐ Sources of information and support

116 Influenza

Avoiding the flu

Urge your patient to get a flu shot before the flu season is under way, typically between December and March in the northern hemisphere.

Inform the patient that epidemics tend to occur every 2 to 3 years (pandemics, every 10 years). Explain that flu spreads through a community in about 3 weeks and subsides in 3 to 4 weeks.

During these periods, 15% to 25% of those living in large communities and more than 40% of those living in closed populations are infected with the virus.

How flu viruses multiply

Does your patient know how flu invades the body? Tell him that the answer lies in the flu virus's makeup.

Classified as type A, B, or C, an influenza virus contains only a portion of nucleic acid (RNA or DNA) on which are strung the genes that carry the instructions for viral replication. The fragmentation of the genetic material accounts for its ability to undergo genetic mutations.

Having only a partial genetic component, the virus can't reproduce or carry out chemical reactions on its own. It needs a host cell. And once your patient inhales this airborne virus, that's what it finds. Inside the respiratory tract, the flu virus attaches itself to a healthy host cell. In an attempt to destroy the invader, the healthy cell engulfs the virus and sends chemicals to dissolve the virus cell's wall. This attempt at destruction releases the virus's genetic material into the healthy cell.

Here, the genes of the virus find fertile conditions in which to replicate, arranging themselves into identical bundles. These new viruses—up to 1,000 reproduced within 6 hours—burst forth to invade other healthy cells. The viral invasion destroys the host cells, impairing respiratory defenses, especially the mucociliary transport system, and predisposing the patient to secondary bacterial infection.

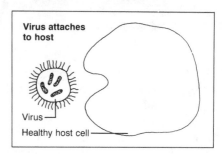

Virus attaches to host

Virus

Healthy host cell

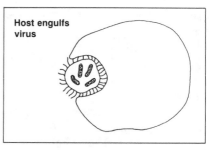

Host engulfs virus

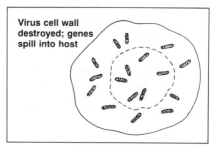

Virus cell wall destroyed; genes spill into host

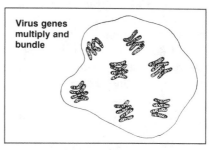

Virus genes multiply and bundle

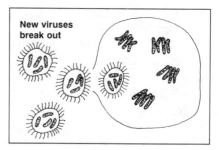

New viruses break out

Complications

Emphasize that the flu virus decreases the patient's resistance to secondary bacterial and viral infections. For this reason, he needs to consult a doctor if his symptoms last more than a week, become more severe, or localize in his throat, lungs, or ears. Also advise him or family members to seek medical attention if he begins to vomit or experience behavioral changes. Inform the patient that pneumonia, tracheobronchitis, acute sinus infection, and middle ear infections are the leading flu complications.

Describe the diagnostic workup

Inform the patient that diagnosis usually hinges on an evaluation of symptoms—especially during an epidemic or during flu season. Although available, laboratory studies (such as cultures) are rarely done. When they're used, cultures of pharyngeal and nasal secretions obtained early in the illness can identify influenza viruses. Tell the patient that serologic test results may show elevated antibody levels, which indicate infection.

If a complication follows the flu, the patient may need additional tests, depending on his symptoms (chest X-rays, for example), for diagnostic and treatment purposes.

Teach about treatments

Because influenza is self-limiting, treatment aims to relieve symptoms by limiting activity (rest), maintaining hydration (fluids), and taking medication (aspirin or acetaminophen). Advise patients in certain high-risk categories to obtain a yearly flu vaccine.

Activity

Tell the patient to stay in bed and rest while he has a fever and for 1 to 2 days after the fever subsides. Warn him that increasing his activity prematurely may lead to recurrent fever and other flu symptoms.

Diet

Advise the patient to drink at least 2 to 3 qt (2 to 3 liters) of fluid daily. Explain that he needs this amount to replace fluid lost from rapid breathing and fever. Also tell him that increasing his fluid intake will help liquefy his respiratory secretions, making them easier to expel by coughing.

Medication

Tell the patient that drug therapy aims to relieve flu symptoms with such medications as analgesics and cold and flu remedies, including antihistamines, antitussives, or expectorants. The doctor may recommend a vaccine or antiviral drugs to prevent influenza. Emphasize that antibiotics have no effect against viral infections. These drugs help only when secondary bacterial infections occur.

Analgesics. To relieve headache, fever, and achiness, advise

Understanding Reye's syndrome

Although affecting fewer than 3 youngsters of every 100,000 who've had the flu, Reye's syndrome is extremely serious. Linked to *viral illnesses,* such as chicken pox, the flu, and measles, and *aspirin use* in patients under age 18, the disorder causes liver changes, brain swelling, heart damage, coma, and sometimes death.

Signs and symptoms

Urge parents to seek medical attention at once if their child has these early warning signs of Reye's syndrome:
- vomiting
- violent headaches
- listlessness
- irritability
- delirium
- disturbed breathing
- stiff arms and legs
- coma.

No cure exists so early treatment is crucial. Statistical findings show that mortality from Reye's syndrome drops from 80% to 20% when treatment starts early.

Taking precautions

As a precaution against Reye's syndrome, advise parents to avoid giving aspirin to children who have the flu, measles, or chicken pox.

Urge parents (and adolescents, too) to scrutinize the labels of over-the-counter cold or flu remedies to make sure that they don't contain aspirin (also known as ASA or acetylsalicylic acid). Recommend an aspirin substitute, such as acetaminophen (Tylenol), to control fever or to ease flu-related achiness.

---

the patient to take acetaminophen or aspirin—as long as he doesn't have GI problems or isn't taking an anticoagulant. Warn parents not to give aspirin to a child or an adolescent because of the danger of Reye's syndrome (for more information, see *Understanding Reye's syndrome*).

Cold and flu remedies. Inform the patient that he may use an antihistamine to dry up congested respiratory passages and relieve watery eyes, a runny nose, and sneezing. Explain, however, that this drug usually provides more effective relief when symptoms are associated with an allergy rather than the flu. Tell the patient that he may also try antitussives (cough suppressants) and expectorants (see *Teaching about drugs to relieve flu symptoms*). Add that oral and nasal decongestants may offer brief relief, although using nasal decongestants for more than 2 or 3 days may cause a "rebound effect," resulting in nasal congestion.

Vaccine. Suggest that the patient at risk for influenza discuss flu vaccination with his doctor. Provide a copy of the patient-teaching aid *Learning about immunization for the flu,* page 122. The vaccine contains either an inactivated or an attenuated virus, and it creates immunity within about 2 weeks. Because immunity

Teaching about drugs to relieve flu symptoms

DRUG	ADVERSE REACTIONS	TEACHING POINTS
Antihistamines		
azatadine (Optimine) **brompheniramine** (Dimetane) **chlorpheniramine** (Chlor-Trimeton, Teldrin) **clemastine** (Tavist) **dexchlorpheniramine** (Polaramine)	• Watch for fever, hallucinations, severe drowsiness, severe dry mouth or throat, sore throat, unusual bleeding or bruising, and unusual fatigue or weakness. • Other reactions include anorexia; blurred vision; insomnia; irritability; mild drowsiness; mild dry nose, mouth, or throat; thickened bronchial secretions; and tremors.	• Warn the patient not to take this drug with alcohol. The combination may increase central nervous system (CNS) depression. • Explain also that many over-the-counter cough and cold medicines contain antihistamines or alcohol. Because these may further increase CNS depression, he should avoid taking them if he's already taking an antihistamine. • Caution him that the drug causes drowsiness, so he should proceed carefully when using power tools, walking up and down stairs, and driving a motor vehicle. • Advise him to take the drug with food or milk to avoid gastric upset. • Suggest that he chew sugarless gum or suck ice chips or sugarless candy to help relieve mouth and throat dryness. • Advise him also to drink extra fluids.
astemizole (Hismanal) **terfenadine** (Seldane)	• Watch for sweating; visual disturbances; wheezing; and yellow skin, mucous membranes, and sclera. • Other reactions include dizziness, dry mouth and throat, mild drowsiness, and nausea.	• Tell the patient that this drug usually causes less drowsiness than other antihistamines. • Advise him to take the drug with food or milk to avoid gastric upset. • Suggest that he chew sugarless gum or suck ice chips or sugarless candy to help relieve mouth dryness.
Antitussives		
codeine	• Watch for confusion, dizziness, respiratory difficulty, and sedation. • Other reactions include constipation, drowsiness, dry mouth, and nausea.	• Tell the patient to consult his doctor if his cough becomes productive. • Advise against taking this drug with alcohol or over-the-counter cough and cold medicines that contain alcohol or antihistamines. These may increase CNS depression. • Warn him that prolonged use of codeine, a controlled substance available only by prescription, can lead to drug tolerance and dependence. • Instruct him to use caution when operating a motor vehicle, heavy machinery, or power tools because this drug can impair mental and physical function. • Suggest that he chew sugarless gum or suck ice chips or sugarless candy to relieve mouth and throat dryness.
dextromethorphan (Benylin DM, Comtrex, Coricidin Cough Syrup, DM Cough, Novahistine DMX, NyQuil, Robitussin-DM, Triaminicol, Vicks Children's Cough Syrup)	• Watch for insomnia, irritability, nervousness, and unusual excitement. • Other reactions include dizziness, drowsiness, and gastric upset.	• Because dextromethorphan is usually given in combination with antihistamines, sympathomimetics, or other drugs, emphasize that the patient must check with his doctor or pharmacist before taking any other flu remedies. • Advise him against taking this drug with alcohol, which may increase CNS depression. • Caution him to avoid driving a car, operating heavy machinery, or using power tools if the drug makes him drowsy. • Suggest that he chew sugarless gum or suck ice chips or sugarless candy to relieve mouth dryness.
Expectorants		
guaifenesin (Coricidin Cough Syrup, Novahistine DMX, Robitussin, Triaminic)	• Watch for nausea and vomiting. • Other reactions include diarrhea, drowsiness, and mild gastric upset.	• If not contraindicated, encourage the patient to drink as much water as possible to help thin his mucus. • Advise him to avoid unintentional double-dosing by checking with his doctor before taking any other cough-syrup-type flu remedies.

lasts from 3 to 6 months, November is the best month for persons living in the northern hemisphere to receive the vaccine.

Inform the patient that he'll need a flu vaccine yearly because immunity is short-lived and the flu virus changes (mutates) every year. If your patient is a child, urge his parents to consult the doctor about a flu shot for the child.

Take time to clarify that the yearly flu vaccine differs from the *Haemophilus* B vaccine that the child should receive at age 15 months. Explain that the *Haemophilus influenzae* type B (HIB) bacterium causes HIB infection, whereas a virus causes influenza. Point out that some parents mistakenly think HIB infection (which is highly contagious and produces serious flulike symptoms) and the flu are the same disease.

Antiviral agents. Tell the patient that an antiviral drug, such as amantadine (Symmetrel) or rimantadine (an investigational drug), may prevent or alleviate symptoms caused by the type A flu virus. Antiviral drugs may help patients in the high-risk category who can't receive the influenza vaccine because of an allergy.

Taken as soon as possible after initial exposure and continued for 24 to 48 hours after symptoms disappear, amantadine shortens the duration of the illness. But to prevent the flu, the patient must take the medication every day for the entire 6 to 8 weeks of the flu epidemic. Assure him that the drug is 70% to 90% effective if taken according to directions. Caution him, however, that some persons who take amantadine—between 7% and 10%—experience depression, dizziness, nausea, and sleep disturbances. Inform elderly patients and those with kidney disease that the doctor may lower their dosage because their bodies may not readily excrete the drug. Tell pregnant and breast-feeding patients that the drug's safety for a fetus or an infant hasn't been established.

Other care measures

Suggest that the patient may feel more comfortable if he humidifies his environment with a vaporizer. Explain that by adding moisture to the air he breathes, he may avoid the drying effects of the flu. As appropriate, provide the patient-teaching aid *Tips for using a humidifier or vaporizer safely,* page 130.

Demonstrate proper hand-washing technique to prevent transmitting the flu virus, and offer the patient the teaching aid *Tips for proper hand washing*, page 114. Explain that when he rubs his eyes or touches his mouth with his hands, he risks giving or getting the flu. Instruct him to cover his nose and mouth with a tissue when he sneezes or coughs. Remind him to dispose of contaminated tissues by wrapping them in a plastic bag or by flushing them down the toilet.

Inform the patient that another way to avoid spreading or getting the flu virus is to stay out of crowds and away from persons with known illness during the flu season.

Sources of information and support

American Public Health Association
1015 Fifteenth Street, NW, Washington, D.C. 20005
(202) 789-5600

Centers for Disease Control
1600 Clifton Road, NE, Atlanta, Ga. 30333
(404) 332-4551 (provides special influenza information between
October and May)

The National Institute of Allergy and Infectious Diseases
9000 Rockville Pike, Building 31, Room 7A-03, Bethesda, Md. 20892
(301) 496-5717

U.S. Department of Health and Human Services
Public Health Service
National Institutes of Health
9000 Rockville Pike, Bethesda, Md. 20892
(301) 443-2403

Further readings

Ackerman, S.J. "Flu Shots: Do You Need One?" *FDA Consumer* 23(8):8-
11, October 1989.
Bryan, C.S. "Serious Infections in the Elderly: Preventing Pneumonia and
Influenza Deaths in 1989-1990," *Consultant* 29(11):25-28, 31, Novem-
ber 1989.
Fedson, D.S. "Prevention and Control of Influenza in Institutional Settings,"
Hospital Practice 24(9A):87-91, 94-96, September 30, 1989.
Fekety, R., et al. "Prophylaxis for Children and Travelers," *Patient Care*
23(9):104-08, 111-14, May 1989.
Haeuber, D. "Recent Advances in the Management of Biotherapy-related
Side Effects: Flu-like Syndrome," *Oncology Nursing Forum* 16(6):35-41,
November-December 1989.
"Influenza: The Cardiac Effects," Part 2. *Emergency Medicine* 21(17):75-
76, October 15, 1989.
"Influenza: The Deadly Potential," Part 1. *Emergency Medicine* 21(17):61-
72, October 15, 1989.
"Influenza: Now Is the Time to Vaccinate," Part 3. *Emergency Medicine*
21(17):84-86, October 15, 1989.
Pachucki, C.T., et al. "Influenza A Among Hospital Personnel and Patients:
Implications for Recognition, Prevention, and Control," *Archives of Inter-
nal Medicine* 149(1):77-80, January 1989.
Scheifele, D.W., et al. "Evaluation of Adverse Events After Influenza Vaccination in Hospital Personnel," *Canadian Medical Association Journal*
142(2):127-30, January 15, 1990.

PATIENT-TEACHING AID

Learning about immunization for the flu

Dear Patient:

During flu season, you may hear many people discussing the pros and cons of flu immunization. As a result, you may wonder whether you should have a flu shot. Use the following information to help answer your questions.

Do flu shots really work?
Yes. The Centers for Disease Control reports that the vaccine reduces your chance of coming down with the flu by 60% to 80%. Even if you were to catch the flu, you would experience fewer and milder symptoms.

Should I get a flu shot?
Depending on the specific flu virus and the risk of a widespread flu outbreak, your doctor will probably recommend vaccination if you fall into one of the following categories:
• persons over age 65
• persons with chronic lung diseases, such as asthma or emphysema
• persons with heart disease, kidney disease, diabetes, or severe anemia
• persons suffering from cancer or taking a drug that interferes with the body's immune system
• persons who run a high risk of exposure to the flu virus
• children and teenagers who are receiving long-term aspirin therapy and may be at risk for Reye's syndrome if they develop the flu
• pregnant women due to deliver in the winter months.

When is the best time to get a flu shot?
In the fall. Immunization usually consists of one dose of vaccine. Children under age 9 who've never been vaccinated may need two injections, given 1 month apart.

Immunity develops about 2 weeks after vaccination and lasts for 1 year only. This is so because the flu virus changes, and different strains usually are responsible for epidemics from year to year.

I'm allergic to eggs. Can I still get a flu shot?
That depends on your symptoms when you eat eggs. Because the vaccine may contain egg protein, you shouldn't have a flu shot if eggs or egg-containing foods cause swelling in your face or tongue, hives, or wheezing.

However, if you experience only stomach cramps or gas after eating eggs, you can probably receive the vaccine safely.

Can a flu shot give me the flu?
No. The vaccine contains inactive or weakened virus, so it can't produce the flu. When you receive the vaccine, your body responds by creating antibodies to the virus. These antibodies then fight the virus when you're exposed to it.

About 30% of the people vaccinated experience mild soreness and swelling at the injection site. A few others suffer from muscle and joint aches and a low-grade fever (less than 100° F. [37.8° C.]).

Croup

A common illness in infants and young children, croup produces a barklike cough and sometimes respiratory distress that can evoke alarm, even terror, in parents. Your first teaching priority is to reassure and calm the whole family; croup may worsen when a child is upset or anxious.

Because croup is usually mild and self-limiting, most parents can manage the child's illness at home. You'll teach them what signs herald croup and its complications. Then you'll help them master effective home-care methods, such as monitoring the child's respiratory status, providing adequate fluids, and using a humidifier or vaporizer.

Next, you'll teach parents how to recognize signs of respiratory distress. Croup can cause complete laryngeal obstruction—a medical emergency calling for immediate treatment. Occasionally, a child with croup requires hospitalization. If so, you'll inform the parents about diagnostic tests, possible drug therapy, and other treatments to improve the child's breathing.

In all of your teaching about croup, you'll focus on reducing the family's fear and increasing their control of the illness. This will help them manage recurrence.

Discuss the disorder

Inform the parents that croup syndrome refers to infections of the epiglottis, larynx, trachea, and bronchi that cause severe inflammation and narrowing of the upper airway. Croup usually stems from a viral infection, although bacteria may cause it, too. Its major signs are a distinctive cough (that sounds brassy or like a barking seal), breathing difficulty, a hoarse cry, and stridor. Explain that breathing difficulty results from laryngeal constriction caused by inflammatory swelling and spasms of the larynx (see *How croup affects the upper airway*, page 124).

Identify the child's form of croup—acute laryngotracheobronchitis, acute spasmodic croup, or acute epiglottitis. Then discuss his specific illness (see *Comparing croup syndromes*, page 125).

If the child has *acute laryngotracheobronchitis*, the most common form, tell the parents that this syndrome usually occurs several days after an upper respiratory tract infection. The infection spreads first to the larynx and then rapidly descends to the trachea and the bronchi. As the infection descends, the child expe-

Paula A. Campagna, RN, MSN, and **Kathleen Heverley, RN, MS,** contributed to this chapter. Ms. Campagna is a nursing instructor at Frankford Hospital School of Nursing, Philadelphia. Ms. Heverley is an educational nurse specialist at the Children's Hospital of Philadelphia.

CHECKLIST

Teaching topics in croup

☐ Explanation of the three major croup types: acute laryngotracheobronchitis, acute spasmodic croup, and acute epiglottitis
☐ Physical examination, X-rays, and blood studies to confirm diagnosis
☐ Importance of bed rest and sitting or semi-Fowler's position in bed
☐ Dietary modifications
☐ Emergency procedures to open an obstructed airway: tracheostomy and nasotracheal intubation
☐ Evaluation of the child's respiratory and hydration status
☐ Ways to humidify the environment
☐ Source of information and support

How croup affects the upper airway

When teaching about croup, help the child's parents understand how the illness causes breathing difficulty. Explain that in croup inflammatory swelling and spasms constrict the larynx, thereby reducing air flow. The drawing at left represents a normal upper airway. The drawing at right shows the upper airway changes caused by croup. Here, inflammatory changes almost completely obstruct the larynx (which includes the epiglottis) and significantly narrow the trachea.

NORMAL UPPER AIRWAY   **INFLAMED UPPER AIRWAY**

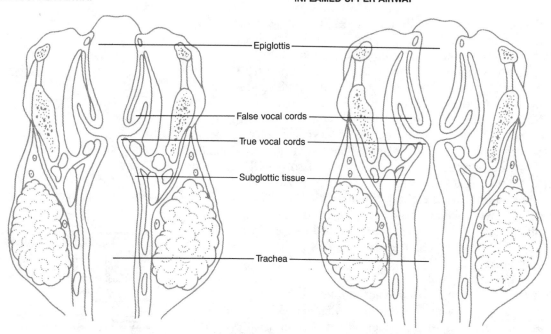

Epiglottis

False vocal cords

True vocal cords

Subglottic tissue

Trachea

riences greater difficulty breathing and labored, prolonged exhalation. He may appear extremely restless and frightened.

The main signs of *acute spasmodic croup* are sudden breathing difficulty in the evening or at night with noisy inspirations and a barking, brassy cough. Explain that the child may seem anxious, frightened, and extremely tired but that he won't have a fever. The severe nocturnal signs usually diminish in several hours. The next day he may appear well except for hoarseness and a cough. Encourage the parents to keep the child calm and quiet, which may help to ease his breathing. These episodes usually occur nightly for several nights, diminishing in intensity. Anxious or excitable children are more prone to this syndrome.

If the child has *acute epiglottitis,* inform the parents that this potentially life-threatening form of croup requires immediate medical attention. Resulting from acute inflammation of the epiglottis (the leaf-shaped flap that covers the entrance to the voice box during swallowing), acute epiglottitis may block the airway, causing death. Reassure the parents that with prompt medical treatment, this syndrome usually lasts for only 2 to 3 days. Tell them that a child with acute epiglottitis typically goes to bed feeling well but awakens at night with a high fever, drooling, and moderate to severe respiratory distress, sometimes with stridor. (See *Recognizing respiratory distress in infants*, page 126.)

Complications
Teach the parents that close attention to their child's symptoms and early treatment may prevent complete laryngeal obstruction. Such obstruction blocks the airway and prevents ventilation. Stress the importance, too, of carefully watching for symptoms and providing early treatment for other common complications, including middle ear infection, bronchitis, bronchiolitis, and pneumonia.

Describe the diagnostic workup
Tell the parents (and the child, if appropriate) that the child will need a physical examination. Before the doctor can diagnose croup, he must rule out other possible causes of respiratory distress, such as foreign body obstruction of the airway. He'll also require a complete medical history.

Explain that the doctor may order an X-ray of the child's neck to pinpoint areas of upper airway narrowing and swelling. X-ray films of acute epiglottitis show a swollen epiglottis, whereas in acute laryngotracheobronchitis, they show a normal epiglottis but swollen subglottic tissue. But the doctor won't attempt a visual inspection of an enlarged epiglottis because this may trigger immediate airway obstruction.

Inform the parents that blood tests may distinguish between viral and bacterial causes of croup. Tell them that their child may have a test called pulse oximetry. Explain that a small probe is attached to a finger or toe and connected to a machine that measures oxygen level, heart rate, and strength of pulse.

Teach about treatments
Because croup may be treated at home or in the hospital, you'll need to tailor your teaching accordingly. In either situation, discuss with the parents the need for bed rest, a liquid diet, possible drug therapy, and other measures to keep the child hydrated and breathing more easily.

Activity
If the child is at home, tell the parents that bed rest is essential to conserve his energy and limit oxygen needs. To ease the child's breathing, advise them to use pillows to prop him into a sitting or semisitting (semi-Fowler's) position. An infant may sit in an infant seat in a crib with the side rails up. Warn the parents never to rest a child (or an infant) flat on his back. It's easier for the child to breathe when he's semi-upright. Advise them that keeping him quiet and comfortable will reduce his oxygen needs and that holding him as often as possible will soothe and comfort him.

If the child is in the hospital, tell the parents that similar measures apply. Bed rest is necessary, and the child probably will

Comparing croup syndromes

Use this guide to help parents distinguish the three major croup syndromes.

Acute laryngotracheobronchitis
Commonly caused by a virus but sometimes by bacteria, this form of croup occurs in children ages 3 months to 3 years. It's usually mild and self-limiting, but it can be severe in infants.

Symptoms, which accompany an upper respiratory tract infection, develop over 1 to 3 days. They include a barklike cough, dyspnea, edema, fear, hoarseness, inflammation, laryngospasm, low fever, restlessness, and stridor. Symptoms tend to recur with subsequent respiratory infections.

Acute spasmodic croup
Of unknown cause, acute spasmodic croup may be related to allergens, infection, or stress. It affects children ages 1 to 3.

Symptoms emerge suddenly, become increasingly severe, peak during the night, and usually resolve by morning. They include a barking, brassy cough, dyspnea, edema, hoarseness, inflammation, laryngospasm, restlessness, and stridor. Fever is absent.

Acute epiglottitis
Requiring immediate intervention, acute epiglottitis strikes children ages 3 to 7 and sometimes affects older children and adults as well. Its cause is bacterial, usually *Haemophilus influenzae* (type B).

In acute epiglottitis, a mild upper respiratory tract infection precedes (by 24 hours) the sudden onset of a bright red epiglottis, drooling, dysphagia, dyspnea, edema, high fever (over 101.3° F. [38.5° C.]), inflammation, mouth breathing with hyperextended neck, muffled voice, restlessness, sore throat, and stridor. A cough is absent.

Recognizing respiratory distress in infants

Because infants can't verbalize their symptoms, you'll need to teach parents how to recognize the signs of infant respiratory distress. Using the illustrations below, show them how to evaluate three cardinal signs of breathing difficulty: a visible rib cage as the infant inhales (retractions), flared nostrils, and a grunting sound on expiration. These signs are graded to measure the severity of respiratory distress as follows.

	RIB CAGE DURING INHALATION	NASAL FLARING	GRUNTING DURING EXHALATION
Grade 0 The infant breathes normally, with no visible or audible respiratory distress signs.	Not visible	None	None
Grade 1 The infant shows some respiratory distress. Important signs include a slightly visible rib cage as the infant inhales and slightly flared nostrils. Instruct the parents to watch the infant closely and to begin measures to help him breathe more easily.	Just visible	Slight	Audible by stethoscope only
Grade 2 The infant has pronounced respiratory distress. His rib cage is quite visible on exhalation, his nostrils flare widely, and he grunts as he exhales. Tell the parents to call the doctor immediately and to continue measures to make breathing easier.	Markedly visible	Marked	Audible by unaided ear

Adapted with permission from Silverman, W.A., and Anderson, D.H. "A Controlled Clinical Trial of Effects of Water Missed on Obstructive Respiratory Signs: Death Rates and Necropsy Findings Among Premature Infants," *Pediatrics* 17(1):1, January 1956.

be positioned in a sitting or semisitting position. Again, warn the parents not to place the child on his back, and encourage them to make him feel as loved and secure as possible.

Diet

If the parents are treating the child at home, stress the importance of keeping the child hydrated by giving him plenty of fluids. Give the parents a copy of the teaching aid *Checking your child's fluid balance,* page 129. Suggest clear, high-calorie liquids (such as Gatorade), flavored gelatin dissolved in water, or ginger ale with the bubbles stirred out, given at room temperature. Tell them to avoid thicker, milk-based fluids because they may thicken secretions. To relieve sore throat, suggest fruit sorbet or ice pops. Instruct the parents to withhold solid foods until the child can breathe and swallow more easily. Inform them that the child may have little or no appetite until he feels better.

Explain that the hospitalized child will be hydrated with I.V. fluids if he can't be hydrated orally. Tell the parents that this step is necessary to conserve the child's energy and prevent him from aspirating fluids. Reassure them that once the danger of aspiration passes, he'll start a clear-liquid diet.

Medication

Warn the parents not to give the child aspirin because of its link to Reye's syndrome. If the child has a fever of 101° F. (38.5° C.) or higher, instruct them to call their doctor. He may order a non-aspirin substitute, such as acetaminophen (Tylenol), to reduce the fever.

Explain to the parents that the hospitalized child may receive racemic epinephrine by an aerosol mist. Describe how this drug makes breathing easier by opening constricted airway passages. Tell the parents that the child will be placed on a cardiorespiratory monitor to watch for signs of tachycardia, a possible adverse effect from the drug. Other adverse reactions include dizziness, headache, and nausea. Point out that the child will receive an antibiotic for acute epiglottitis.

Emergency procedures

Inform the parents that a child with acute epiglottitis will require insertion of an artificial airway to allow him to breathe. If a tracheostomy is ordered, explain that this surgical procedure opens the airway externally. The doctor makes a horizontal incision in the child's neck and then inserts a tracheostomy tube into the trachea. If nasotracheal intubation is ordered, explain that the doctor inserts a flexible tube that extends up the child's nose, down the larynx, and into the trachea.

If the child has severe laryngotracheobronchitis or acute spasmodic laryngitis, advise the parents that nasotracheal intubation or tracheostomy also may be necessary. Inform them that these procedures are used only when the child has severe respiratory distress despite appropriate treatment. They're usually done in the

INQUIRY

Questions parents ask about croup

My child's barking cough at night sends me into a panic. What can I do right away to help him breathe better?
One of the best ways to relieve a croupy spell is to turn your bathroom into a temporary steamroom. Take your child into the bathroom, close the door, and turn on the hot water in the shower. Then sit outside of the shower with him while steam fills the room. Let your child breathe in the steam for a few minutes. Don't let him lie on his back, which may obstruct his airway.

You can also take your child out into the cool, night air—weather permitting and with proper clothing. The cool air may relieve his distress. If his barking cough occurs during the day, however, call the doctor.

Can I do anything to prevent my child from getting croup again?
Unfortunately, you can't. Once a child has croup, he's likely to get it again with subsequent upper respiratory infections. But you can take steps to control croupy spells. At the first sign of a cold, use a humidifier or vaporizer to help minimize airway irritation and break up congestion. Then, closely watch your child for signs of respiratory distress, and report any problems to his doctor right away.

Will he outgrow these attacks?
Yes. Usually by age 3, or slightly older, a child is no longer susceptible to the most common form of croup, acute laryngotracheobronchitis. This form tends to recur in children age 3 months to 3 years, usually in the late fall or winter.

operating room if time permits; the tubes remain in place for only a few days.

Other care measures

Teach the parents how to use a cool-mist humidifier. Explain that maintaining a high humidity level makes breathing easier and helps to liquefy secretions. Show them how to create a mist tent by securing a bedsheet over the top of the child's crib while running the humidifier. Warn them not to use plastic, which could smother the child. Although a humidifier is preferred, tell the parents that they also may use a steam-producing vaporizer. Warn them, however, to follow safety precautions when using steam to prevent accidental burns. Emphasize that they shouldn't use steam in a mist tent. Give them a copy of the teaching aid *Tips for using a humidifier or vaporizer safely,* page 130, for future use.

If the child is hospitalized, tell the parents that he may be placed in a cool-mist tent, with or without oxygen, to provide high humidity. An infant will be placed in a mist tent, too. Encourage the parents to bring familiar toys to help the child feel secure. Warn them, however, not to bring sharp objects that might puncture the tent or toys that could cause sparks (for example, metal trucks or cap guns), which could ignite a nearby oxygen source. Caution them to leave fuzzy toys at home because they may become damp and breed bacteria.

Discuss with parents and other family members how to recognize when the child's breathing and hydration status are worsening. Stress the importance of reporting earache, productive cough, high fever, or increasing shortness of breath. Instruct them to monitor the child's temperature by taking an axillary or rectal temperature. (Give them a copy of the teaching aid *How to take a temperature correctly,* pages 112 and 113.) Caution them never to take an oral temperature in a child with croup because closing the mouth may cause complete airway obstruction.

Source of information and support

American Lung Association
1740 Broadway, New York, N.Y. 10019
212-315-8700

Further readings

Branson, P.S. "Fever, Dysphagia, and Raspy Cough in a Child," *Respiratory Care* 32(9):808-9, September 1987.
Gagliano, N. "Coping with Croup," *Patient Care* 22(15):89-91, 94, September 30, 1988.
Huston, C.J. "Action STAT! Epiglottitis," *Nursing88* 18(4):59, April 1988.
Mastropietro, C. "The Potentially Difficult Airway," *Journal of the American Association of Nurse Anesthetists* 56(1):25-35, February 1988.
Nemes, J., et al. "Epiglottitis: ED Nursing Management," *Journal of Emergency Nursing* 14(2):70-75, March-April 1988.

Checking your child's fluid balance

Dear Parents:

While your child has croup, take extra care to make sure he doesn't become dehydrated. Croup may cause him to lose body fluids. Perhaps he can't swallow enough liquids because of a sore throat. Or, if he's breathing through his mouth, his mouth and throat may dry out. If he has a fever, he'll need more fluids than usual. Use this checklist to help you decide if your child is well hydrated.

• Inspect the insides of your child's mouth and lower eyelids. Do the tissues look pink and moist?

☐ Yes　　☐ No

• Watch your child closely the next time he has a crying spell. Are his eyes producing plenty of tears?

☐ Yes　　☐ No

• Watch for changes in the amount of your child's urine and bowel movements. Does the amount increase when your child drinks more fluids?

☐ Yes　　☐ No

• Pinch your child's skin *gently*. Does his skin quickly spring back to normal?

☐ Yes　　☐ No

• Weigh your child daily. Is he maintaining his normal weight?

☐ Yes　　☐ No

• If he's a baby, observe his fontanelles (the soft spots on top of his head). Do they appear flat, not sunken or bulging?

☐ Yes　　☐ No

If you answered "yes" to all these questions, your child probably is well hydrated. If you answered "no" to any questions, don't be alarmed, but do call your doctor immediately and discuss the symptoms with him. Remember, dehydration can cause serious problems because it upsets the body's balance of salt and fluids. If your child is dehydrated, follow your doctor's advice for treating the condition.

PATIENT-TEACHING AID

Tips for using a humidifier or vaporizer safely

Dear Parent:

A humidifier or vaporizer may help your child breathe easier. These devices add moisture to dry air, helping to soothe an irritated airway and break up congestion.

To ensure safety, most health professionals recommend using a cool mist humidifier. However, if you use a vaporizer, you need to take precautions to prevent accidental steam burns. To use either unit, follow these guidelines.

1 Read the manufacturer's directions carefully. Check the unit, especially the power cord, for signs of damage.

2 Fill the unit's water tank to the right level with cool, clean tap water or distilled water. Assemble the unit as directed in the instruction booklet.

3 If you use a humidifier, place the unit on a flat surface, several feet away from the child.

If you use a vaporizer, place the unit on the floor—not on a table or chair, where it might be knocked over and spill hot water. Also, don't point the steam vent directly at the child.

4 Before plugging in either unit, make sure the power cord lies safely away from such objects as radiators or heaters. And make sure no one can step on or trip over it.

5 With either unit, periodically check to make sure it's working properly. Refill the water tank as necessary. Also, at least every hour, make sure your child's bed linen isn't damp with excess moisture. If it is, change the sheets, and move the unit slightly farther away from your child.

6 Unplug the power cord when you're not using the humidifier or vaporizer. And never move or tilt a unit without first turning it off and unplugging it.

7 Empty and clean the humidifier or vaporizer daily. In a humidifer, germs can breed and thrive in any remaining water. In a vaporizer, mineral deposits from hard water may build up and block steam flow. Follow the manufacturer's directions for cleaning your unit. Then wipe it dry after each use.

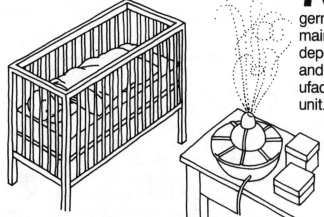

3

Neurologic Conditions

Contents

Cerebrovascular accident

The most common cause of neurologic deficits, a cerebrovascular accident (CVA) poses difficult but not insurmountable challenges for patient teaching. First of all, you'll need to teach the patient about his disorder. You'll also need to prepare him for the diagnostic workup and help him understand treatment, such as drug therapy or surgery. To support his sense of independence, you'll need to discuss how he can compensate for any temporary or permanent neurologic deficits.

At times, the CVA patient may feel depressed about his condition and the prospects of a lengthy rehabilitation. During times like these, it's up to you to provide encouragement for him and his family as you explain the benefits of rehabilitation and a lifestyle plan to avoid CVA's risk factors.

Discuss the disorder

Explain to the patient that CVA is often, but not necessarily, associated with atherosclerosis. Inform him that CVA (also known as stroke) follows an interruption of cerebral blood supply. For example, a blood clot or plaque can occlude an artery, producing tissue *ischemia* and *infarction*. Or a vessel may rupture, causing increased intracranial pressure from *hemorrhage* and, possibly, brain herniation.

Explain your patient's type of CVA. In an *ischemic cerebral* infarction, partial or complete arterial occlusion impairs cerebral perfusion, halting delivery of oxygen, glucose, and other nutrients to affected brain cells, which therefore stop functioning. Transient ischemia may last from a few minutes to 24 hours. This focal neurologic deficit, called a *transient ischemic attack (TIA),* resolves completely without permanent damage. A reversible ischemic neurologic deficit may also be called reversible ischemic neurologic event or stroke with full recovery. It is identical to a TIA except that recovery takes longer than 24 hours. Stroke-in-evolution means that the neurologic deficits are worsening, and a completed stroke indicates that the deficits are stable, neither increasing nor dramatically resolving.

In an *intracerebral hemorrhage,* a ruptured intracerebral artery, usually resulting from hypertension, produces a focal area of bleeding into brain tissue.

Explain that neurologic deficits can be specific or wide-

CHECKLIST

Teaching topics in CVA

☐ An explanation of the type of CVA: ischemic or hemorrhagic
☐ Risk factors in CVA
☐ Preparation for diagnostic tests, such as a CT scan and cerebral angiography
☐ If necessary, an explanation of the type of surgery: craniotomy, carotid endarterectomy, extracranial intracranial bypass, or ventricular shunt
☐ Importance of rehabilitation in minimizing neurologic deficits
☐ A balanced program of activity and rest
☐ Communication tips for the patient and his family
☐ Dietary adjustments, such as semisoft foods for dysphagia
☐ Assistive feeding devices
☐ Use of a cane or a walker, if needed
☐ Home safety tips
☐ Sources of additional information and support

Janette R. Yanko, RN, MN, CNRN, who wrote this chapter, is a neuroscience clinical nurse specialist practicing at Allegheny General Hospital in Pittsburgh, Pennsylvania.

Understanding sites and signs of neurologic deficits

A cerebrovascular accident (CVA) can leave one patient with mild hand weakness and another with complete unilateral paralysis. In both patients, the functional loss reflects damage to the brain area normally perfused by the occluded or ruptured artery. But the damage doesn't stop there. The resulting hypoxia and ischemia produce edema that affects distal parts of the brain, causing further neurologic deficits.

Most CVAs occur in the anterior cerebral circulation and cause middle cerebral artery syndrome, internal carotid syndrome, or anterior cerebral artery syndrome. CVAs can also occur in the posterior circulation. These originate in the vertebral arteries and result in vertebral-basilar artery syndrome and posterior cerebral artery syndrome, causing higher mortality. The illustrations show arterial circulation and the brain sites that control various body functions.

Middle cerebral artery syndrome
The most common deficits include contralateral motor or sensory deficits or both, aphasia, homonymous hemianopsia, neglect of paralyzed size (with nondominant hemisphere involvement), apraxia, agnosia, and paralysis of conjugate gaze.

Anterior cerebral artery syndrome
This least common syndrome produces contralateral motor or sensory deficits or both, urinary incontinence, flat emotional affect, and gait apraxia.

Internal carotid syndrome
Similar to the middle cerebral artery syndrome, this syndrome causes contralateral motor or sensory deficits or both, altered level of consciousness, neglect, and apraxia. It also causes homonymous hemianopsia, ipsilateral blindness, and aphasia.

Vertebral-basilar artery syndrome
Impaired vertebrobasilar circulation causes motor or sensory deficits or both on the same side of the body as the lesion, on both sides, or in all extremities; nystagmus; vertigo with nausea and vomiting; diplopia and lateral and vertical gaze palsies; visual field deficits; ataxia; dysphagia; dysarthria; coma; and vital sign instability.

Posterior cerebral artery syndrome
This syndrome results in visual field deficits, blindness (if bilateral involvement), and sensory loss on one side.

SITES OF CEREBRAL FUNCTION

Frontal lobe
Voluntary muscle movements, motor area for speech (Broca's area), emotional behavior, and complex intellectual abilities

Parietal lobe
Sensations of pain, cold, pressure, size, shape, and texture; location and intensity of stimuli; awareness of body parts

Temporal lobe
Hearing, taste, and smell; interpretation of sounds

Occipital lobe
Visual stimuli

MAIN CEREBRAL ARTERIES

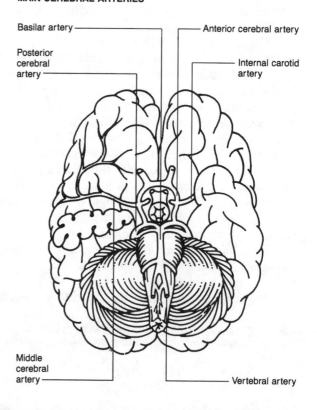

Basilar artery
Posterior cerebral artery
Anterior cerebral artery
Internal carotid artery
Middle cerebral artery
Vertebral artery

spread, depending on the brain area affected. (See *Understanding sites and signs of neurologic deficits.*) Tell the patient that the deficits may be temporary if brain cells were only injured or permanent if they were destroyed.

Complications
Let the patient know that his participation in a rehabilitation program, including range-of-motion exercises and speech and language therapy, is important for maximum recovery. Point out that immobility heightens the risk of infection. Also point out he may have another CVA if he fails to address risk factors. (See *Who's at risk for CVA?*)

Describe the diagnostic workup
Prepare the patient for angiography, scanning tests, or other tests to identify abnormalities and evaluate cerebral blood flow. Blood tests may be performed to evaluate clotting.

Before any test, tell the patient who will perform it and when and where it will be done. Before any radiologic test, tell the patient to remove all metallic objects, such as jewelry, from the test site. Also tell him to report any possible adverse reactions, especially for tests using contrast media, or radiopaque dye (see *Recognizing adverse reactions to contrast media*).

Angiography
If the patient will be undergoing cerebral angiography or digital subtraction angiography (DSA), explain the purpose of the test and what will happen before, during, and after it.

Cerebral angiography. Inform the patient that this test (also called cerebral arteriography) highlights the brain's blood vessels on an X-ray as a dyelike substance circulates through them. It detects disruption or displacement of the cerebral circulation by occlusion or hemorrhage.

Tell the patient that the test takes about 2 hours, that he'll need to lie still during it, and that he may feel discomfort from this prolonged motionlessness. Also tell him that a technician will shave and cleanse the injection site—the carotid or femoral artery—and may also immobilize the patient's head with tape or straps. If the carotid artery is used, inform the patient that he may have his face covered with a drape and his arms immobilized to maintain a sterile field.

Explain that during the test he'll lie on an X-ray table. Then the doctor will inject a local anesthetic and insert a catheter at the appropriate site for injection of the dye. During the injection, the patient may sense pressure, warmth, a transient headache, nausea, or a salty taste. Tell him to report any of these sensations to the doctor. Immediately after the injection, he'll hear clacking sounds as the X-ray equipment takes pictures. Explain that multiple injections of the dye may be required to completely visualize the blood vessels. Instruct him to lie still to avoid blurring the films. Of course, he should comply if the doctor tells him to move an arm or a leg.

Inform the patient that after the test, the catheter is removed.

Who's at risk for CVA?

Cerebrovascular accident (CVA) can strike people of any age, but mostly it affects older adults. In young adults, CVA can stem from I.V. drug abuse and congenital problems, such as sickle cell disease. It occurs more frequently in men than in women and in blacks more frequently than in whites.

Risk factors for CVA include age, family history of cerebrovascular disease, cardiovascular disease, diabetes mellitus, and smoking. Use of oral contraceptives and phenylpropanolamine-containing appetite suppressants also heighten CVA risk.

Recognizing adverse reactions to contrast media

Teach the patient to report these signs and symptoms when they occur during or after diagnostic tests using contrast media:
• restlessness
• tachypnea and respiratory distress
• tachycardia
• facial flushing
• urticaria (hives)
• nausea and vomiting.
To treat a mild reaction, administer diphenhydramine (Benadryl), as ordered. To treat a severe reaction (which can cause hypotension and respiratory arrest), start an I.V. of dextrose 5% in water and administer epinephrine, as ordered; begin cardiopulmonary resuscitation, if necessary.

How DSA works

If your patient will be undergoing digital subtraction angiography (DSA), you'll need to be sufficiently familiar with the test so you can explain it to him. First of all, the test uses video equipment and computer-assisted image enhancement to examine cerebral vessels. Unlike conventional angiography, DSA involves taking radiographic images both before and after injection of a contrast medium. A computer converts these images into digital information and then "subtracts" the first image from the second, eliminating most information (mainly soft tissue and bone) common to both images. The result is an improved, high-contrast view of blood vessels without interfering images or shadows.

Each DSA image can be recalled for review and stored on magnetic tape or a videodisk.

Then pressure is applied to the puncture site for about 15 minutes, followed by a pressure dressing and an ice pack. Tell the patient that his pulses will be checked frequently to monitor his circulation. Instruct him to hold his head and neck (for the carotid approach) or leg (for the femoral approach) straight for 4 to 12 hours. Tell him he can resume his usual diet.

DSA. Inform the patient that this test evaluates the patency of cerebral vessels and identifies their position in his head and neck (see *How DSA works*). It also detects and evaluates lesions and vascular abnormalities. The test takes 30 to 45 minutes. Instruct the patient to fast for 4 hours before the test.

Explain that during the test the patient will be positioned on an X-ray table and a catheter will be inserted in a blood vessel to deliver a radiopaque dye (which may give him a feeling of warmth or a metallic taste). He should report immediately any discomfort or shortness of breath. He'll be instructed to lie still while a series of X-ray images are taken.

If the I.V. route was used, the patient can resume his normal activities. For the intra-arterial route, he'll need to restrict movement in his arm or leg for 4 to 12 hours.

Scanning tests

If appropriate, teach the patient about scanning tests, such as computed tomography (CT), positron emission tomography (PET), single photon emission computed tomography (SPECT), and magnetic resonance imaging (MRI).

CT scan. Inform the patient that a CT scan uses X-ray images to detect structural abnormalities, edema, and lesions, such as nonhemorrhagic infarction and aneurysms. Mention that the test takes 30 to 60 minutes and causes little discomfort, although he may feel chilled because the equipment requires a cool environment. Explain that he won't be allowed food or fluids for 4 hours before the scan if the test requires use of a dye.

Explain that during the test a technician will position him on an X-ray table and place a strap across the body part to be scanned, to restrict any movement. The table then slides into the tubelike opening of the scanner. If a dye is ordered, the infusion will take about 5 minutes. Instruct the patient to report immediately any discomfort or a feeling of warmth or itching. (The technician can see and hear him from an adjacent room.) Then describe noises he'll hear from the scanner as it revolves around him.

Advise the patient that immediately after the test he can resume his usual activities and diet. Urge him to drink additional fluids for the rest of the day to help eliminate the dye, if used.

PET scan. Inform the patient that this test measures how rapidly tissue consumes radioactive isotopes. (For more information, see *Comparing PET and SPECT*.) Prepare the patient by telling him that the test takes about 1 hour, is painless, and involves minimal radiation exposure.

Explain that during the test, the patient will lie on a moving table with his head immobilized and placed inside a ring-shaped opening in the machine. He'll be given a radioactive tracer either by *inhalation* or by *I.V. injection*. If the doctor chooses the inhalation method, tell the patient he'll inhale a radioactive tracer through a mask. Tell him to breathe normally; he won't smell or taste anything odd. If the doctor uses the I.V. method, tell the patient that he may feel a warm sensation during the injection. Advise him to report any discomfort. In both methods, tell the patient he'll have a dome-shaped hood placed over his head and face to prevent the exhaled tracer from circulating in the room. Stress the importance of lying still to avoid blurring the images.

If the I.V. method was used, explain that the doctor will remove the needle after the test and collect a blood sample. Then the patient can resume his normal activities.

SPECT scan. Tell the patient that this test studies cerebral blood flow, helping to diagnose cerebral infarctions. The test takes about 1 hour. Inform the patient that before the test he may receive a dose of salty-tasting Lugol's solution (depending on the tracer agent) and an I.V. amine tracer. Mention that he'll lie on a narrow metal table.

Explain that during the test he'll feel the table move and will see a large disklike machine moving around his head as it makes images of the tracer agent flowing through the brain. Stress the importance of lying still to ensure accurate results. Tell the patient that he can resume his usual activities after the test.

MRI scan. Explain that MRI evaluates the brain's condition by providing clear images of blood vessels. It allows imaging of multiple planes, including direct sagittal and coronal views, in regions where bone normally hampers visualization. Inform the patient that this test involves no radiation exposure, but does involve exposure to a strong magnetic field. Therefore, he should tell you if he has any metal objects in his body (such as a pacemaker, aneurysm clip, hip prosthesis, or implanted infusion pump), which could make him ineligible for the test. The test takes about 1 hour. Mention that he may feel some discomfort from being enclosed within the large cylinder. Ask him if he's claustrophobic.

Explain that during the test the patient will be positioned on a table that slides into a large cylinder that houses the MRI magnets. Tell him that his head, chest, and arms will be restrained to help him remain still. Stress that lying still prevents blurring the images. Also explain that a technician can see and hear him from an adjacent room. Tell the patient he'll hear a loud knocking noise while the machine operates. If the noise bothers him, he may be given earplugs or pads for his ears. A radio encased in the machine or earphones may help block the sound (but he will still hear some noise). Tell the patient that he can resume his normal activities after the test.

Other tests

Teach the patient about other tests the doctor may order to evaluate a CVA, including cerebral blood flow studies, oculoplethysmography (OPG), neuropsychological tests, and transcranial Doppler studies.

Cerebral blood flow studies. Explain that these studies measure blood flow to the brain and help detect abnormalities. Inform

Comparing PET and SPECT

Acronyms like PET and SPECT provide easy ways to remember high-tech tests. But these verbal shortcuts often don't come in handy when it's time to teach your patient about these tests—or to explain why he's receiving one test instead of another. Let's look at the differences between PET and SPECT.

A PET scanner detects the gamma rays produced as brain tissue absorbs a radioisotope. A computer then translates these gamma rays into cross-sectional images that portray the brain's metabolic activity.

A close cousin of PET, SPECT is less costly because it uses commercially available radioisotopes. Unlike PET, SPECT detects only one emitted gamma ray, so it provides less data for evaluation. It's also less accurate than PET, but can still portray evidence of cerebral infarction before it can be identified by computed tomography scan.

138 Cerebrovascular accident

Tips on managing daily activities

Use these commonsense tips to help the patient and his family relearn ways to manage his daily activities.

• To help distinguish left from right, suggest that the patient wear a watch or bracelet on the left wrist as a "landmark." Or, he can mark the left shoe sole with an *L* or tag the inside left trouser leg or sweater sleeve with a colored tape to differentiate left from right.

• If the patient has problems with spatial relations, suggest maps or colored dots to mark a daily route. Advise the family to keep the environment as uncluttered as possible—for example, keeping only a few items on the nightstand. Also suggest *pointing* to objects to give verbal clues, such as "*in* the wastebasket" or "*under* the desk."

• If the patient's apraxia makes dressing himself difficult, recommend buttoning shirts (or blouses) from the bottom up. Some patients find it easier to match buttonholes that way.

• Whatever the task, urge the family to praise the patient's efforts. Discouragement can be disabling in itself. A patient with a right-side lesion will understand encouraging words; a patient with a left-side lesion may respond to nonverbal encouragement, such as a pat on the back.

the patient that the test takes about 30 minutes. It's painless and exposes him to less radiation than a chest X-ray.

Tell the patient that he'll lie still on a table during the test, and that he'll have a frame placed around his head. He may inhale xenon, a radioactive gas, through a mask or mouthpiece for about 10 minutes. Or he may receive an I.V. injection of xenon, technetium, or krypton and breathe through a mask or dome while the isotope-sensitive detector probes measure the blood flow rate. Explain that he can resume his usual activities immediately after the test.

OPG. Explain that OPG indirectly evaluates carotid blood flow. Before the test, instruct the patient to remove any contact lenses. Inform him that he'll receive anesthetic eyedrops, which may cause burning. The test takes only a few minutes.

Explain that during the test his head will be placed in a frame; he'll have eyecups placed on his eyes (held in place with light suction) and photoelectric cells clipped to his earlobes. He'll have to remain still and avoid blinking during the test. If he's also having ophthalmic artery pressure studies, mention that he'll briefly lose his vision when suction is applied to his eyes.

Tell the patient that the doctor will remove the eyecups and head frame after the test. Advise him not to rub his eyes or replace his contact lenses for at least 2 hours. Also tell him to blink and to protect his eyes until the effects of the anesthetic drops wear off.

Neuropsychological tests. Explain that this battery of tests evaluates simple to complex mental and verbal abilities and also includes a personality inventory. Inform the patient that it's used to evaluate cognitive function and takes 1 to 2 hours.

Tell the patient that he may be asked to make calculations, solve problems, and answer questions about current events. Tell the family that after the test, the patient with memory loss may show increased confusion and restlessness.

Transcranial Doppler studies. Explain to the patient that these studies examine the size of intracranial vessels and the direction of blood flow. Inform him that the test takes about 30 minutes and is painless. Mention that he'll lie on a table or in his bed and that he'll rest his head on a foam cushion.

Explain that during the test, the technician will apply gel in front of his ear, over his eye, or on the back of his head. Tell him to expect light pressure in that area as the technician places a microphone-like probe against his head; he'll hear a swishing sound as the probe senses the blood flowing through the vessels. Stress the importance of lying still to ensure accurate results. Tell the patient that he can resume his normal activities after the test.

Teach about treatments

Provide instruction about CVA treatments. These commonly include physical rehabilitation, dietary and drug regimens to help decrease risk factors, possibly surgery, and care measures to help the patient adapt to specific deficits, such as speech impairment or paralysis (see *Tips on managing daily activities*).

Activity
Urge the patient to follow the prescribed exercise program. Then teach him to perform range-of-motion exercises for the arm or leg affected by the CVA. Or teach a family member to perform passive range-of-motion exercises. Advise frequently interrupting exercise with rest periods. Reinforce the importance of wearing slings, splints, or other prescribed devices to prevent complications and ensure safety.

Diet
If the patient is obese or has elevated serum levels of cholesterol, lipoproteins, or triglycerides, you may need to explain a weight-reduction diet or one low in saturated fats. If the patient has dysphagia or one-sided facial weakness, tell him to eat semisoft foods and to chew on the unaffected side of his mouth.

Instruct the patient to sit upright when eating and to tilt his head slightly forward. Recommend preparing solid foods in a blender and freezing liquids to a slush or mixing them with other foods. If the patient has partial arm paralysis, suggest feeding aids, such as specially adapted plates with rims and built-up utensils. Give the patient and his family a copy of the patient-teaching aid *Making eating easier,* pages 143 and 144.

Medication
Teach the patient about the schedule, dosage, and adverse effects of prescribed medications, including antiplatelet drugs, such as aspirin and dipyridamole, and vasodilators, such as isoxsuprine.

Aspirin. If the patient is taking large doses of aspirin for a prolonged period to prevent blood clotting, tell him to watch for adverse reactions. (See *Teaching aspirin precautions.*)

Dipyridamole. Explain that dipyridamole (Persantine, Pyridamole) prevents blood clotting. Instruct the patient to be alert for any adverse reactions, such as signs of bleeding, bruising, rash, tinnitus, hearing loss, nausea, vomiting, diarrhea, headache, dizziness, weakness, flushing, or fainting.

Isoxsuprine. Tell the patient that the vasodilator isoxsuprine (Rolisox, Vasodilan) helps peripheral circulation. Instruct him to report adverse reactions, such as vomiting and GI upset. Advise him to stop taking the drug and call his doctor if a rash develops.

Surgery
Depending on the CVA's cause and extent, the patient may undergo a craniotomy to remove a hematoma, endarterectomy to remove atherosclerotic plaques, or extracranial-intracranial bypass to circumvent an artery that's blocked completely by occlusion or stenosis. Possibly, he may need a ventricular shunt to drain cerebrospinal fluid. (See *Teaching about ventricular shunts,* page 140.)

Craniotomy. If you're preparing the patient for a craniotomy, explain that his head will be shaved and scrubbed and that he'll be given a general anesthetic. Reassure him that his hair will grow back.

Explain that during the operation, the surgeon will make an inci-

Teaching aspirin precautions

Commonly prescribed to prevent blood clots in cerebrovascular accident, aspirin can cause severe reactions, especially among the elderly. To minimize such reactions, instruct the patient to:
• Watch for bruising, rashes, tinnitus, hearing loss, nausea, vomiting, or GI upset.
• Be alert for petechiae, bleeding gums, and signs of GI bleeding, and maintain adequate fluid intake if he's taking large doses for an extended duration.
• Take aspirin with food, milk, an antacid, or a large glass of water to reduce GI effects.
• Crush aspirin and mix it with soft food or liquid if he has difficulty swallowing. (Don't crush enteric-coated aspirin.) He should ingest it immediately because the drug isn't stable in solution.
• Avoid alcohol because it can potentiate the bleeding effect of the aspirin and cause GI upset.
• Avoid interactions by consulting his doctor or pharmacist before using any other drug.

Teaching about ventricular shunts

A ventricular shunt involves insertion of a flexible tube through a small hole in the skull and then into a ventricle to drain cerebrospinal fluid and relieve pressure.

The procedure

The surgeon places one end of the shunt in a ventricle and the other end in a cavity large enough to absorb additional fluid, such as the abdominal cavity, a vessel leading to the heart, or, rarely, a space at the back of the head. Placement in the back of the head is temporary; in the other areas, it's permanent. The shunt extends from the ventricle to the scalp, where it's tunneled under the skin to the appropriate cavity.

The patient can usually resume activities the day after shunt insertion.

Aftercare

Tell the patient to avoid putting pressure on the shunt (for example, not wearing eyeglasses). Also tell him to report any signs of infection (fever or inflamed skin at the shunt site) or malfunction (drowsiness, headache, restlessness, nausea, or vomiting) to the doctor.

If the doctor recommends pumping the ventricular shunt, tell the caregiver to follow these steps:

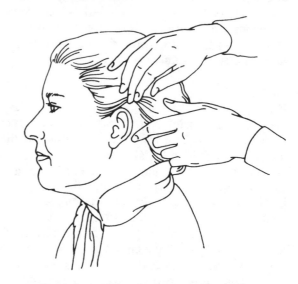

• Locate the pump by feeling for the device's soft center under the skin behind the ear, as shown here.
• Depress the device's center with the forefinger and then release it slowly.
• Pump only as many times as the doctor orders.

sion in his scalp to open the skull over the damaged area. (The size of the skull opening varies from a small hole, which later fills with new bone, to a larger flap, which will be positioned back in place at the completion of surgery.)

Tell the patient that after surgery, his head will be bandaged. If he had a supratentorial craniotomy, the head of his bed will be raised about 30 degrees. Or, if had an infratentorial craniotomy, he may lie flat in bed or with the head elevated. Tell him he can turn from side to side, but caution him to avoid coughing, which may increase intracranial pressure. Instruct him to ask for medication if he has a headache after surgery.

After the patient recovers from surgery, tell him that the surgeon will remove the sutures within 7 days. Also, mention that he'll be given a cap to wear after removal of the bandages. Before discharge, tell him he may wash his hair but should gently pat the incision area until dry; warn against scrubbing or rubbing it.

Endarterectomy. If you're preparing the patient for a carotid endarterectomy, tell him that the skin on his neck will be thoroughly cleansed and shaved. If he receives a cervical block anesthetic, tell him he'll be awake during surgery. Or, if he receives a general anesthetic, he'll sleep during surgery.

Mention that dressings will cover the incision after surgery and that he may experience numbness and tightness in the incision area, a transient numbness in his earlobe, and soreness or a lump in his throat. Reassure the patient that these effects of swelling should resolve in a few days. Tell him that he'll be able to resume his usual daily activities the day after surgery, barring complications. Mention that the doctor will remove any sutures before the patient's discharged from the hospital.

Extracranial-intracranial bypass. If you're preparing the patient for this surgery, tell him that part of his head will be shaved and scrubbed and that he'll receive a general anesthetic.

Explain that the surgeon makes an incision in the scalp above the ear. Then through an opening in the skull, the surgeon splices one end of the dissected artery to an artery on the brain's surface, bypassing the impaired area and restoring blood flow.

Inform the patient that after surgery, he'll have a bulky dressing over the incision; he may also have a mild headache, caused by swelling that normally occurs in the surgical area. Caution him not to put pressure on the surgical site, and tell him to avoid lying on the affected side. If he wears eyeglasses, suggest that he adjust the temple piece that extends over the surgical site. Assure him that he can probably resume most activities the day after surgery.

Before discharge, instruct him to avoid wearing hats, scarves, or wigs that exert pressure over the suture line, thus causing potential blockage of the anastomosed artery.

Other care measures

Involve both the patient and his family in supporting his recovery and boosting his efforts to attain self-sufficiency. Also teach the patient how to prevent another CVA.

Alternate communication methods. If the patient has a *speech deficit,* recommend other communication methods, such as writing or using a picture board. Review his prescribed speech and language therapy; reinforce the importance of continuing it.

Instruct the family to speak slowly to the patient in normal tones. Recommend that they use gestures to clarify their message if the patient has receptive aphasia. (See *Major aphasia types.*) Tell them to give the patient short, simple directions, cues, and lists. Warn them that the patient may overestimate his abilities, claiming he can perform tasks (for example, driving a car) that in fact he cannot. Explain the importance of carefully monitoring the patient's abilities without frustrating his efforts for independence. Tell them to allow the patient to try most activities—short of those that could injure him or others or could cause excessive frustration or fatigue. Also mention to the family that the patient may be *emotionally labile,* crying or laughing at seemingly inappropriate times. Explain that he can't control these reactions.

Safety measures. Recommend installing grab bars near the toilet and bathtub, removing throw rugs, and securing carpets—or removing them entirely if the patient uses a walker or wheelchair. If the patient needs to use a walker or cane, give him a copy of the appropriate patient-teaching aids (see pages 145 to 154). Also, if the patient has sensory losses, suggest lowering the water heater's temperature to prevent burns.

Established routines. To prevent confusing the patient who has *difficulty generalizing,* tell the family to follow a routine and minimize changes. For example, a patient who has learned to feed

---

Major aphasia types

Broca's, Wernicke's, global, and anomic make up the major types of aphasia.

• Broca's aphasia, a motor or expressive aphasia, affects the patient's ability to communicate (speak, write, or gesture).

• Wernicke's aphasia, a sensory or receptive aphasia, affects the patient's ability to understand oral or written communication.

• Global aphasia affects the patient's ability to understand and communicate.

• Anomic aphasia, also called amnestic aphasia or verbal amnesia, affects the patient's ability to name objects.

himself at home may have difficulty eating in a restaurant. One solution: Take his utensils to the restaurant rather than risk his social withdrawal.

Further compensatory measures. If the patient has a *one-sided deficit,* encourage him to bathe and dress the affected side first. Suggest calling attention to that side with a watch or a ring. If the patient has *homonymous hemianopsia,* tell him to scan his environment by carefully looking from side to side.

CVA prevention. Teach the patient and his family about correcting any risk factors. For example, if the patient smokes, refer him to a stop-smoking program. As appropriate, teach him to maintain his ideal weight; to follow his prescribed diet, exercises, and stress-reduction program; and to check with the doctor before taking any nonprescription drugs. If the patient's a woman of childbearing age, tell her to avoid using oral contraceptives.

Encourage the patient and his family to contact a local support group and to obtain additional information from the local branch of one of the organizations listed below. In addition, urge the patient to obtain a medical identification bracelet or necklace if he's taking anticoagulants or antiplatelet drugs.

Sources of information and support

American Heart Association
7320 Greenville Avenue, Dallas, Tex. 75231
(214) 373-6300

National Easter Seal Society, Inc.
70 East Lake Street, Chicago, Ill. 60601
(312) 726-6200

National Institute of Neurological and Communicative Disorders and Stroke
9000 Rockville Pike, Bethesda, Md. 20892
(301) 496-9746

Further readings

Hahn, K. "Left vs. Right: What a Difference the Side Makes in Stroke," *Nursing* 17(9):44-47, September 1987.

Kernich, C., and Robb, G. "Development of a Stroke Family Support and Education Program," *Journal of Neurosurgical Nursing* 20(3):193-97, June 1988.

Mitchell, P., et al., eds. *AANN's Neuroscience Nursing: Phenomena and Practice, Human Responses to Neurologic Health Problems.* East Norwalk, Conn.: Appleton & Lange, 1988.

Pimental, P. "Alterations in Communication: Biopsychosocial Aspects of Aphasia, Dysarthria, and Right Hemisphere Syndromes in the Stroke Patient," *Nursing Clinics of North America* 21(2):321-27, June 1986.

Rocker, J. "Promoting Occupational Therapy by Using a Simulated Hemiplegic Arm to Demonstrate Dressing Technique," *American Journal of Occupational Therapy* 42(2):123-26, February 1988.

Making eating easier

Dear Patient:

Special glasses, cups, plates, and utensils can make eating easier and more enjoyable. Here are some tips on ways to use these devices.

Glasses and cups

If you have trouble holding a glass, use an unbreakable plastic tumbler instead. Plastic is lighter and less slippery than glass. Or use terry cloth sleeves over glasses to make them easier to grasp.

You can also choose from many specially designed cups. For instance, you can use a cup with two handles, which is easier to keep steady than a cup with one handle. You can try a pedestal cup or a T-handle cup, which is

T-HANDLED CUP WITH WEIGHTED BASE

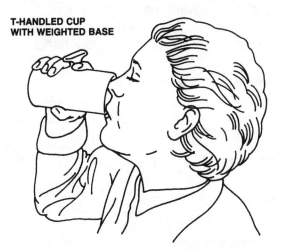

easy to grasp. You can also try a cup with a weighted base, which helps prevent spills.

If you have a stiff neck, use a cup with

CUP WITH V-OPENING

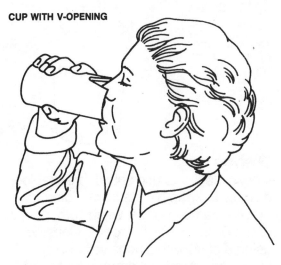

a V-shaped opening on its rim. You can easily tip this cup to empty it without bending your neck backward.

If your hands are unsteady, you may find it easier to hold a cup with a large handle. Or drink from a lidded cup with a lip to help decrease spills. If you have decreased sensation or feeling in your hands, use an insulated cup or mug to avoid burning yourself.

HANDLED CUP WITH LID AND LIP

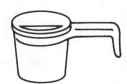

Drinking straws

Flexible or rigid straws, either disposable or reusable, come in several sizes. Some straws are wide enough for you to drink soups and thick liquids

continued

Making eating easier—*continued*

through them. To hold the straw in place, use a snap-on plastic lid with a slot for the straw.

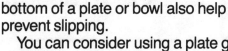

STRAW SECURED BY SLOTTED LID

Dishes

If possible, try to use only unbreakable dishes. To keep a plate from sliding, place a damp sponge, washcloth, paper towel, or rubber disk under it. Consider using a plate with a nonskid base or place mats made of dimpled rubber or foam. Suction cups attached to the

DISH WITH SIDES AND SUCTION CUPS

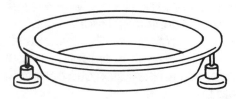

PLATE GUARD

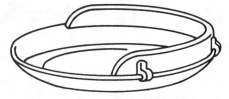

SCOOPER PLATE

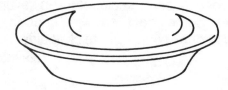

bottom of a plate or bowl also help prevent slipping.

You can consider using a plate guard. This helpful device blocks food from falling off the plate, so it can be picked up easily with a fork or spoon. Attach the guard to the side of the plate opposite the hand you use to feed yourself.

A scooper plate has high sides that provide a built-in surface for pushing food onto the utensil. Eating from a sectioned plate or tray may also be convenient.

Flatware

If your hand is weak or your grip is shaky, you may want to try ordinary flatware with ridged wood, plastic, or cork handles—all easier to grasp than smooth metal handles. Or try building up the handles with a bicycle handlebar, a foam curler pad, or tape (this also works for holding pens and pencils, toothbrushes, or razors). You can also try strapping the utensil to your hand.

WAYS TO BUILD UP HANDLES

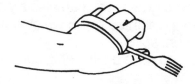

Bicycle handlebar

Foam curler pad

Tape

UTENSIL WITH STRAP

Learning about canes

Dear Patient:

The doctor may order a cane if you have weakness on one side of your body or if you have poor balance. Either the doctor or physical therapist will help you select the cane that's best for you.

Hold the cane in the hand opposite your weaker side, and flex your elbow at a 30-degree angle. If the cane's made of aluminum, you can adjust it by pushing in the metal button on the shaft and raising or lowering the shaft. If the cane's wooden, you or a helper can remove the rubber safety tip, saw off any excess wood, and replace the tip. Available in several types, canes can be standard, straight-handled, or broad-based.

Standard canes
The doctor will recommend a standard cane if you'll be going up and down stairs often. Made of wood or metal, a standard cane commonly comes in 34- to 42-inch (86 to 107 cm) sizes. It features a single foot and a half-circle handle. It's usually inexpensive, easy to use, and hooks onto your belt or arm when you're going up or down stairs and onto the back or arm of a chair when you sit down.

Choose a cane with a wooden or plastic handle rather than a metal one. If your hand perspires, you may lose your grip on a metal handle. Besides, a metal handle may feel uncomfortable in cold weather.

Straight-handled canes
The doctor will recommend a straight-handled cane if your hand is weak. Made of wood, plastic, or metal, a straight-handled cane has easy-to-hold handgrips and a rubber safety tip. If you're selecting one, make sure the handgrip isn't too thick or too thin for you to hold comfortably and that the cane is the proper height. Because this cane doesn't hook over railings or chair arms, you can place it on the floor near you when you sit down.

Broad-based canes
This lightweight, metal cane has three or four prongs or legs that provide a sturdy supportive base. The height can be adjusted, and extra-long handles and child sizes are also available. A broad-based cane stands upright when not in use.

Cane bases range from narrow to wide. A narrow broad-based cane fits on the standard stair step in the normal cane position, whereas a wide broad-based cane fits on the step if you turn the cane sideways. Usually, the narrower the cane's base, the less you tend to rely on it for support.

Openings for height adjustment

Locking button for height adjustment

Walking with a cane

Dear Patient:

You can use the following guidelines for walking with a cane if your *left* leg is weaker. If your *right* leg is weaker, start with the cane on your left side, and adapt the instructions. You may want to draw the step patterns for yourself.

1 First, be sure you're wearing nonskid, flat-soled, supportive shoes, and check that they fit securely (loose laces can be hazardous). Avoid wearing sandals or clogs because they do not support your weight properly. Next, check your cane's rubber tip to be sure it has no cracks or tears and is wearing evenly. Also, make sure the tip fits securely and evenly on the cane's end.

If possible, remove throw rugs and avoid walking on slippery, wet, or waxed floors or on gravel driveways. Also, try to walk close to a wall, so you have something to lean against if you drop your cane.

2 Now, position the cane about 4 inches (10 cm) to the side of your stronger leg, as shown. Distribute your weight evenly between your feet and your cane.

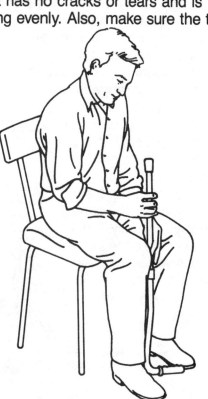

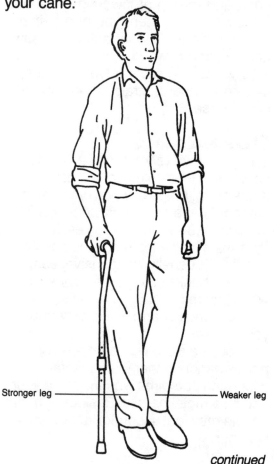

Stronger leg ——————— ——————— Weaker leg

continued

Walking with a cane—*continued*

3 Shift your weight to your stronger leg and move the cane about 4 inches (10 cm) in front of you.

Cane tip

Weaker leg —————— ————— Stronger leg

4 Now you're ready to move your weaker foot forward so it's even with the cane.

5 Shift your weight to your weaker leg and the cane. Now, move your stronger leg forward, ahead of the cane. If you've done this step correctly, your heel will be slightly beyond the tip of the cane.

6 Next, move your weaker foot forward, so it's even with your stronger foot. Then move your cane in front of you about 4 inches (10 cm).
   Repeat these steps. As you proceed, remember to keep your head erect, shoulders back, and back straight. Your abdomen should be in, and your knees slightly flexed.

PATIENT-TEACHING AID

Learning about walkers

Dear Patient:

The doctor will order either a stationary or a reciprocal walker for you, depending on your needs.

STATIONARY WALKER

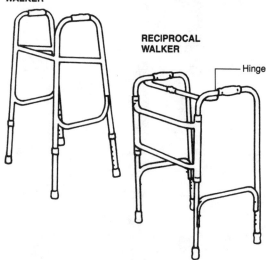

RECIPROCAL WALKER

Hinge

Stationary walker
Usually lightweight, inexpensive, and very stable, a stationary walker consists of an adjustable metal frame with handgrips and four legs. Most stationary walkers have no movable parts, although some models are available with small front wheels. Some models also fold up for travel and easy storage.

Reciprocal walker
This type of walker consists of a metal frame with handgrips, four legs, and a hinge mechanism that allows one side to be advanced ahead of the other. Its height is usually adjustable from 27 to

37 inches (69 to 94 cm), and some models fold up for storage and travel. The reciprocal walker is flexible and "walks" with you.

Feeling comfortable with your walker
Put on the shoes you'll be wearing when you use the walker. Then stand up straight with your feet close together. Relax your shoulders, and put the walker in front of and partially around you. Now, grasp the sides of the walker and look at the position of your elbows—they should be nearly straight. If they're not, adjust the

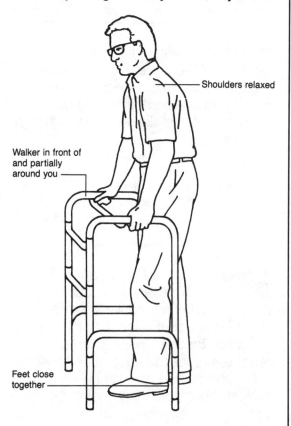

Shoulders relaxed

Walker in front of and partially around you

Feet close together

continued

Learning about walkers—*continued*

walker's height by pushing in the button on each of the walker's legs and sliding the tubing up or down as appropriate. Make sure that the button locks back into place and that you've adjusted the legs to the same height.

Now, try the walker. You should be able to move it without bending over. If you still don't feel comfortable, try adjusting the height again.

Coping with a fall

If you fall while using a walker, first call for help before you try to get up. If no help is available, use the following method to help yourself up.

1 Look around the room for a low, sturdy piece of furniture, such as a coffee table. Inch backward toward the table by pushing your hands down on the floor and lifting your buttocks up. As you do this, pull the walker with one hand.

2 When you get to the table, place your walker near it. Then reach

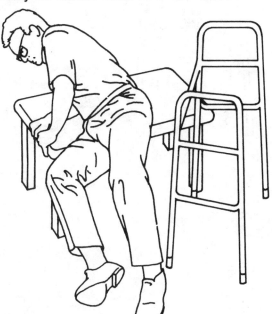

back and place both hands on the table top. Next, press down on the table top and lift your buttocks onto the table.

3 Place the walker in front of you and raise yourself to a standing position by pushing your hands down on the handgrips.

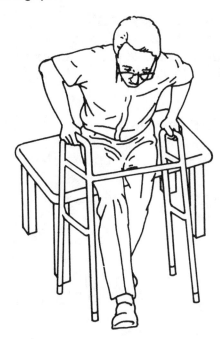

Remember: It's normal to feel a little dizzy when you first stand up. Take a moment to gain your balance before walking. If dizziness doesn't go away or seems excessive, lower yourself back onto the table and call for help. Or you may wish to sit for a while before attempting to stand up.

How to use a two-point gait

Dear Patient:

The doctor has recommended a two-point gait for you. Follow these steps for using this gait with your walker:

Positioning the walker

1 Stand the walker in front of and partially around you. Keep your weight evenly distributed between your legs and the walker.

Moving forward

2 Simultaneously advance the walker's right side and your left foot.

Next, advance your walker's left side and your right foot. Continue in this manner.

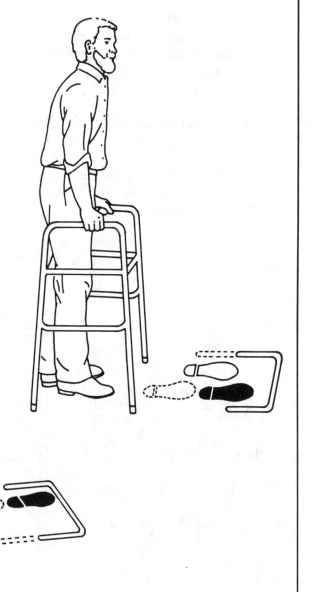

MOVING RIGHT FOOT AND LEFT SIDE OF WALKER

MOVING LEFT FOOT AND RIGHT SIDE OF WALKER

How to use a two-point gait with swing through

Dear Patient:

The doctor has recommended a two-point gait with swing through for you. Follow these steps for using this gait with your walker:

Shifting your weight

1 Stand with the walker in front of and partially around you. Then, distribute your weight evenly between the walker and your stronger leg. Hold your weaker foot off the floor. Now, simultaneously shift your weight to your stronger leg as you lift and advance the walker about 8 inches (20 cm). Don't put any weight on your weaker leg.

Moving forward

2 Swing your stronger leg about 8 inches (20 cm) forward while you support your weight on the walker. Repeat these steps, moving first the walker and then your stronger leg. Remember, don't put any weight on your weaker leg.

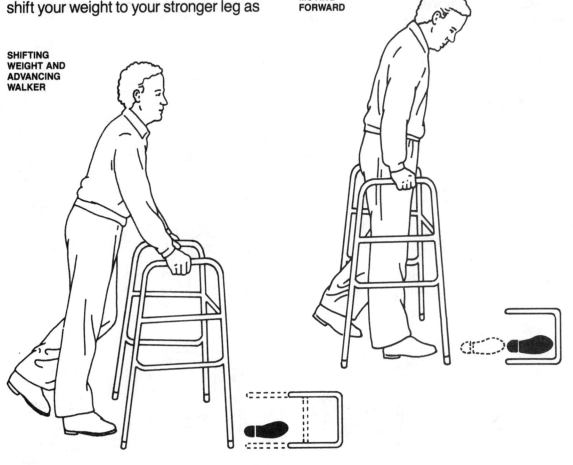

SHIFTING WEIGHT AND ADVANCING WALKER

MOVING FORWARD

How to use a three-point gait

Dear Patient:

The doctor has recommended a three-point gait for you. Follow these steps for using this gait with your walker:

Moving your weaker leg

1 Place the walker slightly in front of you. Distribute most of your weight between your stronger leg (footstep shown in solid black) and the walker, but try to support some weight on your weaker leg as well. Now, shift all of your weight to your stronger leg while you lift and advance your weaker leg (patterned footstep) and the walker as far as 8 inches (20 cm).

Moving your stronger leg

2 Next, shift your weight to your weaker leg and the walker while you move your stronger leg as far as 8 inches (20 cm) forward.

Repeat these steps, moving first the walker and your weaker leg and then your stronger leg. Never attempt to put all of your weight on your weaker leg.

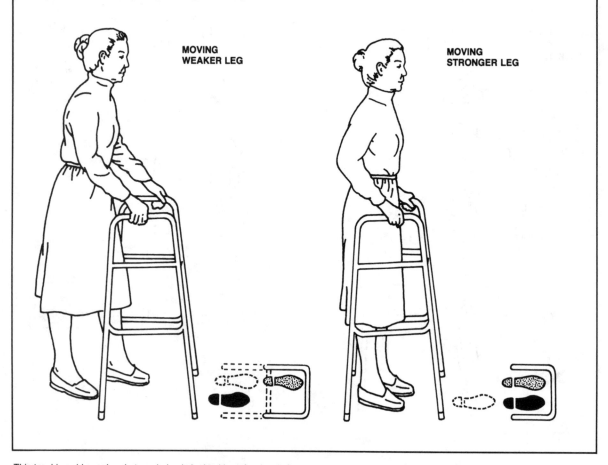

MOVING
WEAKER LEG

MOVING
STRONGER LEG

How to use a four-point gait

Dear Patient:

The doctor has recommended a four-point gait for you. Follow these steps for using this gait with your walker:

Moving your left foot forward

1 Stand the walker in front of and partially around you. Distribute your weight evenly between the walker and

your legs. Then, move the right side of the walker forward. Now, move your left foot forward.

Moving your right foot forward

2 Move the left side of the walker forward. Then, move your right foot forward to complete the four-point gait.
Repeat both procedures to continue walking.

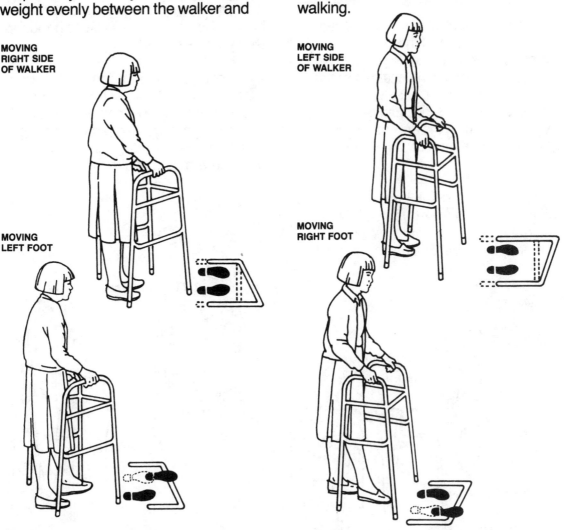

MOVING RIGHT SIDE OF WALKER

MOVING LEFT FOOT

MOVING LEFT SIDE OF WALKER

MOVING RIGHT FOOT

Sitting down and getting up with a walker

Dear Patient:

Follow these directions to help you sit down in a chair and then stand up.

Sitting down

1 Begin by choosing a sturdy armchair. Stand with your back to the chair and with the walker directly in front of you.

2 Place the back of your stronger leg against the seat of the chair. Carefully lift your weaker leg slightly off the floor. Now grasp the chair's armrest with the hand on your weak side. Shift your weight to your stronger leg and the hand grasping the armrest. Then grasp the other armrest with your free hand.

3 Balancing yourself between both arms, gently lower yourself into the chair and slide backward. After you're seated, place the walker beside your chair.

Getting up

1 Pull the walker in front of you. Slide forward in the chair.

2 Place the back of your stronger leg against the seat. Then move your weaker leg forward. Now, placing both hands on the armrests, push yourself to a standing position. Support your weight with your stronger leg and the opposite hand. Then grasp the walker's handgrip with your free hand.

3 Grasp the free handgrip with your other hand. Now, distribute your weight evenly between your hands and your stronger leg. Take a moment to get your balance. Steady yourself, take a deep breath, and you're off.

GRASPING
THE HANDGRIP

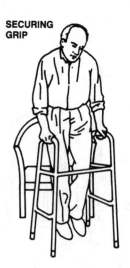

SECURING
GRIP

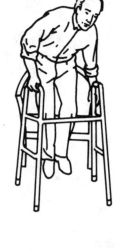

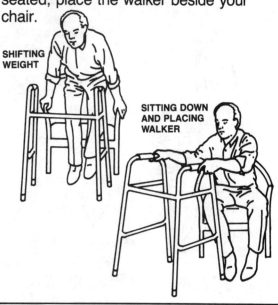

SHIFTING
WEIGHT

SITTING DOWN
AND PLACING
WALKER

Seizures

In a seizure disorder, the patient's prospects of leading a productive life may hinge on your success in teaching him about seizure-triggering factors and the importance of strict compliance with long-term drug therapy. You'll need to point out that his drug therapy may change, depending on his symptoms and the rate at which he metabolizes the drug. What's more, you'll need to teach him about possible activity restrictions, precautions for an imminent seizure, preparation for diagnostic tests, and, if ordered, surgery.

Remember to include the family in your teaching, too. They'll need to know how to help the patient during a seizure and promote his pursuit of a normal life.

Discuss the disorder

Explain to the patient that a seizure is a sudden change in normal brain activity that causes distinctive changes in behavior and body function. Mention that epilepsy is a condition characterized by recurrent seizures.

Inform the patient that the cause of seizures can't always be determined. Tell him that seizures result from the rapid, uncontrolled discharge of central nervous system (CNS) neurons. The site of this cerebral hyperactivity determines the patient's signs and symptoms.

Explain the patient's type of seizure: generalized convulsive; generalized nonconvulsive; simple partial; complex partial; or partial, secondarily generalized (for more information, see *Comparing seizure types*, page 156).

A *generalized convulsive* seizure, such as a tonic-clonic (or grand mal) seizure, involves the entire brain and, therefore, the entire body in convulsive activity. *Generalized nonconvulsive* seizures include atonic and absence (petit mal) seizures.

Partial seizure activity occurs in one part of the brain. A *simple partial* seizure usually has one associated manifestation, such as a jerking motion of a leg. *Complex partial* seizures have more than one manifestation, such as a jerking motion of an arm and loss of consciousness. Some types of partial seizures may spread and thereby become *secondarily generalized*.

Tell the patient that he may experience more than one type of seizure. Also tell him that during the initial seizure phase he may notice an aura—a sensory phenomenon, such as seeing stars or smelling roses—but that not every seizure victim experiences one.

Janette R. Yanko, RN, MN, CNRN, wrote this chapter. Ms. Yanko is a neuroscience clinical nurse specialist at Allegheny General Hospital, Pittsburgh.

CHECKLIST

Teaching topics in seizures

☐ How the brain's abnormal electrical activity leads to seizures
☐ The patient's type of seizure: generalized convulsive; generalized nonconvulsive; simple partial; complex partial; or partial, secondarily generalized
☐ Preparation for diagnostic tests, such as EEG and CT scan, to help determine the seizure's cause
☐ Importance of diet in providing energy for normal neuron function
☐ Drugs and their administration, including the risks of overmedication and undermedication
☐ Preparation for craniotomy, if necessary
☐ Trigger factors, including fatigue and hypoglycemia
☐ Precautions for an imminent seizure
☐ How the family or other caregivers should manage a seizure
☐ Importance of wearing a medical identification bracelet
☐ Sources of information and support

Comparing seizure types

Once the doctor has diagnosed the patient's seizure, help the patient and his family understand what type he has. Some common seizure types and their clinical manifestations are listed below.

Generalized seizures (convulsive)
• *Tonic-clonic (grand mal).* In the tonic phase, all muscles are contracted. The clonic phase, occurring less than a minute later, consists of rapid, jerking movements. Both phases include loss of consciousness, increased salivation, dilated pupils, and abnormal breathing.
• *Tonic.* In a tonic seizure, all muscles are contracted, pupils are dilated, and the patient loses consciousness.
• *Clonic.* This seizure type consists of rapid, jerking motions, dilated pupils, and loss of consciousness.
• *Myoclonic.* A myoclonic seizure is characterized by short, abrupt contractions of the extremity muscles and a brief loss of consciousness.

Generalized seizures (nonconvulsive)
• *Absence (petit mal).* A blank stare and rapid eye-blinking with altered awareness (lasting for 5 to 30 seconds) distinguishes this seizure. Lip smacking may also occur.
• *Atonic (drop attacks, astatic).* This seizure is characterized by abrupt loss of muscle tone and, usually, consciousness.

Partial seizures (simple)
• *Motor.* In a motor seizure, convulsive movement occurs in an arm, a leg, the face, or in all three body parts at the same time. Convulsive movement may progress (jacksonian march); consciousness remains unimpaired.
• *Somatosensory.* Sensory symptoms in this type of seizure involve hallucinations, flashing lights, tingling sensations, a foul odor, or vertigo.
• *Autonomic.* Epigastric sensations, sweating, flushing, tachycardia, pupillary dilation, and piloerection characterize an autonomic seizure.
• *Psychic.* Manifestations of a psychic seizure include déja vu, jamais vu, fear, anger, time distortion, and illusions.

Partial seizures (complex)
• *Simple with (or followed by) impaired consciousness.* Manifestations are the same as those of a simple partial seizure with (or followed by) impaired consciousness.
• *Automatisms.* This seizure type involves repetitions, such as ripping paper or buttoning and unbuttoning a shirt. Consciousness is impaired.

Partial seizures (secondarily generalized)
• *Simple to general, complex to general, or simple to complex to general.* Symptoms of partial seizures evolve to those of generalized seizures.

Complications
Emphasize the need for strict adherence to the drug regimen to prevent overmedication or undermedication. Overmedication may cause increased adverse reactions. In contrast, undermedication can increase the duration, frequency, and number of seizures. The result: an increased risk of injury.

Emphasize to the patient that he can seriously injure himself and others if he has a seizure while driving a car or operating machinery.

Describe the diagnostic workup
Teach the patient about blood tests to monitor anticonvulsant drug levels and to detect any blood dyscrasias resulting from drug therapy. As appropriate, prepare the patient for the following diagnostic tests to help identify the cause of seizures.

Electroencephalography (EEG)
Explain to the patient that the EEG records the electrical activity of his brain. Assure him that the test is painless and that the elec-

trodes won't give him an electric shock. Tell him who will perform the test and where, and that it takes about 45 minutes.

Depending on the type of EEG (such as sleep, sleep deprivation, or photic stimulation), explain the necessary restrictions. Then instruct the patient to wash his hair 1 to 2 days before the test to remove hair spray, cream, or oil.

Explain that during the test the patient will be comfortably positioned in a reclining chair or on a bed. After lightly abrading the patient's skin to ensure good contact, a technician will apply paste and attach electrodes to the patient's head and neck. Instruct the patient to remain still throughout the test. Review the activities that he may be asked to perform, such as breathing deeply and rapidly for 3 minutes (hyperventilating) or sleeping, depending on the type of EEG.

After the test, the technician will remove the electrodes. He'll also remove the paste, using acetone. (Mention that this may sting where the skin was scraped.) Tell the patient to wash his hair to remove residual paste; then he can resume his usual activities.

Closed-circuit television electroencephalography

Explain to the patient that if the routine EEG produces insufficient information, the doctor may request more extensive monitoring over an extended period. Tell him that a log may be kept to help determine what triggers his seizures. Mention that the monitoring is painless and won't give him an electric shock. Tell him who will perform the test, where it will take place, and how long monitoring will last. If the test will use special scalp electrodes, instruct the patient to wash his hair.

Explain how special electrodes will be inserted, if they are to be used. Fluoroscopy will help guide transsphenoidal electrode insertion. A trocar will be used to pass a very thin wire through the pterygoid fossa. Tell the patient to expect some discomfort, and mention that he'll have a wire extending from his upper cheek area. Subdural or depth electrodes require surgical insertion, involving an open flap craniotomy or burr holes. The electrodes will then extend from the patient's skull. Explain that heavy, cast-like dressings will protect them from dislodgement.

Tell the patient that he may have bathroom privileges, but otherwise, he'll be confined to an area within the videocamera's range (usually in bed). Reassure him that after the electrodes are removed, he can resume his normal activities.

Computed tomography (CT) scan

Inform the patient that a CT scan uses X-ray images to detect structural abnormalities, edema, and lesions, such as nonhemorrhagic infarction and aneurysms, and tumors, which may cause seizures. Tell the patient that the test takes 30 to 60 minutes and causes little discomfort, although he may feel chilled because the equipment requires a cool environment. Explain that he won't be allowed food or fluids for 4 hours before the scan if the test requires a dye.

Explain that during the test a technician will position him on an X-ray table and place a strap across the body part to be scanned, to restrict any movement. The table then slides into the tubelike opening of the scanner. If a dye is ordered, the infusion will take about 5 minutes. Instruct the patient to report immediately any discomfort or a feeling of warmth or itching. (The technician can see and hear him from an adjacent room.) Then describe noises he'll hear from the scanner as it revolves around him.

Advise the patient that immediately after the test he can resume his usual activities and diet. Urge him to increase his fluid intake for the rest of the day to help eliminate the dye, if used.

Positron emission tomography (PET) scan
Inform the patient that this test measures how rapidly tissue consumes radioactive isotopes. Prepare the patient by telling him that the test takes about 1 hour, is painless, and involves minimal radiation exposure.

Explain that during the test, the patient will lie on a moving table with his head immobilized and placed inside a ring-shaped opening in the machine. He'll be given a radioactive tracer either by *inhalation* or by *I.V. injection*. If the doctor chooses the inhalation method, tell the patient he'll inhale a radioactive tracer through a mask. Tell him to breathe normally; he won't smell or taste anything odd. If the doctor uses the I.V. method, tell the patient that he may feel a warm sensation during the tracer's injection. Advise him to report any discomfort to the technician. In both methods, tell the patient he'll have a dome-shaped hood placed over his head and face to prevent the exhaled tracer from circulating in the room. Stress the importance of lying still to avoid blurring the images.

If the I.V. method is used, explain that the doctor will remove the needle after the test and collect a blood sample. Then the patient can resume his normal activities.

Single photon emission tomography (SPECT) scan
Explain to the patient that SPECT studies cerebral blood flow and can help determine the cause of seizures. The test takes about 1 hour.

Inform the patient that before the test, he may receive a dose of salty-tasting Lugol's solution (depending on the tracer agent) and an I.V. amine tracer. Mention that he'll lie on a narrow metal table.

Explain that during the test, he'll feel the table move and will see a large disklike machine moving around his head as it makes images of the tracer agent flowing through the brain. Stress the importance of lying still to ensure accurate results. Tell the patient that he can resume his usual activities after the test.

Magnetic resonance imaging (MRI) scan
Inform the patient that MRI evaluates the brain's condition by providing clear images of the brain. It allows imaging of multiple

planes, including direct sagittal and coronal views, in regions in which bone normally hampers visualization. This test, like the others, helps determine a seizure's cause.

Explain that this test involves no radiation exposure, but does involve exposure to a strong magnetic field. Therefore, he should report any metal objects in his body (such as a pacemaker, aneurysm clip, hip prosthesis, or implanted infusion pump), which could make him ineligible for the test. The test takes about 1 hour. Mention that he may feel some discomfort from the loud noise and from being enclosed within the large cylinder. Ask him if he is claustrophobic.

Explain that during the test, the patient will be positioned on a table that slides into a large cylinder that houses the MRI magnets. Tell him that his head, chest, and arms will be restrained to help him remain still. Stress that lying still prevents blurring the images. Also explain that a technician can see and hear him from an adjacent room. Tell the patient he'll hear a loud knocking noise while the machine operates. If the noise bothers him, he may be given earplugs or pads for his ears. A radio encased in the machine or earphones may help block the sound (but he will still hear some noise). Tell the patient that he can resume his normal activities after the test.

Cerebral blood flow studies

Explain that these studies measure blood flow to the brain and help detect abnormalities. Inform the patient that the test takes about 30 minutes. It's painless and exposes him to less radiation than a chest X-ray.

Tell the patient that he'll lie still on a table during the test, and he'll have a frame placed around his head. He may inhale a radioactive gas, such as xenon, technetium, or krypton. Or he may receive an I.V. injection of the radioactive substance and breathe through a mask or dome while the isotope-sensitive detector probes measure the blood flow rate. Explain that he can resume his usual activities immediately after the test.

Wada (amobarbital) test

Teach the patient that the Wada test determines hemispheric dominance for speech, memory, and other specific activities, which can help decide the cause of a seizure. Tell him who will perform the test and where. Inform him that the test takes 1 to 2 hours, depending on whether both sides of the brain are tested.

Explain that the patient will be positioned on an X-ray table. The doctor will insert a catheter into the femoral artery and, aided by fluoroscopy, guide it to the carotid artery. He will then inject the amobarbital and ask the patient to perform tests related to memory, speech, and cognitive functions. Drug effects disappear in about 20 minutes. If the other cerebral hemisphere is to be tested, the doctor will reposition the catheter to the other carotid artery and repeat the drug infusion and performance tests.

After the test, instruct the patient to lie in bed for 2 to 12 hours with his leg kept straight; he may have an ice pack over the catheter insertion site.

160 Seizures

Preventing seizures

Teach the patient to control factors that can precipitate a seizure.
• Instruct him to take his *exact* dose of medication at the times prescribed. Missing doses, doubling doses, or taking extra doses can cause a seizure.
• Stress the importance of good nutrition. Advise him to eat balanced, regular meals. Explain that low blood glucose levels (hypoglycemia) and inadequate vitamin intake can lead to seizures.
• Teach him to be alert for odors that may trigger an attack. Advise him and his family to note any strong odors they notice at the time of a seizure and inform the doctor.
• Caution the patient to limit his alcohol intake. He should check with the doctor to find out whether he may drink *any* alcoholic beverages.
• Urge him to get enough sleep. Excessive fatigue can precipitate a seizure.
• Tell him to treat a fever early during an illness. If he can't reduce a fever, he should notify the doctor.
• Help him learn to control stress. If appropriate, suggest learning relaxation techniques, such as deep-breathing exercises.
• Tell the patient to avoid his trigger factors; for example, flashing lights, hyperventilation, loud noises, heavy musical beats, video games, and television.

Teach about treatments

Emphasize strict compliance with the patient's anticonvulsant medication regimen to control seizures. Also explain the significance of a balanced diet and regular meals to prevent seizures. If necessary, prepare the patient for a craniotomy: Explain its purpose, what happens during surgery, and preoperative and postoperative care. Be sure to educate the patient and his family about seizure triggers and what to do if a seizure occurs.

Diet

Instruct the patient to eat regular meals and to check with the doctor before dieting. Maintaining adequate blood glucose levels provides the necessary energy for CNS neurons to work normally. Skipping meals or dieting may lead to decreased glucose levels (hypoglycemia). This can cause unstable neurons to malfunction, thus triggering a seizure. Teach the patient to recognize the symptoms of hypoglycemia, so he can eat a snack when needed (see *Preventing seizures*).

Medication

Make sure the patient understands that anticonvulsant drugs can't cure his seizures, but they will control them. Advise him to take his medication exactly as ordered—both undermedication and overmedication can cause seizures. Explain that the doctor will regulate drug dosage according to his blood levels, so the dosage may periodically change (for example, with age or illness). If illness prevents the patient from taking his medication, tell him to have a family member or other caregiver contact the doctor immediately. The doctor may decide to administer medication by another route.

Tell the patient what to do if he misses a dose. Caution him, however, not to apply missed dose instructions for an anticonvulsant drug to any other drug he's taking because instructions will vary according to each drug's half-life. Stress that withdrawal seizures are possible if he abruptly stops taking his anticonvulsant drug.

Explain that he'll be taking medication as long as he needs it to control his seizures. Even if he doesn't have a seizure for years, he shouldn't stop taking it unless ordered by the doctor. The length of time he'll require an anticonvulsant drug (a few years or for life) depends on many factors, such as the cause of his seizures and his age (see *Teaching patients about anticonvulsants*).

Surgery

Prepare the patient for a craniotomy, if ordered. Explain that this surgery can remove a structure or lesion that can cause seizures, or it can sever a structure that allows abnormal electrical discharges to spread to other unstable neurons. Tell him that the success rate of craniotomy varies, but that this surgery may decrease

Teaching patients about anticonvulsants

DRUG	ADVERSE REACTIONS	TEACHING POINTS
carbamazepine (Tegretol)	• Watch for blurred vision, bradypnea, confusion, dark urine, depression, easy bruising or bleeding, edema of the legs or ankles, fever, hives, itching, jaundice, mouth ulcers, nightmares, nystagmus, palpitations, paresthesias, rash, sore throat, unusual tiredness or weakness, and urine retention. • Other reactions include abdominal pain, aching muscles or joints, ataxia, constipation, diarrhea, diaphoresis, dizziness, drowsiness, dry mouth, glossitis, headache, and nausea.	• If the patient misses a dose, tell him to take it as soon as he remembers, unless it's almost time for the next dose. Warn him not to double-dose. He should call the doctor if more than one dose a day is missed. • Advise him to take the drug with food to reduce nausea. If he experiences dry mouth, tell him to suck on ice chips or sugarless candy or to chew sugarless gum. • Warn him to operate machinery cautiously and to avoid driving if he experiences dizziness, drowsiness, or ataxia. • Because the drug may make him more sensitive to ultraviolet light, tell him to avoid using sunlamps and to wear a sunscreen, sunglasses, and protective clothing in the sun. • Stress the importance of keeping appointments for blood and eye tests. • Tell him that before any surgery, he should inform his doctor or dentist that he's taking this drug. • Inform the diabetic patient that this drug may affect urine glucose levels. • If he's taking the liquid form of the medication, instruct him to store it at room temperature in the original container. He should not refrigerate it. • Caution him not to abruptly discontinue the drug without first checking with his doctor.
clonazepam (Klonopin)	• Watch for ataxia, aphasia, behavior changes, chest congestion, choreiform movements, "glassy-eyed" look, hallucinations, hyperactivity, lymphadenopathy, muscle weakness, nystagmus, rash, and tremors. • Other reactions include alopecia, anorexia, constipation, diarrhea, double vision, drowsiness, hirsutism, increased appetite, increased salivation, insomnia, slurred speech, and sore gums.	• If the patient misses a dose, instruct him to take it only within 2 hours of the scheduled administration time. Warn him not to double-dose. • Warn him that abrupt cessation of the drug may cause withdrawal seizures. • Caution him to avoid operating machinery or driving if he feels dizzy, drowsy, or unsteady. • Stress the need for regular follow-up blood tests and medical visits. • Instruct him to avoid drinking alcoholic beverages and taking medications containing central nervous system (CNS) depressants. • Tell him that before any surgery, he should inform his doctor or dentist that he's taking this drug.
ethosuximide (Zarontin)	• Watch for abdominal pain, aggressiveness, ataxia, blurred vision, depression, epigastric distress, hematuria, hyperactivity, muscle weakness, rash, swelling of the tongue, and vaginal bleeding. • Other reactions include alopecia, constipation, diarrhea, dizziness, drowsiness, gum hypertrophy, hiccups, hirsutism, inability to concentrate, lethargy, nausea, periorbital edema, photophobia, and vomiting.	• If the patient misses a dose, instruct him to take it only within 2 hours of the scheduled administration time. Warn him not to double-dose. • Warn him that abrupt cessation of the drug may cause withdrawal seizures. • Caution him to avoid operating machinery or driving if he feels dizzy, drowsy, or unsteady. • Instruct him to avoid alcohol and medications that contain CNS depressants. • Stress the need for follow-up blood tests and medical visits. • Teach him that before any surgery, he should inform his doctor or dentist that he's taking this drug. • Tell the female patient that ethosuximide can decrease the effectiveness of estrogen and oral contraceptives. • If he's taking the liquid form of the medication, instruct him to store it at room temperature in the original container. Tell him not to refrigerate this medication.

continued

162 Seizures

Teaching patients about anticonvulsants — *continued*

DRUG	ADVERSE REACTIONS	TEACHING POINTS
ethotoin (Peganone) **mephenytoin** (Mesantoin) **phenytoin** (Dilantin)	• Watch for ataxia, blurred vision, confusion, easy bruising or bleeding, fever, gingival hyperplasia (with phenytoin), gingivitis (with ethotoin), hallucinations, jaundice, joint pain, lymphadenopathy, nystagmus, rash, seizures, severe abdominal pain, slurred speech, and sore throat. • Other reactions include constipation, diarrhea, drowsiness, headache, hirsutism, insomnia, mild dizziness, muscle twitching, nausea, urine discoloration, and vomiting.	• If the patient misses one daily dose at the scheduled time, tell him to take it as soon as he remembers, unless it is close to his next dose. If he's taking several daily doses, tell him to take a missed dose as soon as he remembers. • If he's using a liquid form, teach him to shake it *well* and to use a measuring spoon, not a household teaspoon. If he's taking the chewable form, he *must* chew or crush the tablets. • Advise him to take this drug with food if he develops nausea. • Warn him to operate machinery cautiously and to avoid driving if he feels dizzy (more common with ethotoin and mephenytoin). • Tell him to avoid regular consumption of alcohol and large doses of salicylates. Instruct him not to take vitamins containing folic acid without first consulting his doctor. • Advise him not to take antacids within 3 hours of taking his anticonvulsant. • Stress the importance of good oral hygiene and dental care to the patient taking phenytoin. • Explain that these drugs may turn his urine pink or reddish brown. • Warn him that changing brands or abruptly stopping the drug may result in seizures. • Stress the importance of keeping follow-up blood test and doctors' appointments. • Tell him that before any surgery, he should inform his doctor or dentist that he's taking this drug. • Inform the diabetic patient that this drug may affect his urine and blood glucose levels.
phenobarbital (Luminal)	• Watch for ataxia, bradycardia, bradypnea, confusion, depression, easy bleeding or bruising, fever, hives, hyperexcitability, insomnia, jaundice, joint or muscle pain, rash, severe drowsiness or weakness, shortness of breath, slurred speech, and sore throat. • Other reactions include anxiety, dizziness, drowsiness, headache, irritability, nausea, nightmares, and vomiting.	• If he misses a dose, tell the patient to take it as soon as he remembers unless it's almost time for the next dose. Warn him not to double-dose. • Caution him never to abruptly stop the drug because withdrawal seizures could occur. • Warn him to take the drug as ordered to prevent possible dependence on it. • Warn him not to crush, chew, or break extended-release capsules. • Tell him to avoid alcohol and hay fever, allergy, cold, and sleeping medications that contain CNS depressants, such as antihistamines. • Instruct him to operate machinery cautiously and to avoid driving if he feels dizzy or drowsy. • Explain that before any surgery, he should inform his doctor or dentist that he's taking this drug.
primidone (Mysoline, Sertan)	• Watch for ataxia, confusion, difficulty breathing, easy bruising or bleeding, facial edema, hives, itching, nervousness, rash, restlessness, sore throat, unusual tiredness, and visual changes. • Other reactions include anorexia, decreased libido, dizziness, drowsiness, headache, nausea, unsteadiness, and vomiting.	• If the patient misses a dose, tell him to take it only within 2 hours of the scheduled administration time. Warn him not to double-dose. • Instruct him never to abruptly stop the drug, because seizures are possible. • If he's taking the suspension form, teach him to shake the bottle *well* before pouring and to use a measuring spoon (not a household teaspoon). • Tell him to avoid cold, hay fever, allergy, or sleeping medications containing CNS depressants, such as antihistamines. Tell him also to avoid drinking alcoholic beverages — also a CNS depressant. • Advise him to take this drug with meals if he develops nausea. • Warn him to operate machinery cautiously and to avoid driving if he feels dizzy, drowsy, or unsteady. • Stress the need for regular follow-up blood tests and medical visits. • Tell him that before any surgery, he should inform his doctor or dentist that he's taking this drug.

continued

Teaching patients about anticonvulsants — *continued*

DRUG	ADVERSE REACTIONS	TEACHING POINTS
valproic acid (Depakene)	• Watch for dark urine, depression, easy bruising or bleeding, jaundice, nausea, nightmares, rash, seizures, severe abdominal pain, visual changes, and vomiting. • Other reactions include constipation, diarrhea, dizziness, drowsiness, indigestion, mild abdominal pain, and transient alopecia.	• If the patient misses a dose, tell him to take it when he remembers. But if his next scheduled dose is within 6 hours, tell him not to take the missed dose. Warn him not to double-dose. • Caution him never to stop the drug abruptly because withdrawal seizures may occur. • Instruct him never to chew the drug because it will irritate his mouth and throat. • Advise him to take this drug with meals (but not with milk) if he experiences GI distress. • Warn him to operate machinery cautiously and to avoid driving if he feels drowsy. • Caution him to avoid taking hay fever, allergy, cold, or sleeping medications containing CNS depressants, such as antihistamines. Warn him not to drink alcohol, which is also a CNS depressant • Advise him to avoid taking aspirin, which may increase the risk of bleeding and bruising. • Stress the importance of regular follow-up blood tests and medical visits. • Tell him that before any surgery, he should inform his doctor or dentist that he's taking this drug. • Inform the diabetic patient that this drug may produce false urine ketone results.

the number and severity of seizures. Inform the patient that he may still require anticonvulsant drugs after surgery.

Advise the patient to wash his hair on the day before surgery, if possible. Tell him that a technician will shave his head at the incision site. (Reassure him that his hair will grow back and that the surgery won't affect his memory, his feelings, or his ability to think.) Explain to the patient that after he receives an anesthetic, the surgeon will open part of the skull to expose the brain tissue. The size of the opening varies from a small burr hole to a larger open flap. The burr hole later fills in with bone growth; the large bone flaps are put back or replaced by synthetic material.

Inform the patient that after surgery, he'll have a bandage over his head, and that the head of his bed will be elevated about 30 degrees (for a supratentorial craniotomy) or kept flat (for an infratentorial craniotomy). Caution him to avoid changing the bed's position; tell him, however, that he can turn from side to side. Also tell him to avoid coughing, which could increase intracranial pressure. Remind him to ask for medication if he develops a headache.

Explain that the doctor will remove his skin sutures within 7 days, and that he'll wear a cap to keep his head warm after removal of the bandages. (Tell him that the size of the scalp incision doesn't necessarily reflect the size of the skull opening.)

Before the patient is discharged from the hospital (usually 7 to 10 days after surgery), remind him to keep his head warm. Tell him he may wash his hair (but should avoid scrubbing around the incision), gently patting the incisional area dry. Instruct him to re-

164 Seizures

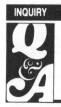

Questions patients ask about seizures

How will seizures interfere with my normal activities?
Once your seizures are under control, you'll be able to continue your normal activities—with some safety considerations. Avoid swimming alone and working at heights. (For example, don't climb a ladder to paint your house.) If you drive, contact your state's motor vehicle department. Most states prohibit you from driving a motor vehicle until you're seizure-free for a certain time period, possibly up to 1 year.

What will happen if I have a seizure in a public place?
To make sure you're cared for correctly, you should always wear a medical identification bracelet or necklace stating that you have a seizure disorder. This will alert others to your condition. If you feel a seizure coming on, find a safe spot and lie down. (Of course, you should be aware of your trigger factors and avoid them, if possible.)

Will I lose my job?
You shouldn't lose your job because you have seizures. If you're honest with your employer about your disorder, you're protected by the equal opportunity laws. However, keep in mind that your exact job description may change, depending on the position's requirements and on liability considerations.

port any signs of infection (redness, warmth, or drainage) or separation of the incision. Inform him that he can resume most routine activities, but that he'll require the doctor's permission to return to work or to engage in strenuous activities, such as running or contact sports.

Other care measures
Help the patient identify factors that can trigger a seizure (see *Preventing seizures,* page 160). Stress that seizures can be triggered even if the patient is taking his anticonvulsant medication as prescribed.

Encourage the patient to pursue his normal activities if possible, but remind him of safety considerations. Tell him what to do if he feels a seizure coming on (see *Questions patients ask about seizures*).

Make sure the patient's family knows what to do if a seizure occurs (see *Helping a seizure victim*). If the patient's a child, instruct the parents to notify day care or school authorities of their child's condition (see *Seizures and your child,* page 166).

Stress the importance of wearing a medical identification bracelet or necklace at all times. Also encourage the patient to contact the Epilepsy Foundation of America for additional information. Refer him to a local support group.

Sources of information and support
Epilepsy Concern Service Group
179 Allyn Street #304, Hartford, Conn. 06103
(203) 246-6566

Epilepsy Foundation of America
4351 Garden City Drive, Landover, Md. 20785
(Hotline) (301) 459-3700

Further readings
Austin, J.K., et al. "Parental Attitude and Coping Behaviors in Families of Children with Epilepsy," *Journal of Neuroscience Nursing* 20(3):174-79, June 1988.
Callanan, M. "Epilepsy: Putting the Patient Back in Control," *RN* 51(2):48-56, February 1988.
Dreifuss, F.E., et al. "Epilepsy: Management by Medication," *Patient Care* 22(7):52-58, April 15, 1988.
Freidman, D. "Taking the Scare out of Caring for Seizure Patients," *Nursing88* 18:53-59, February 1988.
Richard, A. "Self-Help for Seizures," *Medical Self-Care* 3:44-51, May-June 1988.

Helping a seizure victim

Dear Caregiver:

A person with a seizure disorder may have an attack at any time, in any place. During a seizure, he may lose consciousness and fall down. You can prepare yourself to help him by reading the following instructions.

During the seizure

1 Turn the person on his side and remove hard or sharp objects from the area. Loosen restrictive clothing, such as a collar or a belt, and place something soft and flat under the person's head.

  Never force anything into the person's mouth, especially your fingers. Ask onlookers to leave the area.

2 If you suspect the person has swallowed his own vomit, call a doctor immediately.

After the seizure

1 Allow the person to lie quietly. As he awakens, gently call him by name, and reorient him to his surroundings and to recent events.

2 If the person has an injury, such as a badly bleeding tongue, take him to the doctor's office or to the hospital emergency department.

3 Write an accurate description of the seizure as soon as you can. The doctor may request certain information, including the seizure's duration and the victim's activity immediately before, during, and after the seizure.

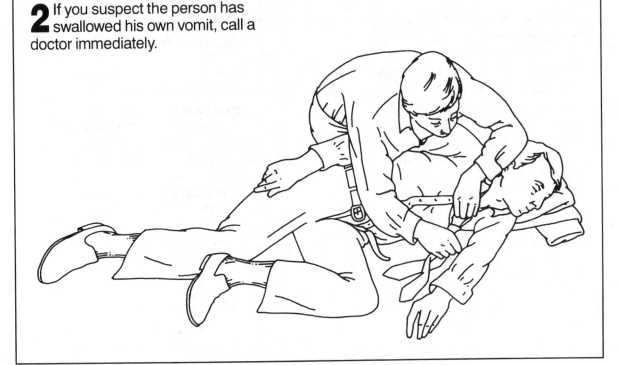

Seizures and your child

Dear Parent:

You probably have many questions about seizures and how to help your child lead a normal life. Here are some answers.

What causes seizures?

Seizures may follow a birth injury, a head injury, a high fever, or a disease that affects your child's nervous system, such as meningitis and encephalitis.

However, the cause of many seizures is never known. Rest assured, though, that they aren't contagious. No one gave them to your child, and no one can catch them from him, either.

Taking medication

Follow your doctor's instructions *exactly* for the dose of medication to give your child and when to give it. Taking medication exactly as the doctor prescribes will help control your child's seizures. *Remember:* Missing doses of medication could lead to a seizure.

When your child begins taking medication for seizures, he may seem less alert or his behavior may change. If these side effects interfere with his activities and school work, tell your doctor. He may adjust the dose or change the medication.

Restricting activities

Has the doctor placed any restrictions on your child's activities? If so, follow his instructions. If not, take the same precautions as you would with any other child. For example, caution him to wear a helmet when he's skateboarding or bicycling. And don't let him swim alone.

Providing support

Help your child deal with people who have misguided ideas about seizures. If you have other children, help them understand their brother's or sister's condition. Explain what they should do if their brother or sister has a seizure.

Telling others

Enlist the support of your child's teacher. Tell her about your child's seizures, and explain what to do if he has one in school. She can help your child's classmates accept him as being just like them — except that he has seizures. She can also help his classmates deal emotionally with a seizure if he has one in school.

Ask the school nurse to help if your child must take medication during school hours. Also inform camp counselors, babysitters, and any other people who care for your child about his seizures and how to handle them.

Getting more information

Contact the Epilepsy Foundation of America for free information for you, your child, the rest of your family, and your child's friends. You can also call your doctor if you have questions.

Guillain-Barré syndrome

A frightening disease, Guillain-Barré syndrome (GBS) may considerably alter the patient's mobility and disrupt his life. So you'll need to marshall all your teaching skills as you instruct and counsel the patient affected by this rapidly progressing—*but reversible*—neurologic disease. At best, GBS causes mild muscle weakness; at worst, complete paralysis.

Your teaching efforts may be complicated by the patient's intense anxiety should the disease progress to paralysis. You'll need to prepare him for worsening symptoms and for possible complications. You'll reassure him repeatedly that most patients recover fully. If he has a family or close friends, you'll include them as you teach about the treatments and assistance he'll need with activities of daily living. Once he starts to recover, you'll help him relearn old skills during a slow, possibly difficult, rehabilitation.

Discuss the disorder

Inform the patient and his family that GBS causes inflamed, swollen peripheral nerves, producing numbness, tingling, and burning sensations. It also causes bilateral muscle weakness and possible paralysis.

Outline how the disease progresses through acute, plateau, and recovery stages. In the acute stage, the patient usually experiences symptoms that begin in the lower legs and progress upward for 2 to 3 weeks before they peak. As the disease enters the plateau stage, which lasts from several days to 2 weeks, his symptoms may not change. Then gradually, during the recovery stage, he may experience some pain and discomfort, resulting from neural edema or regeneration of peripheral nerve tissue. Explain that recovery can take 2 to 3 years.

Typically preceded by a viral illness or an immunization, GBS is thought to be an autoimmune response. The illness or the immunization may stimulate a T-cell attack on the nerve's myelin sheath. This prevents the normal transmission of electrical impulses along sensorimotor nerve routes and results in paresthesia, weakness, and motor dysfunction. (For more information, see *Understanding sensorimotor nerve degeneration in GBS,* page 168.)

Complications

Explain that throughout the disease the patient's inability to use his muscles may cause complications, including thrombophlebitis, pressure sores, contractures, muscle wasting, respiratory infec-

Ellie Z. Franges, RN, MSN, CCRN, CNRN, wrote this chapter. Ms. Franges is head nurse in the central nervous system unit of the Allentown Hospital-Lehigh Valley Hospital Center, Allentown, Pa.

CHECKLIST

Teaching topics in Guillain-Barré syndrome

☐ Explanation of how neural swelling and inflammation affect movement
☐ The stages and complications of Guillain-Barré syndrome (GBS)
☐ Preparation for diagnostic tests, such as cerebrospinal fluid analysis, electromyography, and nerve conduction studies
☐ Activity to maintain joint and muscle function, minimize muscle wasting, and prevent pressure sores and other complications
☐ Dietary measures to promote adequate nutrition
☐ Medications, such as prednisone, to reduce nerve swelling, and aspirin or propoxyphene, to relieve pain
☐ Plasmapheresis to retard GBS
☐ Breathing assistance by mechanical ventilation
☐ Alternative communication techniques
☐ Psychological considerations

Understanding sensorimotor nerve degeneration in GBS

If your patient asks, "Why do I feel so numb and weak?"or "Why can't I move my arms and legs right?" explain that Guillain-Barré syndrome (GBS) attacks the peripheral nerves so that they can't transmit messages correctly to the brain. Here's what goes wrong:

In GBS, the myelin sheath degenerates for unknown reasons. This sheath covers the nerve axons and conducts electrical impulses (messages) along the nerve pathways. With degeneration comes inflammation, swelling, and patchy demyelination. As GBS destroys myelin, the nodes of Ranvier (at the junctures of the myelin sheaths) widen. This delays and impairs impulse transmission along both the dorsal and the ventral nerve roots.

Because the dorsal nerve roots handle sensory function, the patient experiences sensations, such as tingling and numbness, when the nerve root's impaired. Similarly, because the ventral nerve roots are responsible for motor function, impairment causes varying weakness, immobility, and paralysis.

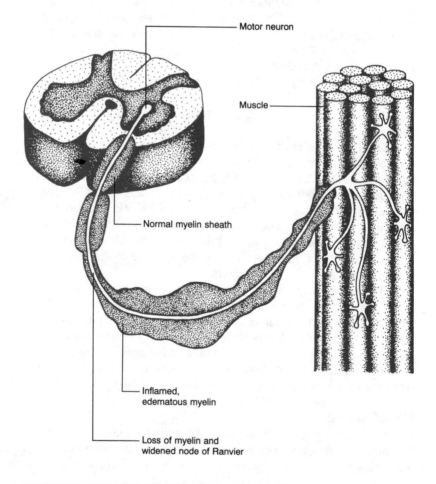

Motor neuron

Muscle

Normal myelin sheath

Inflamed, edematous myelin

Loss of myelin and widened node of Ranvier

tions, and life-threatening respiratory and cardiac compromise. During its peak period the health care team will take measures to prevent most complications. Warn the patient that during recovery he must actively comply with therapy—especially exercise, rest, and dietary measures—to promote recovery and prevent complications or a possible relapse.

Describe the diagnostic workup

Tell the patient that no definitive test can detect GBS. The doctor bases diagnosis on the patient's muscle weakness and progressive symptoms. He'll also check for a precursor disease or event, such as a flulike illness, an immunization, or surgery. To confirm the diagnosis and rule out other neurologic diseases, however, the doctor may order cerebrospinal fluid (CSF) analysis, electromyography (EMG), and nerve conduction studies.

CSF analysis

Explain that this test involves extracting and analyzing spinal fluid to detect elevated protein levels and CSF pressure in GBS. Tell the patient that the test takes about 15 minutes and that the doctor will obtain the sample by lumbar or cisternal puncture. Although the site will be numbed with a local anesthetic, warn the patient that he may feel some pressure when the doctor inserts the needle to withdraw CSF.

To prepare the patient for a *lumbar puncture,* describe how he'll lie on his side near the edge of the bed, with his knees drawn up to his abdomen and his chin resting on his chest. Tell him to report any tingling or sharp pain when the doctor injects the local anesthetic. Then, inform him that the doctor will insert a hollow needle into the subarachnoid space surrounding the spinal cord. Urge him to stay motionless so that he won't dislodge the needle. Add that the doctor may ask the patient to breathe deeply or to straighten his legs and that the doctor may also apply pressure to his jugular vein. After obtaining the fluid sample, the doctor will remove the needle and apply an adhesive bandage.

He'll instruct the patient to lie flat on his back for 4 to 24 hours to prevent a headache. Caution the patient to keep his head even with or below hip level. Reassure him that although he mustn't raise his head, he can turn his body from side to side. Advise him to increase his fluid intake for the rest of the day to help replenish his spinal fluid and to help prevent a headache.

Explain that with a *cisternal puncture,* the patient will need to restrict food and fluids for 4 hours before the test, as ordered. Tell him that he'll lie on his side at the edge of the bed with a small pillow placed beneath his head, which he'll bend forward. Inform him that after cleansing and possibly shaving the upper neck area, the doctor will inject a local anesthetic. Then, he'll insert a hollow needle into the midline of the vertebral column below the occipital bone and withdraw some CSF. Caution him to remain as still as possible during the needle insertion. Then tell him that after the test he should lie flat on his abdomen until the puncture site seals, usually in 6 to 8 hours.

Neuromuscular tests

If the doctor orders electromyography (EMG), nerve conduction studies, or both, inform the patient that these similar tests measure different processes. Explain that EMG measures the electrical activity of specific muscles, whereas nerve conduction studies measure the speed with which electrical impulses travel along a nerve. Tell him that these tests aid the doctor in determining the type and site of nerve damage, which helps rule out other disorders.

When preparing your patient for these tests, warn him that they may cause discomfort. Explain that during testing, which may take about an hour, he'll lie down or sit up, depending on the muscle or nerve being tested. Instruct him to stay still (except when asked to contract or relax a muscle) because movement may affect the accuracy of test results. Inform him that the technician will cleanse the skin over the test area and insert shallow needle electrodes either in the muscle or in the area near the distal nerve ending. Next, the technician will place another electrode on the test area. This electrode delivers a mild charge to stimulate each muscle or nerve and measure its response.

If the patient's undergoing EMG studies, reassure him that the amplified crackling sounds he hears are normal. These sounds occur whenever a muscle moves. Also describe the muscle movement patterns he may see on the EMG monitor.

Teach about treatments

Tell the patient that supportive treatment aims to maintain his body systems at an optimal level while the disease progresses so that he'll have a smoother recovery. As needed, the health care team will exercise his weakened arms and legs to keep them mobile, promote circulation, and prevent complications. What's more, they'll ensure adequate nourishment—feeding him through tubes if the disease prevents him from swallowing. Inform him that he may receive medications or undergo plasmapheresis to decrease nerve swelling and inflammation. Explain that depending on his condition he may need intensive care and breathing assistance with mechanical ventilation. If vocal communication becomes impossible, reassure him that you'll implement alternate means of communication. During teaching sessions, urge his family to plan some activities to lessen boredom and prevent depression.

Activity

Tell the patient that during the acute GBS stage the health care team will monitor the range of his mobility. Acknowledge that these checks may annoy him, but that they're necessary to help the team plan his care and anticipate his needs. Assure him that as his muscles grow weaker (and while they're paralyzed, if they are), the nurses and physical therapists will frequently reposition him and perform range-of-motion exercises. These activities will help maintain muscle tone, preserve joint and muscle function, prevent contractures, and relieve pain. Add that he may have splints applied to his arms and legs, which can maintain joint function, provide support, promote rest, prevent contractures, and ensure proper body alignment.

Advise him, too, that he may lie in a movable bed (Roto-bed) that allows frequent repositioning and turning from side to side—another way to help maintain joint and muscle function. If his vital signs are stable and his condition permits, he'll be allowed out of the bed to sit in a chair for some time each day.

Explain that during the patient's recovery the physical therapist will recommend an exercise program to strengthen and retrain weakened muscles. Advise him to follow instructions precisely because overdoing the exercise can enhance demyelination and worsen his symptoms or cause a relapse. Tell him to expect aching joints and muscles as his strength increases.

Stress the benefits of the exercise program, explaining that normal daily activity won't be enough to challenge his muscles. The physical therapist may recommend hydrotherapy at first because water promotes buoyancy, which makes exercising easier and more effective. What's more, the moist heat will soothe his pain and promote circulation.

Depending on the patient's progress and needs, show him how to use a walker or a cane to increase and support his mobility. As appropriate, give him patient-teaching aids related to assistive devices (see pages 145 to 154).

If the patient feels discouraged with his progress, remind him that strengthening and retraining muscles is always slow and tedious. Cite the progress that he's already made. And suggest that he take one day and one step at a time.

Diet
Inform the patient that while GBS progresses he may need tube feedings—especially if he loses his gag reflex or can't swallow enough food by mouth.

However, during recovery, encourage him to consume a high-calorie diet to help restore his strength. Explain that the dietitian may recommend five small meals daily rather than three larger ones to ensure that he gets the required number of calories. She may also suggest that he start with thicker fluids, such as pudding or yogurt. To help him avoid choking, advise him to rest before meals, eat slowly, and remain in an upright rather than a reclining position.

Medications
Tell the patient that the doctor may prescribe corticosteroids to relieve GBS symptoms. These drugs decrease neural inflammation and swelling. He may also prescribe pain relievers: nonnarcotic analgesics, such as aspirin; narcotic analgesics, such as propoxyphene (Darvon); or other drugs, such as carbamazepine (Tegretol).

If the doctor prescribes a corticosteroid (for example, prednisone or dexamethasone), warn the patient that GBS symptoms may worsen before they get better. And because the drug can cause fluid and salt retention, advise him to report swollen hands and feet. Other reactions to corticosteroid therapy include blurred vision, dizziness, nausea and vomiting, nervousness, and rash. If the drug causes GI irritation, suggest that he take it with food or with an antacid. Also caution him to follow dosage instructions exactly and not to stop taking the drug abruptly. Explain that his doctor will withdraw the corticosteroid slowly to allow his body to begin producing the naturally occurring hormones suppressed by the drug therapy.

Teach the patient to take pain medication before pain becomes intolerable. If the doctor recommends *aspirin* or *acetaminophen,* explain that possible adverse reactions may include abnormal bleeding, itching, rash, ringing in the ears, and stomach upset.

If the doctor prescribes *propoxyphene,* tell the patient that this drug is a mild narcotic, so he shouldn't exceed the recommended dosage. Nor should he use alcohol with this drug because it may cause or increase central nervous system or respiratory depression. Caution him to watch for adverse reactions, such as dysrhythmias, hypersensitivity, or seizures. Other reactions include constipation, dizziness, drowsiness, headache, indigestion, lightheadedness, minor visual disturbances, nausea and vomiting, rashes, and weakness.

If the doctor prescribes *carbamazepine* to relieve neuralgia, caution the patient to watch for abdominal pain, bleeding, drowsiness, GI distress, mouth ulcers, sore throat, incoordination, and fluid retention. To avoid or minimize possible stomach upset, advise the patient to take the drug with meals.

Encourage the patient to report the effectiveness of all pain medications so that the doctor can assess their value and make adjustments accordingly.

Procedures

If appropriate, explain to the patient that plasmapheresis aims to stop or slow the disease's progression by removing harmful antibodies from his blood. These are the antibodies suspected of attacking the nerves and causing muscle weakness. Explain that the process takes several hours, every 2 to 3 days, for 2 to 4 weeks.

Inform the patient that he'll recline throughout the procedure. To begin, a technician will insert a catheter into a vein. The catheter leads to a machine called a cell separator. Then blood is withdrawn from the patient's body and circulated through the cell separator, which separates the plasma from the other blood components, filters the attacking antibodies from the plasma, and returns the plasma and other blood components to the patient.

Reassure him that the entire process should cause only minimal discomfort. Mention that the procedure cannot reverse symptoms that have already occurred.

Other care measures

Depending on the severity of GBS, prepare the patient for intensive care, mechanical ventilation, and nonverbal communication and entertainment. (See *Talking boards.*)

Talking boards

If your patient has a tracheostomy to assist her breathing during the acute stage of Guillain-Barré syndrome, show her and her family board devices that promote communication without speech.

Letter-number board
Show the patient and her family a letter-number board like the one shown here. Arrange four rows of letters alphabetically and one row of numbers zero through nine. Tell the patient to stare at the board when she wants to use it. Then, ask her if she wants the first, second, third, fourth, or fifth row. By blinking once for yes and twice for no, she can answer which rows and then which letters she wants to spell out a message.

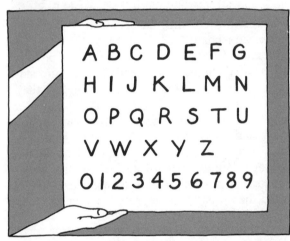

Phrase board
Another helpful tool, the phrase board concisely lists the patient's most common communications, such as *rub my back* or *turn on the TV.*

Number each column; then number each phrase. Fill each column with 10 phrases. Then, by blinking yes or no, as above, the patient can signal which message she wants to convey.

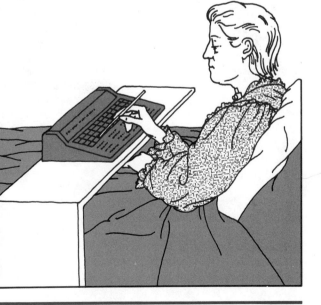

1	2	3
1. TURN ME TO THE RIGHT	11. PLEASE CHECK THE VENTILATOR	21. PULL THE SHADE DOWN
2. TURN ME TO THE LEFT		22. PUT ON MY GLASSES
3. PULL ME UP IN BED	12. ADD AIR TO MY TRACH CUFF	
4. RAISE MY HEAD	13. BEND MY KNEES	
5. TURN OFF THE LIGHTS	14. PROP UP MY FEET	
6. SUCTION MY MOUTH	15. STRAIGHTEN MY SHEETS	
7. SUCTION MY TRACH	16. I'M TOO HOT	
8. RUB MY BACK	17. I'M TOO COLD	
9. PUT A PILLOW UNDER MY HIPS	18. PLEASE READ TO ME	
10. OPEN THE WINDOW	19. TURN THE TV ON/OFF	
	20. TURN THE RADIO ON/OFF	

Powered communicator board
If your hospital has a powered communicator board, teach the patient how to use it. Assuming she has enough strength, she can use a straw or a stick to press letters and numbers to spell out a message on a display panel. Or she can press preprogrammed buttons on the keyboard to convey frequent requests, such as *turn me,* without having to fashion the message letter by letter.

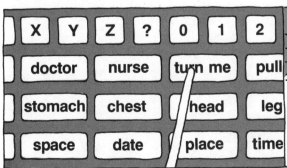

Intensive care. Describe the intensive care environment, should the patient need it. Tell him that his heart and respiratory rate will be monitored. Explain that a nurse will check on him frequently and that she can see him from a central location. Inform him that he may hear and see unfamiliar sounds and sights—for example, suction equipment and chest tubes.

Mechanical ventilation. Should the patient's muscles become so weak that he cannot breathe adequately, describe how he will breathe through a temporary endotracheal tube. The tube will be inserted through an opening created in his throat and connected to a machine. Encourage him to express his feelings about this body change and about having a machine breathe for him.

Nonverbal communication. Because he won't be able to talk, help him develop another way to communicate while he has a tracheostomy. For example, suggest he can answer questions by blinking once for yes and twice for no. For more complex communications, show him and his family how to design and use a letter-number board and a phrase board. Or demonstrate how to use a powered communicator board.

Entertainment. Because GBS doesn't weaken thought processes, encourage the patient's family and friends to help him stay mentally alert, fight boredom, and avoid depression. Suggest they borrow videos or books on tape from the library—if the patient likes films or reading. While he's in the hospital, they can supply a list of his favorite TV and radio programs. Warn them that depression and feelings of helplessness are common for the patient and the family. Encourage them to air these feelings so that they can overcome their fears and promote understanding. Praise their efforts to cope. Remind them that slow progress is common.

Further readings

"A Man Alone... and Afraid: Caring for a Patient with Guillain-Barré Syndrome," *Nursing87* 17(12):44-48, December 1987.

Fawcett, M. "Lessons from a Patient," *AD Nurse* 2(6):11-13, November-December 1987.

Sica, S., et al. "Immobility Syndrome: Use It or Lose It!" *AD Nurse* 2(6):6-10, November-December 1987.

Uprichard, E., et al. "Guillain-Barré Syndrome... Patients' and Nurses' Perspectives," *Intensive Care Nursing* 2(3):123-34, 1987.

Head injuries

Your teaching about head injuries will range from simple to complex. For example, the patient with a mild concussion may need only a few home care instructions. But severe head trauma can affect every human response and change all aspects of the patient's life. For this patient, you'll design a complex teaching plan that encompasses the care of many body systems.

Begin your teaching with an explanation of the patient's injury and the diagnostic workup. If the patient is severely compromised and unable to communicate, focus your teaching on his family. When the patient's condition stabilizes, address such treatment measures as activity and dietary guidelines, medications, and procedures to monitor and reduce increased intracranial pressure (ICP). If the patient has a moderate to severe head injury, teach him and his family about rehabilitation and long-term care.

Discuss the disorder

The term *head injury* refers to various traumatic insults to the skull and brain—not to a distinct disease process. Tell the patient (or his caregiver, if appropriate) that head injury can involve the skull, the entire brain, or specific brain areas. The mechanism of injury depends on the forces applied to the brain on impact. The skull's inner surface has many irregular projections. Jostled across these projections, the brain's soft tissue can be bruised, torn, or entrapped.

Inform the patient and his family that his signs and symptoms depend on which areas of the brain were injured. In a simplified manner, discuss brain structure and function with him, correlating his dysfunctions with specific brain areas. (See *Teaching about brain structures and functions,* page 176.)

Next, discuss his type of injury and its classification. (See *Classifying head injuries,* page 177.) If necessary, clarify the doctor's explanation of the patient's injury and discuss its implications.

Complications

Inform the patient (or his caregiver) that a brain injury raises the body's metabolic rate, increasing all organs' need for oxygen. Without supportive treatment, hypoxia can develop, causing further brain damage, permanent disability, and even death. Other possible complications include systemic hypotension, hypercapnia, sustained increased ICP, cerebral edema, respiratory problems, and infections.

Julie N. Tackenberg, RN, MA, CNRN, who wrote this chapter, is a clinical nurse specialist at the University Medical Center in Tucson, Ariz.

CHECKLIST

Teaching topics in head injuries

☐ Explanation of head injuries and their classification
☐ Preparation for diagnostic tests, such as computed tomography scan, evoked potential studies, and neuropsychological testing
☐ Complications, such as hypoxia and increased intracranial pressure (ICP)
☐ Activity measures
☐ Dietary adjustments, including fluid restrictions and semisoft foods for dysphagia
☐ Prescribed medications to reduce ICP or prevent seizures
☐ Preparation for procedures, such as ICP monitoring or barbiturate coma
☐ Explanation of craniotomy, if necessary
☐ Importance of rehabilitation in minimizing neurologic deficits; need for family involvement in rehabilitation
☐ Other care measures, such as adapting to neurologic deficits, home safety tips, and post-concussion instructions
☐ Source of information and support

Teaching about brain structures and functions

How can a head injury impair so many body functions? This question may puzzle your patient and his family. Explain that the brain acts as the body's control center—receiving messages from the senses and controlling motor function and thought processes. Then review major sites of brain function, and explain that functional losses depend on which part of the brain is injured.

The cerebrum
Head trauma typically impairs the *cerebrum*, the largest part of the brain and the center for many higher functions, including sensory interpretation (hearing, vision, touch, and smell), movement (individual and group muscle function), consciousness, emotion, language, and memory.

The brainstem
The *medulla oblongata,* the *pons,* and the *midbrain* constitute the brainstem, which controls cardiac, vasomotor, respiratory, auditory, and visual reflexes.

The cerebellum
Responsible for the skeletal muscles, the *cerebellum* controls coordination, balance, and posture.

The diencephalon
Located between the cerebrum and the midbrain, the diencephalon contains the *thalamus* and the *hypothalamus.* The thalamus relays sensory impulses, and the hypothalamus controls involuntary activities, such as glandular function, wakefulness, appetite, and body temperature.

CROSS-SECTION OF THE BRAIN

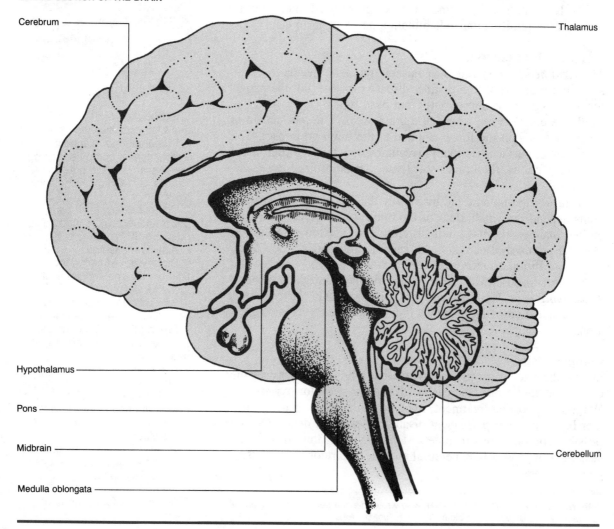

Cerebrum

Thalamus

Hypothalamus

Pons

Midbrain

Medulla oblongata

Cerebellum

Classifying head injuries

Point out to the patient and his family that health care professionals use varying classification systems for head injuries.

Explain that classification may be based on the severity of injury (mild, moderate, severe); the type of injury (concussion, contusion, laceration); the mechanism of injury (direct impact, acceleration, deceleration); or skull integrity (open or closed). As shown in the following illustrations, head injury may be also be classified by cerebral involvement—focal or diffuse.

Focal head injury

If the patient has a focal head injury, inform him that cerebral damage, which usually results from direct impact, is well delineated. Examples include hematomas, concussions, contusions, and skull fractures. Focal injuries can cause permanent deficits. However, complications may be moderated if the patient's injury (for example, from a skull fracture) also falls in the open head trauma class because the open skull accommodates cerebral swelling.

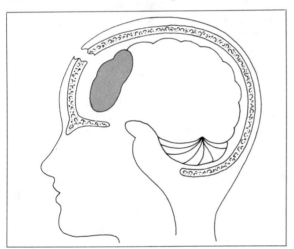

Diffuse head injury

Many brain areas are damaged in a diffuse injury. Typical causes include an indirect blow to the head or a combination of direct and indirect impacts. Examples are concussions and diffuse axonal injuries, in which axons tear as the brain jostles against the skull. These injuries are associated with closed head injury and rarely cause outward signs of trauma. However, generalized swelling and increased intracranial pressure may occur inside the skull.

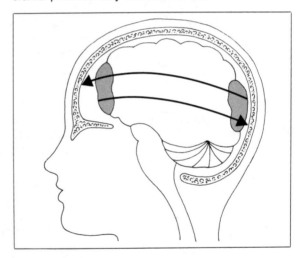

Add that head trauma can cause diabetes insipidus and syndrome of inappropriate antidiuretic hormone (SIADH). Point out that these complications affect the entire body by disrupting fluid and electrolyte balances.

For patients who need prolonged convalescence, review common complications of immobility: contractures, pressure sores, pneumonia, and atelectasis.

Describe the diagnostic workup

Prepare the patient for several phases of tests—first to evaluate his injury and later to measure his recovery. Baseline studies may include X-rays of the skull and cervical spine, computed tomography (CT), and possibly, magnetic resonance imaging (MRI) and evoked potential studies. Explain that these tests help determine the extent of the patient's injury. Mention that neuropsychological testing may be ordered once his condition stabilizes.

Skull and cervical spine X-rays

Tell the patient (or his caregivers) that this test detects skull fractures and vertebral displacement in the cervical spine. X-ray studies may also detect or monitor increased ICP, brain infections, and bleeding.

Explain that a technician will take X-ray films of the skull and cervical spine from various angles. Reassure the patient (if responsive) that the procedure, which takes 15 to 30 minutes, causes no pain. If he's wearing dentures, jewelry, or metal objects, he'll have to remove them to prevent distorting the images.

Inform the patient that he'll lie on a table, and a technician will change his position several times to obtain different views of his head (see *Preparing for routine skull X-rays*). Instruct him to remain still to avoid blurring the X-ray images. Also explain that a head board, foam pads, or sandbags may be used to immobilize or steady his head and make him more comfortable.

CT scan

Inform the patient that CT uses X-rays and a computer to scan the brain for structural damage, edema, and lesions such as hematomas. Reassure him that the test causes no pain, but he may feel chilled because the equipment must be kept cool. Tell him that the test may take from 30 to 60 minutes. If the doctor has ordered an infusion of contrast medium to enhance the images, instruct the patient not to eat or drink anything for 2 hours before the test.

Teach the patient that during the test a technician will position him on an X-ray table and secure him with a strap to ensure that accidental movement won't blur the test results. Then the table will slide into the scanner's circular opening. If appropriate, tell him that the I.V. infusion of contrast medium takes about 5 minutes and that he may experience a sensation of warmth, which should subside. Instruct him to tell the technician immediately if he has any discomfort or symptoms of hypersensitivity, such as itching or hives. Mention that the technician can see and hear him from an adjacent room. Tell him that he'll hear noises from the scanner and may notice the machine revolving around him.

Magnetic resonance imaging

Inform the patient that MRI produces a detailed and clear image of the brain's soft tissue, its blood supply, and fluid spaces, making MRI more useful than a CT scan in detecting diffuse axonal and brainstem injuries. Because he'll be exposed to a strong magnetic field, caution the patient to report any metal objects in his body, such as a pacemaker or a hip prosthesis.

Explain that he'll lie on a small table that will move into a cylindrical chamber. Reassure him that the test causes no pain and that it usually takes between 30 and 40 minutes. Prepare him, however, for close quarters and for possible claustrophobic feelings. Inform him that his head may be taped or strapped in position to help him lie still. Stress that lying still prevents blurring the images. Also describe the loud noises that the machine will make as the equipment rotates around him.

Preparing for routine skull X-rays

The idea of having skull X-rays may make your patient anxious. To help dispel his anxiety, describe what happens during this routine test. Show him how the technician will position his head to obtain several images as follows:

Right lateral and left lateral positions

Tell the patient that he'll lie with his right and then his left cheek parallel to the X-ray film. His fist or a folded towel will support his chin. The sagittal plane is parallel to the tabletop and the film, so the X-ray results will show both halves of the mandible directly superimposed.

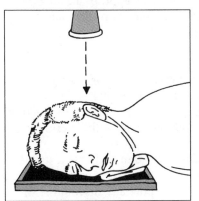

Posteroanterior (Caldwell) position

Explain that the patient will lie facedown with his fist or a folded towel supporting his chin and his forehead and nose touching the X-ray film. The sagittal plane and the canthomeatal line are perpendicular to the tabletop and the film. The X-ray beam will be angled 15 degrees toward the patient's feet.

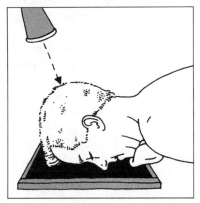

Anteroposterior (Towne's) position

Inform the patient that he'll lie on his back with his chin flexed toward his neck. With the canthomeatal line perpendicular to the tabletop and the film, the X-ray beam will be angled 30 degrees toward the patient's feet.

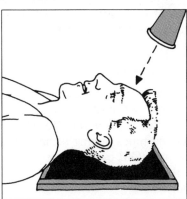

Axial (base) position

Tell the patient that he'll lie prone with his chin fully extended. Further explain that his head will be positioned so that his profile will be perpendicular and the canthomeatal line will be parallel to the tabletop and the X-ray film.

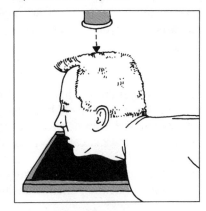

Evoked potential studies

Tell the patient that these studies may further pinpoint his injury to provide an early prognosis. Explain that these tests measure the nervous system's electrical response to visual, auditory, or sensory stimuli.

Reassure him that the tests cause no pain and may take about 1 hour. Inform him that his hair will be washed 1 or 2 days before the test. Then during the tests he'll be positioned on a bed, a table, or a reclining chair. Emphasize the need to lie still. Tell him that a technician will cleanse his scalp and apply paste and electrodes to his head and neck. Prepare him for the noises from the test equipment.

Explain that he'll be asked to perform various activities, such as gazing at a checkerboard pattern or a strobe light or listening through headphones to a series of clicks. Or he may have electrodes placed on an arm and leg and be asked to respond to a tapping sensation. Mention that the technician will remove the electrodes and paste after the tests. Then, as appropriate, the patient can resume his usual activities. Reassure him that shampooing will remove any residual paste.

Neuropsychological testing

Once the patient begins recovering, prepare him for neuropsychological testing to evaluate cognitive function. Explain that these tests may determine whether his head injury impaired his thinking ability. Emphasize that they have nothing to do with determining sanity.

Explain that he'll take a battery of written and oral tests lasting for several hours. Forewarn him that these tests may produce fatigue and frustration. Instruct him to report any discomfort to the test administrator because fatigue and frustration can alter the test results. A short rest period is usually all that's needed before testing can continue. Mention that the doctor will explain the test results.

Teach about treatments

Discuss the treatment plan with the patient and his family or caregivers. Instruct them about physical rehabilitation, dietary measures, and drug regimens. If necessary, prepare the patient for cranial surgery or for such procedures as ICP monitoring or barbiturate coma. Review other care measures to help compensate for neurologic deficits.

Activity

Inform the patient (or his caregiver) that his activity level will depend on his condition. If he's unstable and seriously impaired, his activities may be limited to turning and range-of-motion (ROM) exercises. Show his caregiver turning and repositioning techniques and passive ROM exercises. Explain that ROM exercises help to prevent muscle atrophy and provide the brain with important information about the patient's position.

If the patient's paralyzed, teach his caregiver how to position him to maintain proper body alignment and prevent musculoskeletal problems. If the patient's allowed out of bed, prepare him for some initial discomfort. Reassure him that physical activity will help him sleep better and prevent pulmonary complications. Explain that head trauma can interfere with the brain's sleep-control center. Physical activity will make him tired, helping to induce normal sleep.

When the patient can sit in a chair or ambulate, show the family proper transfer and ambulation techniques. Stress the importance of proper body mechanics to prevent patient falls and injury to the caregiver. If the doctor orders physical therapy, reinforce the program's principles and instructions. Motivate the patient to work hard in physical therapy, reminding him that his efforts will pay off in increasing strength and motor control.

Diet
Point out that head injury induces a hypermetabolic state that depletes the body's store of glycogen and protein. Inform the patient and his family that this condition can induce muscle wasting because the muscles are used as an energy source. Instruct the patient to eat high-calorie, protein-rich meals. Reinforce the dietitian's instructions.

Advise the patient to sit upright and tilt his head slightly forward when eating. If he has dysphagia or facial weakness on one side, recommend that he eat semisoft foods and chew on the unaffected side of his mouth. Suggest preparing solid foods in a blender and freezing liquids to a slush or mixing them with other foods. If appropriate, teach him how to use feeding aids, such as utensils with built-up handles. Also offer him and his caregivers a copy of the patient-teaching aid *Making eating easier,* pages 143 and 144.

If the patient has severe head trauma, he may be unable to eat. Explain to the family that nutrition will be provided intravenously by total parenteral nutrition or by tube feeding through a nasogastric or gastrostomy tube. If any of these feeding methods will continue at home, instruct the caregivers on their use.

The patient with high ICP may have to restrict his fluid intake. Teach him (or his caregiver) how to measure and record how much fluid he takes in and how much he eliminates. Provide a copy of the patient-teaching aid *How to measure fluid intake and output,* page 302.

Medication
If the patient's condition is critical, teach his family about drugs he'll take to control his symptoms and prevent complications. Explain that he may receive high doses of a corticosteroid, such as dexamethasone, to reduce brain swelling. If he experiences increasing ICP, his doctor may order an osmotic diuretic, such as mannitol. Explain that this I.V. medication helps to reduce ICP by moving fluid out of the cells and into the vascular system where it can be eliminated as urine.

For the patient with a moderate-to-severe head injury, discuss anticonvulsants, if ordered. Explain that a common anticonvulsant, such as phenytoin, may prevent seizures. Also discuss how head trauma can reduce the brain's seizure threshold, causing potentially serious complications. Then offer a copy of the patient-teaching aid *Learning about phenytoin*, page 187.

Procedures

If appropriate, teach the patient and family about ICP monitoring to detect early signs of this potentially dangerous complication. If he requires barbiturate coma to treat increased ICP, prepare him for this procedure.

ICP monitoring. Tell the patient and family that this procedure measures the pressure exerted by brain tissue, blood, and cerebrospinal fluid against the skull. Explain that monitoring can detect small increases in ICP before clinical danger signs develop.

Discuss which of the three types of monitoring he'll undergo. In *ventricular catheter monitoring,* he'll have a small polyethylene catheter inserted into the lateral ventricle. In *subarachnoid screw monitoring,* he'll have an ICP screw and transducer wick introduced into the subarachnoid space. In *epidural sensor monitoring*—the least invasive method—he'll have a fiber-optic sensor placed in the epidural space. In all three procedures, pressure readings appear on a display monitor or chart recorder.

Clarify measures the doctor may order to reduce increasing ICP, typically medication adjustments or decreased fluid intake. Or he may attach a catheter to the monitoring device to drain excess cerebrospinal fluid, thereby decreasing pressure.

Barbiturate coma. If the patient has a sustained increase in ICP that can't be corrected by conventional treatments, the doctor may order a barbiturate coma. If the patient's deteriorating condition limits communication with him, inform his family that the procedure reduces the patient's metabolic rate and cerebral blood flow, which helps to relieve increased ICP.

Tell the family that the patient will receive a loading dose of a barbiturate, then a continuous I.V. infusion of the drug. Warn them that he'll be unresponsive once the coma's induced. Prepare them for observable—and, to them, quite disturbing—changes in the patient's status resulting from decreased respiration, hypotension, and loss of muscle tone during therapy. Reassure them that this procedure includes careful monitoring and necessary supportive care. Inform them that the doctor will discontinue this therapy as soon as appropriate.

Surgery

Prepare the patient for cranial surgery, if necessary. Explain that a craniotomy involves creating a surgical incision in the skull. This exposes the brain for many possible treatments. For instance, it may be done to repair a depressed or comminuted skull fracture, evacuate a hematoma, remove bony fragments, or repair a tear in the dura mater. Alternatively, the neurosurgeon may drill a burr hole in the patient's skull. Using this technique, he can aspirate an epidural hematoma with a fluid clot.

Review preoperative procedures. Tell the patient that his hair will be washed with an antimicrobial shampoo the night before surgery. In the operating room, his head will be shaved and he'll be given a general anesthetic.

For a *craniotomy,* explain that the surgeon will make an incision in the patient's scalp, then open the skull over the damaged area. The opening may range from a small hole, which eventually will fill in with new bone, to a larger open flap, which may later be replaced with a metal plate. If the surgeon plans to drill a *burr hole,* mention that new bone growth will gradually fill the hole.

Prepare the patient for postoperative recovery. Tell him that he'll awaken from surgery with his head bandaged to protect the incision or burr hole. Mention that the head of his bed will be elevated if he's had a supratentorial craniotomy or a burr hole drilled. If he's had an infratentorial craniotomy, tell him that he'll lie flat in bed, although he can turn from side to side. Warn him to avoid coughing, which may increase ICP. Reassure him that he'll receive medication to relieve his headache after surgery. After the doctor removes the bandages, inform the patient that he'll wear a special cap. Tell the craniotomy patient that the doctor will remove the sutures within 7 days.

Other care measures
Involve both the patient and his family in supporting the patient's recovery. Before discharging a patient with a concussion, make sure he has a responsible adult accompanying him. List symptoms that call for medical attention, and review whom to call if his condition worsens. Also, give the patient's caregiver a copy of the teaching aid *Caring for a patient after a concussion,* page 188.

If the patient has a serious head injury resulting in permanent neurologic deficits, prepare him and his family for a lengthy recovery. Help them to cope by explaining proposed rehabilitation programs. (See *Recovering from head injury: A family affair,* pages 184 and 185.)

Coping with speech and visual deficits. If the patient has a speech deficit, assist him to communicate in other ways, such as writing or using a picture board. Instruct the family to speak slowly to him in normal tones. Recommend that they use gestures to clarify their message if he has receptive aphasia. Advise them to give the patient short, simple directions, cues, and lists.

If the patient has a vision deficit, show him how to scan his environment. Teach family members how to approach him to avoid startling him. For example, if he's lost peripheral vision, advise family members to approach him from the front, not the side. Demonstrate how they can set up his meal trays and living environment for optimal visualization.

Managing cognitive deficits. Explain that cognitive deficits may become more evident as the patient spends more time at

184 Head injuries

Recovering from head injury: A family affair

Don't overlook the most valued players on your patient's rehabilitation team—his family, friends, and other caregivers. To promote recovery, the patient and his supporters need to work closely together and with the hospital staff. Ideally, you'll share rehabilitation objectives to ensure a consistent approach to care.

Teach the patient and his family what to expect during each recovery stage, and discuss how to modify care accordingly. This chart, adapted from the Ranchos Los Amigos Scale of Cognitive Levels, provides a framework for your teaching. Remind the patient and his family that not all patients go through every rehabilitation stage. Nor do they progress at the same pace. Tell them to continue to focus on realistic expectations for recovery.

REHABILITATION STAGE	PATIENT BEHAVIOR	TEACHING POINTS
I	No response to stimuli.	• Inform the family that the patient needs skilled care to monitor his body functions and prevent complications. • Update the family on the patient's status, and explain the purpose of procedures. • Reinforce and clarify, as needed, the doctor's explanation of the injury. • Encourage family caregivers to talk to and try to stimulate the patient even when he doesn't respond. • Advise them to refresh themselves by spending some time away from the patient's bedside.
II	Nonpurposeful and inconsistent response to stimuli. This may include posturing and reflex responses, such as opening the eyes, wandering eye movements, facial grimacing, and arm and leg movements.	• Reassure the family that the patient's responses are a small sign of improvement. Explain, however, that he's not yet aware of himself or his surroundings. • Instruct the family to inform you if they notice new signs of patient awareness. • Ask them to anticipate possible causes of patient discomfort and to call them to your attention. • If the patient's condition is stable, show family caregivers how to bathe and turn him. Also show them how to perform passive range-of-motion exercises.
III	Localized and purposeful response to stimuli, including inconsistent ability to follow commands. Mostly, patient responds to immediate physical needs or discomfort—exhibiting, for example, restlessness from a full bladder.	• Show the family how to stimulate the patient's senses during a given task. For example, tell them to try rousing him with his favorite scent, photographs, or music. • Instruct them to eliminate background distraction, such as television or radio, when working with the patient. • Encourage them to meet their own needs for rest and diet once the patient's condition stabilizes.
IV	Confused and bizarre behavior, resulting from impaired information processing. The patient has a short attention span and short-term memory loss. He's dependent on others for his care, and he's unable to learn new tasks or perform previously learned ones. His safety is a major concern.	• Teach the family to simplify the patient's environment to prevent sensory overload. Instruct them to limit periods of concentrated effort to 5 to 10 minutes. • Advise them to speak to the patient in quiet tones and keep instructions simple and brief. • Prepare them for aggressive outbursts, acting out, uninhibited behavior, and confusion. • Help them to recognize how the patient's agitation relates to his stress level. • Instruct them to check for physical discomfort as a cause of agitation and inappropriate behavior. • Discuss safety measures to prevent accidents. • Encourage family and friends to plan quiet, restful periods for themselves and the patient. This will relieve their fatigue and frustration. Encourage them to take occasional breaks.

continued

Recovering from head injury: A family affair — *continued*

REHABILITATION STAGE	PATIENT BEHAVIOR	TEACHING POINTS
V	Easily distracted, but with direction and assistance, can perform simple, previously learned tasks. However, the patient's performance deteriorates without supervision or with more difficult tasks.	• Explain that the patient will continue to be agitated. However, he should be encouraged to participate in simple self-care tasks. • Emphasize the need for supervised psychomotor activities, such as walking or using a rocking chair, to help the patient release and channel his pent-up energy. • Advise family caregivers to use restraints prudently because they may increase his agitation. • Tell them to give the patient plenty of time to participate in an activity. Show them how to give him directions by breaking down a task into simple steps. • Suggest using distraction to divert the patient's attention from agitating situations.
VI	Completes simple, previously learned tasks without assistance, but still needs supervision. The patient's thought processes are less concrete; he's aware of memory problems. His awareness may leave him feeling frustrated or depressed.	• Explain that the patient is still confused, so the family should continue to simplify his environment and supervise tasks. • Advise them to help him build up his memory cues. For example, suggest showing him a photograph of himself to help him remember his name. Other cues may include schedules and calendars. • Tell them to encourage his independence and initiative within the limits set by the nursing staff.
VII	Starts and completes tasks and routines. Consistently oriented, the patient's more aware of himself and others. However, he lacks sound judgment and insight, he can't solve problems well, and his safety is still a concern.	• Tell the family to encourage the patient to complete tasks without supervision. • Advise them to let him initiate previously learned tasks. • Tell them to supervise the introduction of new tasks. New tasks should be added one at a time to reduce patient stress.
VIII	Capable of learning new tasks. The patient is more responsible for himself. He's also more aware of his deficits. He finds new situations stressful, performing best within a routine.	• Encourage the family to let the patient be responsible for all his personal care. Explain that he needs to practice these skills in the safety of the hospital environment. • Stress that the patient needs to be as self-sufficient as possible. • Tell the family to encourage the patient to socialize and show awareness of others. • Advise them to meet with the rehabilitation team to help the patient plan goals and activities after discharge. • Help them accept permanent neurologic deficits, if necessary. Discuss vocational planning, rehabilitative training, and continued speech and physical therapy, as indicated. • Review safety in the home.

home. Reassure the patient and his family, though, that cognitive deficits don't constitute an emergency although they may hinder the patient's ability to work and his social behavior. Help the family appreciate that the patient isn't being lazy or manipulative; rather, he isn't capable yet of performing in any other way.

Warn the family that the patient may overestimate his abilities, claiming that he can perform tasks (for example, drive a car) that in fact he cannot. Discuss ways to monitor the patient's abili-

Reviewing cognitive deficits

After recovering from head injury, the patient may look fine to his family and friends, but he may not act like his old self. That's because a serious head injury can cause cognitive deficits—intangible symptoms, such as memory lapses or poor concentration, that initially may baffle those around him.

Teach the family to recognize and accept such symptoms as:
• short-term memory loss—the patient can't remember a conversation he had an hour earlier
• diminished learning ability—he can't learn new work skills, even less complex ones than he performed previously
• difficulty concentrating—he leaves many projects unfinished
• language misuse—he names items and people incorrectly
• confusion and inability to act—he's easily overwhelmed and becomes immobilized in a complex environment or in situations that require decisions
• egocentricity—he's preoccupied with his own feelings and needs and less aware of others' needs
• mood swings—he's happy one minute and depressed the next without obvious cause
• diminished insight—he doesn't recognize the implications of his words and actions
• lack of initiative and motivation—he falters at starting or completing projects without urging and supervison from others
• increased fatigue.

ties without frustrating his efforts toward independence. Suggest allowing the patient to try most activities—short of those that could injure him or others or could cause excessive frustration or fatigue. Make sure to forewarn the patient and his family or other caregivers that he may be emotionally labile, crying or laughing at seemingly inappropriate times. Explain that he can't control these reactions. For more information, see *Reviewing cognitive deficits*.

Using mechanical assistance. If the patient needs a walker or a cane, reinforce his efforts to use these devices safely, and give him a copy of the appropriate patient-teaching aids, pages 145 to 154. For safety's sake, recommend installing grab bars near the toilet and bathtub, removing throw rugs, and securing carpets. Also, if he has sensory losses, suggest lowering the water heater's temperature to prevent burns.

If the patient's injury impairs his cough reflex, show his caregivers how to perform oral suction. Inform them that this will make the patient more comfortable and will help keep him from gagging on his own secretions.

If the patient experiences hypertonic movements after head trauma, discuss any splints and serial casts that may help him maintain a functional position.

Source of information and support

The National Head Injury Foundation
333 Turnpike Road, Southborough, Mass. 01772
(508) 485-9950

Further readings

Davidson, L. "The Forgotten Injury: Head Injury," *Nursing Times* 85(4):31-32, December 25-31, 1989.
Eames, P. "Behavior Disorders After Severe Head Injury: Their Nature and Causes and Strategies for Management," *Journal of Head Trauma and Rehabilitation* 3(3):1-6, September 1988.
Gordon, V.L. "Recovery from a Head Injury: A Family Process," *Pediatric Nursing* 15(2):131-33, March-April 1989.
Hannegan, L. "Transient Cognitive Changes After Craniotomy," *Journal of Neuroscience Nursing* 21(3):165-70, June 1989.
Kozak, G.S. and Ira, H. "A Comparison of Teaching Methods for ED Discharge Instruction After Head Injury," *Journal of Emergency Nursing* 15(1):18-22, January-February 1989.
Lee, S. "Intracranial Pressure Changes During Positioning of Patients with Severe Head Injury," *Heart and Lung* 18(4):411-14, July 1989.
Reimer, M. "Head-Injured Patients: How to Detect Early Signs of Trouble," *Nursing89* 19(3):34-42, March 1989.
Sbordone, R.J. "Assessment and Treatment of Cognitive-Communicative Impairments in the Closed-Head-Injury Patient: A Neurobehavioral Approach," *Journal of Head Trauma and Rehabilitation* (2):55-62, June 1988.

Learning about phenytoin

Dear Patient:

The medication that the doctor prescribed for you is called phenytoin. (The label may say Dilantin or Diphenylan). This medicine can help to prevent seizures.

How to take this medicine
● Take phenytoin exactly as the doctor directs. If you're taking one daily dose, take it at the same time every day. If you're taking several daily doses, take a missed dose as soon as you remember, but don't double the dose without checking with the doctor.
● If you're taking liquid medicine, shake it well. Then measure your dose in a standard measuring spoon — not a household teaspoon.

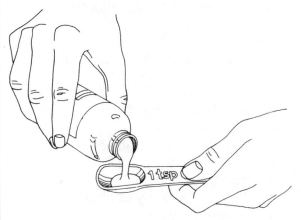

● If you're taking a chewable medicine, chew or crush the tablet thoroughly.
● Take this drug with meals or milk to prevent stomach upset.
● Avoid activities that require alertness until you know how you react to this drug. It may make you feel drowsy.
● Also avoid alcohol, which reduces phenytoin's effectiveness.

When to call the doctor
Call the doctor right away if any of these problems develop: blurred vision, dizziness, confusion, headache, jerky eye movements, sluggishness, rash, unsteadiness, twitching, and unusual bleeding or bruising.

Also call him if you lose weight inexplicably, notice a loss of taste or appetite, feel sick to your stomach, vomit, or become constipated.

Special instructions
● Take good care of your gums and teeth. And see your dentist regularly because phenytoin may promote gum overgrowth.
● Use one brand of medicine consistently. Don't switch from brand to brand. And don't abruptly stop taking this drug without your doctor's advice. Observing these precautions is important to prevent seizures.

Reminders
● Keep appointments with your doctor for follow-up exams and for blood tests. This is a way to make sure you're getting the right amount of the drug.
● Carry medical identification stating that you take phenytoin. Be sure to tell your other doctors, including your dentist, that you're taking it too.

PATIENT-TEACHING AID

Caring for a patient after a concussion

Dear Caregiver:

Although a concussion isn't a serious brain injury, it can temporarily disrupt normal activities.

Your patient can continue recovering at home—as long as you watch him for the next 24 hours and call for medical help if necessary.

Here are some guidelines:

Observe the patient
Set an alarm clock to wake the patient every 2 hours during his first night home. Ask him his name. Ask him where he is. Ask whether he can identify you. If he won't wake up or if he can't answer your questions, take him to the hospital right away.

Review medical instructions
Help the patient follow the instructions given by the nurse for the first 48 hours after discharge. Tell him to:
• take it easy and return gradually to his usual activities.
• avoid medicine stronger than acetaminophen (Tylenol) for a headache. Avoid aspirin. It can intensify any bleeding caused by the accident.
• try relieving a headache by lying down but raising the head slightly with pillows.
• eat lightly, especially if nausea or vomiting occurs. (Occasional vomiting isn't unusual, but it should subside in a few days.)

Call for medical help
Call the doctor or return to the hospital at once if the patient experiences:

• increasing irritability or personality changes
• increasing sluggishness
• confusion
• convulsions
• persistent or severe headache, unrelieved by acetaminophen
• forceful or constant vomiting
• blurred vision
• abnormal eye movements
• staggering gait.

Recognize delayed symptoms
Although the patient may feel fine in a few days, new symptoms may emerge later. Called postconcussion syndrome, these symptoms may occur up to a year after the injury.

Tell him to to watch for:
• headache that gets worse with emotional stress or physical activity
• lack of usual energy
• occasional double vision
• dizziness, giddiness, or light-headedness
• memory loss
• emotional changes (feeling irritable or easily upset, especially in crowds)
• feelings of tension and nervousness
• difficulty concentrating
• reduced sex drive
• easy intoxication by alcohol
• loss of inhibitions
• difficulty relating to others
• noise intolerance.

These symptoms should subside. If they get worse or last longer than 3 months, urge the patient to seek medical advice.

Trigeminal neuralgia

More common in women than in men, trigeminal neuralgia causes paroxysmal attacks of facial pain after stimulation of a trigger zone. The pain may become so intense that it disrupts your patient's life-style, causing complications ranging from weight loss to social isolation. To help the patient cope with the disorder, you'll need to identify the stimuli that set off her attacks, and then teach her how to avoid them.

First, though, you'll need to prepare the patient for the diagnostic workup, which may include skull radiography, computed tomography (CT), and magnetic resonance imaging (MRI). You'll also need to provide instructions about various pain relief measures, such as medications. If she reports particularly severe symptoms, you'll need to clarify any proposed procedures to destroy trigeminal nerve fibers.

Discuss the disorder

Inform the patient that trigeminal neuralgia usually affects the branches of the fifth cranial (trigeminal) nerve. Explain that this nerve controls chewing movements and sensations of the face, scalp, teeth, and mouth. Mention that most experts think these painful attacks result from a blood vessel compressing a nerve at the brain's base. Occasionally, trigeminal neuralgia results from a demyelinating disorder, such as multiple sclerosis, or from a viral infection.

Point out that attacks follow stimulation of a trigger zone—an especially sensitive facial area. Then, together with the patient, try to identify the stimuli that may set off attacks, such as a light touch, a draft of air, exposure to heat or cold, eating, smiling, talking, or drinking a hot or cold beverage. Explain that the particular stimuli that trigger her attacks indicate which nerve branch of the trigeminal nerve is involved. For example, attacks that follow eating or talking indicate mandibular branch involvement. Those that follow a light touch or temperature changes point to maxillary or ophthalmic branch involvement. (For more information, see *Mapping the trigeminal nerve,* page 190.)

Discuss the disorder's sporadic nature. Explain that the frequency of attacks varies from many times daily to several times monthly. Between attacks, most patients have no pain, although remissions remain unpredictable in frequency and duration. Mention that the disorder occurs mostly in people over age 40 and affects the right side of the face more often than the left.

Julie Tackenberg, RN, MSN, CNRN, who wrote this chapter, is a clinical specialist at the University Medical Center in Tucson, Ariz.

CHECKLIST

Teaching topics in trigeminal neuralgia

☐ Explanation of the disorder
☐ Trigger factors that precipitate sudden attacks of facial pain
☐ Distribution of the trigeminal nerve and symptoms associated with each branch
☐ Preparation for skull radiography, computed tomography, and magnetic resonance imaging
☐ Activity and dietary modifications to prevent attacks
☐ Medications and their administration
☐ Procedures to provide permanent pain relief
☐ Oral hygiene and other self-care measures

Mapping the trigeminal nerve

In trigeminal neuralgia, the exact location of facial pain depends on which trigeminal nerve branch is involved. With three branches—the ophthalmic, the maxillary, and the mandibular—the trigeminal nerve can distribute pain across several facial areas.

Identify for the patient which nerve branch produces pain. Then, use a simple illustration or model to map the nerve's course and the area innervated (see the illustration). This may help the patient visualize where pain travels within a trigger zone.

Pain around the eyes
The *ophthalmic branch* carries sensory fibers to the skin on the forehead, upper eyelids, and parts of the scalp and nose. It also innervates the eyeballs, the cornea, and the mucosa of the frontal and nasal sinuses.

Pain around the temples
The *maxillary branch* carries sensory fibers to the skin on the temples, lower eyelids, upper cheeks and lip, and part of the nose. It also innervates the gums, the molar and premolar canine teeth, and the mucosa of the mouth, nose, and maxillary sinus.

Pain around the cheeks and chin
The *mandibular branch,* the largest of the three, carries both sensory and motor fibers. The motor fibers control the muscles involved in chewing. The sensory fibers innervate the skin on the cheeks, chin, lower jaw, lower teeth and gums, the oral mucosa, and part of the ear.

TRIGEMINAL NERVE

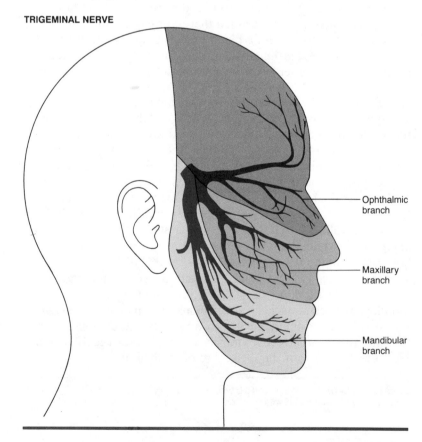

Ophthalmic branch

Maxillary branch

Mandibular branch

Complications

During attacks, your patient may be so overwhelmed by pain that she neglects to comply completely with therapy. Emphasize that failure to take prescribed medications or to follow other treatment measures may cause continued pain leading to secondary complications, such as extreme weight loss, depression, and social isolation. If she's neglecting regular oral hygiene and dental care to avoid triggering an attack, caution her about risking tooth decay and mouth infection. If she's not eating, warn her about excessive weight loss and malnutrition.

Describe the diagnostic workup

Tell the patient that her pain history forms the basis for diagnosing trigeminal neuralgia because the disorder produces no objective clinical or pathologic changes. Explain, however, that she may undergo various tests to rule out other disorders that cause similar pain (see *Recognizing conditions that cause facial pain,* pages 192 and 193).

Prepare her for skull radiography, intracranial CT, or MRI. Explain that these tests will scan the base of her skull, where the trigeminal nerve emerges from the brain stem. Tell her that the images may also show whether other processes (a tumor or demyelination, for example) may be causing pain. Reassure her that these noninvasive tests should cause no discomfort and require only that she lie quietly for awhile.

Skull radiography

Explain that this test involves taking several X-ray images of the head from various angles. Reassure the patient that this painless procedure takes about 15 minutes. Before the test, ask her to remove any dentures, eyeglasses, jewelry, and metal objects so they won't obscure the X-ray image.

Tell the patient that during the test she'll be positioned on the X-ray table or seated in a chair. Remind her to lie or sit still while the technician takes the X-rays. Mention that a headband, foam pads, or sandbags may be used to steady her head to produce an unblurred image.

Intracranial CT

Inform the patient that this test produces a series of cross-sectional images of the brain. Reassure her that a CT scan causes no pain and takes from 15 to 30 minutes. If the doctor orders a contrast medium to enhance the images, instruct the patient not to eat or drink for 4 hours before the test. Ask her if she's ever experienced an allergic reaction to shellfish or to iodine or other contrast media. If the study doesn't use a contrast medium, tell her not to restrict food and fluids.

Inform the patient that she'll lie on her back on an X-ray table with her head gently steadied by straps. Reassure her that her face will remain uncovered. The head of the table will move into the scanner, which will rotate around her head and make clicking sounds.

If the doctor injects a contrast medium, tell the patient that two sets of X-rays will be taken, one before and one after the in-

Recognizing conditions that cause facial pain

When you discuss trigeminal neuralgia, inform the patient that various conditions (both neurologic and nonneurologic) can cause extreme facial pain. Ask the patient to describe the pain. For example, on which side of the face does the pain occur? How long does the pain last? What symptoms accompany the pain? Compare the patient's description with the information below to supplement your assessment.

CONDITION	SEX	PAIN PATTERN	CHARACTERISTICS
Trigeminal neuralgia 	Affects more women than men	Unilateral	• Jabbing, shocklike bursts of pain, interposed with pain-free periods • Intermittent, with 30-second refractory periods between attacks • Usually affects patients between ages 45 and 60
Cardiac pain 	Affects more men than women	Usually unilateral (left side more often than right)	• Aching, tingling, or burning in the lower third of the face or angle of the mandible • Burning sensation in throat • Acute onset
Cluster headache 	Affects more men than women	Unilateral	• Intermittent, intense penetrating pain lasting 5 minutes to several hours, accompanied by increased lacrimation, facial flushing, and swelling • Pain episodes occur in clusters, with remissions lasting days to years
Dental pain 	Affects both sexes equally	Unilateral to bilateral	• Constant, aching pain that may be diffuse or well defined • Soft-tissue swelling may accompany pain • Usually acute onset
Paranasal sinus pain 	Affects both sexes equally	Unilateral to bilateral	• Dull, constant throbbing pain, possibly accompanied by fever and vertigo • Positional change, such as lowering head, may increase pain • Acute onset

continued

Recognizing conditions that cause facial pain — *continued*

CONDITION	SEX	PAIN PATTERN	CHARACTERISTICS
Temporal arteritis	Affects more men than women	Unilateral to bilateral	• Constant throbbing or aching over blood vessels • Pain accompanied by swelling, redness, and warmth • Usually occurs between ages 50 and 60
Temporomandibular joint syndrome	Affects more women than men	Unilateral to bilateral	• Pain and stiffness with jaw movement • Pain increases during the day with jaw movement, such as talking and eating • Insidious, chronic onset

jection. Instruct her to notify the technician immediately if she feels a burning sensation at the injection site.

Magnetic resonance imaging

Tell the patient that MRI produces cross-sectional images of the brain without using ionizing radiation or injected contrast agents. Instead, MRI relies on a strong magnetic field to produce images. By showing the soft tissues in detail, MRI can help to diagnose or rule out nerve fiber demyelination as the cause of painful attacks. Discuss who will perform the test and where. Stress that although MRI causes no pain, the test may take up to 90 minutes.

Explain that the patient will be positioned on a narrow bed and slid into a large cylinder that houses the MRI magnets. Because the strong magnetic field can damage watches and other jewelry, and because these objects can produce distorted images, ask her to remove all metal objects before the test. Also tell her to report any metal objects in her body, such as a hip prosthesis, pins, bullet fragments, a pacemaker, or aneurysm clips. Stress that lying still promotes an unblurred image. Tell her she'll hear a loud knocking noise while the machine runs. Suggest that she ask for earplugs if the noise bothers her. Mention that she can resume her usual activities after the test.

Teach about treatments

Keep two objectives in mind as you teach the patient about treatments: preventing a neuralgia attack and implementing pain relief measures to minimize complications. Discuss ways to modify diet and activities to avoid stimulating trigger zones. At the same time, point out how adequate nutrition and regular physical activity may help her cope with pain. Then discuss analgesics and, possibly, procedures to destroy trigeminal nerve fibers.

Activity
Show the patient how to modify activities that cause her pain. For example, demonstrate how she can minimize facial movement by supporting her jaw with her hand while she talks. Encourage her to stay as active as possible, which will improve her sense of well-being and help her cope with pain.

Diet
If the patient fails to eat and loses weight because of pain, discuss her diet and food preferences. Help her select foods that are high in calories and nutrients so that she can get more nourishment with less chewing. Suggest that she eat many frequent, small meals instead of three large ones. Add that small meals may help to eliminate nausea, which can accompany certain medications. To minimize jaw movements during chewing, suggest that she puree or finely mince foods and eat soft or liquid foods, such as soups, custards, and stews.

Medication
Inform the patient that drug therapy may temporarily relieve or prevent pain, but it can't offer a cure. Her medication regimen may include carbamazepine, phenytoin, or narcotic analgesics.

Carbamazepine. If your patient's taking carbamazepine, explain how to increase the dose for effective pain relief. Also give her a copy of the patient-teaching aid *Learning about carbamazepine,* page 196, for future reference.

Phenytoin. If the patient's taking phenytoin (Dilantin), tell her that this drug may reduce neuralgia attacks by decreasing inflammation around the trigeminal nerve. Advise her to report such adverse reactions as double vision, loss of coordination, rash, slurred speech, and yellowish skin or mucous membranes. To minimize GI upset, suggest that she take the drug with food or milk. If the drug makes her drowsy, caution her to avoid activities (such as driving) that require physical and mental alertness. Remind her to check with her doctor before taking phenytoin with any other prescription or nonprescription drugs.

Narcotic analgesics. In some instances, the patient may receive narcotic analgesics temporarily to relieve pain until a therapeutic level of the primary treatment drug is reached. Advise her to ask for such an analgesic before her pain becomes too severe. Mention that a narcotic drug will make her feel sleepy. Because she may also experience constipation, suggest that she take a stool softener, if ordered. Also explain that she may need to do deep-breathing and coughing exercises to keep her lungs clear.

Procedures
Explain neurosurgical procedures that may provide relief if drug therapy fails or neuralgia attacks increase or become more severe. Tell the patient about radiofrequency gangliosis. This simple and most commonly performed procedure relieves pain by partially

destroying the trigeminal nerve root. Prepare her for an overnight hospital stay. Inform her that she'll receive a local anesthetic for the 30- to 90-minute procedure. Explain that a needle will be placed into her cheek and inserted into the affected part of the trigeminal nerve. Then a small portion of the nerve will be destroyed with heat. Although the procedure causes few complications, advise the patient to discuss its risks and benefits carefully with her doctor.

In a variation on this procedure, trigeminal nerve fibers are destroyed with extreme cold. Tell the patient that a needle will be inserted through her cheek and into the nerve. Then a chemical that produces intense cold will be injected into the trigeminal branch that carries sensory fibers. Mention that she'll receive a local anesthetic for this procedure, which causes few complications.

Surgery

If the patient has severe symptoms, her doctor may suggest brain surgery to relieve pressure around the trigeminal nerve root. Tell her that this major surgery is performed only after extensive presurgical evaluation. Explain that the surgery frees the nerve from arteries that may be wrapped around it, thus eliminating the pain source. Tell her the surgery takes 4 to 5 hours. Although more successful than less invasive techniques, the surgery may cause serious complications—among them, infection.

Counsel the patient on the importance of careful decision making. Advise her to review her options with her doctor and to ask about potential complications, such as facial numbness or paralysis.

Other care measures

Tell the patient how to ward off neuralgia attacks. For instance, she can protect her trigger zones from such stimuli as wind or temperature changes by wearing a scarf or turning up her coat collar. Because many patients neglect oral hygiene if jaw movement triggers pain, discuss ways other than brushing to promote dental health. For example, suggest she use a water-powered dental device to stimulate gums and teeth, yet reduce jaw movement.

Further readings

Burchiel, K.J., et al. "Long-term Efficacy of Microvascular Decompression in Trigeminal Neuralgia," *Journal of Neurosurgery* 69(1):35-38, July 1988.

Goodkin, R. "Trigeminal Neuralgia: Helping Patients to Understand Treatment Options," *Consultant* 27(2):51-53, 56, 59, February 1987.

Headley, B. "Historical Perspective of Causalgia: Management of Sympathetically Maintained Pain," *Physical Therapy* 67(9):1370-74, September 1987.

Loeser, J.D., and McLean, W.T. "When the Complaint Is Facial Pain," *Patient Care* 22(7):75-78, 79-81, 84+, April 15, 1988.

Weinberg, A.D. "The Etiology, Evaluation and Treatment of Head and Facial Pain in the Elderly," *Journal of Pain Symptom Management* 3(1):29-38, Winter 1988.

PATIENT-TEACHING AID

Learning about carbamazepine

Dear Patient:

Your doctor has prescribed carbamazepine to help relieve your facial pain. Read over the information below to help you get the greatest benefit from this medication.

Follow instructions exactly

Take carbamazepine exactly as your doctor directs you. This will lower your chances of having unwanted side effects. Don't take more of it—and don't take it more often—than your doctor directs.

Report side effects

Call your doctor if you notice any unusual bleeding, bruising, or abdominal pain. Also call him if you have dark-colored urine, fever, chills, a sore throat or mouth ulcers, a rash, unusual mood changes, or a loss of coordination.

Watch what you eat and drink

Avoid spicy or acidic foods while you're taking this drug. They may upset your stomach. Also avoid alcoholic beverages, but do drink lots of other fluids.

Be cautious about other drugs

Talk to your doctor or pharmacist before you take any other prescription or over-the-counter medications. Other medications may interact with carbamazepine, causing unwanted side effects or changing effectiveness.

Special instructions

• Remember, carbamazepine is not an ordinary pain reliever. Use it only as your doctor prescribes. Don't take it for any other pains.
• Avoid driving if this medication makes you feel drowsy or dizzy or if you have blurred vision. And don't operate machinery or take part in activities that require alertness.
• Some people who take carbamazepine become more sensitive to sunlight. Until you know how you'll react, wear a sunscreen and sunglasses outdoors. Avoid both too much sun and sunlamps.
• If you feel nauseated, try taking your medication with meals.
• Don't stop taking carbamazepine without checking first with your doctor.
• Keep all appointments with your doctor so he can check your progress.
   You may need certain tests to see if you're getting the right amount of carbamazepine or if the medication is causing certain side effects without your knowing it.

A few reminders

• Store your medication in a cool, dry place (not the bathroom medicine chest) because heat and humidity may cause it to break down.
• Let no one else take your medication. It's intended only for you.
• Discard your medication on its expiration date unless your doctor tells you otherwise.

Immune and Hematologic Conditions

Contents

Anaphylaxis

A severe allergic reaction, anaphylaxis can be a life-threatening emergency, causing acute respiratory failure and vascular collapse. Even a milder reaction can understandably trigger panic.

Typically, you'll be teaching a patient who has already had anaphylaxis or one who is at risk. To help your patient guard against complications, you'll need to teach him to respond quickly to the earliest signs of anaphylaxis. You'll demonstrate how to use the supplies in an emergency anaphylaxis kit. And above all, you'll discuss how to prevent further reactions by avoiding exposure to known antigens, such as insect stings or certain foods. You'll also encourage him to carry medical identification naming his allergy. This will alert caregivers to his condition should he be unconscious or otherwise unable to speak.

Discuss the disorder
Begin by explaining that anaphylaxis is a severe allergic reaction that occurs after second or subsequent exposures to an antigen. Tell the patient that the first exposure produces no symptoms but causes his body to recognize the foreignness of the antigen and to create antibodies against it. At some subsequent exposure, his body will undergo a major allergic—or anaphylactic—reaction, potentially much more serious than the watery eyes or itchy nose commonly associated with allergies.

Point out the signs and symptoms that signal an anaphylactic reaction. Usually, initial indications include vague feelings of uneasiness and anxiety, headache, dizziness, numbness, or disorientation. Skin signs and symptoms usually begin with generalized itching followed by redness and, possibly, wheals or hives. Initially, the patient's skin feels clammy, but as redness and swelling develop, he's likely to feel warm and uncomfortable. Swelling may affect his eyelids, lips, tongue, palms, and soles. Explain that he may feel as though he has a lump in his throat or have trouble breathing. He also may experience hoarseness, coughing, sneezing, and wheezing.

Mention that most reactions occur within 30 minutes after exposure. Less typically, they can occur within seconds or up to an hour after exposure. Point out that the greater the sensitivity to the antigen, the more rapid and severe the reaction. For more information, see *What happens in anaphylaxis*, page 200.

Review common antigens and the routes through which they enter the body. Explain, for example, that an antigen may be inhaled, ingested, or injected. Mention that people who react to one

Patricia L. Carroll, RN,C, MS, CEN, RRT, who wrote this chapter, is the owner of Educational Medical Consultants in Middletown, Conn., and staff nurse, emergency department, Manchester Memorial Hospital, Manchester, Conn.

CHECKLIST

Teaching topics in anaphylaxis

☐ Explanation of anaphylaxis and its signs and symptoms
☐ Common causes of anaphylaxis
☐ Complications, including respiratory failure and cardiovascular collapse
☐ Skin testing and elimination diet to identify allergens
☐ Importance of immediate treatment after exposure
☐ How to use an anaphylaxis kit
☐ How to apply a tourniquet
☐ Avoiding known antigens
☐ Using a medical identification service
☐ Sources of information and support

What happens in anaphylaxis

Inform the patient that the severity of anaphylaxis depends on the allergen's entry route, the amount and speed of allergen absorption, and his degree of hypersensitivity. Usually, a sensitized person notices warning signs—for example, a hivelike reaction at the site of a bee sting—before experiencing severe systemic symptoms.

Explain that the most severe anaphylactic responses typically occur within minutes of exposure to the offending antigen. The victim may experience chest tightness or sense impending doom—possibly without preceding symptoms.

Or generalized skin signs—diffuse erythema, flushing, urticaria, and periorbital and mouth angio-

edema—may precede rapidly progressive respiratory distress (triggered by laryngeal edema and bronchospasm). For instance, the posterior pharynx, vocal cords, and uvula swell to obstruct the airway. Meanwhile, auscultation of the lungs reveals diffuse wheezes and prolonged expirations. Hypotension and other signs of shock may follow—although such signs sometimes occur first.

Changes in level of consciousness usually parallel respiratory effects: initial alertness gives way to decreased responsiveness as the patient's arterial oxygen (PaO$_2$) level or cerebral perfusion declines.

Review the following graphic representation of anaphylaxis with your patient.

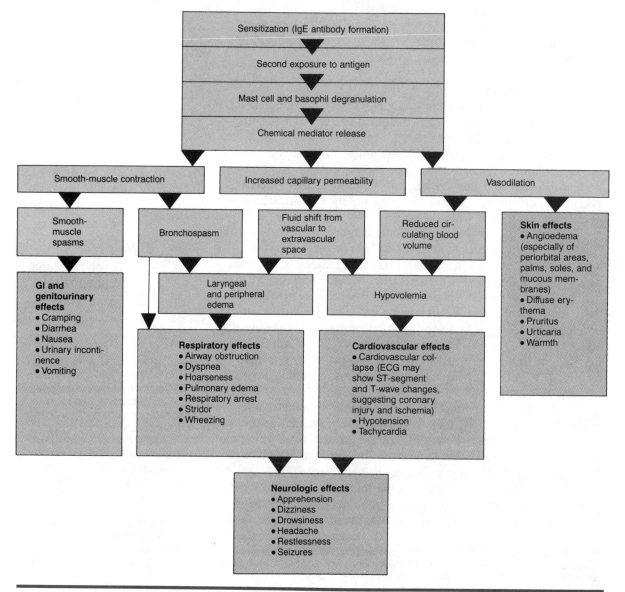

antigen are more likely to react to similar or other substances (for more information, see *Avoiding common antigens*).

Complications
Stress that prompt treatment of the earliest symptoms may prevent potentially fatal complications. Warn the patient that an unchecked reaction can lead to respiratory failure or cardiovascular collapse. Total airway obstruction, caused by swollen upper airway structures, remains the most common cause of death from anaphylaxis. Severe, prolonged bronchospasm also may cause respiratory failure. Cardiovascular failure may result if chemical mediators released during anaphylaxis cause capillary leakage. Then fluids leave the blood vessels and enter the tissues, and the blood volume drops, causing hypotension, shock, and cardiac arrest.

Describe the diagnostic workup
Explain that no test can diagnose anaphylaxis (although certain tests can identify antigens). Instead, the doctor bases diagnosis on the patient's signs, symptoms, and health history. Advise the patient to give a thorough accounting of previous reactions and potential exposures. Tests that may be done to evaluate his condition during an attack include blood studies, an ECG, and chest X-rays.

If appropriate, teach the patient about skin testing and an elimination diet, which may be ordered to screen for sensitivity to various antigens. Reassure him that his reaction to possible antigens will be monitored. Explain that the most common positive reaction is a raised, red, itchy area where his skin was exposed to the antigen.

Skin testing
Inform the patient that some sensitivities and antigens may be obvious without testing. For example, if hives and breathing problems occur after he plays with a kitten, he can conclude that cat dander triggers his reaction. In other situations, however, skin testing may be necessary to identify the offending substance.

Intradermal skin testing. Tell the patient that the doctor will inject antigens into the patient's skin at spaced intervals on his forearm or interscapular area. At the same time, the doctor will inject a control substance (which should cause no reaction). After 15 to 30 minutes, he'll inspect the injection sites for wheals and surrounding erythema—a positive reaction. Intradermal testing detects allergies to pollen, feathers, animal dander, and dust.

Scratch testing. Describe this alternative to intradermal testing. First, the doctor cleans areas of the patient's skin with alcohol. When the skin dries, the doctor will use an instrument to make a superficial scratch (about 1 to 4 mm long) on the patient's skin. Then he'll apply an extract containing the test antigen. After waiting 30 minutes, he'll check for erythema at the site.

Patch testing. If the doctor suspects allergies to fibers, detergents, perfumes, or cosmetics, patch testing may be in order. He'll saturate a 1″ × 1″ gauze pad with the suspected antigen and tape the square to the patient's skin. After 48 hours, he'll remove the patch, inspect the skin, and grade the response. A + signifies

Avoiding common antigens

Review common antigens with your patient, and discuss how he can avoid those that may trigger an anaphylactic response. If he has a severe reaction to one antigen, warn him that he'll react to it in all forms and by all routes. For example, if a penicillin tablet triggers an anaphylactic response, so will a penicillin injection. If peanuts produce an anaphylactic response, so will peanut butter. Review the following list of the most common antigens to help your patient compose his own list of antigens to avoid.

Food
- beans, including soybean products
- chocolate
- eggs
- fruit, especially strawberries and citrus fruits
- milk
- nuts and seeds
- seafood, especially shellfish

Drugs
- analgesics, such as aspirin and indomethacin
- antibiotic agents, especially penicillin and its derivatives
- diuretics
- insulin and other hormones
- iodine-based radiographic contrast media
- serum proteins, such as gamma globulin
- vaccines

Other antigens
- animal dander
- bites and stings from insects (such as ants, bees, hornets, and wasps), jellyfish, snakes, and spiders
- grass and ragweed pollens
- mold spores
- tartrazine (yellow dye #5), used to color foods and drugs

erythema only; + + indicates erythema and papules; + + + indicates erythema, papules, and vesicles; + + + + signifies erythema, papules, vesicles, and bullae or ulceration.

Elimination diet
Tell the patient that this procedure helps identify food allergies. First he'll keep a record of everything he eats for at least a week. Next, he'll remove potentially antigenic foods, such as eggs, milk, and wheat, from his diet. Once his symptoms subside, he'll reintroduce these foods—one at a time—to his diet. A reaction after he consumes this food—occurring either immediately or over time—identifies the offending substance.

Teach about treatments
Anaphylaxis is always an emergency. Instruct the patient to minimize activity during a reaction. Show him how to use the medications and tourniquet in an anaphylaxis kit. Finally, discuss ways to avoid exposure to the antigens that cause anaphylaxis.

Activity
Caution the patient not to move around if he's been exposed to an antigen that could cause anaphylaxis. For example, if he's allergic to bee stings, advise him to sit down and minimize all activity if he's stung. Explain that physical activity stimulates blood flow, which can hasten the anaphylactic response.

Diet
Advise the patient with a food allergy to avoid the offending food in any form. Urge him to read labels to avoid antigens, for example, nuts or dyes, hidden in food. Remind him to ask about ingredients, especially when eating away from home. Advise children to check with an adult about ingredients of new or unfamiliar foods.

Medication
Demonstrate how to use an emergency kit to treat anaphylaxis. Give the patient the teaching aid *How to use an anaphylaxis kit,* pages 204 and 205. Explain that the kit contains alcohol swabs, a tourniquet, a syringe, and two medicines: epinephrine and an antihistamine.

Epinephrine. This injectable drug, also known as Adrenalin, counteracts anaphylaxis by raising blood pressure and dilating breathing passages. It also inhibits histamine release and offsets the effects of circulating histamine. Alert the patient to possible blurred vision, excitability, eye irritation, headache, hypertension, light-headedness, nausea, restlessness, sweating, or vomiting.

Chlorpheniramine maleate. Also known as Chlo-Amine and Chlor-Trimeton, this antihistamine helps control symptoms associated with anaphylaxis. Advise the patient to contact the doctor if he experiences blurred vision after taking this drug. Add that he may experience constipation, dry mouth and throat, or impaired motor function. Inform him that antihistamines may cause drowsiness, so caution him to avoid activities that require physical or mental alertness.

Other care measures

Remind the patient that a prompt response after exposure to the offending antigen can save his life. If the doctor wants him to use an emergency kit, tell him to follow its instructions as soon as he's exposed to the antigen. If his condition doesn't improve within 10 minutes, he should call an ambulance for immediate transport to the hospital. If he lives far from an emergency department, tell him to call the ambulance before starting the self-treatment.

If the patient's allergic to insect stings, offer him a copy of the teaching aid *Insect stings: How to avoid them,* page 206. If an insect should sting him, however, instruct him to apply ice packs to the site, if possible. Tell him not to place the ice directly on his skin. Instead, he should wrap the ice in a cloth and then apply it to the affected area. Explain that ice will decrease blood flow around the sting and slow his reaction to the antigen.

If he's allergic to a medication, remind him to tell his doctor or other caregivers before drugs are prescribed or administered. Point out that if he's allergic to one drug, he's probably sensitive to all drugs in the same family. Tell him to speak up about drug allergies if he's having diagnostic tests that require use of contrast media. Also suggest he wear medical identification, such as a Medic Alert bracelet or necklace, to alert caregivers in emergency situations when he may be unable to communicate (for more information, see *The Medic Alert service*).

Sources of information and support

American Allergy Association
P.O. Box 7273, Menlo Park, Calif. 94026
(415) 322-1663

Asthma and Allergy Foundation of America
1717 Massachusetts Avenue, Suite 305, Washington, D.C. 20036
(202) 265-0265

Further readings

"Anaphylaxis from Lubricant Jelly," *Nurses Drug Alert* 13(3):24, March 1989.
Cason, D. "Anaphylactic Shock," *Journal of Emergency Medical Services* 14(2):42-46, 51-52, February 1989.
"Cinoxacin-Induced Anaphylaxis," *Nurses Drug Alert* 13(2):15-16, February 1989.
"Clinical Presentation of Anaphylaxis," *Hospital Medicine* 23(9):182, September 1987.
Dickerson, M. "Anaphylaxis and Anaphylactic Shock," *Critical Care Nursing Quarterly* 11(1):68-74, June 1988.
Hammond, E. "Anaphylactic Reactions to Chemotherapeutic Agents," *Journal of the Association of Pediatric Oncology* 5(3):16-19, 1988.
Murdock, R.T., et al. "Hymenoptera Stings: A Warm-Weather Hazard," *Physician Assistant* 12(8):65-66, 68, 73+, August 1988.
Segal, M. "Anaphylaxis: An Allergic Reaction That Can Kill," *FDA Consumer* 23(4):21-23, May 1989.
Steinberg, P. "Anaphylaxis Avoidance: 22 Commonsense Ways to Prevent the (Largely) Preventable," *Consultant* 29(8):52-53, 57-58, August 1989.
Vanselow, N.A. "Minutes to Counter Anaphylaxis," *Emergency Medicine* 20(15):121-23, September 15, 1989.

The Medic Alert service

After your patient recovers from anaphylaxis, tell him about Medic Alert. In an emergency, this nonprofit, 24-hour medical identification service alerts caregivers to a subscriber's special medical needs.

How the service works
A patient wears a Medic Alert necklace or bracelet to identify a special health condition — for example, allergies.

The engraved emblem (available in stainless steel, silver, or gold) contains the patient's personal identification number, and Medic Alert's 24-hour hot line number.

By calling the hot line and identifying the patient by his identification number, the caregiver has access to crucial medical information.

The service also records the names and phone numbers of the doctor and persons to contact in a crisis.

Who needs medical identification?
Patients with:
• allergies to drugs, venoms, or other substances
• conditions, such as diabetes, heart disease, or asthma
• medication regimens, such as insulin for diabetes
• devices, such as contact lenses or a pacemaker
• special instructions (organ donation, for example).

How to obtain medical identification
Your patient can obtain more information by writing or calling Medic Alert
Turlock, Calif. 95381-1009
(800) ID-ALERT

How to use an anaphylaxis kit

Dear Patient:

Because you could have a severe reaction from insect stings or other substances, your doctor has prescribed an anaphylaxis kit for you to use in an emergency. The kit contains everything you need to treat an allergic reaction:
- a prefilled syringe containing 2 doses of epinephrine
- alcohol swabs
- a tourniquet
- antihistamine tablets.

If an insect stings you, use the kit as follows. Also, notify the doctor immediately, or ask someone else to call him.

Getting ready

1 Take the prefilled syringe from the kit and remove the needle cap. Hold the syringe with the needle pointing up. Then push in the plunger until it stops. This will expel any air from the syringe.

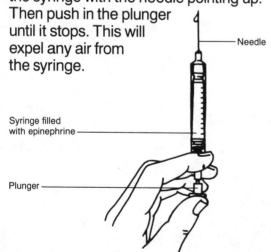

Needle

Syringe filled with epinephrine

Plunger

2 Next, clean about 4 inches of the skin on your arm or thigh with an alcohol swab. (If you're right-handed, clean your left arm or thigh. If you're left-handed, clean your right arm or thigh.)

Inject the epinephrine

Rotate the plunger one quarter turn to the right so it's aligned with the slot. Insert the entire needle—like a dart—into the skin.

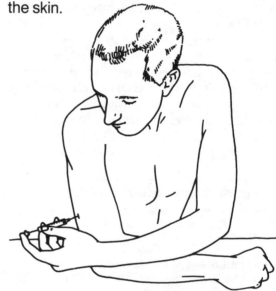

Push down on the plunger until it stops. It will inject 0.3 ml of the drug for an adult or a person over age 12. Withdraw the needle.

Note: The dose and administration for babies and for children under age 12 must be directed by the doctor.

Remove the stinger (if you can)

Quickly remove the insect's stinger if you can see it. Use a dull object, such as a fingernail or tweezers, to pull it straight out. Don't pinch, scrape, or squeeze the stinger. This may push it

continued

How to use an anaphylaxis kit — *continued*

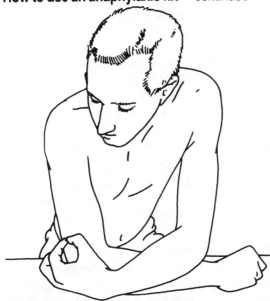

farther into the skin and release more poison. If you can't remove the stinger quickly, stop trying. Go on to the next step.

Apply the tourniquet

If you were stung on your *neck, face,* or *body,* skip this step and go on to the next one.

If you were stung on an *arm* or *leg,* apply the tourniquet between the sting site and your heart. Tighten the tourniquet by pulling the string.

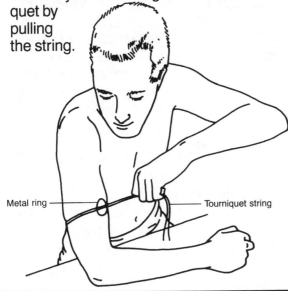

Metal ring ———————— Tourniquet string

After 10 minutes, release the tourniquet by pulling on the metal ring.

Take the antihistamine tablets

Chew and swallow the antihistamine tablets. (For children age 12 and under, follow the dose and administration directions supplied by your doctor or provided in the kit.)

What to do next

Next, apply ice packs — if available — to the affected area. Avoid exertion, keep warm, and see a doctor or go to a hospital immediately.

Important: If you don't notice an improvement within 10 minutes, give a second injection by following the directions with your anaphylaxis kit. If your syringe has a preset second dose, don't depress the plunger until you're ready to give the second injection. Proceed as before, following the instructions to inject the epinephrine.

Special instructions

● Keep your kit handy to ensure emergency treatment at all times.
● Ask your pharmacist for storage guidelines. Find out whether the kit can be stored in a car's glove compartment or whether you need to keep it in a cooler place.
● Periodically check the epinephrine in the preloaded syringe. Pinkish brown solution needs to be replaced.
● Make a note of the kit's expiration date. Then renew the kit just before that date.
● Dispose of used needle and syringe safely and properly.

Insect stings: How to avoid them

Dear Patient:

Because you're allergic to insect stings, you need to take special precautions when you spend time outdoors. By following the guidelines below, you may be able to prevent an insect sting.

Protect yourself
• Cover up. Wear long sleeves, slacks, shoes, and socks when you hike in open fields or wooded areas.
• Don't walk barefoot (don't even wear sandals). Lots of stinging insects live in underground burrows hidden by grass.
• Wear smooth fabrics in low-intensity colors—greens, tans, and whites, for instance. Floral hues attract insects.
• Avoid scented toiletries. Soaps, perfumes, after-shave, hair sprays, deodorants—and even some sunscreens—attract stinging insects.
• Inspect the borders of your windows, doors, shutters, and eaves for insect hives or nests. Then have them removed. *Don't* try to remove them yourself.
• Consider giving up lawn mowing, gardening, and other yard work.

Get to know the enemy
Of course you can't spend your life indoors, so learning about the traits and habitats of stinging insects can help you avoid them. In general, steer clear of hedges, flower gardens, wildflower fields, and picnic grounds. Here are some traits of common pests:

• With a fat, fuzzy, black and yellow body, the *bumblebee* flies slowly and buzzes loudly. If you don't hear a bumblebee, you're likely to see one hovering about alfalfa, clover, and vivid flowers.
• The *honeybee* has a tan and black body and a smooth abdomen. Usually, this insect won't harm you unless you sit or step on it.
• *Yellow jackets, hornets,* and *wasps* are more aggressive than the honeybee. In fact, the yellow jacket will sting without provocation. Yellow and black, this insect commonly feeds on rotting fruit in orchards and garbage sites. It lives under sod and rocks and behind siding on barns or other dwellings.

Like the yellow jacket, the hornet has yellow (or white) and black markings. Unlike the yellow jacket, however, the hornet lives high above ground suspended in a lantern-shaped nest.

Black with white, red, or yellow specks, the wasp has a narrow waist, a long abdomen, and almost no fuzz. Its nest looks like a honeycomb.
• The bright red *imported fire ant* lives in loose dirt mounds. Once disturbed, fire ants may swarm, stinging an unwitting victim over and over and causing severe reactions and, possibly, death.

Act immediately
Seek immediate medical attention should you be stung despite the precautions you take. Or if your doctor has provided an emergency treatment kit, follow the instructions. Then get medical help right away.

Aplastic anemia

Because aplastic anemia can lead to life-threatening complications, your teaching will emphasize the need for compliance with prescribed treatment. However, the disorder's early clinical features are vague, so your initial teaching will involve preparing the patient for the diagnostic workup, including blood studies and a bone marrow biopsy. After diagnosis, you'll help him understand the pathophysiology of this disorder. Describe the three major blood cell types—red blood cells (RBCs), white blood cells (WBCs), and platelets—and explain the function of each. Then encourage compliance with supportive treatment: restricting activity, maintaining a proper diet, taking prescribed medications, and avoiding infection. As appropriate, prepare the patient for a splenectomy or a bone marrow transplant. Throughout your teaching, underscore the importance of remaining alert for developing complications, such as infection, bleeding, and worsening anemia.

Discuss the disorder

Inform the patient that aplastic anemia results when the bone marrow fails to produce or suppresses all three blood cell lines: RBCs, WBCs, and platelets (for more information, see *Understanding bone marrow's role,* page 208). Explain that RBCs carry oxygen from the lungs to the rest of the body, WBCs fight infection, and platelets initiate clotting to stanch bleeding.

Tell the patient that signs and symptoms relate directly to blood cell shortages. For example, too few RBCs cause anemia and subsequent weakness, fatigue, and shortness of breath on exertion. A deficiency of WBCs (leukopenia) may result in fever, malaise, and areas of red, swollen, tender skin. Specific shortages of such WBCs as basophils, eosinophils, and especially neutrophils (neutropenia) significantly increase the patient's risk for infection. Thrombocytopenia, a platelet deficiency, commonly results in bruising, superficial bleeding, and petechiae. A deficiency in all of these blood cells (pancytopenia) results in aplastic anemia.

Aplastic anemia usually begins with nonspecific symptoms, such as fatigue, headache, pallor, and shortness of breath. As it progresses, severe—even life-threatening—infection, congestive heart failure, or hemorrhage may occur. The disorder's rate of progression and severity are unpredictable and related to the degree of bone marrow damage.

Scott L. C. Baker, RN, BSN, who wrote this chapter, is a clinical nurse specializing in bone marrow transplantation at Johns Hopkins Hospital in Baltimore.

CHECKLIST

Teaching topics in aplastic anemia

☐ The roles of bone marrow, red and white blood cells, and platelets in aplastic anemia
☐ Complications, such as organ damage, serious infection, and massive bleeding
☐ Diagnostic studies, including blood tests and bone marrow aspiration and biopsy
☐ Activity restrictions and dietary guidelines
☐ Drug therapy, including androgens, corticosteroids, immunosuppressants, and experimental drugs, such as colony-stimulating factors
☐ Blood transfusions
☐ Surgery, such as splenectomy and bone marrow transplantation
☐ Preventing infection with isolation, hand washing, and other personal hygiene practices
☐ Preventing injury and reducing stress
☐ Sources of information and support

Understanding bone marrow's role

Review bone marrow function with your patient. Explain that marrow is soft connective tissue found mostly in the cavities of long bones, such as the femur, humerus, and sternum. Inform him that marrow, which comes in two types (red and yellow), produces the body's blood cells.

Red marrow, which is found mostly in the cancellous (spongy) tissue at the epiphyses, produces red blood cells, white blood cells, and platelets. Yellow marrow, which replaces red marrow as the patient ages, is mostly inactive connective tissue. It lies in the cancellous tissue at the epiphyses and in a canal that runs centrally through the bone.

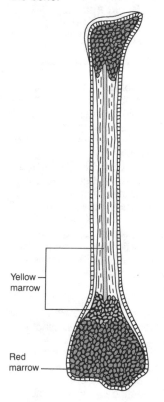

Yellow marrow

Red marrow

Explain that aplastic anemia may be congenital or acquired (for more information, see *What causes aplastic anemia?*).

Complications
Point out that untreated aplastic anemia can result in life-threatening complications. Inform the patient that a decreased number of RBCs reduces the amount of oxygen available to major organs, possibly leading to confusion, angina, myocardial infarction, and renal damage. Also point out that a deficiency of WBCs will increase his susceptibility to bacterial, viral, or fungal infections. Finally, explain that a reduction in platelets can precipitate massive bleeding, leading to organ damage or hemorrhagic shock.

Describe the diagnostic workup
Tell the patient that blood studies will help to differentiate aplastic anemia from other blood abnormalities, such as leukemia. Add that a bone marrow biopsy is used to confirm the diagnosis.

Blood studies
The doctor will order a complete blood count—including an RBC count, total hemoglobin and hematocrit values, RBC indices, WBC count, and WBC differential count—and a platelet count. Inform the patient that repeated blood studies will be used to monitor the course of his illness and to measure his response to treatment. The frequency of these tests will range from daily to monthly, depending on the severity of the illness and the treatment regimen. Tell him that blood test results usually are available within a few hours.

Bone marrow biopsy
This microscopic examination of a bone marrow sample allows the doctor to evaluate the bone marrow's production of RBCs, WBCs, and platelets. Forewarn the patient that he may experience some discomfort from the biopsy procedure, but reassure him that local anesthesia will minimize his pain. The test usually takes about 10 to 20 minutes. Additional bone marrow biopsies may be required later to monitor treatment effectiveness. Offer the patient more detailed information with the teaching aid *Preparing for bone marrow aspiration and biopsy,* page 213.

Teach about treatments
Inform the patient that treatment will help to prevent complications and make him more comfortable. However, it won't cure the disorder. Also explain that even if the cause of aplastic anemia is successfully treated, recovery may take months.

Tell the patient that his treatment regimen will depend on the disorder's severity and may include drug therapy, blood transfusions, activity restrictions, and a nutritious diet. Occasionally, spontaneous remission occurs with supportive care; more commonly, the disorder progresses, and the doctor recommends bone marrow transplantation or splenectomy.

Activity

To maintain cardiovascular health, encourage the patient to engage in regular, moderate exercise, such as walking. Remind him to avoid contact sports and other traumatic activities. Advise him to pace his daily activities to conserve his energy and avoid shortness of breath.

Diet

Because bone marrow requires iron and B vitamins to produce blood cells, advise the patient to maintain a diet rich in these nutrients to help boost the number of circulating blood cells. As for food preparation, direct the patient to cook meats thoroughly, to keep perishable food refrigerated, and to discard food (especially dairy products) still on hand after the expiration date. Following these precautions may help him to avoid infections, such as food poisoning from salmonella.

Medication

Tell the patient that aplastic anemia may respond to several medications—for example androgens, corticosteroids, and immunosuppressants. Explain that the doctor may order androgens and corticosteroids to stimulate bone marrow function. The medications may be taken orally (daily) or I.M. (weekly). Emphasize that 2 to 3 months may pass before the patient notices improvement.

Inform the patient that the doctor may prescribe immunosuppressants (given I.V.) in severe anemia for patients not considered suitable candidates for bone marrow transplantation. Combined with supportive therapy, immunosuppressants may induce partial or complete hematologic remission.

As needed, the patient may receive supportive drug therapy, such as antibiotics to control infection or acetaminophen to control fever.

Warn the patient to avoid taking aspirin, aspirin-containing products, and certain nonsteroidal anti-inflammatory drugs, such as ibuprofen. Explain that these agents may decrease platelet aggregation and cause GI irritation, thereby increasing his risk for bleeding. For safety's sake, urge him to read all nonprescription drug labels carefully.

Androgens. Tell the patient that androgens—for example, fluoxymesterone (Halotestin), oxymetholone (Anadrol), and nandrolone decanoate (Deca-Durabolin)—are forms of male hormones. Therefore, female patients taking androgens may experience a change in voice or menstrual irregularities. Effects of androgens in male patients may include enlarged breasts, frequent or persistent erections, or shrunken testicles. Both sexes may experience headache, nausea and vomiting, swollen arms and legs caused by fluid retention, and weight gain.

What causes aplastic anemia?

If your patient is the 1 person in 200,000 affected by aplastic anemia, tell him that in about one-half of all cases, the cause is unknown. In the rest, the cause may be drugs, industrial chemicals, a virus, a congenital abnormality (for example, Fanconi's syndrome), or environmental factors, such as radiation.

Temporary aplastic anemia can follow treatment with chemotherapeutic agents, such as adriamycin, cyclophosphamide (Cytoxan), cytosine arabinoside (ARA-C), and nitrogen mustard. Scan the list below for a sampling of causes.

Drugs
- acetazolamide
- carbamazepine
- chloramphenicol
- cimetidine
- diphenylhydantoin
- gold compounds
- mephenytoin
- metazolamide
- methsuximide
- oxyphenbutazone
- phenylbutazone
- quinacrine
- sulfonamides
- trimethadione

Industrial chemicals and toxins
- benzene
- chlordane
- chlorophenothane
- hexachlorocyclohexane
- lindane
- trinitrotoluene

Viral agents
- Epstein-Barr virus
- hepatitis A, B, and C antigens
- infectious mononucleosis

Miscellaneous
- paroxysmal nocturnal hemoglobinuria
- pregnancy
- radiation exposure

Direct the patient to report any of these changes to the doctor, who may adjust the dosage. Advise him that he'll need regular blood tests (to detect imbalances such as hypercalcemia) while he's receiving androgen therapy.

Corticosteroids. Teach the patient about corticosteroids, such as prednisone (Deltasone, Meticorten, Sterapred). Warn him that the drug's effects include acne, euphoria, and a puffy face. Advise him to report any of these signs, as well as any other adverse reactions to this drug. Emphasize that he must never abruptly stop taking the medication after he starts therapy; corticosteroids must be discontinued gradually to avoid serious complications. Mention that he'll need regular blood pressure monitoring (to detect hypertension) and blood studies (to detect hyperglycemia) during therapy.

Immunosuppressants. Antilymphocyte globulin and lymphocyte immune globulin (Atgam) are examples of immunosuppressant drugs used in aplastic anemia. Tell the patient that he'll be hospitalized for I.V. administration of these medications for up to 10 days. Warn him that adverse reactions to therapy may include serum sickness (chills, fever, flushing, and malaise). Reassure him, however, that simultaneous treatment with a steroid drug—prednisone, for example—will minimize his discomfort. Advise him that he may also receive acetaminophen (Tylenol)—not aspirin—to control fever. Emphasize that his response to immunosuppressive therapy won't be immediate, so he'll require supportive care during and after treatment.

Experimental drugs. Explain that if standard drug therapy fails, the doctor may suggest medications to stimulate blood cell production. Widely available through research centers, these medications known as colony-stimulating factors include granulocyte colony-stimulating factors (G-CSF), granulocyte-monocyte colony-stimulating factors (GM-CSF), monocyte colony-stimulating factors (M-CSF), interleukin 1 (IL-1), and interleukin 3 (IL-3). The patient may receive these medications I.V., I.M., or S.C. (researchers are still determining the most effective dosage and administration method).

Tell the patient that he'll probably enter the hospital during treatment. He'll have frequent blood tests and bone marrow biopsies. Warn him that common adverse reactions to colony-stimulating factors include anorexia, bone pain, chills, diarrhea, fever, headache, malaise, myalgias, nausea, and vomiting. Less common reactions include dysrhythmias with ischemia, hepatic dysfunction, peripheral edema, pruritus, rash, and shortness of breath.

Procedures

When aplastic anemia causes disability or life-threatening bleeding, the doctor will probably order blood transfusions. Explain that RBC and platelet transfusions may relieve some symptoms temporarily. If indicated, give the patient a copy of the teaching aid *Learning about blood transfusions,* pages 214 and 215. Also see *Questions patients ask about treating aplastic anemia.*

Surgery

A splenectomy may be recommended if the doctor suspects that the spleen is destroying normal RBCs and platelets. Lying behind and to the left of the stomach, the spleen normally filters old, damaged, and abnormal blood cells from the circulation. Removing the spleen allows older, still-functioning blood cells to survive longer, which increases the number of circulating cells. After a splenectomy, other lymphatic tissue takes on the task of removing dead blood cells but does so at a slower rate.

Bone marrow transplantation is the treatment of choice for severe aplastic anemia. The ideal patient is under age 40 and free from sensitization by excessive blood transfusions. He requires a donor, usually a sibling, who is human leukocyte antigen matched. Explain that tissue typing and matching require a blood sample from both the patient and the potential donor. Once a match is found, the doctor will collect healthy bone marrow from the donor's iliac crest in the operating room. The marrow cells will then be purified and diluted with heparin. Next, the new bone marrow will be infused into the patient through a special catheter that has been placed under his collarbone (Hickman catheter). For more information, give the patient the teaching aid *Learning about bone marrow transplantation,* page 216.

Cover general preoperative and postoperative procedures, and advise the patient that he'll be hospitalized for 2 to 3 months. Clarify the risk of graft rejection, graft-versus-host disease (GVHD), and serious infection. Point out that he'll undergo long-term follow-up and treatment with oral immunosuppressants to control GVHD and ensure long-term survival.

Other care measures

Inform the patient with a low WBC count that he may require isolation to prevent infection. If he's in the hospital, this may encompass special airflow rooms, protective isolation techniques, or simply hand washing. Recommendations vary because of controversy over the mechanism of infection acquisition. If he requires only protective isolation, he should expect visitors to wear masks in addition to washing their hands thoroughly.

If the patient is caring for himself at home, stress the importance of following strict personal hygiene practices and minimizing exposure to infection. Teach him to take his temperature two to three times daily. Instruct him to report signs of infection, including chills, fever, and red, swollen, tender areas on his skin. Also advise him to report any severe anemia symptoms, such as headache, ringing in the ears, and light-headedness. Urge him to report any chest pain at once or to go to the nearest emergency room.

INQUIRY

Questions patients ask about treating aplastic anemia

Why do I need so many red blood cell and platelet transfusions?
Transfusions help to replenish the blood cells that your bone marrow fails to produce or suppresses. Blood cells are living cells with a limited life span. Red blood cells usually live for 120 days, whereas platelets live only for 8 to 10 days. Normally, bone marrow produces replacements for the cells that die.

Why can't I have a transfusion of white blood cells?
White blood cells have a short life span. They don't survive long enough to be helpful when given by transfusion.

Why can't I just take antibiotics to prevent infections?
Taking antibiotics to prevent an infection may encourage the growth of resistant strains of bacteria. Remember, infections sometimes come from germs existing in your own body. Preventive treatment with antibiotics will kill this "normal flora" and encourage the growth of bacteria resistant to treatment. You're safer practicing standard hygiene (such as washing your hands before eating) and avoiding crowds and people that you know are sick.

Because of the blood's decreased ability to clot, caution the patient to avoid injury—for example, by using an electric razor and by avoiding sharp instruments or tools. Urge him to be especially careful when trimming his nails. Remind him to inspect his surroundings for safety. Then suggest that he clear hallways of clutter, install lights on stairways, discard slippery throw rugs or doormats, and install grab bars in the bathroom.

Finally, because of the intensity of aplastic anemia treatments, offer emotional support to the patient and his family. Encourage the patient to practice stress-reduction and relaxation techniques, such as deep breathing, guided imagery, and biofeedback.

Sources of information and support

Aplastic Anemia Foundation of America
P.O. Box 22689, Baltimore, Md. 21203
(301) 955-2803

National Marrow Donor Program
100 South Robert Street, St. Paul, Minn. 55107
(612) 291-4612

Further readings

Alkire, K., and Collingwood, J. "Physiology of Blood and Bone Marrow," *Seminars in Oncology Nursing* 6(2):99-108, May 1990.

Anderson, K., and Braine, H. "Specialized Cell Component Therapy," *Seminars in Oncology Nursing* 6(2):140-49, May 1990.

Bonato, J. "Blood Transfusions: Are They Safe?" *Critical Care Nurse* 9(7):40-42, 44, 46, July-August 1989.

Flynn, J.C. "Perioperative Autotransfusion: Avoiding Donated Risks," *Today's OR Nurse* 12(7):20-23, July 1990.

Ford, R., and Eisenberg, S. "Bone Marrow Transplant: Recent Advances and Nursing Implications," *Nursing Clinics of North America* 25(2):405-22, June 1990.

Froberg, J.H. "The Anemias: Causes and Courses of Action," Part 1. *RN* 52(1):24-30, January 1989.

Froberg, J.H. "The Anemias: Causes and Courses of Action," Part 2. *RN* 52(3):52-57, March 1989.

Froberg, J.H. "The Anemias: Causes and Courses of Action," Part 3. *RN* 52(5):42-50, May 1989.

Griffin, J.P. *Hematology and Immunology: Concepts for Nursing.* East Norwalk, Conn.: Appleton & Lange, 1986.

Pavel, J.N. "Red Blood Cell Transfusions for Anemia," *Seminars in Oncology Nursing* 6(2):117-22, May 1990.

Shahidi, N.T., ed. *Aplastic Anemia and Other Bone Marrow Failure Syndromes.* New York: Springer-Verlag, 1989.

Wilke, T., et al. "Bone Marrow Transplant: Today and Tomorrow," *American Journal of Nursing* 90(5):48-58, May 1990.

PATIENT-TEACHING AID

Preparing for bone marrow aspiration and biopsy

Dear Patient:

Your doctor has ordered a bone marrow aspiration and biopsy. This test will evaluate your bone marrow, which is the soft tissue inside your bone.

An *aspiration biopsy* involves withdrawing a fluid sample containing bone marrow particles from the marrow. A *needle biopsy* involves removing a core of solid cells from the marrow. Either test will take about 10 to 20 minutes.

The bone marrow sample will be examined under a microscope to determine whether the marrow produces enough normal blood cells and how mature they are. You'll usually know the results in 1 or 2 days.

Before the test
• You may continue your usual diet and fluid intake. But you may wish to eat lightly before the test.
• Expect to have a blood sample taken.
• You may be given a mild sedative an hour before the test to help you relax.

During the test
The most common biopsy site is the back of the hip (called the posterior superior iliac crest). Other sites include the spine, a leg bone (epiphysis), or the breastbone.

If the doctor takes a marrow sample from the back of the hip, you'll lie on your stomach as still as you can. The doctor will drape the skin around the site and clean the skin with an antiseptic solu-

tion. Then he'll inject a local anesthetic, which may cause brief discomfort before the area becomes numb.

For *aspiration biopsy:* Using a twisting motion, the doctor will insert the marrow aspiration needle through the skin, the tissue below, and the cortex of the bone. Then he'll remove the metal core from the needle and draw a bone marrow sample into the syringe.

For *needle biopsy:* The doctor will insert the biopsy needle through the skin and underlying tissue and into the bone. Next, he'll remove the core of the needle. Then he'll advance and rotate the needle in both directions, forcing a tiny core of bone into the needle.

As the doctor collects the bone marrow sample, you'll feel a pulling or grinding sensation or a brief, sharp pain. After he withdraws the needle, he'll apply pressure to the biopsy site for several minutes to stop any bleeding. Then he'll dress the wound with a sterile bandage.

After the test
• Rest for several hours.
• Report any bleeding that completely soaks the dressing or bleeding that continues for more than 24 hours.
• Reinforce the dressing as the doctor directs, but don't remove it for at least 24 hours.
• If you have discomfort, take medication as directed by your doctor.
• Continue to inspect the biopsy site daily until it heals. Notify your doctor without delay if you notice swelling or pus at the site or if you feel severe pain.

Learning about blood transfusions

Dear Patient:

Your doctor wants you to have a blood transfusion to help treat your medical problem.

How will a transfusion help?
A blood transfusion will help your body maintain its normal functions. Keep in mind that blood is composed of red blood cells (RBCs), white blood cells (WBCs), and platelets. Also remember that blood carries food, oxygen, and other important substances for growth and repair of your body's tissues.

Your body needs a certain number of RBCs, WBCs, and platelets. When the number of blood cells (blood count) circulating in your body gets too low, your body can't function properly.

For example, too few RBCs impairs your body's ability to carry oxygen, eliminate waste products and poisons, keep warm, and maintain blood pressure. Too few WBCs affects your ability to fight infection. And if you don't have enough platelets, your blood can't clot properly.

That's when your doctor will order a transfusion containing the needed cells. The new blood you receive may contain just one cell type or a mixture.

How will I know when my blood count is low?
Your doctor will tell you when your blood count is low enough to warrant a blood transfusion. Notify him if you experience symptoms that may indicate a low RBC count, such as:

- short-windedness or constant, rapid breathing
- unusually pale skin
- difficulty staying warm
- dizziness.

Also contact the doctor if you have symptoms that suggest a low platelet count, such as:
- easy bruising
- tiny purple or red spots on your skin
- bleeding gums
- blood-tinged urine or bowel movements
- persistent bleeding from a cut.

What happens during a transfusion?
Before your transfusion, a technician will collect a sample of your blood to determine your blood type and match it to donor blood. This may be done the day before the transfusion. On the day of the transfusion, a nurse or another trained specialist will insert an I.V. line (tubing connected to a needle) in your arm.

Once you're ready for the transfusion, two nurses (or a nurse and a doctor) will carefully check and double-check the information on the blood bag to make sure that the blood is specifically for you. This may require that they examine your identification bracelet, too.

They'll hang the bag above your bed. Then the infusion will begin. (You may also receive an infusion of a clear saline solution before and after the blood transfusion.)

Expect to have your temperature,

continued

Learning about blood transfusions — *continued*

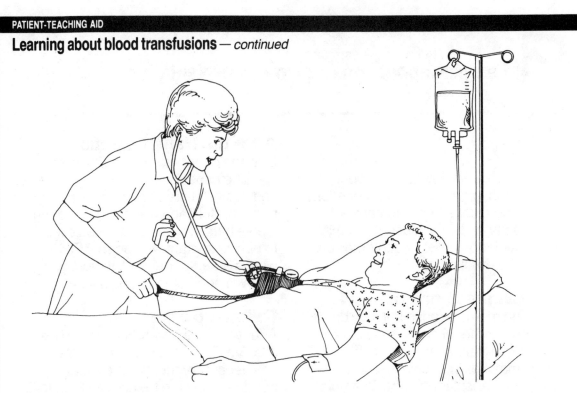

pulse rate, blood pressure, and breathing rate taken before and frequently during the infusion. A transfusion of RBCs takes from 2 to 4 hours. A platelet transfusion takes 15 to 45 minutes.

What are the risks of a transfusion?
Your greatest risks are infection and allergic reaction — and these risks are low.

Your risks for *infection* are low because of careful blood and donor screening procedures. Your chance of getting hepatitis from a blood transfusion is about 1 in 10,000. The chance of getting acquired immunodeficiency syndrome (AIDS) is about 1 in 40,000. (For comparison, your risk of dying in a car accident is 1 in 20,000.)

Occasionally, a transfusion may trigger an *allergic reaction.* Symptoms include fever, chills, and hives during or after the transfusion. If this happens during the procedure, your nurse will stop

the transfusion and return the remaining blood to the blood bank along with a sample of your blood. Then the blood will be examined to determine the cause of your reaction.

If you have an allergic reaction, you'll be given medications, such as acetaminophen (Tylenol) and diphenhydramine (Benadryl), to ease your symptoms.

Rarely, a reaction to a blood transfusion is severe. If you experience any of the following symptoms during or after your transfusion, notify your doctor or nurse immediately:
- a feeling of warmth or flushing
- redness (especially of your face and chest)
- a rash or itching
- aching muscles
- pain at the infusion site
- chest pain
- severe headache
- brown urine or pain when you urinate.

Learning about bone marrow transplantation

Dear Patient:

The doctor wants you to have bone marrow transplantation. This procedure will replace diseased bone marrow with healthy cells. Because bone marrow forms blood cells, healthy marrow is essential for life.

Obtaining the bone marrow

Your bone marrow transplant may come from your brother or sister, mother or father, or another donor whose marrow closely matches your own. In some cases, the transplant may be a sample of your own marrow, which the doctor previously removed and froze.

Preparing for transplantation

Before the transplantation, you may receive chemotherapy and total-body radiation to destroy your diseased marrow and to suppress your immune system so that the transplanted marrow can become part of you, or "engraft," with minimal complications.

Infusing the bone marrow

Once the doctor obtains and processes the bone marrow, he'll infuse it through intravenous tubing or through a special intravenous catheter that has been placed near your collarbone.

After circulating through your bloodstream, the transplanted cells will eventually lodge in your bone marrow spaces. Here the transplanted cells will grow and produce healthy blood cells in 2 to 4 weeks.

After the transplantation

Until the donor marrow grafts itself, you'll be especially vulnerable to infection. Hospital precautions may range from careful hand washing to wearing sterile hats, gowns, and shoe covers to minimize contact with germs. For 3 to 4 weeks after the transplantation, you also will need blood transfusions.

Follow-up care

After you're discharged from the hospital, you'll need regular medical checkups because your immune system needs a long time to recover. Plan to stay away from work or school for 9 months to a year after the transplantation.

Understanding the risks

The most serious complication of a bone marrow transplant is graft-versus-host disease (GVHD). In this condition, the transplanted bone marrow works against you. The disease may be acute (occurring anywhere from 1 week to 50 days after transplantation), or it may be delayed (occurring about 100 days after transplantation).

Protect yourself by learning and reporting suspicious symptoms, including signs of infection (breathing problems, dry cough, fatigue, and fever) or bleeding, especially from your nose or gums.

Contact your doctor immediately if you develop abnormally dry eyes, diarrhea, a rash, or skin changes. Follow his instructions for any medication therapy to help prevent GVHD.

Thrombocytopenia

In teaching your patient about this congenital or acquired bleeding disorder, you'll need to emphasize the importance of taking precautions against accidental bleeding—without unduly frightening the patient. You'll also need to explain just what platelets are and how they function before you discuss implications and treatment options. Understanding this disorder will help the patient and his family to cope with its limitations, to take realistic but not excessive precautions, and to respond to treatment recommendations.

Discuss the disorder

Explain that thrombocytopenia—or a shortage of platelets (thrombocytes) needed for normal blood clotting—may have several causes. Then identify the cause or causes of the patient's case, if known. These include decreased or defective platelet production in the bone marrow, abnormal platelet sequestration (collection) in the spleen, and increased platelet destruction in the bloodstream. Mention that the disorder also may result from conditions related to infection, certain drugs, a primary immune disorder, vitamin deficiency, or other disease (see *What causes thrombocytopenia?* page 218).

Reassure the patient that in many instances, thrombocytopenia—the most common bleeding disorder—resolves spontaneously. Then discuss the role of platelets. Explain that these blood cells are essential for normal blood clotting, and describe the normal clotting process. When a cut occurs, explain that the blood vessels constrict in an attempt to stop the bleeding. Platelets rush to the injured area, stick to the edges of the torn vessels, and clump together, forming a plug that temporarily stops the bleeding until a clot can form. Tell the patient that a clot then builds within the platelet plug; without the platelet plug, a clot cannot form. Even when the patient isn't injured, platelets help maintain vascular integrity by filling small gaps in blood vessel walls. This prevents blood from leaking out of vessels.

In thrombocytopenia, decreased platelet function not only impairs blood clotting after a vascular injury but also allows red blood cells to escape from the circulatory system through small gaps in undamaged vessels. This produces the petechiae, ecchymoses, and mucous membrane bleeding that's common with this

Regina B. Butler, RN, Maribel J. Clements, RN, MA, and **Brenda Shelton, RN, MS, CCRN, OCN,** contributed to this chapter. Ms. Butler is a hemophilia coordinator and hematology nurse specialist at Children's Hospital of Philadelphia. Ms. Clements is a clinical associate at Puget Sound Blood Center in Seattle. Ms. Shelton is a critical care instructor at Johns Hopkins Oncology Center in Baltimore.

CHECKLIST

Teaching topics in thrombocytopenia

☐ Explanation of platelets and their role in clotting
☐ Possible causes of thrombocytopenia
☐ Severity of thrombocytopenia
☐ Signs and symptoms of reportable bleeding
☐ Identifying purpuric lesions
☐ Bleeding complications
☐ Platelet counts and other diagnostic tests
☐ Activity restrictions
☐ Platelet infusions and possible reactions
☐ Immunosuppressive agents
☐ Treatment of local bleeding
☐ Explanation of splenectomy, if performed
☐ Bleeding precautions
☐ Source of information and support

What causes thrombocytopenia?

Inform your patient that certain disorders, medications, and toxic agents can cause thrombocytopenia—or that the cause may never be known. The following are the most prominent causes.

Disorders
- aplastic anemia
- chicken pox, measles, and mumps
- Hashimoto's thyroiditis
- Hodgkin's or non-Hodgkin's lymphomas
- leukemia
- mononucleosis
- myasthenia gravis
- sarcoidosis
- scleroderma
- smallpox
- systemic lupus erythematosus
- thyrotoxicosis
- tuberculosis
- viral hepatitis
- vitamin deficiencies, for example, folic acid and B_{12}

Medications
- carbamazepine (Tegretol)
- cimetidine (Tagamet)
- digoxin (Lanoxin)
- famotidine (Pepcid)
- gold salts
- heparin calcium (Calciparine)
- indomethacin (Indocin)
- methyldopa (Aldomet)
- phenylbutazone (Azolid)
- quinidine gluconate (Duraquin)
- quinine (Quine)
- rifampin (Rifadin)
- sulfonamides
- thiazide diuretics

Toxic agents
- insecticides
- organic arsenicals
- radiation exposure
- vinyl chloride

disorder (see *Identifying purpuric lesions*). The severity of these signs varies with the degree of thrombocytopenia.

Inform the patient that a normal platelet count ranges between 150,000 and 400,000 platelets/μl of blood. Usually, though, abnormal bleeding won't occur, even with surgery, unless the platelet count drops below 100,000/μl.

Review the severity of the patient's disorder and describe the symptoms of abnormal bleeding. If, for example, his platelet count falls between 30,000 and 50,000/μl, tell him to expect bruising with minor trauma.

If his platelet count drops further—between 15,000 and 30,000/μl—warn him to expect spontaneous bruising and petechiae, most prominently on his arms and legs. (A woman with a platelet count in this range may have menorrhagia.)

If the patient's platelet count dips under 15,000/μl, tell him that he may experience spontaneous bruising or—after minor trauma—mucosal bleeding, generalized purpura, epistaxis, hematuria, and GI or intracranial bleeding.

Without alarming the patient, emphasize the symptoms of intracranial bleeding—persistent headache, mood change, nausea, vomiting, and drowsiness. Instruct him to report any of these symptoms immediately, even if he hasn't suffered a head injury. Additionally, capillary or mucosal bleeding may lead to GI bleeding, epistaxis, menorrhagia, or gingival or urinary tract bleeding. Explain the significance of black, tarry stools or "coffee-ground" emesis. Tell the patient that by reporting bleeding signs promptly, he may prevent serious blood loss from a tiny ulcer or another internal lesion.

Complications
Urge the patient to comply with treatment recommendations and activity restrictions to avoid the dangers of abnormal bleeding. Warn the patient that severe thrombocytopenia can cause acute hemorrhage, which may be fatal without immediate therapy. The most common sites of severe bleeding include the brain and the GI tract, although intrapulmonary bleeding or cardiac tamponade also can occur.

Describe the diagnostic workup
Advise the patient with thrombocytopenia that he may need to provide frequent blood samples. For example, he may have his *platelet count* evaluated often. Although this relatively simple test requires only a small venous blood sample, *platelet antibody studies* require a larger blood sample. If the patient needs these additional tests, explain that antibody studies can help to determine why his platelet count is low and may help to direct treatment.

Occasionally, a patient will need *platelet survival studies*. These tests help the doctor differentiate between ineffective platelet production and inappropriate platelet destruction. (Platelet production disorders may occur after radiation exposure, medication

Identifying purpuric lesions

Clarify the terms that the patient's doctor may use to refer to what the patient calls a rash or a bruise. Tell the patient that the purpuric lesions (purplish discoloration from blood seeping into the skin) associated with spontaneous bleeding in thrombocytopenia include petechiae, ecchymoses, and hematomas.

Petechiae
Painless, round, and as tiny as pinpoints (1 to 3 mm in diameter), these red or brown lesions result from leakage of red blood cells into cutaneous tissue. Inform the patient that petechiae usually occur on dependent portions of the body, appearing and fading in crops and sometimes grouping to form ecchymoses.

Ecchymoses
Another form of blood leakage and larger than petechiae, these purple, blue, or yellow-green bruises vary in size and shape. Tell the patient that these bruises can occur anywhere on the body as a result of traumatic injury. In patients with bleeding disorders, ecchymoses usually appear on the arms and legs.

Hematomas
If your patient has a palpable ecchymosis that's painful and swollen, he has a hematoma. Usually the result of traumatic injury, superficial hematomas are red, whereas deep hematomas are blue. Although their size varies widely, hematomas typically exceed 1 cm in diameter.

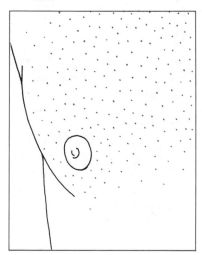 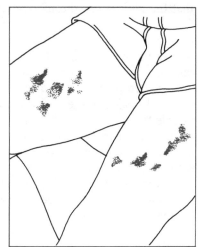 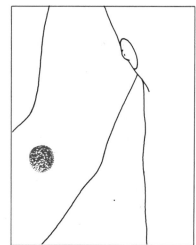

ingestion, or an infectious disease. They also may occur idiopathically. Inappropriate platelet destruction may occur with splenic disease and platelet antibody disorders.)

Patients with severe thrombocytopenia usually have a *bone marrow study* to determine the number, size, and cytoplasmic maturity of the megakaryocytes (the bone marrow cells that release mature platelets). This information may identify ineffective platelet production as the cause of thrombocytopenia and rule out a malignant disease process at the same time. If appropriate, explain that this test, which takes 5 to 10 minutes to perform, evaluates the blood cells produced by the bone marrow. Tell the patient that before the test, the skin over the bony protrusion just above his buttock (the iliac crest) will be cleaned with an antiseptic solution and anesthetized. Then the doctor will introduce a hollow needle containing a stylet into the bone marrow cavity. Next, the doctor will remove the stylet, attach a syringe to the needle apparatus and aspirate a small amount of blood and marrow.

If the patient is also having a biopsy, tell him that the doctor will make a small incision in the same area so that he can insert a larger hollow needle to remove a tiny core of bone marrow. Forewarn the patient that he may feel brief discomfort when the doctor aspirates the marrow. With the procedure completed, the doctor will apply pressure to the puncture site for 10 to 15 minutes to stop residual bleeding. Advise the patient to expect slight soreness over the puncture site. Instruct him, however, to report severe pain or bleeding.

Teach about treatments
Explain that typical treatment for thrombocytopenia includes activity restrictions to prevent injury and medications to depress the immune response. Additional therapy may involve platelet transfusions or surgery, such as splenic excision. Emphasize self-care measures to prevent bleeding episodes. These include performing meticulous oral hygiene and informing all health care providers that the patient has thrombocytopenia.

Activity
Advise the patient that the lower his platelet count falls, the more cautious he'll have to be in his activities. If the patient has severe thrombocytopenia, instruct him to avoid sports and other strenuous physical activities in which he might twist a joint, strain a muscle, sustain hard blows or kicks, or traumatize vital organs. Explain that even minor bumps or scrapes may result in bleeding. In extreme situations, spontaneous hemorrhage may occur. If this is the case for your patient, suggest that a family member or other caregiver provide supervision and assistance to prevent injury and to monitor for bleeding. Also provide the patient with a copy of the teaching aid *How to avoid excessive bleeding,* page 224.

Medication
Inform the patient that corticosteroids may be prescribed to suppress his immune response if his disorder doesn't resolve spontaneously. Typical drugs include betamethasone, cortisone, dexamethasone, hydrocortisone, prednisolone, prednisone, and triamcinolone. Remember to point out whether therapy will be brief or long-term. Also describe possible adverse effects. Tell women to inform their doctor if they are pregnant, suspect they're pregnant, plan to become pregnant, or are breast-feeding. Tell women and men patients *never* to stop taking the medication without consulting the doctor. Because abrupt drug withdrawal may cause serious adverse effects, the doctor will recommend tapering the dose before stopping the drug.

If the patient is receiving high doses of corticosteroids, forewarn him about possible cushingoid effects. Reassure him that the effects typically subside after therapy ends. For safety's sake, recommend that he wear medical identification describing his condition and treatment. Also instruct him to keep his medicine away from children and to dispose of unused medication properly.

Suggest that he calculate his caloric intake to prevent weight gain (common with corticosteroid therapy). And encourage him to take the drug with meals to prevent GI upset. Remind him to inform health care providers that he's taking a corticosteroid before he undergoes any vaccinations, skin tests, surgery, or treatment for serious injuries or infections. Also inform the patient that he's at increased risk for infection.

Advise the patient how to handle a missed dose. If he's on an every-other-day schedule, tell him to take the missed dose—if he remembers—early in the day and then to continue as scheduled. If he remembers late in the day, tell him to take his medication the next morning and skip the following day, returning to the every-other-day schedule.

If he's on a daily schedule, advise him to take the missed dose as soon as he remembers and to continue the schedule. If he doesn't remember until the next day, tell him not to double the dose. Instruct him to skip the missed dose and continue with the schedule.

If he should take medication several times daily, tell him to take the missed dose as soon as he remembers. If it's nearly time for the next dose, inform him that he may take both doses.

Tell the patient to avoid alcohol and sodium-containing foods or drugs while taking corticosteroids and also to avoid ephedrine, aspirin, and nonsteroidal anti-inflammatory drugs, such as ibuprofen, which can cause bleeding. Warn the patient that the effects of corticosteroid therapy may continue for some time after treatment stops.

If corticosteroid therapy fails to increase the platelet count, inform the patient that other immunosuppressive agents, such as cyclosporine, may be tried. Explain, however, that this treatment remains investigational.

Remember to teach all patients with thrombocytopenia about agents used to control bleeding episodes (for more information, see *Controlling local bleeding,* page 222).

Procedures

Tell the patient that he may need to receive an I.V. infusion of platelets to stop episodic abnormal bleeding caused by a low platelet count. (If platelet destruction results from an immune disorder, however, platelet infusions may have only minimal effect and may be reserved for life-threatening bleeding.)

Besides platelet infusions, discuss experimental treatments, such as I.V. immune globulin, if appropriate. Mention that this treatment achieves moderate success in some patients who have immune thrombocytopenia.

Tell the patient who receives repeated platelet infusions that he may produce antibodies to the white blood cells contained in the platelets. If this reaction produces fever and chills, reassure him that these symptoms aren't serious, just uncomfortable. Advise him that acetaminophen (Tylenol) may decrease or prevent

Controlling local bleeding

Tell your patient about agents used at home or in the hospital to control local bleeding and capillary oozing.

Agents for home use
Let your patient know about preparations, such as absorbable gelatin sponges (Gelfoam), ice packs, or dicresulene polymer (Negatan), that the doctor may recommend to control persistent bleeding.

If the doctor recommends *gelatin sponges* to stop bleeding — from a puncture wound (venipuncture or a tooth extraction), for example — tell the patient to saturate this foamlike wafer with an isotonic saline or a thrombin solution. Instruct him to place the sponge on the bleeding site and apply pressure for 10 to 15 seconds. Advise him to keep the sponge in place after the bleeding stops. Explain that this agent, which holds many times its weight in blood, can be systemically absorbed so the patient can leave the sponge in place.

If the patient bleeds from a blood vessel or into a joint (hemarthrosis), instruct him to elevate the bleeding part and apply an *ice pack* to the site until the bleeding subsides.

Inform the patient that *dicresulene polymer (Negatan)* — an astringent and protein denaturant — may be applied to oral ulcers. Tell him first to clean and dry the ulcer and then to apply the preparation for 1 minute. Next, he should neutralize the area with large amounts of water. Because the agent burns or stings, some patients apply a topical anesthetic first.

Agents for hospital use
Reassure the patient — especially the surgical patient — that bleeding can be controlled with such agents as the following: oxidized cellulose (Surgicel), microfibrillar collagen hemostat (Avitene), or thrombin (Thrombinar).

Tell him that *oxidized cellulose,* for instance, helps to control surgical bleeding or external bleeding at open wounds. Explain that the agent may remain in place for a while before the caregiver irrigates it (to prevent fresh bleeding) and then removes it with sterile forceps.

Another agent, *thrombin,* may be used during surgery or for GI bleeding. The caregiver mixes thrombin with sterile isotonic saline solution or sterile distilled water and applies it to the wound. Or she mixes thrombin with milk, which the patient drinks to control GI bleeding. As appropriate, mention that some patients react to thrombin with hypersensitivity and fever.

---

his discomfort. Besides fever and chills, the patient may develop antibodies to plasma proteins. This reaction typically results in hives. Explain that he may be given an antihistamine before a platelet infusion to prevent this reaction.

Inform the patient that he may need to provide a blood sample for a blood count after a platelet infusion—especially if he's received repeated infusions. Explain that test results will reveal whether his condition is responding to infusion therapy or whether the platelets are being destroyed.

Surgery
Splenectomy may be necessary to correct thrombocytopenia caused by platelet destruction. Because the spleen acts as the primary site of platelet removal and antibody production, a splenectomy usually significantly reduces platelet destruction. Indications that hypersplenism causes thrombocytopenia include abdominal pain, nausea, vomiting, and an enlarged, tender spleen.

Tell the patient scheduled for this surgery where the spleen is located and what type of incision to expect. Warn him that he may have a fever and abdominal distention postoperatively. Explain that he'll receive antipyretics to relieve fever. To relieve abdominal distention, he may need a rectal tube, an abdominal binder, or an antiflatulent.

Other care measures

Encourage good dental hygiene to avoid bleeding by preventing the need for tooth extractions or restorations. Advise the patient to use a soft toothbrush. Also demonstrate proper flossing technique. The patient should avoid using a sawing motion that cuts the gums. (If his platelet count drops below 30,000/μl, he may have to stop flossing altogether.) Also tell him to avoid using toothpicks.

If the patient experiences frequent nosebleeds, instruct him to use a humidifier at night. Suggest also that he moisten his inner nostrils twice a day with an anti-infective ointment, such as Neosporin Ointment.

Advise the patient to carry medical identification to alert others that he has thrombocytopenia. Finally, teach the patient to monitor his condition by examining his skin for ecchymoses and petechiae.

Ideally, he should make sure that someone else checks skin areas that he has difficulty seeing. Tell him to report any bleeding from the mucous membranes or GI tract, as well as any new petechiae or ecchymoses.

Show the patient how to test his stools for occult blood. If the patient is a female, instruct her to report increased menstrual flow to her doctor.

Source of information and support

Children's Blood Foundation
424 East 62nd Street, Room 1045, New York, N.Y. 10021
(212) 644-5790

Further readings

"Danazol-related Thrombocytopenia," *Nurses Drug Alert* 10(12):94-95, December 1986.
Hrozencik, S.P., and Connaughton, M.J. "Cancer-associated Hemolytic Uremic Syndrome," *Oncology Nursing Forum* 15(6):755-59, November-December 1988.
Knuppel, R., et al. "The Pregnant Patient with Medical Disease," *Hospital Medicine* 23(3):94, 96-97, 101-05+, March 1987.
Reynolds, M.S. "Role of Immune Globulin in the Treatment of Idiopathic Thrombocytopenic Purpura," *Journal of Pediatric Health Care* 3(2):109-12, March-April 1989.
Thomas, G.A., et al. "Idiopathic Thrombocytopenic Purpura in Children," *Nurse Practitioner* 12(4):24, 26-27, 30, April 1987.

How to avoid excessive bleeding

Dear Patient:

Because you have a tendency to bleed easily and for a longer time than normal, you may need to change your daily activities and modify your living habits. Observe these general do's and don'ts to help you function safely and avoid excessive bleeding.

Do's
- Use an electric razor.
- Wear gloves when washing dishes, raking, or gardening.

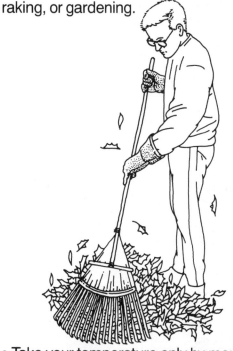

- Take your temperature only by mouth.
- Wear socks and shoes that fit properly. Footwear that's too large can cause abrasions. Footwear that's too small can pinch the blood vessels in your feet.
- Regularly check your urine, stools, and sputum for blood.

- Use a thimble while sewing on a button or stitching a hem.
- Wear a medical identification necklace or bracelet that identifies your bleeding disorder.
- Inform all health care workers of your condition before undergoing any procedure—including routine dental care.
- Use a nasal spray containing normal saline solution or run a vaporizer to moisturize your breathing passages and prevent nosebleeds.
- Use a soft toothbrush and floss gently unless your doctor advises otherwise.
- Take stool softeners, as needed. Eat sensibly to avoid constipation and subsequent straining and bleeding.
- Keep your head elevated when lying down.

Don'ts
- Avoid shaving, cutting paper, or removing paint with a straight-edged razor blade.
- Never go barefoot. Always protect your feet with shoes.
- Avoid leaving knives, scissors, thumbtacks or other sharp objects on countertops or tables where they could accidentally cut you. Store them in protective containers instead.
- Steer clear of contact sports and general roughhousing.
- If possible, turn down intramuscular or subcutaneous injections.
- Avoid plucking your eyebrows.
- Reject substances that increase your risk for bleeding—for example, alcohol, nicotine, caffeine, or products containing aspirin or ibuprofen.

5

Gastrointestinal Conditions

Contents

Peptic ulcer disease

Because peptic ulcer disease can lead to life-threatening complications, the thrust of your teaching will be to underscore the need for compliance with prescribed treatment. Begin by helping the patient understand the disease's causes and aggravating factors.

One obstacle to your teaching may be the patient's intermittent pain. During painful episodes, the patient may not be receptive to learning. And, as his pain abates, he may lose some of his motivation to learn. Keeping this in mind, emphasize to him that peptic ulcer disease can recur. Encourage him, however, that by recognizing ulcer symptoms, following the prescribed medication regimen, and reducing stress, he may prevent or delay recurrence.

Because ulcer disease may be hereditary, include the patient's family in your teaching sessions.

Discuss the disorder

Although your patient already knows that a peptic ulcer causes intense pain, he may not know that an ulcer is an erosion of the stomach lining caused by contact with acidic gastric secretions (pepsin or hydrochloric acid). Explain that a peptic ulcer may be located in the duodenum or stomach. Regardless of location, the ulcer develops in the same way (see *How a peptic ulcer forms and develops,* page 228). Mention that typically, the gnawing, burning, or aching pain in the epigastric area subsides when food, milk, and antacids neutralize stomach acid.

As appropriate, explain which factors contribute to ulcer formation. These may include trauma or illness, stress, hereditary predisposition, alcohol, caffeine, and tobacco. Such medications as aspirin, hormones, indomethacin, and corticosteroids can also contribute to ulcers.

Complications

Explain that an unchecked, unhealed ulcer can produce life-threatening complications as it erodes the layers of stomach lining: the mucosa, submucosa, muscularis, and serosa.

While slow bleeding from mucosal erosion may go unnoticed, life-threatening hemorrhage can result when a major blood vessel erodes. Even if the patient doesn't bleed to death, the ulcer can penetrate and then perforate the stomach wall, allowing gastroduodenal contents to leak into the peritoneum and cause peritonitis, hemorrhage, and septic or hypovolemic shock.

Another complication—obstruction—may be caused by scar

Catherine K. Foran, RN, and **Susan M. Hart, RN, MSN,** wrote this chapter. Ms. Foran is an independent consultant from Cherry Hill, N.J. Ms. Hart is a medical-surgical nursing instructor at Our Lady of Lourdes School of Nursing, Camden, N.J.

CHECKLIST

Teaching topics in peptic ulcer disease

☐ Definition of a peptic ulcer
☐ Explanation of the two types of peptic ulcer disease: duodenal and gastric
☐ Warning signs of such complications as hemorrhage, perforation, peritonitis, and intestinal obstruction
☐ Preparation for diagnostic tests, such as barium swallow and upper GI and small-bowel series, to confirm and evaluate ulcer disease
☐ Dietary modifications to neutralize acid and reduce gastric motility and secretions
☐ Medications to relieve symptoms: antacids, anticholinergics, histamine$_2$-receptor antagonists, and antianxiety agents
☐ Possible surgical procedures, such as gastroenterostomy and vagotomy
☐ Managing dumping syndrome
☐ Therapeutic rest, exercise, stress management, and smoking cessation
☐ Sources of information and support

How a peptic ulcer forms and develops

What is a peptic ulcer? How does it start? You've probably heard these questions before from your ulcer patients. Although no one knows the answers for sure, researchers think that a peptic ulcer results from excessive acid or pepsin secretion, from inadequate production of protective mucus, or from a breakdown in the mucosal membrane that bars gastric acid from the stomach muscles and adjacent structures. Identify which of the two peptic ulcer types—duodenal or gastric—your patient has and describe how it forms and develops.

Duodenal ulcer

A duodenal ulcer may begin with increased gastric motility, causing gastric contents to empty into the duodenum so rapidly that gastric acid remains unneutralized by the food it's digesting. Consequently, the excess acid goes to work eroding the duodenal lining. The result: inflammation and erosion. Duodenal ulcers usually affect the pylorus.

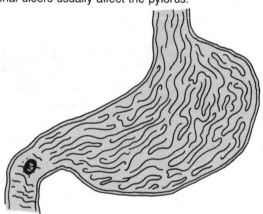

Gastric ulcer

A gastric ulcer, on the other hand, probably results not from excessive acid but from inadequate mucus production or a breakdown in the stomach's protective mucosal lining. This allows acid to permeate, inflame, and erode underlying tissues.

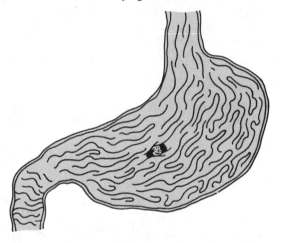

How erosion occurs

Once inflammation occurs, the body responds by releasing histamine. Histamine, in turn, stimulates acid secretion, which increases capillary permeability to proteins (pepsin), leading to mucosal edema and possible obstruction.

Unchecked, the ulcer erodes the layers of the stomach lining, damaging blood vessels in the submucosa and causing hemorrhage and shock. Further erosion into the muscularis and serosa results in perforation, peritonitis, and possibly death.

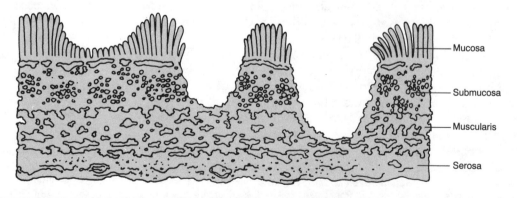

Mucosa

Submucosa

Muscularis

Serosa

tissue, edema, inflammation, or pyloric spasms. This causes the stomach to distend with food and fluid and may cause an abdominal or intestinal infarction.

Describe the diagnostic workup
Prepare the patient for diagnostic tests to confirm or evaluate peptic ulcer disease, including basal gastric secretion test, upper GI endoscopy, and barium swallow or upper GI and small-bowel series (see *Explaining barium tests,* page 230). Possibly, the doctor may order a gastric acid stimulation test.

Basal gastric secretion test
Tell the patient that this 90-minute test helps evaluate epigastric pain and measures how much acid his stomach secretes when he's fasting. Tell him to refrain from eating for 12 hours and from drinking fluids or smoking for 8 hours before the test. Because certain ulcer medications neutralize or inhibit acid secretion, instruct him to withhold antacids, anticholinergics, cholinergics, cimetidine, reserpine, adrenergic blockers, or adrenocorticosteroids, as ordered, for 24 hours before the test.

Inform the patient that the doctor will pass a flexible tube through the nose into the stomach. Assure him that the tube will be lubricated to ease its passage; however, he may feel some discomfort and may cough or gag as the tube advances. When the tube's in place, he'll lie in various positions as the doctor withdraws stomach content samples through the tube. The samples will be analyzed for acid content. Assure him that this part of the test won't hurt.

Explain that after the test his throat may feel sore from the tubing. Tell him that he may resume his normal diet and, as ordered, his medications.

Upper GI endoscopy
Tell the patient that this 30-minute test identifies ulcers. Explain that the doctor advances an endoscope through the mouth and into the stomach or small intestine.

Inform him that he won't be allowed food or fluid for at least 6 hours before the test, but he can take his medicines, as ordered. If the test is done in an emergency, tell the patient that he'll have his stomach contents suctioned to permit better visualization.

Describe to the patient how he'll lie on an X-ray table as a nurse takes his vital signs and inserts an I.V. line into his hand or arm to administer medications, if needed, during the test. Inform him that he'll be awake, but because the procedure may produce discomfort, he'll receive a sedative to help him relax.

Before the doctor inserts the endoscope, he'll numb the patient's throat with an anesthetic spray. Advise him that the spray tastes unpleasant. What's more, his mouth will feel swollen and numb, causing swallowing difficulty. Tell him he'll be positioned so that saliva safely drains from the side of his mouth, and he'll receive a mouthguard to protect his teeth. He'll have no difficulty

Explaining barium tests

If your patient's scheduled for a barium swallow or an upper GI and small-bowel series, you'll need to teach him about these tests and their effects. The barium swallow takes about 30 minutes and can detect an ulcer near the esophagus. An upper GI and small-bowel series takes up to 6 hours and can identify a gastric or duodenal ulcer. Each test uses barium to outline internal structures and X-ray films to record the findings.

Review restrictions
Explain that the clearer the GI tract, the clearer the X-ray images. So, before a barium swallow, remind the patient to stop taking antacids (if ordered) for 24 hours and to restrict food and fluids after midnight before the test.

Before an upper GI and small-bowel series, advise the patient to maintain a low-residue diet for 2 to 3 days and then to fast and stop smoking after midnight before the test. Tell him he'll receive a laxative the afternoon before the test and up to three cleansing enemas the evening before or the morning of the test. Because the test consists of a series of X-ray images taken hours apart, advise the patient to bring a book or a radio to help pass the time.

Mention that for either test, he'll wear a hospital gown, but no jewelry, hairclips, or other objects that can obscure details on the X-ray films.

Describe barium and its effects
Prepare the patient for barium's taste, consistency, and aftereffects. First describe the solution's chalky flavor and milkshake-like consistency. Explain that for a barium swallow he'll drink a thick solution and then a thinner one. For an upper GI series, he'll sip the solution several times through a perforated straw (to allow air to enter the GI tract, thereby adding contrast to the X-ray images). After either test he'll receive a laxative or enema to help him expel the barium. Explain that retained barium can harden, causing obstruction or impaction. Caution him that barium will lightly color his stools for 24 to 72 hours after the test.

Explain the procedure
Tell the patient that for either test he'll lie on a movable X-ray table. As the barium outlines the digestive system, the doctor will tilt the table so he can take films of the GI tract from various angles. For the upper GI series, this will occur several times as the barium reaches various structures. Make sure to mention that the doctor may compress the patient's abdomen to make sure the barium coats the stomach well.

Discuss aftercare
Assure the patient that he may resume his normal diet and medication, as ordered, after the test. If the patient underwent an upper GI series, he may want to rest after the test.

breathing, but he won't be able to speak with the tube in position.

Next, explain that the doctor may advance the tube while the patient sits, lies down, or alternates each position. In either position, he'll feel abdominal pressure and fullness or bloating as the doctor gently introduces air to view internal structures better.

Inform the patient that after the test, a nurse will monitor his vital signs for about 8 hours. Then mention that he can resume

Questions ulcer patients ask

Should I drink milk to heal my ulcer?
Maybe yes, maybe no. Milk's role in ulcer therapy remains controversial, so your best bet is to consume milk in moderation, unless your doctor recommends otherwise. Here's why. In the past, milk was the mainstay of an ulcer diet. Then a few years ago, experts found that although milk relieves pain, it stimulates acid production. The latest findings show that milk neutralizes acidity and contains substances (prostaglandins and growth factors) that protect the stomach lining.

My doctor says smoking will aggravate my ulcer. Why?
Smoking irritates the stomach lining and the duodenum by altering pancreatic secretions that help neutralize stomach acid. Smoking also increases gastric motility, making food pass more quickly into your duodenum. When that happens, excess (and irritating) gastric acid passes too. Both of these effects can delay ulcer healing.

I know that my high-pressure job isn't good for my ulcer, but I can't quit. Does this mean I'll have an ulcer forever?
Try to modify your routine to diminish stress. Start by trying to reduce your workload. Failing that, plan your work schedule more realistically. If your workplace is noisy, listen to soothing music through earplugs. Install soft lighting or rearrange your workspace to provide more privacy. If possible, take short breaks.

At night, get enough sleep to refresh you for the next day. Engage in relaxing activities and exercise moderately (avoid strenuous activity because it increases acid secretion). Possibly, consult a therapist or attend a stress management workshop.

eating when his gag reflex returns, usually in about 1 hour. Inform him that he may have a sore throat for several days.

Gastric acid stimulation test
Explain that this 1-hour test helps diagnose a duodenal ulcer by determining whether the stomach secretes acid normally.

Instruct the patient to stop taking antacids, anticholinergics, cholinergics, cimetidine, reserpine, adrenergic blockers, or adrenocorticosteroids, as ordered, 24 hours before the test. Also tell him not to eat, drink, or smoke after midnight before the test.

Describe how the doctor advances a lubricated, flexible tube through the patient's nose into his stomach. Caution him that he may feel discomfort and may cough or gag. After positioning the tube, the doctor will inject pentagastrin subcutaneously to stimulate acid secretion. Advise the patient to report abdominal pain, nausea, vomiting, flushing, dizziness, faintness, or paresthesias in his extremities at once. Next, the doctor withdraws several stomach content samples for laboratory analysis. Inform the patient that he may have a sore throat after the test. He may resume his normal diet and medication, as ordered.

Teach about treatments
Inform the patient that treatment focuses on resting the stomach so that the ulcer heals. Specific measures include dietary changes (see *Questions ulcer patients ask*) and medication (see *Teaching about drugs for peptic ulcer disease,* pages 232 and 233). Another
continued on page 234

Teaching about drugs for peptic ulcer disease

DRUG	ADVERSE REACTIONS	TEACHING POINTS
Antacids		
Calcium-containing antacids (Dicarbosil, Titralac, Tums)	• Watch for abdominal cramps, anorexia, constipation, dysuria, frequent urination, joint pain, mood or mental status changes, muscle pain, muscle twitching, nausea, nervousness, restlessness, vomiting, and weakness. • Other reactions include belching, chalky taste, confusion, and mild constipation.	• Explain to the patient that this drug helps relieve heartburn and acid stomach. • Instruct him to chew the tablet well before swallowing and to follow the dose with a full glass of water. • Caution him about acid rebound if he takes this drug for more than 2 weeks. Explain the dangers of self-medication, and advise him to consult his doctor before making any changes in the medication regimen. • Tell him to take a missed dose as soon as possible, then resume his schedule. He must never double-dose. • Advise him to contact the doctor if constipation's a problem. The doctor may prescribe an alternate antacid, combination therapy, or a stool softener. • Tell him to take antacids 1 to 3 hours after meals and at bedtime. • Instruct him to space doses of these antacids and iron preparations, tetracyclines, digoxin (Lanoxin), indomethacin (Indocin), and other drugs 2 hours apart, to prevent decreased absorption.
Magnesium-containing antacids (Maalox, Mylanta, Riopan)	• Watch for anorexia, dizziness, dysuria, headache, irregular heart rate, mood changes, and weakness. • Other reactions include abdominal pain, diarrhea, nausea, vomiting, white specks in stools.	• Explain to the patient that this drug helps relieve heartburn and acid stomach. • Instruct him to chew the tablet well before swallowing and to follow the dose with a full glass of water. • Tell him to shake the liquid form of this drug well before taking. • Suggest mixing the tablet and liquid forms with fluids or food if preferred. • Instruct him to take a missed dose as soon as possible. If it's almost time for his next dose, he should skip the missed dose and resume his schedule. He must never double-dose. • Warn him about the dangers of self-medication. Advise him to consult his doctor before making any changes in the medication regimen. • If he has diarrhea, tell him that the doctor may prescribe an alternative antacid or combination therapy. • Tell him to take antacids 1 to 3 hours after meals and at bedtime. • Instruct him to space doses of these antacids and iron preparations, tetracyclines, digoxin (Lanoxin), indomethacin (Indocin), and other drugs 2 hours apart to prevent decreased absorption.
Anticholinergics		
atropine	• Watch for blurred vision, confusion, dizziness, dyspnea, eye pain, flushing, rash, seizures, tachycardia, unusual tiredness or weakness. • Other reactions include constipation; decreased sweating; drowsiness; dry mouth, nose, and throat; dysuria, headache, nausea, photophobia, and vomiting.	• Explain to the patient that this drug helps relieve abdominal cramps. Point out that it's used with other drugs to treat ulcers, and may also prevent nausea, vomiting, and motion sickness. • If the patient misses a dose, instruct him to take the missed dose as soon as possible. If it's almost time for his next dose, he should skip the missed dose and resume his schedule. He must never double-dose. • Inform him that this drug may reduce sweating, allowing body temperature to rise. To prevent heat stroke, caution him to avoid becoming overheated during exercise or hot weather. • Explain that this drug may make his eyes more sensitive to light. Suggest wearing sunglasses. • Advise him to be sure his vision is clear before driving or performing other activities that require good eyesight. • Suggest that he chew sugarless gum or ice chips to relieve dry mouth. • Advise him to separate doses of atropine from doses of antacids and of kaolin- or pectin-containing antidiarrheals, to prevent decreased effectiveness of atropine. • Instruct him to take this drug 30 minutes to 1 hour before meals, as ordered. • Tell him to avoid alcohol and central nervous system (CNS) depressants to prevent adverse reactions.

continued

Teaching about drugs for peptic ulcer disease—*continued*

DRUG	ADVERSE REACTIONS	TEACHING POINTS
Anticholinergics—*continued*		
methantheline bromide (Banthine) **propantheline bromide** (Probanthine)	• Watch for constipation, difficult urination, eye pain, rash, and tachycardia. • Other reactions include confusion, decreased sweating, dizziness, drowsiness, dry mouth, fatigue, headache, nausea, photophobia, and vomiting.	• Explain that this drug helps relieve abdominal cramps and acid stomach. • If he misses a dose, instruct him to skip the missed dose and resume his schedule. He must never double-dose. • If this drug makes him feel drowsy, caution him to avoid driving, operating machinery, or performing other activities that require alertness. • Explain that this drug may make his eyes more sensitive to light. • Inform him that this drug may reduce sweating, allowing body temperature to rise. To prevent heat stroke, caution him not to become overheated during exercise or hot weather. • Suggest chewing sugarless gum or ice chips to relieve dry mouth. • Instruct him to take this drug 30 minutes to 1 hour before meals, as ordered. • Advise him that antacids and kaolin- or pectin-containing antidiarrheals may decrease these drugs' effectiveness. He should separate doses by 1 hour. • Instruct the patient to avoid alcohol and other CNS depressants (increased adverse reactions possible).
Histamine₂-receptor antagonists		
cimetidine (Tagamet) **pepcid** (Famotidine) **ranitidine** (Zantac)	• Watch for confusion and unusual bleeding, bruising, tiredness, or weakness. • Other reactions include decreased libido, diarrhea, dizziness, gynecomastia, headache, muscle cramps or pain, and rash.	• Explain that this drug relieves symptoms by decreasing gastric secretion. • Instruct him to take the drug with or immediately after meals. Food delays absorption and prolongs drug effect. • Advise him to separate doses of the drugs and antacids by 1 hour (decreased absorption possible). • If he misses a dose, instruct him to take the missed dose as soon as possible. However, if it's almost time for his next dose, tell him to skip the missed dose and resume his regular schedule. He must never double-dose. • Tell him smoking interferes with this drug's effect. Advise him to stop smoking at least after taking the evening dose to prevent interfering with drug control of nocturnal gastric acid secretion.
Miscellaneous		
sucralfate (Carafate)	• Reactions include backache, constipation, diarrhea, dizziness, dry mouth, light-headedness, indigestion, nausea, rash, sleepiness, and stomach cramps.	• Explain to the patient that this drug helps relieve ulcer symptoms and promotes healing. • Advise him to take the drug with a full glass of water. • If he misses a dose, instruct him to take the missed dose as soon as possible. However, if it's almost time for his next dose, tell him to skip the missed dose and resume his regular schedule. He must never double-dose. • Tell him to separate doses of this drug and antacids by 1 hour, to prevent decreased effectiveness of sucralfate. • Inform him that this drug may reduce absorption of fat-soluble vitamins A, D, E, and K. He should take them separately. • Suggest that he take the drug 1 hour before meals for best results. • Advise him to separate doses of this drug and tetracycline (Tetracyn) or phenytoin (Dilantin) by 2 hours, to prevent decreased absorption.
misoprostol (Cytotec)	• Watch for abdominal pain, constipation, cramps, diarrhea, dysmenorrhea, dyspepsia, flatulence, hypermenorrhea, miscarriage, nausea, spotting, and vomiting. • Another reaction includes a headache.	• Explain to the patient that this drug helps prevent ulcers induced by nonsteroidal anti-inflammatory drugs. (In Canada, it's also used to relieve ulcer symptoms and promote healing.) • Warn the female patient of childbearing age not to become pregnant while taking misoprostol. This drug may cause miscarriage, possibly with life-threatening bleeding. Discuss contraception, and tell the patient that she must have a negative serum pregnancy test 2 weeks before therapy. Therapy won't begin until the 2nd or 3rd day of her next menstrual period.

treatment measure is stress reduction or life-style changes. If these measures fail or if complications develop, explain that the doctor may recommend surgery.

Diet

Until the patient's ulcer heals, the doctor may direct the patient to eat six small meals daily, rather than three regular meals. Possibly, small hourly feedings may relieve his symptoms. Frequent feedings prevent complete stomach emptying and reduce distention, which reduces gastric acid secretion and gastric motility. Once healing occurs, the patient can eat three balanced meals a day.

During the acute ulcer phase, make sure the patient understands his prescribed diet. If the doctor orders the Sippy diet, inform the patient that he'll have small amounts of milk and antacids alternately every 30 minutes. Gradually, he'll add frequent, small amounts of bland foods, such as cooked cereals, toast, and soft-boiled eggs. He won't be able to eat high-fiber foods, such as cabbage, or irritating foods, such as soups and gravies. If constipation develops, the doctor may prescribe laxatives. Reassure the patient that eventually he'll resume a normal diet, but usually he'll remain on the restricted diet until he has a follow-up X-ray that demonstrates healing. If the dietary regimen requires changes in cooking methods, be sure to include the family or significant others in your teaching.

As the acute phase subsides, advise the patient to avoid large meals, extremely hot or cold foods, and high-fiber, gas-forming, and spicy foods that cause him pain. Advise him to eliminate fruit juices, carbonated beverages, caffeine, and broth, because these substances increase gastric secretions. He should avoid alcohol, or at least limit it to 2 ounces or less a day—and never drink it on an empty stomach. Stress that *when* he eats is more important than *what* he eats because any food acts as an acid-neutralizing agent.

Advise the patient to eat slowly, to chew thoroughly, to have small snacks between meals if this relieves pain, and to try to avoid stress at mealtimes and immediately afterward.

Medication

Point out that symptoms usually diminish before the ulcer heals completely. This means that even though he feels well, he must follow his medication regimen to completion (usually at least 8 weeks) to prevent complications or recurrent symptoms.

As appropriate, explain the drugs the doctor may prescribe, such as antacids to reduce gastric acidity, histamine$_2$-receptor antagonists to reduce gastric secretion, and anticholinergics to reduce gastric activity. As appropriate, explain how the prescribed drug works and what adverse reactions should be reported. Mention that the doctor may prescribe antianxiety drugs to promote rest and relaxation.

Instruct the patient to read the labels of nonprescription medications. He should avoid preparations that contain corticosteroids, aspirin (acetylsalicylic acid), or other nonsteroidal anti-inflammatory drugs (NSAIDs), such as ibuprofen (Motrin). Explain that these drugs inhibit mucus secretion and, therefore, leave the GI lining vulnerable to injury from gastric acid. Advise him, if needed, to use alternative analgesics, such as acetaminophen (Tylenol). Caution him to avoid systemic antacids, such as sodium bicarbonate, because they're absorbed into the circulation and can cause acid-base imbalance.

If the patient smokes, inform him that smoking interferes with the effect of *all* peptic ulcer drugs. Encourage him to quit or at least cut down. If he can't quit, discourage him from smoking after he takes his evening medication, which controls nocturnal gastric acid secretion.

Surgery

Inform the patient that surgery may be necessary if conservative treatments fail or if complications develop. As appropriate, explain the surgery he'll have. For example, if the doctor recommends *gastroenterostomy*, explain that the surgeon will make an opening in the stomach and attach a segment of the small intestine around the opening, thus allowing excess gastric acid to drain from, rather than accumulate in, the stomach. Point out, however, that because the surgery doesn't decrease acid secretion, the surgeon may also perform *vagotomy*, which retards acid secretion by partially severing the nerves that signal acid production. Other surgical procedures include pyloroplasty and gastrectomy. For more information, see *Types of peptic ulcer surgery*, page 236.

If the patient must have emergency surgery (usually to stop hemorrhage), inform him that preparations include X-rays and immunohematologic studies. Explain, as appropriate, the various pain-relief and life-saving procedures he'll undergo, such as nasogastric suctioning and iced saline lavage.

If the patient undergoes planned surgery, inform him that he'll have cleansing laxatives and enemas the evening before and a nasogastric tube inserted on the morning of surgery. Explain that both measures prevent complications.

Tell the patient that the nasogastric tube will prevent distention by draining the GI tract until his bowels begin to function in 2 to 3 days. Inform him that he'll have a drain at the incision site for 1 or 2 days after surgery to remove any accumulated fluid. What's more, he may be fed through a gastrostomy tube. He'll probably resume eating several days after surgery, beginning with clear liquids and gradually advancing to solid foods. If he's not allowed to eat for more than a week, he'll receive total parenteral nutrition.

Explain to the patient that although coughing and deep breathing will cause incisional pain, he must try to do them to prevent postsurgical complications. Tell him he'll go home in 1 to

Types of peptic ulcer surgery

SURGERY		INDICATIONS	EFFECTS
Vagotomy Truncal (total abdominal vagotomy)		• Recurrent ulcer disease • Acid reduction	• Completely severs both vagus nerves at the esophageal base • Destroys gastric, intestinal, and gallbladder motility • Stops acid production • Causes impaired emptying and diarrhea
Selective vagotomy		• Recurrent ulcer disease • Acid reduction	• Severs vagus nerve • Destroys vagal innervation of stomach (but retains abdominal innervation) • Reduces acid production • Impairs gastric motility
Highly selective (parietal cell vagotomy)		• Recurrent ulcer disease • Acid reduction	• Severs only the parietal cell branches of vagus nerve • Denervates acid-producing cells, but doesn't affect motility
Pyloroplasty		• Pyloric stricture or obstruction (may be combined with vagotomy to reduce gastric secretion and motility)	• Enlarges pylorus by removing sphincter • Gives stomach and duodenum free communication • Facilitates neutralization without inhibiting gastric secretion • Increases gastric emptying
Gastrectomy Billroth I (gastroduodenostomy, hemigastrectomy)		• Gastric ulcer • Pyloric obstruction • Hemorrhage	• Resects antrum and connects gastric remnant to proximal duodenum • Destroys antral function and pyloric sphincter • May cause bile reflux • Reduces gastric secretion • Increases gastric emptying • May cause steatorrhea, dumping syndrome, weight loss, vomiting, and anemia
Billroth II (gastrojejunostomy)		• Duodenal ulcer • Pyloric obstruction	• Resects antrum and attaches gastric remnant to proximal jejunum (retains duodenum) • Destroys antral function • Allows digestive secretions of liver and pancreas to mix in duodenum • Duodenum serves as afferent loop; proximal jejunum as efferent loop • Reduces gastric secretion • Increases gastric emptying • Commonly causes steatorrhea, dumping syndrome, weight loss, vomiting, and anemia
Total gastrectomy (esophagojejunostomy)		• Ulcer disease • Perforation • Gastric cancer	• Resects stomach from lower esophageal sphincter to duodenal bulb; anastomoses duodenum and esophagus • Destroys gastric function; ingested materials pass from esophagus to duodenum
Gastric resection (antrectomy)		• Recurrent ulcers • Perforation	• Removes stomach portion • Effects depend on stomach portion removed (for example, antrectomy alters digestive function)

2 weeks and that he'll probably resume normal activities 2 to 4 weeks later. Remind him to continue avoiding poorly tolerated foods, to adhere to his medication schedule, to follow stress management techniques, and to abstain from smoking. If appropriate, describe the signs and symptoms of dumping syndrome and teach the patient to minimize or prevent this problem by properly managing his diet (see *Understanding the dumping syndrome*).

Other care measures
Discuss necessary life-style changes. Bear in mind that the patient may be assertive and independent, and changes may be difficult for him to accept. Inform him that emotional tension can precipitate an ulcer attack and prolong healing. Advise him and his family to identify stressors and explore ways to eliminate them or reduce their impact.

Instruct the patient to notify the doctor immediately if he has any sign of life-threatening complications—hemorrhage, obstruction, or perforation. Give him a copy of the patient-teaching aid *Recognizing warning signs of ulcer complications,* page 238. Then urge him to schedule regular appointments with his doctor.

Sources of information and support
Digestive Disease National Coalition
511 Capital Court, NE, Suite 300, Washington, D.C. 20002
(202) 544-7499

National Digestive Diseases Information Clearinghouse
Box NDDIC, Bethesda, Md. 20892
(301) 468-6344

National Ulcer Foundation
675 Main Street, Melrose, Mass. 02176
(617) 665-6210

Further readings
Brasitus, T.A., and Foster, E.S. "Peptic Ulcer Update: Approaches to Treatment," *Physician Assistant* 12(4):71-72, 77-78, 83, April 1988.
"Erosive Gastritis and 'Stress Ulcer,'" *Hospital Medicine* 23(10):200, 203-04, October 1987.
Konopod, E., and Noseworthy, T. "Stress Ulceration: A Serious Complication in Critically Ill Patients," *Heart & Lung* 17(4):339-48, July 1988.
Marshall, B.J. "Peptic Ulcer: An Infectious Disease?" *Hospital Practice* 22(8):87-96, August 15, 1987.
Modeland, V. "Ulcers: Screaming or Silent, Watch Them with Care," *FDA Consumer* 23(5):14-17, June 1989.
Olsen, K.M., and Barton, C.L. "Peptic Ulcer Disease," *Journal of Practical Nursing* 37(4):20-27, December 1987.

Understanding the dumping syndrome

If the patient's had a gastric resection with pyloric removal, prepare him for dealing with dumping syndrome, which may begin about 2 weeks after surgery and typically occurs between 15 and 30 minutes after eating. Lasting about 1 hour, the syndrome causes abdominal cramps, diaphoresis, diarrhea, palpitations, syncope, tachycardia, and weakness.

What causes the problem
Explain that after gastric resection, food and fluid, which the stomach can no longer store, empty rapidly and in large amounts into the small intestine. To accommodate the onrush, the bowel draws fluid from the vascular system. Then, the jejunum distends with food and fluid; intestinal peristalsis and motility increase.

Managing symptoms
To minimize or prevent symptoms, suggest the patient:
• eat four to six small meals a day
• maintain a normal intake of fats and proteins; they leave the stomach more slowly and attract less fluid into the intestine
• avoid foods with concentrated carbohydrates; they attract more fluid into the intestine·
• avoid drinking fluids with meals; rather, take them between meals
• avoid overly hot or cold foods and fluids
• lie down for 30 minutes to 1 hour after eating
• take medications to slow intestinal motility, if ordered.

Reassure the patient that the syndrome usually resolves within a year after surgery. However, a few patients may have long-term problems and require reconstructive surgery.

PATIENT-TEACHING AID

Recognizing warning signs of ulcer complications

Dear Patient:

You shouldn't have any serious complications from your ulcer if you follow your treatment plan. But just in case, get to know the warning signs of complications. Make sure you get prompt medical attention if any of these signs occur.

Signs of bleeding

If you've ever bumped a scab off a cut finger, you know it can bleed. At times, an ulcer can affect the blood vessels in your stomach lining in much the same way.

Contact your doctor or go to the hospital if you have:
- bloody or black, tarry stools
- vomit that looks like coffee grounds
- chills or sweating, or both
- dizziness
- paleness
- restlessness and anxiety
- breathing problems.

Signs of perforation

If you've ever stepped on a nail or a pin, you know it hurts and leaves a little hole in your skin. An ulcer can leave a hole and hurt, too. What's more, the hole lets what's in your stomach leak out to cause infection or other problems.

Contact your doctor or go to the hospital if you have:
- severe pain in your stomach or shoulders (or both) that's relieved if you bend at your waist or pull your knees up to your chest

- a rigid, boardlike stomach
- a flushed, sweaty sensation
- fever and dizziness
- breathing problems.

Signs of obstruction

If you've ever had a plumbing problem—perhaps your sink backed up or your washing machine overflowed—you know that an obstruction must be fixed to allow normal function again. Likewise, an obstruction that results from an ulcer needs attention.

Contact your doctor or go to the hospital if you have:
- a swollen stomach or an extremely full feeling that gets worse after meals or at night
- wavelike stomach tremors that you can see
- constipation
- a foul taste in your mouth and on your tongue
- loss of appetite, nausea, and foul-smelling vomit
- unusual thirst
- weight loss.

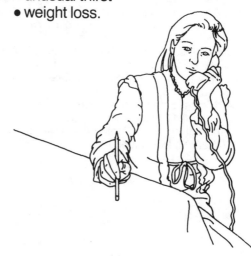

Hepatitis

Because hepatitis can result in permanent liver damage, you'll stress the need for strict compliance with treatment. Your first priority, though, may be to demystify the disease for the patient and his family. Because viral hepatitis is contagious and must be reported to the local public health authorities, many people erroneously associate it only with unsanitary conditions or with socially unacceptable behavior. Reassure the patient that having hepatitis doesn't mean that he's dirty or immoral. In teaching some patients with viral hepatitis, however, you'll be challenged to remain objective and nonjudgmental.

You'll explain to the patient how hepatitis is diagnosed, in particular, by liver function tests. During recovery, you'll emphasize the importance of rest and good nutrition in healing the liver. What's more, you'll teach him how to reduce the risk of spreading the disease. Finally, you'll urge him to remain under medical supervision until he is completely well and free of infection.

Discuss the disorder

Inform the patient that hepatitis is an inflammation of the liver, which interferes with normal hepatic function and causes his symptoms. Confirm that initial symptoms of hepatitis include malaise, fever, anorexia, nausea, headache, and abdominal pain. As the disease progresses, jaundice usually develops—a yellowish discoloration of the skin and the whites of the eyes—as well as itching, dark urine, and light-colored stools.

Explain that fever, malaise, and abdominal pain reflect the presence of an infection. Headache, anorexia, and nausea may result from the build-up of a toxin—either a chemical released from the damaged liver or a substance that it can no longer detoxify. Jaundice and abnormally colored urine and stools occur when the liver fails to adequately eliminate bilirubin (a bile pigment produced during the breakdown of red blood cells) from the blood.

Inform the patient that hepatitis may result from a viral infection or, less commonly, alcohol, drugs, or an unrelated disease, such as leukemia (see *What causes hepatitis?* page 240). Explain that the term "viral hepatitis" denotes hepatitis caused by a virus, most commonly hepatitis virus A, B, C (also known as non-A, non-B), or D.

Complications

Emphasize that strict adherence to the treatment plan is essential for liver regeneration. Explain that incomplete regeneration can

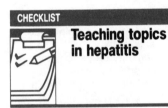

CHECKLIST

Teaching topics in hepatitis

☐ How hepatitis affects the liver
☐ Causes of hepatitis
☐ Types of viral hepatitis: A (HAV); B (HBV); C (HCV); and D (HDV)
☐ Symptoms, transmission, and complications, including chronic hepatitis
☐ Preparation for diagnostic tests, such as liver function studies, hepatitis profile, and liver biopsy
☐ The importance of rest and diet
☐ Restrictions on alcohol and drug consumption
☐ The use of immune globulin and vaccination to prevent hepatitis in exposed persons
☐ Proper hygiene and other measures to prevent the spread of viral hepatitis
☐ Sources of information and support

Brenda L. W. Hagan, RN,C, MSN, who wrote this chapter, is director of clinical services for Liberty Healthcare Corporation in Philadelphia.

What causes hepatitis?

The most common cause of hepatitis is infection by one of several hepatitis viruses. Hepatitis can also result from other viruses or drugs. Note that drug toxicity can be idiosyncratic or dose-related. Other causes include alcohol consumption and certain diseases. Use this list of causes to help pinpoint the patient's source of hepatitis.

Viral infections
• Hepatitis A, B, C, and D viruses
• Epstein-Barr virus
• Cytomegalovirus
• Adenoviruses
• Echoviruses
• Yellow fever virus
• Rift valley fever virus
• Lassa fever virus
• Hemorrhagic fever virus
• Marburg monkey virus

Selected hepatotoxic drugs
• Analgesics (acetaminophen and salicylates)
• Antianxiety drugs (chlordiazepoxide and diazepam)
• Anticonvulsants (phenytoin and mephenytoin)
• Antidepressants (monoamine oxidase inhibitors and tricyclic antidepressants)
• Antimicrobial drugs (erythromycin estolate, griseofulvin, nitrofurantoin macrocrystals, rifampin, sulfonamides, and tetracycline)
• Antipsychotic drugs (haloperidol and phenothiazines)
• Cardiovascular drugs (methyldopa and quinidine sulfate)
• Hormone derivatives (antithyroid drugs, oral contraceptives, and oral hypoglycemic drugs)

Alcohol

Diseases
• Leukemia
• Lymphomas
• Wilson's disease

lead to cirrhosis—progressive destruction of the liver, characterized by scarring, fibrosis, and fatty deposits. Point out that cirrhosis can, in turn, result in conditions that can lead to hemorrhage, coma, and even death.

Even with satisfactory compliance during convalescence, viral hepatitis, especially hepatitis B, can still lead to complications. About 10% of patients with hepatitis B remain infected with the virus 6 months after the initial infection. These patients are said to have chronic hepatitis. For more information, see *Tracing the course of hepatitis B*. Furthermore, hepatitis C is associated with an increased risk of liver cancer. Explain that the development of these complications is influenced by the patient's age when first infected, his immune status, and the severity of the acute infection.

Describe the diagnostic workup
Inform the patient that a diagnosis of hepatitis relies on his symptoms and a number of studies that reflect the functional status of the liver. If viral hepatitis is suspected, diagnosis may also include a hepatitis profile.

Liver function tests
Advise the patient that several tests will be performed on blood and urine samples to assess his liver function. Such tests include serum and urine bilirubin, urine and fecal urobilinogen, serum enzymes and proteins, and prothrombin time. Explain that some studies, particularly serum enzymes, will be repeated every 2 to 6 weeks (depending on the severity of his illness) until laboratory values return to normal.

Hepatitis profile
If viral hepatitis is suspected, tell the patient that a blood sample will be analyzed to identify the specific virus responsible for his disorder. (See *Comparing types of viral hepatitis*, pages 242 and 243, for diagnostic tests used to confirm viral hepatitis. Also refer to this chart to compare transmission modes, incubation periods, prophylaxis, high-risk individuals, and isolation precautions.)

Liver biopsy
Inform the patient that the doctor may perform a liver biopsy if serum enzyme levels remain elevated for more than 6 months. Tell him that this test will determine if the persistent enzyme abnormality is associated with chronic active hepatitis. Explain that the doctor will obtain a small tissue sample from the liver.

Instruct the patient to avoid food and fluids for at least 4 hours before the test. Inform him that he'll be awake during the 15-minute test. Although the test causes discomfort, assure him that he'll receive medication to help him relax.

Explain that the doctor will drape and cleanse an area on the patient's abdomen and then inject a local anesthetic, which may cause some brief stinging and discomfort. The patient will then be asked to hold his breath and lie still while the doctor inserts the biopsy needle into his liver. Tell the patient that the needle insertion may cause a sensation of pressure and discomfort in his upper right back. Assure him that the needle will remain in his liver for only about a second.

Inform the patient that the nurse will monitor his vital signs for several hours after the test. Explain that he must remain in bed on his right side for 2 hours and then rest in bed for 24 hours. He may experience pain for several hours. Tell him that he may resume a normal diet immediately.

Teach about treatments

Educate the patient about the importance of rest and a proper diet to help the liver heal and minimize complications. Explain that the liver takes 3 weeks to regenerate and up to 4 months to return to normal functioning. If the patient has viral hepatitis, emphasize measures to prevent spreading the disease.

Activity

Encourage the patient to rest as much as possible. In the early stages, fatigue will motivate him to rest. As he begins to feel better, rest is still important, so you may need to urge him to curtail unnecessary activity. Help him find ways to minimize employment demands, food shopping, child care, and stair climbing. Explain that he'll need to reduce his schedule for at least 3 weeks, depending on the severity of his illness. Emphasize that exertion and stress during recovery can lead to complications or relapse.

Diet

Explain that good nutrition will promote liver regeneration. Because the patient may experience anorexia, nausea, or vomiting, help him build an appealing meal plan based on frequent small meals. Inform him that a well-balanced diet can meet his nutritional needs.

Encourage the patient to consume at least 4 liters of fluid a day. If he is anorectic, drinking sufficient fluids may be especially difficult. Suggest that he try fruit juices or soft drinks containing ice chips. Stress that alcohol consumption is strictly forbidden.

Advise the patient to weigh himself daily. Instruct him to notify the doctor of any weight loss greater than 5 lb.

Medication

Inform the patient that there's no specific drug therapy for hepatitis. If he has viral hepatitis, explain that anyone exposed to the disease through contact with him should receive immune globulin or the hepatitis B vaccine as soon as possible after exposure. (See *Hepatitis B prophylaxis,* page 244.) Help him to identify those at risk.

Advise the patient to check with the doctor before taking any medication, including nonprescription drugs, because some drugs can precipitate a relapse.

Tracing the course of hepatitis B

Inform your patient that most patients with hepatitis B recover fully within 6 months. In these patients, the viral protein hepatitis B surface antigen (HBsAg) can no longer be detected in the blood, indicating that the virus has been eliminated from the body.

Chronic hepatitis B

About 10% of patients continue to have detectable levels of HBsAg in their blood 6 months after the initial infection. These patients remain infected with the hepatitis B virus and have chronic hepatitis B.

Chronic hepatitis is benign in 70% to 90% of cases. Asymptomatic and with no evidence of more serious liver disease, these patients remain carriers of the hepatitis B virus and can infect others.

Chronic active hepatitis affects 10% to 30% of those who develop chronic hepatitis B. This variant may progress to cirrhosis or liver failure. Chronic hepatitis is also associated with an increased risk of hepatocellular carcinoma.

Emphasize that the development of chronic hepatitis depends on factors beyond the patient's control, such as age, immune status, and the severity of the initial infection.

Comparing types of viral hepatitis

Refer to this chart as you begin teaching your patient about his type of hepatitis. First, explain isolation precautions.

If the patient has hepatitis A, the hospital staff will exercise *enteric precautions.*

For example, the patient may have a private room (necessary only for a patient with fecal incontinence or with poor hygiene), and staff members will wear gowns (when fecal soiling's likely) and gloves (for contact with feces or feces-soiled items). They'll double-bag fecally contaminated bed linens in isolation bags and label any fecal specimens "Enteric precautions."

Whenever hospital staff members transport the patient, they'll use added protection (for example, moisture-resistant pads for a fecally incontinent patient).

At home the patient should use meticulous hygiene after a bowel movement—starting with thorough hand washing, for example. Furthermore, the patient shouldn't handle food or share food or hand towels.

If the patient has hepatitis B, C, or D, the hospital staff will observe *universal (blood and body fluid) precautions.* The patient may have a private room (necessary only for a patient with poor hygiene), and staff members will wear gowns and gloves (for direct contact with blood or body fluids).

Staff members will dispose of needles and syringes in prominently labeled puncture-resistant containers and won't recap needles and syringes. They'll double-bag dressings and tissues and dispose of them in the hospital's designated area for contaminated refuse.

If bed linens are contaminated with blood or body fluids, the staff will double-bag them in isolation bags. And they will label specimens "Blood and body fluid precautions." The patient must avoid sexual relations until the doctor confirms there's no danger of contagion.

After discussing isolation measures, educate the patient about the mode of transmission, incubation period, diagnostic tests, prophylaxis, and those at high risk for his type of hepatitis.

HEPATITIS A (HAV)	HEPATITIS B (HBV)	HEPATITIS C (HCV)	HEPATITIS D (HDV)
Transmission modes			
• Fecal-oral route; spread by infected food handlers, sewage, and contaminated water and shellfish • Oral-anal sexual practices (uncommon)	• Blood or blood products or both • Skin or mucous membrane break by inoculation (for example, by needle sticks, cuts or scratches, ear piercing, tattooing, or contaminated drug paraphernalia) • Sexual contact • Infected asymptomatic carrier	• Blood or blood products or both • Sexual contact • Infected asymptomatic carrier	• Blood and blood products • Skin or mucous membrane break by inoculation (for example, by needle sticks, cuts or scratches, ear piercing, tattooing, or contaminated drug paraphernalia) • Sexual contact • Infected asymptomatic carrier • *Note:* HDV can occur only in the presence of HBV (active or chronic).
Incubation period			
• 2 to 6 weeks (average: 4 weeks); also the most contagious period	• 4 weeks to 6 months (average: 12 weeks) • Contagious as long as serum marker (surface antigen) appears • *Note:* Serum marker that remains detectable after 6 months indicates that the person is a carrier or has chronic HBV.	• 2 weeks to 6 months (average: 7 to 8 weeks)	• Occurring with HBV—1 to 6 months • In a chronic HBsAG carrier—1 to 4 months

continued

Comparing types of viral hepatitis — *continued*

HEPATITIS A (HAV)	HEPATITIS B (HBV)	HEPATITIS C (HCV)	HEPATITIS D (HDV)
Diagnostic tests			
• Anti-HAV IgM (hepatitis A antibodies) in serum indicates current infection; antibodies remaining after 4 to 6 weeks indicate immunity • Abnormal liver function tests (LFTs)	• HBsAg (hepatitis B surface antigen) in serum • HBeAg (hepatitis Be antigen) in serum — measures infectivity • Anti-HBc (hepatitis B core antibodies) in serum — diagnoses carrier state • Anti-HBsAg in serum — indicates HBV immunity • Abnormal LFTs • *Note:* HBsAg test has largely replaced Australian antigen test.	• No known diagnostic serum marker • Diagnosis made by ruling out other causes • Abnormal LFTs (specifically, fluctuating ALT, AST activity)	• Positive anti-HD during acute phase • IgM anti-HD indicates progressive HDV; distinguishes HDV from HBV carriers
Prophylaxis			
Immune globulin (IG) before or after exposure or both • Provides passive immunity for 2 to 3 months • Dosage: 0.02 ml/kg I.M. given to household and sexual contacts within 2 weeks of exposure	*HBV vaccine (before and after exposure)* • Provides active immunity • Dosage: 1 ml I.M. for adults; 0.5 ml I.M. for children under age 10 • Booster recommended after 5 years *HB immune globulin (HBIG) after exposure* • Provides passive immunity • Dosage: 0.06 ml/kg I.M.	*Immune globulin before or after exposure or both* • Provides passive immunity for 2 to 3 months • Dosage: 0.02 ml/kg I.M.	*HBV vaccine (before and after exposure)* • Provides active immunity • Dosage: 1 ml I.M. for adults; 0.5 ml I.M. for children under age 10 • Booster recommended after 5 years *HB immune globulin (HBIG) after exposure* • Provides passive immunity • Dosage: 0.06 ml/kg I.M.
High-risk individuals			
• Household members and visitors • Sexual partners	• Household members and visitors • Sexual partners • Dental, laboratory, and medical personnel • Multiple blood transfusion recipients • Prison inmates • I.V. drug abusers • Infants born to infected mothers	• Multiple blood transfusion recipients or recipient of large transfusion (as required by cardiopulmonary bypass) • Sexual partners • Dental, laboratory, and medical personnel (uncommon compared to HBV) • Blood product recipients	• I.V. drug abusers • Hemophiliacs • Hemodialysis patients • Sexual partners • Prison inmates

Other care measures

If the patient has viral hepatitis, teach him and his family how to prevent the spread of the disease. Emphasize the importance of thorough hand washing in all forms of viral hepatitis.

Inform the patient with hepatitis A that he must prevent contamination of food and water with fecal matter to prevent transmitting the virus to others. Give him a copy of the patient-teaching aid *Preventing the spread of hepatitis A,* page 245.

Inform the patient with hepatitis B, hepatitis C, or hepatitis D that he must prevent transmitting the virus by contamination with his blood or any body fluids (which may contain blood).

Hepatitis B prophylaxis

Tell your patient that prophylactic administration of hepatitis B immune globulin or hepatitis B vaccine can prevent or reduce the severity of hepatitis B. Review these guidelines:

Hepatitis B immune globulin
The patient should receive hepatitis B immune globulin (HBIG) soon after he's exposed to hepatitis B virus (HBV).

For *percutaneous exposure* (needle stick or human bite), he should receive HBIG at once. For *perinatal exposure,* the infant should receive HBIG within 12 hours of birth. After *sexual exposure,* the patient should receive HBIG within 14 days of contact. Tell him that he'll need a second dose if he tests HBsAG-positive for 3 months after initial detection.

Hepatitis B vaccine
The three vaccines that can be given before or after exposure to HBV include Heptavax-B and Recombivax-HB and Engerix-B.

The patient should receive *preexposure* prophylaxis in 3 doses. After an initial dose, the second is given in 1 month, and the final dose is given 6 months after the initial dose.

After *percutaneous exposure,* the patient should be vaccinated within 7 days of exposure, with a second dose in 1 month and a third dose 6 months after the initial dose.

For *perinatal exposure,* the infant requires vaccination within 12 hours of birth, with a second dose in 1 month and a third dose 6 months after the initial dose. (The initial dose can be given with HBIG, but at another site.)

Following *sexual exposure,* the patient should be vaccinated within 14 days of contact, with a second dose in 1 month and a third dose 6 months after the initial dose.

Give him a copy of the patient-teaching aid *Preventing the spread of hepatitis B, C, and D,* page 246.

Tell the patient that viral hepatitis is a reportable disease. This means that the doctor will notify the local public health department so that the occurrence can be recorded. An increase in the number of hepatitis cases reported in a particular area may alert public health officials to a potential sewage contamination of the water supply or to contamination of a common food source, such as a restaurant. As a result, the public health authorities may contact him to investigate the circumstances of his infection.

Stress the importance of continued medical care. Advise the patient to see the doctor again about 2 weeks after a diagnosis is made. At this time the doctor will determine if the patient's fluid intake is adequate and perform additional blood tests to evaluate liver function. After this, he'll need a follow-up appointment once a month for up to 6 months. Then if chronic hepatitis develops, the patient must visit the doctor at regular intervals to monitor the course of his disease.

Sources of information and support
American Hepatitis Association
30 E. 40th Street, Room 305, New York, N.Y. 10016
(212) 599-5070

American Liver Foundation
998 Pompton Avenue, Cedar Grove, N.J. 07009
(201) 857-2626

Further readings
Goodlad, J. "Understanding Hepatitis," *Nursing Times* 85(24):69-71, June 14-20, 1989.
Peicher, J., and Schiff, E.R. "Acute Viral Hepatitis," *Hospital Medicine* 24(6):23-26, 29-30, 32-33, June 1988.
Poss, J. "Hepatitis D Virus Infection," *Nurse Practitioner* 14(8):12-16, August 1989.
Stringer, B., and Walker, M. "Hepatitis," *Canadian Nurse* 85(8):38-40, September 1989.
"The Core of Hepatitis Testing," *Emergency Medicine* 21(10):33, 36, May 30, 1989.
"Update: Universal Precautions for Prevention of Transmission of Human Immunodeficiency Virus, Hepatitis B Virus, and Other Bloodborne Pathogens in Health Care Settings," *Journal of the American Medical Association* 260(4):462-65, July 22-29, 1988.
Williams, R. and Fagan, E. "Viral Hepatitis in Hospitals—A Clinical Overview," *Journal of Hospital Infections* 11(Supplement A):142-49, February 1989.

Preventing the spread of hepatitis A

Dear Patient:

The doctor has determined that you have hepatitis A, one of several types of hepatitis.

How you got hepatitis A
This type of hepatitis is spread when fecal material from an infected person contaminates food or water.

This can happen when an infected person handles food after using the bathroom and not washing his hands. Or it can happen when raw sewage contaminates food supplies or the water used to prepare your food.

Common sources of such contamination include infected restaurant workers, sewage leaks into a water supply, or raw shellfish from polluted waters. Shellfish harbor hepatitis A because their beds can become contaminated with raw sewage, and they concentrate the virus in their bodies.

How you can infect others
When you have a bowel movement, some of the hepatitis A virus will pass out of your body into your stool. This infected fecal matter will contaminate any food or water it comes in contact with. In turn, anyone who eats or drinks the contaminated food or water can develop hepatitis A.

Precautions in the hospital
While you're in the hospital, you'll be placed on *enteric precautions.* This means you'll have a warning sign on your door, and your chart will have a special label. These warnings tell health care workers to wear gowns and gloves when they handle items that your stools may have soiled, such as hospital gowns or bed linens.

Precautions at home
When you go home from the hospital, observe the following precautions:
● Wash your hands thoroughly after every bowel movement.
● Wash your hands before handling food or preparing meals.
● Don't share food, eating utensils, or toothbrushes.

Contagious for how long?
Once you develop jaundice—a yellowish discoloration of the skin and the whites of the eyes—you're no longer contagious. If hepatitis A develops in family members or friends after this, they probably didn't get it from you. Instead, both of you may have been exposed to the same virus source.

Preventing hepatitis A after exposure
Family members and others with whom you have close physical contact (such as sexual partners) may already be infected with the virus by the time your hepatitis is diagnosed. These people should receive immune globulin (IG). IG may prevent hepatitis A. Or, if an attack of hepatitis A occurs, IG may make the attack milder.

PATIENT-TEACHING AID

Preventing the spread of hepatitis B, C, and D

Dear Patient:

The doctor has determined that you have hepatitis B, C, or D.

How you got hepatitis
These forms of hepatitis are spread by contact with the blood of an infected person.

How you can infect others
The hepatitis virus is present in your blood and in any of your body fluids that contain visible blood. If any of your blood enters another person's bloodstream (during a blood transfusion, for example), that person can catch hepatitis from you.

If your blood or body fluids come in contact with the mucous membranes of another person's mouth, vagina, or rectum, that person can catch hepatitis from you.

If your blood or body fluids come in contact with a break in another person's skin, such as a cut or rash, that person can also catch hepatitis from you.

Precautions in the hospital
While you're in the hospital, you'll be placed on *universal precautions*. This means you'll have a sign on your door and a special label on your chart.

Universal precautions are warnings that alert health care workers to wear gloves, gowns, masks, and protective eyewear when handling your blood or body fluids or items that may have come in contact with them.

Precautions at home
Observe the following precautions:
- Wash your hands thoroughly and frequently.
- Don't share food, eating utensils, or toothbrushes.
- If you inject drugs, don't share the needle with anyone.
- Because skin forms a natural barrier against the hepatitis virus, try not to cut or injure yourself.
- Don't have sex with anyone.
- Don't donate blood.

Contagious for how long?
If you have hepatitis B or hepatitis D, observe all of the precautions above until the doctor determines that your blood is free of a viral protein known as hepatitis B surface antigen (HBsAg). The doctor can detect this by a blood test.

If you have hepatitis C, no blood test can tell when you are no longer contagious. Observe the precautions outlined above until the doctor says you can safely stop. You may need to do this for as long as 6 months after infection.

Preventing hepatitis after exposure
Anyone who may have been exposed to your blood or body fluids should receive immune globulin (IG), hepatitis B immune globulin (HBIG), or the hepatitis B vaccine. This includes sex partners and anyone who has shared a needle with you. IG, HBIG, or vaccination may prevent hepatitis or lessen its severity.

Cholelithiasis

About 25 million Americans (mostly women) have cholelithiasis, or gallstones, making it the most common biliary tract disorder in the United States. However, for most patients, you'll need to teach about this disorder from "scratch." Why? Despite its prevalence, few patients know much about its causes or its treatments. Even fewer understand how the gallbladder functions. Most express surprise that untreated gallstones can be life-threatening.

What topics will you teach the patient? And where will you begin? Start with the basics—the anatomy and physiology of the biliary system and how gallstones develop. Review signs and symptoms (including biliary colic), risk factors (such as obesity), and possible complications (for example, cholecystitis). Prepare the patient for various diagnostic tests to detect and confirm the disorder, and discuss medications, such as analgesics, antibiotics, and dissolution agents. Finally, cover nonsurgical and surgical procedures to remove the stones or, if necessary, the gallbladder (for more information see *Teaching the patient with acute cholelithiasis,* page 248).

Discuss the disorder

Inform the patient that cholelithiasis refers to stones, or calculi, in the gallbladder. Gallstones reflect a change in bile components. They signal that, for various reasons, the gallbladder has become sluggish, giving cholesterol, calcium bilirubinate, or a mixture of cholesterol and bilirubin pigment a chance to settle and crystallize. Usually pea-sized, the resultant stone can be as tiny as a pinhead or as large as a hen's egg. To better explain how and where gallstones occur, review biliary structures and functions (for more information, see *How the biliary system works,* page 249).

What causes gallstones? Although no one knows for sure, certain contributing factors set the stage for stone formation. At highest risk for cholelithiasis are women—especially obese women over age 40 who've had several pregnancies. Pregnancy causes increased abdominal pressure, which leads to bile flow stasis and subsequent stone formation. Besides, hormonal changes during pregnancy may delay gallbladder emptying, which may also promote stasis. Increased cholesterol levels during the third trimester contribute as well. Other risk factors associated with gallbladder sluggishness include oral contraceptive use, diabetes mellitus, celiac disease, cirrhosis of the liver, pancreatitis, and heredity.

Review the signs and symptoms of cholelithiasis. Explain that about half of all patients are asymptomatic and may not realize

Marlene Ciranowicz, RN, MSN, CDE, and **Joanne Lavin, RN, EdD,** wrote this chapter. Ms. Ciranowicz is an independent nurse consultant in Dresher, Pa. Ms. Lavin is assistant professor of nursing at Kingsborough Community College, Brooklyn, N.Y.

CHECKLIST

Teaching topics in cholelithiasis

☐ Biliary system anatomy and physiology
☐ How gallstones develop
☐ Risk factors for cholelithiasis, including obesity, age, and multiple pregnancies
☐ Signs and symptoms of biliary colic, such as pain, belching, and nausea
☐ Cholecystitis and other complications
☐ Diagnostic tests: biliary ultrasonography, oral cholecystography, endoscopic retrograde cholangiopancreatography (ERCP), and percutaneous transhepatic cholangiography
☐ Drug therapy, including analgesic and antibiotic agents, oral dissolution drugs, and topical solvents
☐ Procedures to remove gallstones, including ERCP, endoscopic sphincterotomy, and extracorporeal shock wave lithotripsy
☐ Surgery, such as cholecystectomy, cholecystostomy, choledochostomy, and laparoscopic cholecystectomy
☐ How to care for a T tube
☐ Importance of follow-up care to detect recurrent gallstones

Teaching the patient with acute cholelithiasis

If anxiety about acute cholelithiasis has caused your patient to postpone medical attention, you may wonder what teaching approach will quiet her fears and ensure her compliance with recommended treatment. To find out how best to accomplish your goals, refer to a standard teaching plan to organize your information. Then adjust the plan to fit your patient's unique needs. Here's how.

What will your assessment reveal?
Mindy Murphy, a widowed, 46-year-old interior designer with three sons, has been hospitalized after a third episode of biliary colic in 6 months. She's jaundiced and dehydrated. If tests confirm gallstones, she's agreed to treatment.

Ms. Murphy's records show that she was scheduled for tests 3 months ago, but she cancelled them. When you ask her why, she confesses, "I felt fine then and hated the thought of losing time in the hospital. And I didn't have anyone to take care of the boys. Besides, I was scared. I just hate hospitals."

When you ask Ms. Murphy what she knows about gallbladder disease, she says, "I really don't want to know—I get nervous just thinking about it."

What does Ms. Murphy need to know?
To help relieve Ms. Murphy's anxiety, the doctor asks you to teach her about scheduled tests and treatments. As a start, compare what she already knows about gallstones with the content of a standard teaching plan, which includes:
• biliary functions and how gallstones form
• signs and symptoms and risk factors for cholelithiasis
• potential complications of cholelithiasis
• diagnostic procedures, such as biliary ultrasonography, oral cholecystography, endoscopic retrograde cholangiopancreatography (ERCP), and percutaneous transhepatic cholangiography
• nonsurgical treatments, including pain relief, antibiotic medications, dissolution therapy, ERCP, lithotripsy, and endoscopic sphincterotomy
• surgical treatments—standard cholecystectomy and laparoscopic cholecystectomy, for example
• T-tube management and self-care, as needed.

From talking to Ms. Murphy, you realize that she knows nothing about what gallstones are and how they form. You need to cover all the topics in the standard teaching plan. First, help her understand that gallstones usually don't disappear without treatment—by nonsurgical measures or surgery.

After describing how gallstones form, review possible complications of untreated gallstones. Then point out the benefits of treatment, but emphasize that she must first cooperate with diagnostic tests. Follow this with a description of test procedures and their purposes. Be sure to offer her every opportunity to express her feelings and fears.

What learning outcomes will you choose?
Together, you compile a list of learning outcomes based on learning needs. Ms. Murphy will be able to:

```
-describe simply how the biliary system works and
how gallstones form
-list the signs and symptoms and risk factors of
cholelithiasis
-describe ordered diagnostic tests and their purposes
-describe the nonsurgical or surgical procedure the
doctor recommends to remove gallstones
-demonstrate how to care for a T tube, if necessary.
```

What teaching tools and techniques will you select?
What teaching tools and techniques will be effective to help Ms. Murphy avoid the pain of biliary colic? You decide to use *discussion and explanation* along with *visual aids* (anatomic diagrams and videotapes) to point out how treatment can increase long-term comfort.

Start with a short description of the biliary system, using pictures or a model of the gallbladder, common bile duct, and liver. Next, show her how gallstones form, where they're located, and what signs and symptoms result when the stones obstruct biliary structures.

Then explain the tests that the doctor has ordered and nonsurgical and surgical procedures and posttreatment care. As appropriate, provide *demonstrations* of postoperative self-care procedures. Schedule plenty of time for Ms. Murphy's questions. Help her retain the information by scheduling your teaching in several short sessions and then reinforcing these sessions with *printed materials,* such as books and pamphlets, for Ms. Murphy to read on her own.

How will you evaluate your teaching?
Were you an effective teacher? Gauge your success—and Ms. Murphy's understanding of cholelithiasis and her degree of motivation—with a *question-and-answer* session. For example, once the doctor confirms the diagnosis and recommends a treatment, quiz Ms. Murphy about the treatment. If she's having surgery and will go home with a T tube in place, use *direct observation* to assess her knowledge of incision and tube care. If she seems knowledgeable and is more cooperative with treatment and less anxious about surgery, you've successfully achieved your learning outcomes.

How the biliary system works

To help your patient understand how and why gallstones interfere with her digestion, describe the biliary system and its functions. Use this illustration to point out common gallstone sites and to reinforce your discussion.

The role of bile
Inform your patient that bile forms in the liver. A greenish-yellow fluid, bile helps the digestive system to break down fats and to absorb fats and fat-soluble vitamins. Bile is concentrated and stored in the gallbladder, a muscular, membranous, pear-sized sac situated just under the liver.

Where bile travels
To reach the gallbladder, bile flows from the liver through the hepatic and cystic ducts. These ducts join to form the common bile duct that connects the gallbladder and the liver.

The common bile duct joins the pancreatic duct, which opens into the duodenum (the beginning of the small intestine). Bile flow into the duodenum is controlled by sphincter muscles. When these sphincters close, bile returns to the gallbladder for storage.

How gallstones impede bile flow
When food enters the duodenum, a hormone stimulates the gallbladder to contract and release stored bile into the common bile duct. At the same time, the pancreas secretes juices, which join the bile as it flows to the duodenum. Both substances aid digestion. Gallstones that form and lodge in biliary structures (either ducts or organs) block bile flow and interfere with digestion.

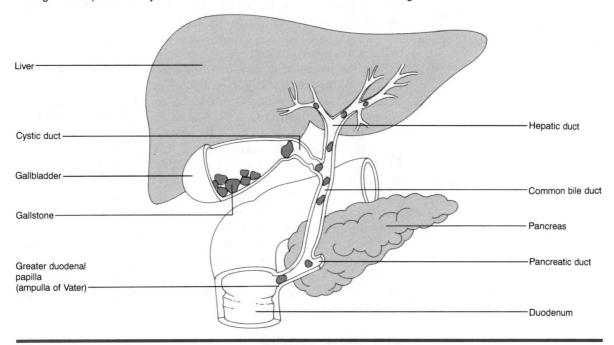

Liver

Cystic duct

Gallbladder

Gallstone

Greater duodenal papilla (ampulla of Vater)

Hepatic duct

Common bile duct

Pancreas

Pancreatic duct

Duodenum

they have gallstones until an X-ray or ultrasonography performed for other reasons detects them. The other half suffer the severe, episodic pain of acute cholelithiasis (also called biliary colic or gallbladder attack). Severe epigastric or right upper quadrant pain commonly radiates to the back and shoulders and lasts up to several hours. Walking or changing position offers no relief. The pain results from a stone lodged in the gallbladder's neck or in the cystic duct. The pain diminishes when the stone dislodges and either slips back into the gallbladder or passes into the intestine. The patient may also experience belching, nausea, vomiting and, in a severe attack, jaundice. After an attack, she usually feels well except for residual tenderness.

Complications

Emphasize that untreated gallstones can cause serious, life-threatening complications. When a gallstone becomes impacted in the cystic duct, acute cholecystitis (inflammation of the gallbladder) can occur, causing prolonged obstruction, inflammation of the gallbladder wall, and risk of infection. One in every ten patients with gallstones develops choledocholithiasis (gallstones in the common bile duct). This occurs when stones that pass out of the gallbladder lodge in the hepatic and common bile ducts, obstructing bile flow into the duodenum. Such an obstruction can result in abscess, necrosis, perforation, and generalized peritonitis.

Describe the diagnostic workup

Tell the patient that several diagnostic studies can detect gallstones. The most commonly performed tests are biliary ultrasonography and oral cholecystography. If these tests fail to reveal gallstones despite symptoms, the doctor may order endoscopic retrograde cholangiopancreatography (ERCP) or percutaneous transhepatic cholangiography (PTC). Also routine laboratory tests may be done to support the diagnosis.

Biliary ultrasonography

Inform the patient that ultrasonography uses sound waves to evaluate the gallbladder and biliary ducts for gallstones. The test takes between 15 and 30 minutes. Advise her to eat a fat-free meal in the evening and then to fast for at least 8 hours before the test.

Tell the patient that during the test she'll lie on an examination table in a slightly darkened room. A technician will apply a conductive gel or oil to the abdominal area. Then the patient may receive an injection of sincalide (a choleretic agent) to stimulate gallbladder contractions. Instruct her to report abdominal cramping, nausea, dizziness, sweating, or flushing. The technician will move a transducer across the gallbladder area.

Explain that the test itself causes no pain. Tell the patient to lie still, relax, breathe normally, and remain quiet because movement will distort the results (the sonogram) and prolong the test. The technician may direct her to hold her breath or inhale deeply. After the test, she may resume her normal diet and activities.

Oral cholecystography

Explain that this test examines the gallbladder through X-rays taken after the patient ingests a contrast medium. The day before the test, the patient will eat a low-fat breakfast and lunch and a fat-free dinner. After dinner, he can have only water and any ordered drug regimen. A few hours after dinner, he'll take as many as 12 tablets, one at a time, at 5-minute intervals. Tell him to report any adverse effects from the tablets: diarrhea, nausea, vomiting, abdominal cramps, or dysuria. The morning before the test he'll give himself an enema. Both the tablets and the enema help outline the gallbladder on the X-ray film.

Inform the patient that during the test he'll lie supine on an X-ray table while films are taken of his gallbladder. After the test, he should drink plenty of fluids to help eliminate the dyelike substance in the tablets from his body.

Diagnostic ERCP

Inform the patient that this procedure can be used both diagnostically and therapeutically. ERCP uses endoscopically administered contrast medium and X-ray films to assess the gallbladder and biliary system for calculi and other abnormalities. The doctor will pass a flexible endoscope through the mouth to the intestine. Describe test preparations and procedures. As needed, provide the teaching aid *Preparing for ERCP,* page 260.

Percutaneous transhepatic cholangiography

Tell the patient that this 30-minute test examines the biliary ducts after an injection of a dyelike contrast medium. She shouldn't eat or drink anything for 8 hours before the procedure but should continue with any prescribed drug regimen. She'll be awake during the test and secured to an X-ray table. The procedure may produce some discomfort, but she'll receive medication to help her relax.

Review how the patient's abdomen will be cleaned and then covered with a sterile drape before the doctor injects the area with a local anesthetic. Mention that the injection will sting briefly. Next, the doctor will inject a contrast medium directly into the liver. (If the patient undergoes PTC postoperatively, the dye will be injected through a T tube inserted into the common bile duct.) Advise the patient to breathe out and then hold her breath during the injection. Warn her that she may sense pressure and right upper back discomfort. Tell her to report any adverse effects immediately, including dizziness, headache, hives, nausea, and vomiting. Instruct her to lie still, relax, breathe normally, and remain quiet as X-ray films are taken of the biliary ducts.

After the test, the nurse will monitor the patient's temperature, pulse rate, and breathing until these vital signs are stable. Advise her that she must lie in bed on her right side for at least 6 hours. Afterward, she may resume her usual diet and activities.

Laboratory tests

Teach the patient that she'll have laboratory tests to help evaluate biliary obstruction. Blood and urine samples will be studied to assess serum and urine bilirubin, total serum cholesterol, cholesterol ester, plasma phospholipid, and serum alkaline phosphatase levels; activated partial thromboplastin time; and white blood cell count. Explain any test preparation, such as fasting.

Teach about treatments

Tell the patient that treatment for cholelithiasis depends on her signs and symptoms. If she's asymptomatic, she doesn't require treatment. If she's had at least one gallbladder attack and test results confirm gallstones, the doctor may recommend their removal. The removal procedure depends on the gallstones' location, their size and number, and potential or confirmed complications, such as acute cholecystitis or choledocholithiasis.

Also explain that medications may be prescribed. If the patient asks whether a special diet can relieve her symptoms, inform her that clinical findings no longer validate diet therapy (see *Questions patients ask about treating gallstones*).

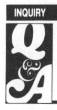

INQUIRY

Questions patients ask about treating gallstones

I just found out that I have gallstones. Will a fat-free diet cure me?
No—this is a common misconception. Your gallstones weren't caused by fatty foods, and a special diet won't make them disappear. They occur when the liver secretes bile that's supersaturated with cholesterol. When the bile reaches the gallbladder—where it's stored—the cholesterol precipitates, forming stones.

Keep in mind, though, that eating fatty foods can cause a gallbladder attack in a person with gallstones. That's because dietary fat triggers a hormone that stimulates gallbladder contractions, forcing stored bile into the duodenum—the opening to the small intestine. If stones block the bile flow, you may experience sudden, severe abdominal pain, nausea, and vomiting.

Suppose the doctor wants to remove my gallbladder. How can I get along without it if it stores bile?
The gallbladder functions to store bile until it's needed in the small intestine to help digest fats. After gallbladder removal, the liver delivers bile directly to the small intestine. So the gallbladder is one of the few organs you can live without.

Once my gallbladder is removed, can I eat what I like—even french fries?
Yes. But not too many fats at first. Follow a low-fat diet for the first few weeks after surgery; then you may increase fats gradually up to 30% of your daily caloric intake. As your body adjusts to not having a gallbladder and as bile flow to the intestine increases, so will your ability to digest fats.

Medication

Review medications to treat gallstones, including analgesics to relieve pain, antibiotics to prevent infections, and drugs to dissolve the stones.

Analgesics. The doctor may prescribe a narcotic analgesic, such as meperidine (Demerol), for the patient with episodic biliary colic and for the hospitalized patient with gallstones complicated by acute cholecystitis. Reassure the patient that pain and inflammation usually subside in 2 to 7 days.

Antibiotics. For the patient with gallstones and acute cholecystitis, the doctor may prescribe a broad-spectrum antibiotic, such as tetracycline, to prevent infection, especially if the patient is elderly, has gallstones in the common bile duct, or has diabetes mellitus or another serious disorder.

Oral dissolution agents. If the patient's gallstones are noncalcified and contain mainly cholesterol, the doctor may recommend oral dissolution therapy. Explain that the bile salts chenodiol (Chenix) and ursodiol (Actigall), alone or in combination, can shrink or dissolve existing gallstones and prevent new formations. She'll take these drugs for about 2 years. During this time, her progress will be monitored by ultrasonography. Caution her that about half of all patients whose stones dissolve completely have a recurrence in 5 to 7 years and require repeat bile salt therapy.

Instruct the patient on how to take these drugs. Because the doctor bases the dosage on body weight, tell the patient to alert the doctor to significant weight gain or loss. Advise her to take the drug with food or milk for best results. If she forgets to take a dose, tell her to take the dose as soon as she remembers. If it's almost time for the next dose, however, she should wait and resume her normal schedule. Direct her not to take a double dose. Urge her to keep scheduled appointments for laboratory tests to monitor how the therapy affects her liver function.

Finally, tell the patient to report these adverse reactions to the doctor immediately: diarrhea and severe abdominal pain (especially in the right upper quadrant), nausea, and vomiting.

Topical solvents. If the doctor prescribes the topical solvent methyl tert-butyl ether (MTBE), explain that this drug can dissolve any size or number of cholesterol stones within hours; however, the stones may recur later. Point out that this solvent must be instilled through a catheter inserted either into the abdomen or through the nose to the hepatic duct, depending on the gallstones' location. Explain that the procedure usually requires a local anesthetic and takes place in the hospital outpatient department. Patient preparation depends on the doctor's approach.

For gallstones in the gallbladder, the doctor may insert a small catheter through the right upper abdomen. He'll use fluoroscopy to guide the catheter into the gallbladder and X-rays to verify its placement. Using a syringe, he'll pump the solvent in and out of the gallbladder until fluoroscopy shows that the stones are completely dissolved. The process may take several hours. Afterward, he'll remove the catheter and place a small dressing over the insertion site.

For gallstones in the hepatic duct, the doctor may insert an endoscope nasally, thread a nasobiliary catheter through it, and verify its placement in the hepatic duct with X-rays. Then he'll instill MTBE through the catheter. Every 30 minutes, he'll aspirate the drug with a syringe, gradually increasing the dose. After 4 hours of this treatment, a second X-ray will confirm whether MTBE has dissolved the stones. When the stones have dissolved, the doctor will remove the endoscope and catheter.

If the doctor instills the topical solvent monooctanoin (Moctanin) immediately after a cholecystectomy to dissolve retained stones, he'll infuse the drug by nasobiliary tube or through a small T tube inserted through an abdominal incision into the common bile duct. The solvent may infuse continuously up to 3 weeks until the stones dissolve. Tell the patient that she'll remain hospitalized during this time. Instruct her to report any abdominal pain, diarrhea, or nausea. When an X-ray shows that the gallstones have dissolved, the doctor will remove the tube.

Procedures

Besides drug therapy to dissolve gallbladder stones, several nonsurgical procedures, such as ERCP, endoscopic sphincterotomy, and extracorporeal shock wave lithotripsy (ESWL), may be used to remove them.

Therapeutic ERCP. During diagnostic ERCP, if the doctor detects gallstones in the common bile duct, he may attempt to remove them at the same time. He'll insert a basketlike device via the endoscope to secure and retrieve them. Reassure the patient that she'll be sedated so she won't experience any discomfort.

Endoscopic sphincterotomy. If the doctor schedules this procedure, explain that he'll use an endoscope and special devices to remove gallstones in the common bile duct. Tell the patient to fast from midnight on before the procedure. She can expect medication to relax her and insertion of an I.V. line in her hand or arm to administer medication. Then a local anesthetic will be sprayed in her throat before an endoscope is inserted. During the procedure, she'll assume various positions to help advance the endoscope for proper placement (for more information, see *Two endoscopic techniques for removing calculi,* page 254).

Tell the patient that afterward her vital signs will be monitored until they're stable. She can eat and drink when her gag reflex returns, but she'll remain in bed for 6 to 8 hours (or overnight in the hospital). Warn her that she'll have a sore throat for several days and may have abdominal discomfort for 1 or 2 weeks. The doctor will prescribe an analgesic to relieve pain.

Extracorporeal shock wave lithotripsy. A noninvasive, painless procedure, ESWL uses high-energy shock waves to shatter gallstones, thereby allowing them to be eliminated naturally. The procedure works best for patients with mild to moderate symptoms and only a few small-diameter stones comprised mainly of cholesterol. Explain that ESWL takes 30 to 60 minutes. Show the patient the lithotriptor or at least a picture of the machine.

Explain that immediately before ESWL the doctor will locate the stones precisely by ultrasonography. To locate stones in the common bile duct, he'll use a contrast medium and X-ray images.

Two endoscopic techniques for removing calculi

If your patient will have an endoscopic procedure to remove his gallstones, explain that the doctor will pass a fiber-optic tube (an endoscope) along the GI tract through the stomach to the duodenum at the ampulla (or papilla) of Vater.

In the technique known as endoscopic sphincterotomy, the doctor advances a cutting wire (called a papillotome) through the endoscope until the device reaches the duodenal papilla. He makes an incision at this site to widen the papilla, allowing the stone to pass into the duodenum and be expelled naturally.

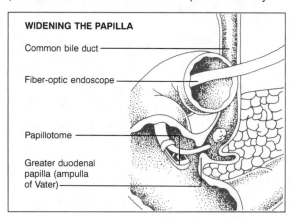

WIDENING THE PAPILLA

Common bile duct

Fiber-optic endoscope

Papillotome

Greater duodenal papilla (ampulla of Vater)

If sphincterotomy fails to advance the stone, the doctor may take another approach. He may insert a Dormier basket through the endoscope and scoop up the stone to remove it.

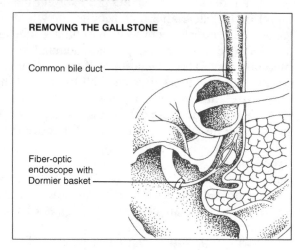

REMOVING THE GALLSTONE

Common bile duct

Fiber-optic endoscope with Dormier basket

If this technique also fails, the doctor may crush the stones mechanically with an accessory device. Afterward, he'll verify stone removal or passage with an X-ray study.

The patient may receive the contrast medium orally, or she may receive it through a nasobiliary catheter or a percutaneous transhepatic catheter. If she'll have a nasobiliary catheter, the doctor will spray the patient's throat with an anesthetic before insertion to prevent gagging. For percutaneous transhepatic catheter administration, tell the patient that she'll lie on her left side, and the doctor will anesthetize her right side. Then he'll insert a rigid catheter through the skin and into the common bile duct.

Next, the patient will have an I.V. line inserted and electrocardiography electrodes attached. She'll receive I.V. narcotics or, occasionally, a general anesthetic.

The patient will be positioned in a semireclining position on the machine's hydraulic stretcher. Then she'll be lowered into the water tank and her position adjusted so that the shock-wave generator focuses directly on the gallstones. Or she'll lie with a water-filled cushion pressed against the area over the gallstones. Next, the lithotriptor will discharge serial shock waves through the water or the cushion to shatter the stones without damaging surrounding tissue. The doctor will synchronize the shock waves with the patient's heart rhythm to prevent dysrhythmias. Tell the patient that her heart activity will be monitored continuously throughout the procedure. Ultrasonic or fluoroscopic devices will monitor the process until the gallstones disintegrate—usually in 1 to 2 hours.

Inform the patient that she won't feel pain but may feel a

fluttering sensation or mild blows. If a catheter has been inserted, the doctor may also inject monooctanoin through the catheter to decrease the stone's size.

After ESWL, tell the patient that her vital signs will be monitored, and she can expect to have liver function studies to make sure her liver sustained no damage from the shock waves. Instruct her to report posttreatment abdominal pain, fever, nausea, or vomiting without delay. The doctor may order narcotic analgesics to relieve pain if stone fragments congest the bile ducts and cause biliary colic. The patient also may require oral bile salt therapy for several months to ensure gallbladder and bile duct patency. However, explain that in the days immediately after ESWL, most of the stones should travel from the gallbladder to the intestine, and she'll excrete them naturally.

Because incompletely pulverized stones can lodge in the biliary tract or pancreas or develop into new calculi, urge the patient to keep scheduled follow-up appointments.

Surgery
When nonsurgical treatments fail or if a complication, such as cholecystitis, develops, surgery may be necessary. Standard gallbladder surgeries include cholecystectomy (the most common), cholecystostomy, and choledochostomy (for more information, see *Reviewing standard gallbladder surgeries,* page 256). Or a relatively new procedure called laparoscopic cholecystectomy may be performed.

Standard gallbladder surgeries. Teach the patient that most gallbladder operations require a general anesthetic before surgery and 1 week recovery time in the hospital. She should consume only clear liquids the day before surgery and nothing after midnight before the operation.

Forewarn the patient that she'll have a nasogastric (NG) tube in place for 1 or 2 days after surgery and a drain at the incision site for 3 to 5 days. She may also have a T tube inserted in the common bile duct to drain excess bile and allow removal of retained stones. If appropriate, explain that the T tube may remain in place for up to 2 weeks, depending on the type of surgery, and that she may be discharged with the tube. Teach her how to perform coughing and deep-breathing exercises to prevent postoperative atelectasis, which can lead to pneumonia. Explain that she can ask for an analgesic before performing these exercises to relieve discomfort.

Finally, prepare the patient for self-care after discharge. If she's going home with a T tube in place, teach her how to perform meticulous tube care. Also teach her how to care for her incision, and direct her to report any signs of infection, such as redness, tenderness, or drainage at the incision site. Also urge her to learn and report the following signs of biliary obstruction: fever, jaundice, pruritus, pain, dark urine, and clay-colored stools. Be sure to provide a copy of the patient-teaching aid *How to care for your T tube,* pages 258 and 259.

Laparoscopic cholecystectomy. Inform the patient that the surgeon may remove her gallbladder through one of four small, slit-

Reviewing standard gallbladder surgeries

If your patient's scheduled for a cholecystectomy or other standard gallbladder surgery, she'll want to know what to expect from the operation itself. Use the information below to review your patient's operation with her.

Cholecystectomy
Explain that this procedure, performed under general anesthesia, removes the gallbladder. The surgeon makes a right subcostal or paramedial incision. Then he isolates the gallbladder from the surrounding organs. After identifying biliary tract structures, he uses X-ray images or ultrasonography to precisely locate the gallstones. Then he inserts a tubular optical instrument called a choledochoscope through the incision to visualize the bile ducts. Through the choledochoscope, he introduces a balloon-tipped catheter to clear the ducts of stones.

After removing the stones, the surgeon ligates and divides the cystic duct and artery and removes the entire gallbladder.

Tell the patient that the surgeon may insert a T tube into the common bile duct. This decompresses the biliary tree and prevents bile peritonitis during healing. He may also insert a drain into the biliary ducts.

Cholecystostomy
In this operation, performed under local anesthesia, the surgeon makes an abdominal incision and inserts a laparoscopic tube with a suctioning apparatus (called a trocar) into the gallbladder. He decompresses the gallbladder and aspirates its contents. Using forceps, he removes any retained gallstones and then inserts a drain.

Choledochostomy
During this procedure, the surgeon incises the common bile duct for exploration and removal of stones. Instead of inserting a T tube, he usually irrigates the duct and closes the incision with sutures.

CHOLECYSTECTOMY

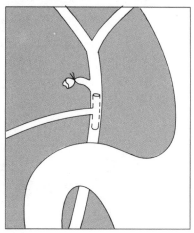

CHOLECYSTOSTOMY

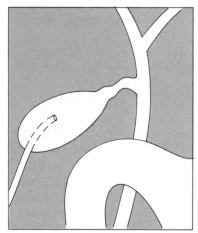

CHOLEDOCHOSTOMY

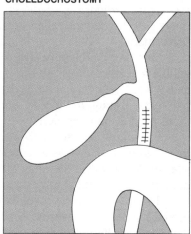

like abdominal incisions. The surgery takes about 90 minutes and requires a general anesthetic. Usually, fewer complications occur following this operation than traditional gallbladder surgery. Tell the patient that she'll probably be admitted to the hospital on the day of surgery and discharged the next day. Instruct her to fast after midnight before surgery. Prepare her for insertion of a urinary catheter and an NG tube just before surgery.

Describe how the surgeon will begin the operation with a small incision above the navel. He'll insert an instrument to inflate the abdominal cavity with carbon dioxide (to improve visibility). Then he'll introduce a narrow, flexible instrument called a laparoscope, which holds a tiny camera. Just below the ribs, he'll make two more incisions to insert a pair of grasping forceps. A fourth incision to the right of the midsection allows insertion of laser equipment. Next, he'll excise the gallbladder with a laser beam and use the forceps to deliver the now-detached gallbladder through one of the incisions. Then he'll remove the laparoscope, suture the incisions, and apply dressings.

Advise the patient that she may experience minor discomfort at the laparoscopic insertion site and mild shoulder pain for up to 1 week—either from diaphragmatic irritation caused by abdominal stretching or from residual carbon dioxide. Reassure her that the doctor will prescribe pain medication. She can resume her normal diet in 24 hours and activities in 48 to 72 hours. Teach her to care for her incisions, and instruct her to report signs of infection to her doctor. Urge her to keep follow-up appointments.

Other care measures

Inform the nonsurgical patient that repeated episodes of biliary colic caused by gallstones may require hospitalization, NG tube insertion, and I.V. therapy for hydration and antibiotic administration. Explain that treatment to remove the stones usually begins soon after the episode subsides.

Encourage the patient to keep all follow-up appointments and to take medications as directed in hopes of avoiding recurrent biliary colic and complications.

Further readings

Adwers, J.R. "Clinical Trials of Gallstone Lithotripsy," *Hospital Practice* 24(7):83-90, July 15, 1989.

Cerrato, P.L. "Would a New Diet Help Your Gallstone Patient?" *RN* 52(7):59-61, July 1989.

Gauwitz, D.F. "Endoscopic Cholecystectomy: The Patient-Friendly Alternative," *Nursing90* 20(12):58-59, December 1990.

Holland, P., et al. "Biliary Lithotripsy: Nonsurgical Treatment of Gallstones," *SGA Journal* 11(3):158-62, Winter 1989.

Jermier, B.J., and Treloar, D.M. "Bringing Your Patient Through Gallbladder Surgery," *RN* 49(11):18-26, November 1986.

Marta, M.R. "Endoscopic Retrograde Cholangiopancreatography: Its Role in Diagnosis and Treatment," *Focus Critical Care* 14(5):62-63, October 1987.

O'Reilly, M., and Mulry, K. "Cholelithotripsy: An Option for Treating Cholelithiasis," *AORN Journal* 49(6):1520-21, 1523-24, 1526-27+, June 1989.

Ransohoff, D.F., et al. "What's New in the Blitz on Gallstones?" *Patient Care* 22(3):111-14, 117-19, 122-24+, February 15, 1988.

Roberts, A. "Senior Systems: Gallstones...Jaundice in the Elderly Patient," Part 19. *Nursing Times* 83(43):55-58, October 28-November 4, 1987.

Willis, D.A., et al. "Gallstones—Alternatives to Surgery," *RN* 53(4):44-51, April 1990.

PATIENT-TEACHING AID

How to care for your T tube

Dear Patient:

Here are some instructions for taking care of your T tube at home. You'll have this tube for 10 to 14 days. During that time, it will drain excess bile so that your incision will heal faster. The tube will also allow passage of any retained gallstones.

Caring for your T tube isn't difficult, but it does take time and planning. Set aside about 20 uninterrupted minutes a day to empty your drainage bag and care for your incision. To help prevent infection and promote healing, carefully follow these directions.

Gathering your supplies
First, assemble these supplies on a table or countertop: a large measuring container, toilet paper, soap, a clean towel, a paper bag, a sterile paper cloth, five sterile 4-inch × 4-inch gauze pads, alcohol, normal saline solution, hydrogen peroxide, povidone-iodine solution, sterile gloves, povidone-iodine ointment, scissors, and adhesive tape.

Emptying the drainage bag
Empty your drainage bag at about the same time each day, or when it's two-thirds full. First, place the large measuring container within easy reach.

1 Sit on a chair, and remove the Velcro belt that secures the drainage bag and connecting tubing to your abdomen. Uncoil the tubing, and position the spout at the bottom of the drainage bag over the measuring container. Don't pull on the connecting tubing, and don't place too much tension on it—you may dislodge the T tube.

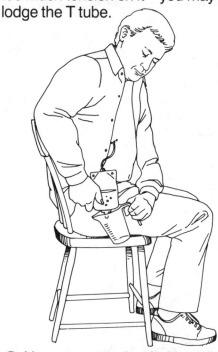

2 Now, to empty the drainage bag, release the clamp on the drainage spout, so that the bile flows freely into the measuring container. When the bag is empty, clean the drainage spout with toilet paper. To reseal the drainage bag, close the clamp.

3 Gently coil the connecting tubing. Then position the drainage bag and tubing *below* the incision site. Secure the bag and tubing with the Velcro belt. *Never* place the drainage bag and connecting tubing higher than your incision. This could cause the draining bile to back up into the common bile duct.

continued

How to care for your T tube — *continued*

4 Finally, note the amount, color, and odor of drainage. Contact your doctor if you notice significant increases or decreases in the amount of drainage or any changes in the color or odor. These may signal complications, such as infection or T-tube obstruction.

Caring for your incision

After you empty and resecure your drainage bag, you're ready to clean and redress the incision site. Just follow these steps:

1 Wash your hands with soap and water and dry them with a fresh, clean towel. Carefully remove the soiled dressing and discard it in the paper bag. Then wash and dry your hands again.

2 Open the package containing the sterile paper cloth. Unfold the cloth, and spread it on a table or countertop. Don't touch the top surface of the cloth.

3 Open the five sterile gauze pads, and drop them onto the sterile cloth.

4 Open the packets of alcohol, normal saline solution, hydrogen peroxide, and povidone-iodine solution, and place them on the table.

5 Put on the sterile gloves. Then pick up a sterile gauze pad with your dominant hand (your "sterile" hand).

6 Pick up the saline solution with your other hand and thoroughly soak the gauze pad.

7 Clean the incision area with the soaked pad. *Wipe outward away from the tube* in a 3-inch circular area.

Repeat this with the hydrogen peroxide and the povidone-iodine solution, again wiping outward. Use a clean pad.

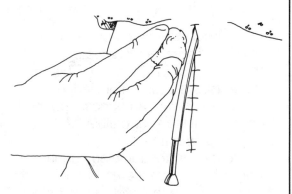

8 Now, soak a clean gauze pad with alcohol, and use it to wipe the first 6 inches of the tube. Start at the incision and wipe toward the drainage bag.

9 Apply a nickel-sized drop of povidone-iodine ointment over the wound site. Cover the ointment with the remaining sterile gauze pad. Be sure to apply the pad so that the slit end faces up and slides under your tube. Then, tape the pad securely to your abdomen.

10 Finally, tape a small segment of the T tube to your abdomen so you won't accidentally dislodge the tube. Discard used supplies in a paper bag.

Watching for complications

Call your doctor if you notice any of the following signs of infection when you're caring for your tubing and incision:
- redness, swelling, or pain
- puslike drainage.
  Also contact him if you have:
- fever
- nausea or vomiting
- clay-colored stools.

PATIENT-TEACHING AID

Preparing for ERCP

Dear Patient:

You're about to undergo endoscopic retrograde cholangiopancreatography—called ERCP for short. This procedure uses a dyelike substance, a flexible tube called an endoscope, and X-rays to outline your gallbladder and pancreatic structures.

Performed in the radiology department, ERCP may take up to 1 hour to complete. Read the information below to help you prepare.

How to get ready
The day before ERCP you can eat and drink as usual. Then after midnight before the procedure, don't eat or drink anything unless your doctor directs otherwise. (He may tell you to continue taking certain medications.) Before you enter the test room, be sure to urinate because ERCP can cause you to retain urine.

What to expect during ERCP
You'll lie on an X-ray table for this test. The nurse will take your temperature, blood pressure, and pulse rate. Then she'll insert an I.V. line in your hand or arm to administer medication. Although you'll be awake, you'll receive a sedative to relax you and to ease the procedure.

The doctor will spray your throat with a bitter-tasting anesthetic. The anesthetic will make your mouth and throat feel swollen and numb. Because you'll have difficulty swallowing, the doctor may give you a device to suction your saliva, or he may tell you to let it drain from your mouth.

Next, the nurse will give you a mouthguard to keep your mouth open and to protect your teeth during ERCP. And though you'll be unable to talk, you'll have no trouble breathing.

When the doctor passes the endoscope down your throat, you may gag a little, but this reflex is normal.

As the tube reaches the duodenum (small intestine), the doctor may inject some air through the tube. You'll also receive medication through your I.V. line. The medication will relax the duodenum. Next, the doctor will insert a thinner tube through the endoscope to the biliary structures and the duodenum.

When the second tube is in place, the doctor will inject dye and quickly take X-ray images from several angles. Then after he views the images, he'll gently remove the endoscope, tube, and mouthpiece.

Aftercare
The nurse will check your blood pressure, pulse rate, and temperature frequently for several hours.

When you regain feeling in your throat and your gag reflex returns, you'll be allowed to have a light meal and liquids. You can resume your regular diet the next day.

Expect to have a sore throat for a few days. Call the doctor if you can't urinate or if you experience chills, abdominal pain, nausea, or vomiting.

Gastroenteritis

In gastroenteritis, the severity of symptoms may compel the patient to seek help and learn about treatment. But he may be less inclined to practice preventive measures after vomiting, diarrhea, abdominal pain, and fever subside. After all, the disorder is usually self-limiting in an otherwise healthy adult, making it easy to ignore or forget preventive measures.

With this in mind, you'll need to emphasize how to prevent recurring bouts of gastric and intestinal inflammation in gastroenteritis. You must persuade the patient to wash his hands thoroughly and often, to handle and prepare food carefully and, if he travels abroad, to avoid suspect foods.

Discuss the disorder

Your patient knows firsthand the abdominal cramping and pain, diarrhea, nausea, vomiting, chills, and fever of gastroenteritis. If he has a severe case, he may experience rectal burning, tenesmus, and bloody, mucoid stools with diarrhea. But he may not know that the severity of his symptoms depends on the identity and amount of the irritant, his resistance, and the extent of GI involvement. And he may not know how he got the disorder or whether it's acute or chronic.

Inform the patient that acute gastroenteritis most commonly results from a viral, bacterial, or parasitic infection—typically from an infected person or from contaminated food or water. Tell him that a viral infection can pass from one person to another and can cause acute, 24- to 72-hour vomiting and diarrhea attacks (known as intestinal flu). Explain that food or water may become contaminated from environmental pollutants or from improper handling, storing, or preparing—allowing harmful bacteria to thrive (see *Major types of food poisoning*, pages 262 and 263). Spicy and greasy foods can also cause gastroenteritis in some people. So can toxic substances, such as those in inedible mushrooms or a rhubarb leaf.

Add that a bacterial change in the GI tract can also cause gastroenteritis. Associated with illness, a dietary change during travel to a foreign country, or antibiotic drugs, this change in bacterial balance allows certain strains to thrive and cause GI upset.

Tell the patient that injury can cause gastroenteritis. For example, radiation treatments may inflame the bowel's mucosal lining and impair absorption. Add that various drugs can cause GI distress, too, by altering the bowel lining.

Vivian Fineman, RN, BS, BSN, CGC, a senior staff nurse in the GI endoscopy suite at the Hospital of the University of Pennsylvania, Philadelphia, wrote this chapter.

CHECKLIST

Teaching topics in gastroenteritis

☐ What causes gastroenteritis
☐ Symptoms and complications
☐ Explanation of diagnostic workup, including patient history and laboratory tests
☐ Dietary guidelines
☐ Medications—for example, antidiarrheals and antiemetics to treat symptoms and antibiotics to fight bacteria
☐ Preventive measures, including travel tips, food handling precautions, and ways to prevent spreading infection
☐ How to manage diarrhea in children

Major types of food poisoning

This chart lists the major types of food poisoning, the foods most often involved, and the symptoms caused by each. Signs and symptoms of most food poisonings are mild—so mild that the poisoning is barely noticed or is passed off as an upset stomach.

However, some types of food poisoning can be dangerous—especially to infants or to elderly or infirm patients.

Use the chart to alert your patient to the dangers of food poisoning and the need to prevent it.

TYPE AND CAUSE	SOURCES	SIGNS AND SYMPTOMS
Amebiasis (amebic dysentery) Caused by *Entamoeba histolytica* (amoebic protozoa)	Found in the human intestinal tract and feces. Can be introduced to food when sewage is used as fertilizer or when food handlers don't wash hands. Chief sources are foods that are handled a lot during preparation.	Tenderness over the colon or liver, loose morning stools, recurrent diarrhea, nervousness, weight loss, and fatigue are common signs and symptoms. Anemia may develop.
Bacterial gastroenteritis Caused by *Yersinia enterocolitica*	Meat, water, raw vegetables, and unpasteurized milk. Bacteria multiply rapidly at room temperature.	Onset is 2 to 5 days after eating with fever, headache, nausea, and diarrhea. Typically mistaken for flu, the disease most commonly strikes children but can strike all ages.
Botulism Caused by *Clostridium botulinum*	These bacteria are everywhere but produce toxins only in an anaerobic (oxygen-free), low-acid environment. Improperly canned low-acid foods (especially home-canned), such as green beans, corn, beets, peppers, mushrooms, spinach, olives, and beef are chief sources.	About 8 hours to 8 days after eating, symptoms may begin with nausea, vomiting, diarrhea, and abdominal cramps followed by weakness, blurred or double vision, headache, difficulty swallowing, slurred speech, drooping eyelids, dilated pupils, and progressive paralysis affecting the respiratory muscles. Symptoms usually last 3 to 6 days and can be fatal. Get help immediately.
Campylobacterosis Caused by *Campylobacter jejuni*	Raw poultry, meat, contaminated water, and unpasteurized milk.	Diarrhea, abdominal cramps, fever, and, sometimes bloody stools develop from 2 to 5 days after eating. Symptoms last 2 to 7 days.
Cereus food poisoning Caused by *Bacillus cereus*	Raw foods; bacteria multiply rapidly at room temperature.	Abdominal pain and diarrhea or nausea and vomiting occur from 1 to 18 hours after eating. Symptoms rarely last longer than 1 day.
Cholera Caused by *Vibrio cholerae*	Fish and shellfish harvested from waters contaminated by human sewage. Chief sources are raw fish and shellfish.	Onset is 1 to 3 days after eating; symptoms range from mild diarrhea to life-threatening dehydration from intense diarrhea. Severe disease requires hospitalization.
Giardiasis Caused by *Giardia lamblia* protozoa	Found in the human intestinal tract and feces. Can be introduced to food when sewage is used as fertilizer or when food handlers don't wash hands. Chief sources include foods that are handled a lot during preparation.	Signs and symptoms include diarrhea, abdominal pain, gas, anorexia, nausea, and vomiting.

continued

Major types of food poisoning — *continued*

TYPE	SOURCE	SIGNS AND SYMPTOMS
Hepatitis A Caused by hepatitis A virus	Shellfish harvested from contaminated waters and foods, such as vegetables, that are handled frequently during preparation and then eaten raw.	Onset takes 2 to 6 weeks. Symptoms include fever, weakness, loss of appetite, and jaundice (yellowing skin and whites of eyes). Severe cases cause liver damage and even death.
Mycotoxicosis Caused by mold toxins	Toxins are produced in foods that contain a lot of moisture, such as beans and grains stored in damp places.	The disease may cause liver or kidney damage.
Parahaemolyticus food poisoning Caused by *Vibrio parahaemolyticus*	Fish and shellfish; caused by bacteria that live in salt water and thrive in warm weather.	Onset — 15 to 24 hours after eating — brings nausea, vomiting, abdominal cramps, diarrhea, and, sometimes, fever, headache, chills, mucoid or bloody stools. Symptoms can last 1 to 2 days and are occasionally fatal.
Perfringens food poisoning Caused by *Clostridium perfringens*	Meat and poultry and foods made with them, including stews, soups, sauces, and gravies. Bacteria multiply rapidly at room temperature; cooking destroys them.	Onset occurs 8 to 22 hours after eating. Stomach pain and diarrhea — sometimes nausea and vomiting — last 24 to 48 hours and are usually mild but can be serious in elderly or infirm patients.
Salmonellosis Caused by *Salmonella*	Raw meats, poultry, eggs, fish, milk, contaminated water, and foods made with them. (Marijuana and small pet turtles are both prime sources of *Salmonella*.) Bacteria multiply rapidly at room temperature.	Onset is 12 to 48 hours after eating (or smoking marijuana or handling a pet turtle) with severe headache, nausea, fever, abdominal cramps, diarrhea, and, sometimes, vomiting. The disease usually lasts 2 to 7 days. It can be fatal in infants and elderly and infirm patients.
Shigellosis (bacillary dysentery) Caused by *Shigella*	Milk and dairy products, poultry, mixed salads (fish, poultry, potato, macaroni, and egg). Can develop in any moist food that isn't thoroughly cooked; bacteria multiply rapidly at or above room temperature.	Symptoms begin 1 to 7 days after eating and include abdominal pain, cramps, diarrhea, fever, and, sometimes vomiting, with blood or mucus in stool. Symptoms can be serious in infants and in elderly and infirm patients.
Staphylococcal ("staph") food poisoning Caused by *Staphylococcus aureus*	Can develop in any food left too long at room temperature. Chief sources are tuna, chicken, potato, and macaroni salads; egg products, custards, cream-filled pastries; and meats, including ham, salami, and poultry.	Onset may occur 1 to 8 hours after eating. Diarrhea, vomiting, nausea, abdominal cramps, and exhaustion last 24 to 48 hours. Usually mild, it's often attributed to other causes, such as the flu.
Viral gastroenteritis Caused by various viruses	Pathogens found in human intestinal tract and feces. Can be introduced to food when sewage is used as fertilizer, when food handlers don't wash hands, and when shellfish are harvested from sewage-contaminated waters.	Onset occurs after 24 hours with diarrhea, nausea, vomiting, and breathing difficulties. Disease usually lasts 4 to 5 days but may go on for weeks.

If your patient suffers from chronic gastroenteritis, explain that he may have allergies to foods, such as tomatoes, berries, eggs and other dairy products, or shellfish. Or he may have a lactose deficiency that causes milk intolerance.

Complications
Although gastroenteritis is usually self-limiting, with recovery in 24 to 36 hours, explain that persistent and untreated gastroenteritis can cause complications. These complications include severe dehydration and crucial electrolyte losses, which can lead to shock, vascular collapse, and renal failure. Typically, infants and elderly or debilitated patients have the greatest risk for complications because of their immature or impaired immune system.

Describe the diagnostic workup
Inform the patient that the doctor will investigate the possibility that contaminated food or water is the source of distress. The doctor will also ask about travel, recent illnesses, radiation or drug therapy, and food allergies. Then he'll look for signs of dehydration by checking the mucous membranes in the patient's mouth and eyes and inspecting the patient's axillae for moisture.

If severe symptoms persist beyond 48 hours, explain that the doctor may order blood tests, including a complete blood count, to detect blood loss and infection and to evaluate electrolyte levels and fluid balance.

Teach about treatments
Tell the patient that treatment aims to relieve symptoms with rest, diet, and medication and to prevent reinfection.

Activity
Advise the patient to rest during bouts of gastroenteritis to help increase his resistance and conserve his strength.

Diet
Recommend drinking plenty of clear fluids until a diarrhea attack subsides. If the attack is severe, advise the patient that the doctor may prescribe an oral rehydration solution of water, salt, and glucose (available from the drugstore without a prescription). Or the patient can make the solution himself from household items (see *A home solution for rehydration*). Suggest that he drink the solution at half-hour intervals until he passes pale yellow urine. Add that he may need to drink several liters of solution in a day before this occurs.

Once the patient's diarrhea subsides, recommend that (as tolerated) he start taking unsweetened fruit juice, tea, bouillon or other clear broths, flavored gelatin, cooked cereal, and bland soft foods, such as rice or applesauce. Instruct him to avoid foods high in roughage, such as raw fruits and vegetables and whole-grain products. And warn him to avoid milk and other dairy products and spicy or greasy foods. These foods can cause recurrent diarrhea. After 2 or 3 days on a bland diet, he can resume a normal diet.

If vomiting persists longer than 24 hours, advise the patient to consume nothing by mouth. If he's dehydrated, the doctor may order an I.V. infusion of dextrose and electrolyte-balanced fluids.

Medication

Tell the patient that the drugs most commonly used for gastroenteritis include antidiarrheals and antiemetics. Occasionally, the patient may receive an antibiotic if he has a bacterial or systemic infection.

Antidiarrheals. Explain that the doctor may recommend such oral agents as bismuth subsalicylate (Pepto-Bismol), camphorated opium tincture (Paregoric), diphenoxylate and atropine (Lomotil), kaolin and pectin (Kaopectate), and loperamide (Imodium) among others.

Mention that many doctors suggest *bismuth subsalicylate* as the first line of defense against diarrhea. In tablet or liquid form, this drug absorbs surplus water and toxins in the bowel and protectively coats the intestinal lining. Tell the patient to chew the tablets or shake the suspension well. Warn him that this medication may temporarily darken his bowel movements and his tongue. Caution him that high doses may cause salicylism (tinnitus, nausea, and vomiting). Advise parents to avoid giving bismuth subsalicylate to feverish children with flulike symptoms because salicylates are associated with Reye's syndrome.

Inform the patient taking such antidiarrheals as *camphorated opium tincture, diphenoxylate and atropine,* and *loperamide* that these drugs may cause anorexia, constipation, dizziness, drowsiness, nausea, rash, stomach pain, and vomiting. *Kaolin and pectin*—another popular antidiarrheal—may cause mild constipation but no other adverse effects.

Individually, *camphorated opium tincture* can trigger depression, dysuria, hypertension, increased sweating, and oliguria. It can also be habit-forming and shouldn't be used with alcohol or cold, allergy, or sleeping medicines. Tell the patient to take a missed dose as soon as possible but not to double-dose.

Diphenoxylate and atropine can cause bloating, blurred vision, depression, dysuria, dry mouth, fever, headache, shortness of breath, and tachycardia. Inform the patient that this drug controls diarrhea by relaxing the intestinal muscles. Then tell him to take a missed dose as soon as possible and the remaining doses for the day at regular intervals. If his diarrhea has stopped, however, he can skip the dose but take the next dose on schedule.

Advise the patient to avoid alcohol, cold and allergy remedies, and sedatives while he's taking this drug. When he stops taking it, instruct him to contact the doctor if he experiences muscle or stomach cramps, nausea or vomiting, shivering or shaking, or increased sweating.

Tell the patient taking *loperamide* that this drug can cause

A home solution for rehydration

If your patient can't get to a drugstore to buy a rehydration solution, give him these recipes so that he can make the solutions at home. Tell him that these solutions contain chloride, potassium, and sodium—essential electrolytes—and glucose, which help the body absorb the electrolytes that he's lost.

Instruct him to prepare both solutions and to take a few sips of one; then equal sips of the other.

Solution 1
Mix 8 oz (1 measuring cup) apple, apricot, orange, or other fruit juice containing potassium with a pinch of table salt (sodium chloride) and 1/2 tsp of corn syrup or honey (glucose).

Solution 2
Mix 8 oz of pure tap water with 1/4 tsp of baking soda (bicarbonate of soda).

Advise the patient to substitute boiled, bottled, or carbonated water for tap water if his water source isn't pure or if his well's contaminated. Suggest that he also drink pure water, carbonated beverages, or tea as desired.

bloating, dry mouth, and fever. If he misses a dose, instruct him to skip it and to take the next dose on schedule. Caution him never to double-dose.

Inform the patient that because all of these drugs may cause drowsiness, he should exercise caution before performing tasks that require alertness. Of course, he should always read the drug label carefully and take the medication as directed by his doctor.

Antiemetics. For severe vomiting, explain that the doctor may prescribe an antiemetic drug to be taken by mouth, by injection, or in suppository form. Commonly used drugs include prochlorperazine (Compazine) and trimethobenzamide hydrochloride (Tigan). Because all antiemetics may cause drowsiness, warn the patient not to schedule activities requiring mental alertness if he feels sluggish. Advise him to avoid taking any other drugs (such as alcohol, tranquilizers, sleeping medications, and narcotic analgesics) that may cause central nervous system depression or drowsiness. Advise a pregnant patient not to take an antiemetic without consulting her doctor. If the doctor prescribes an I.M. injection of the drug, warn the patient that he may feel pain or burning at the injection site.

Antibiotics. Mention that antibiotic treatment for gastroenteritis remains controversial. Antibiotics are restricted to patients who have bacterial diarrhea; the prescribed antibiotic depends on the bacteria identified by the patient's stool culture. For example, *Campylobacter* is treated with erythromycin; *Entamoeba histolytica* and *Giardia lamblia* with ampicillin; and *Shigella* with trimethoprim-sulfamethoxazole.

Caution the patient to report adverse reactions, such as new or increased bouts of abdominal cramps, diarrhea, nausea, and vomiting. Warn him to stop taking the drug and immediately notify the doctor if he experiences a hypersensitivity reaction (reddened skin, rash, hives, and difficulty breathing). Advise him also to notify the doctor if diarrhea persists.

Other care measures

Discuss preventive measures. If your patient expects to be traveling, tell him how to avoid "traveler's diarrhea" or gastroenteritis caused by inadequate sanitation, particularly in developing nations. Inform him that contaminated food and water contain bacteria that attach themselves to the small intestine's lining. These organisms then release a toxin that causes diarrhea and cramps. Advise the patient to pay close attention to what he eats and drinks. For more information, see *Preventing traveler's diarrhea*.

To prevent food poisoning from contamination, discuss proper food handling, storage, and preparation methods (see *Preventing food poisoning,* pages 268 and 269).

Discuss ways to prevent spreading gastroenteritis to family members and other close contacts. Stress that proper hand washing by the patient and others in his household is the best defense against infection. Instruct the patient to use lots of warm, soapy

---

Preventing traveler's diarrhea

If your patient travels, discuss precautions that he can take to reduce his chances of getting "traveler's diarrhea" (also called "Montezuma's revenge" and "Tut's tummy"). Advise him to:
• drink water (or brush his teeth with water) only if it's chlorinated. Chlorination protects the water supply from such bacterial contaminants as *Escherichia coli*.
• avoid beverages in glasses that may have been washed in contaminated water.
• refuse ice cubes made from possibly impure water.
• express a preference for drinks made with boiled water, such as coffee or tea, or beverages contained in bottles and cans.
• sanitize impure water by adding 2% tincture of iodine (5 drops/liter of clear water; 10 drops/liter of cloudy water) or by adding liquid laundry bleach (2 drops/liter of clear water; 4 drops/liter of cloudy water).
• avoid uncooked vegetables, fresh fruits with no peel, salads, unpasteurized milk, and other dairy products.
• beware of foods offered by street vendors in developing nations.

---

water and to wash under his nails, in crevices, between fingers, and under rings (or remove them and wash them, too).

If the doctor suspects sexually transmitted enteric infections, advise the patient to abstain from sexual practices that promote fecal-oral contamination until fecal analysis shows that treatment has arrested the infection.

If the patient has a bacterial or parasitic infection and his occupation involves food handling or contact with people, tell him that local laws may require him to refrain from working until he can document that he's no longer infected.

Instruct the patient with gastroenteritis to contact his doctor at once if he experiences headache and muscle and nervous irritability—signs of dehydration and severe electrolyte imbalances. Finally, teach parents how to care for their children who have diarrhea to prevent such complications as dehydration. For more information, see *Managing diarrhea in children*, page 270.

Further readings

"Are You Allergic to What You Eat?" *Patient Care* 23(13):225-26, August 15, 1989.
Bahna, S.L., et al. "What Food Allergy Is—And Isn't," *Patient Care* 23(13):94-99, 102, 104-06, August 15, 1989.
Bitterman, R.A. "Acute Traveler's Diarrhea," *Emergency Medicine* 21(12):77-80, 85-86, June 30, 1989.
Desmond, M. "Preparing Patients for Travel," *Patient Care* 21(11): 217-19, 223-24, 227+, June 15, 1987.
Dupont, H.L., et al. "Infectious Diarrhea from A to Z," *Patient Care* 21(18):98-101, 104, 109-11+, November 15, 1987.
Hogan, M., et al. "Gastroenteritis in the Home or Hospital," *Irish Medical Journal* 80(12):419-20, December 1987.
Johnson, P.C., et al. "Traveler's Diarrhea: Strategies to Help Decrease the Odds," *Consultant* 27(5):102-04, 106-07, 110, May 1987.
Jong, E.C. "Infectious Disease Problems During International Travel," *Emergency Care Quarterly* 4(3):47-54, November 1988.

Preventing food poisoning

Dear Patient:

You can prevent food poisoning by following a few simple precautions when you handle, store, and prepare food.

Most kinds of food poisoning are caused by bacteria. These bacteria may be living in your food or on your utensils and cutting boards. Or they may pass from your hands to the foods you handle. That's why it's so important to handle food carefully.

What's more, once bacteria get into food, they can grow and thrive if they're not stopped. That's why it's so important to store foods at temperatures that prevent bacterial growth. And that's why it's equally important to prepare them properly and to serve them promptly.

FOOD TEMPERATURE: SAFE OR DANGEROUS?

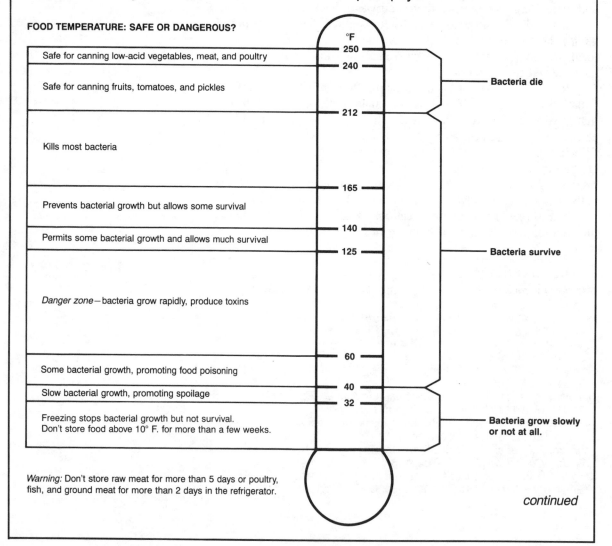

Temperature (°F)	Description	Bacteria status
250	Safe for canning low-acid vegetables, meat, and poultry	Bacteria die
240	Safe for canning fruits, tomatoes, and pickles	Bacteria die
212		Bacteria die
	Kills most bacteria	
165	Prevents bacterial growth but allows some survival	
140	Permits some bacterial growth and allows much survival	
125		Bacteria survive
	Danger zone—bacteria grow rapidly, produce toxins	Bacteria survive
60	Some bacterial growth, promoting food poisoning	
40	Slow bacterial growth, promoting spoilage	Bacteria grow slowly or not at all.
32	Freezing stops bacterial growth but not survival. Don't store food above 10° F. for more than a few weeks.	Bacteria grow slowly or not at all.

Warning: Don't store raw meat for more than 5 days or poultry, fish, and ground meat for more than 2 days in the refrigerator.

continued

PATIENT-TEACHING AID

Preventing food poisoning — *continued*

How to handle food
● Wash your hands thoroughly before you start preparing food — especially if you've just handled money, touched raw foods, used the toilet, changed a baby's diaper, blown your nose, or petted a dog.
● Avoid using your hands to mix foods. Use clean utensils (for example, forks) instead.
● Wear plastic gloves if you have a cut or an infection on your hands.
● Wash dust or dirt off can tops before opening them.
● Wash dishes, cutting boards, work surfaces, and utensils with hot, soapy water before and after using them to prepare raw meat or poultry. Never allow anything that has touched raw meat or poultry to touch uncooked foods, such as salad.

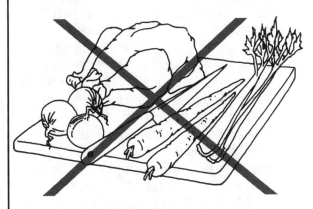

How to store food
● Make food shopping your last errand. Take the food home immediately and put it in the refrigerator right away. This limits the time food bacteria remain at room temperature — an optimal environment for their growth.
● Select meats, frozen foods, and dairy products near the end of your shopping excursion. Don't buy partially defrosted foods or foods in cracked or torn packages.
● Buy perishable foods in small amounts so you won't keep them too long.
● Leave poultry and meat in the plastic wrappings they come in for no more than 1 or 2 days. For longer storage, rewrap them loosely in waxed paper or plastic wrap. To freeze, wrap them tightly and date them. Then use the older items first.
● Throw away food that's moldy, shriveled, or discolored. Also discard any food that has a strange odor.

How to prepare food
● Thaw frozen foods in the refrigerator — not at room temperature. If you're really in a hurry, submerge them in warm water, defrost them in the microwave oven if you have one, or begin cooking them partially frozen.
● Clean poultry thoroughly. If you're stuffing poultry, fill the cavity just before cooking. Allow enough room for heat to penetrate the stuffing and bring it to a temperature of at least 165 degrees.
● Heat food thoroughly to kill bacteria. High heat is especially important when preparing such foods as milk, milk products, eggs, meat, poultry, fish, and shellfish. Use a meat thermometer to be sure the interior is cooked thoroughly.
● Serve hot foods hot and cold foods cold.
● Store leftover hot and cold foods in the refrigerator promptly after eating. Don't leave hot foods out to cool. Reheat leftovers thoroughly. Gravy should be brought to a rolling boil.
● Avoid raw fish, raw meats, and raw (unpasteurized) milk.

Managing diarrhea in children

Dear Parent:

Diarrhea can disrupt essential fluid balance in anyone—and especially in a child. This may make a sick child's recovery take longer.

Observe your sick child carefully. You know he has diarrhea when his bowel movements increase in amount and frequency and they look watery. For example, several loose, runny bowel movements over a few hours signal diarrhea.

Beware of dehydration, which can result from diarrhea. This is a dangerous condition that should be treated right away by your doctor. Here's how to recognize the signs of dehydration, how to know when to call the doctor, and how to restore lost fluids.

Signs of dehydration
Your child may be dehydrated if
• he stops urinating or produces much less urine than usual
• he appears to be losing weight
• his eyes look sunken.

Try this test: Pinch the skin on top of your child's hand and let it go. If the skin remains in the pinched position, instead of returning to its normal position, your child may be dehydrated.

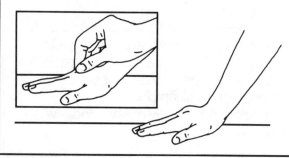

When to call the doctor
Don't delay getting medical care for your child if
• you notice any dehydration signs
• he's younger than 18 months and has watery bowel movements
• he's an older child whose diarrhea continues after 12 hours
• his bowel movement contains blood or mucus or both.

How to restore fluids
• Encourage clear fluids for the first 24 hours after diarrhea starts. Flat soda (stir a carbonated beverage until it stops fizzing), chicken broth, and tea make good choices.
• Offer soft, bland foods—bananas, rice, applesauce—as your child begins to feel better.
• Avoid giving your child milk and other dairy products, such as cheese and ice cream, when he's sick and for a week after he recovers. These foods may trigger a repeated bout of diarrhea.
• Give an oral rehydrating solution if your doctor advises. This is available in powder form from the drugstore. (Or ask your nurse how to mix a homemade one.) Made with pure water, the solution will bring your child's fluid balance back to normal more effectively than an ordinary liquid, such as cola.

Follow your doctor's instructions on how much to give. Don't offer any other fluid but water if you're using this solution.

Inguinal hernia

Sometimes referred to as a "rupture," inguinal hernia is the most common type of abdominal hernia. Because a hernia won't disappear by itself and will only enlarge in time, your most difficult teaching challenge may involve persuading the patient to elect surgery before complications arise.

To do this, you'll educate the patient about the disorder, concentrating on its causes and the risk of complications. Although you'll discuss temporary treatment measures, you'll emphasize that surgery is the only way to repair an inguinal hernia.

If your patient's a child, you'll teach his parents how a hernia occurs and how it's diagnosed and also prepare them for the surgery and provide instructions for postoperative care.

Discuss the disorder

Inform the patient that an abdominal hernia occurs when part of an internal organ bulges through the muscle wall surrounding the abdominal cavity. An inguinal hernia develops in the groin area (see *Common hernia sites,* page 272). In this hernia, the large or small intestine, the surrounding omentum, or the bladder protrudes into the inguinal canal.

Explain that an inguinal hernia may be indirect or direct. An indirect inguinal hernia, the more common form, permits the abdominal viscera to protrude through the inguinal ring, following the spermatic cord (in men) or the round ligament (in women) and extending into the scrotum or labia. A direct inguinal hernia results from a weakness in the fascial floor of the inguinal canal. The viscera protrude through the posterior inguinal wall, extending into the peritoneum.

Describe how an inguinal hernia may be reducible, sliding back easily into place when it's gently manipulated or when the patient lies down.

Tell the patient that hernias occur in both sexes (although they're more common in men) and in all age-groups. Mention that many patients have a family history of hernias. An inguinal hernia can occur in a boy during gestation. In either sex, a hernia can result from weak abdominal muscles caused by congenital malformation, traumatic injury, or aging, or it may be associated with increased intra-abdominal pressure from heavy lifting, exertion, obesity, excessive coughing, or straining with defecation. In women, pregnancy and uterine or ovarian fibroids or tumors are common causes of inguinal hernia.

Point out that an inguinal hernia may appear suddenly, causing a bulge or lump in the groin when the patient stands or strains and disappearing when he lies down. Tension on the herniated

Pamela J. Currie, RN, MSN, CRNP, who wrote this chapter, is a nurse practitioner with Cigna Corporation in Philadelphia.

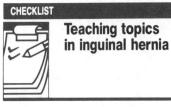

CHECKLIST

Teaching topics in inguinal hernia

☐ Explanation of the type of inguinal hernia: direct or indirect
☐ Causes of inguinal hernia, such as congenital defects, heavy lifting, and obesity
☐ Complications, such as incarceration and strangulation
☐ Diagnosis from a medical history and physical exam
☐ Temporary treatment measures, such as activity restrictions and use of a truss
☐ Herniorrhaphy or hernioplasty to repair an inguinal hernia
☐ Special considerations for inguinal hernia in infants and children
☐ Recognizing signs and symptoms of strangulation

Common hernia sites

Inform the patient that any part of the abdominal wall can rupture. However, most hernias occur in the following areas: through the navel (umbilical hernia), through old surgical incisions (incisional hernia), near the natural openings in the groin area (inguinal hernia), and near the femoral artery (femoral hernia).

Umbilical hernia
Quite common in neonates but also occurring in obese or multiparous women, an umbilical hernia results from abnormal muscle structures around the umbilical cord. Most umbilical hernias in infants close spontaneously, so surgery is necessary only if the hernia persists for more than 4 or 5 years. Until the hernia closes, taping the affected area or supporting it with a truss may relieve symptoms. A severe congenital umbilical hernia, in which the viscera protrude outside the body, requires immediate surgery to prevent incarceration and strangulation.

Incisional hernia
This hernia develops at a site of previous surgery, usually along vertical incisions. It may result from in-

fection or impaired wound healing. Other predisposing factors include poor nutrition, extreme abdominal distention, and obesity. Palpation of the hernia may reveal several defects in the surgical scar. Patients with a large incisional hernia may remain asymptomatic while an intestinal obstruction develops.

Inguinal hernia
An indirect inguinal hernia causes the abdominal viscera to push through the inguinal ring and follow the spermatic cord (in males) or round ligament (in females). A direct inguinal hernia results from a weakness in the fascial floor of the inguinal canal.

Femoral hernia
Typically, in a femoral hernia, part of the peritoneum and bladder protrudes through a hole created by a fatty deposit in the femoral canal.

This hernia appears as a swelling or bulge at the pulse point of the femoral artery. It's usually reducible but often becomes incarcerated or strangulated. Mention that femoral hernias are more common in women.

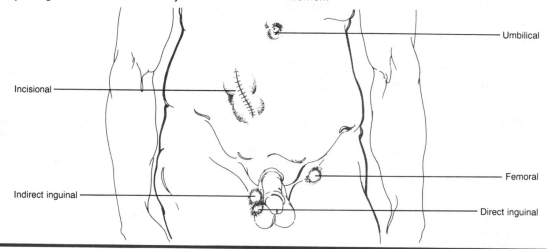

area may trigger a sharp, steady pain that fades when the hernia's reduced. Or the patient may experience an intermittent burning sensation. Mention that he may previously have ignored the condition because his symptoms are episodic rather than constant.

Complications
Emphasize to the patient that an untreated inguinal hernia may become incarcerated if it can't be reduced because adhesions have formed in the hernial sac. Or it may become strangulated if part of the herniated intestine becomes twisted or edematous, cutting off normal blood flow.

Mention that incarceration poses no immediate threat; however, a bowel obstruction may ultimately develop, and further constriction of the hernial sac can lead to ischemia. If strangulation occurs, the blood supply to the bowel segment contained in the hernial sac is cut off, threatening necrosis and necessitating emergency surgical repair.

Point out that treating a hernia on an elective basis is far safer than handling it as an emergency. Warn the patient that a strangulated hernia requires extensive bowel resection, involving a protracted hospital stay and, possibly, a colostomy.

Describe the diagnostic workup

Inform the patient that an inguinal hernia is diagnosed from a medical history and physical examination. Describe how the doctor will palpate the inguinal area while the patient stands and while he lies down. The doctor may ask him to cough or bear down as if he's defecating; if the doctor feels pressure against the fingertip, an indirect hernia exists; pressure felt against the side of the finger indicates a direct hernia.

Explain that the doctor may also order a complete blood count and urinalysis to determine whether the bladder is part of the herniated contents. If so, this may lead to urinary tract infection or urine retention. Suspected bowel obstruction requires abdominal X-rays.

Teach about treatments

Inform the patient that surgery is the treatment of choice for an adult with an inguinal hernia. For infants and children, it's the only option. If the hernia in an adult poses no immediate threat of incarceration or strangulation and the patient wishes to postpone surgery, discuss temporary treatment measures, such as limiting physical activity or wearing a truss.

Give special reassurance and support to a child scheduled for hernia repair. If the child is old enough, encourage him to ask questions, and answer them as simply as possible (see *Inguinal hernias in children,* page 274).

Activity

If the patient chooses to delay surgery, advise him to avoid any activity that increases intra-abdominal pressure, including heavy lifting and straining to defecate. If his job involves strenuous physical activity, explore the need for a temporary job change.

Procedures

Tell the patient that a truss—an elastic, canvas, or metal support—may be used to keep the abdominal contents from protruding into the hernial sac. Stress that wearing a truss won't cure the hernia and that many patients find it quite uncomfortable. Warn him that continued use of a truss after the hernia "outgrows" it can encourage incarceration and strangulation.

Advise the patient to apply a truss only when the hernia's been reduced, preferably before he gets out of bed in the morning. To prevent skin irritation, instruct him to bathe daily and dust the area liberally with cornstarch or baby powder. Caution him against applying the truss over clothing because this reduces the effectiveness of the truss and may cause it to slip.

Inguinal hernias in children

In an infant or child, an inguinal hernia necessitates surgical repair. Because parents will be concerned about any condition requiring surgery, they'll need your reassurance and a clear explanation of the disorder and the procedure for repair. Include the child (if age-appropriate) in your discussion, and answer any questions he has simply and honestly.

How a hernia occurs
Tell the parents of a boy with an inguinal hernia that their son's condition may have occurred during gestation when the peritoneal sac failed to close properly after the testicle descended. This failure leaves an opening through which the intestine can slip.

Explain that an inguinal hernia in either sex can result from weakened abdominal muscles—for example, weakness associated with congenital malformation or previous surgery, such as an appendectomy. Or an inguinal hernia may develop from straining to defecate or from overexertion.

Detecting a hernia
Point out that an inguinal hernia is more difficult to diagnose in a child than in an adult. In particular, a hydrocele (a fluid-filled sac of the spermatic cord) may coexist with or mimic an inguinal hernia in boys.

Describe special maneuvers that may help diagnose a hernia in a child. For example, the doctor may ask the child to jump up and down or to blow up a balloon. These activities make the hernia more prominent and detectable.

Hernia repair
Stress that surgery is the only treatment option in a child. Tell parents that some hernias may become less prominent as the child grows, and thus easier to repair. In an infant, surgery may be delayed until the infant weighs about 10 lb (4.5 kg) or is about age 2 months. If the infant is premature, surgery may be delayed until age 6 months. Mention that incarceration and strangulation are uncommon in infants, but residual testicular damage may occur.

Inguinal hernia repair in an infant or a child is usually straightforward. The procedure takes about 30 minutes, and the child typically returns to school 2 or 3 days later. Advise parents that the child should avoid strenuous activity and contact sports until the doctor says it's okay. While the incision's healing, tell them to dress the child in loose clothing and to change an infant's diaper frequently.

Urge parents to inform any siblings about the surgery, using simple words. After surgery, tell parents to reassure siblings that the child is fine and to show them his incision if they ask.

Occasionally, a hydrocele occurs after surgery. Reassure the parents that this condition may resolve spontaneously within 6 months and rarely requires additional surgery.

Surgery
Explain that herniorrhaphy is the preferred treatment for an inguinal hernia in adults, otherwise healthy older adults, and children. It returns the protruding viscera to the abdominal cavity and then repairs the opening in the abdominal wall. Another effective procedure is hernioplasty, which reinforces the weakened area with plastic, steel mesh, or wire.

Stress that herniorrhaphy and hernioplasty can be performed quickly and produce few complications. A strangulated hernia may, however, need emergency herniorrhaphy or bowel resection.

Preoperative teaching. Inform the patient that, depending on his age, general health, and the extent of the repair, the doctor may recommend general, spinal, or local anesthesia. If the hernia repair is not done as an outpatient procedure, tell the patient that he'll need to remain in the hospital for 2 or 3 days after surgery.

If the patient's scheduled for an outpatient hernia repair, explain that he'll undergo a number of routine tests, such as an electrocardiogram (ECG), several days before surgery. Remind him to comply strictly with any ongoing treatment regimen for a preexisting medical condition (for example, asthma), so he'll be in optimal condition for surgery. Instruct him to restrict food and fluids after midnight the day before the surgery.

Inform the patient that before surgery he'll receive a cleansing enema, a sedative, and the chosen anesthetic. Explain that the surgery itself takes about 30 minutes for children and 60 minutes for adults. After surgery, he'll have no tubes or drains unless surgery has been complicated by a strangulated or incarcerated hernia, but he can expect a dressing over his incision.

Postoperative teaching. Assure the patient that he'll be able to return to work or school within 2 or 3 days and resume normal activities in 2 to 4 weeks. Before the patient goes home, teach him how to care for the incision, minimize discomfort, and recognize signs of infection. Give him a copy of the patient-teaching aid *Recovering from hernia surgery,* page 276.

If the patient's hernia is strangulated or incarcerated, point out that recovery will take longer. He may have a nasogastric tube for several days before he's allowed to eat or get out of bed. He'll go home in 1 or 2 weeks and can return to normal activities in 4 to 6 weeks. Stress the importance of regular follow-up examinations to evaluate wound healing and the success of repair. If his job necessitates heavy lifting or other strenuous activity, help him explore options for a temporary change in responsibilities.

Other care measures

If the patient decides against surgery, ensure that he can recognize signs and symptoms of strangulation: severe, continuous abdominal pain concentrated in the herniated area, severe nausea and vomiting and, possibly, diarrhea. Instruct him to notify the doctor at once if he develops these signs and symptoms. Emphasize that a strangulated hernia may be life-threatening unless it's repaired immediately.

Instruct the patient with an inguinal hernia to check with the doctor before planning any travel. Some doctors discourage traveling because they've noted that it results in an increased incidence of incarceration and strangulation.

Advise the patient that the likelihood that a hernia will recur depends on the success of the surgery and on his overall health and life-style.

Further readings

Ashby, D. "The Pediatric Patient: A Left Inguinal Hernia," *Journal of Post Anesthesia Nursing* 4(2):116-17, April 1989.

Ashby, D. "Susan's First Pregnancy and First Surgery," *Journal of Post Anesthesia Nursing* 4(6):406-08, December 1989.

Donworth, G. "On the Road to Recovery: The Repair of a Right Inguinal Hernia—a Theatre Nursing Care Study," *National Association of Theatre News* 24(1):12-14, January 1987.

"Hernias," *Medical Times* 117(4):77-78, April 1989.

"Inguinal Hernia Repair Simplified by New Surgery Technique," *Same Day Surgery* 13(12):160-62, December 1989.

Kingsley, A.N., et al. "Common Hernias in Primary Care," *Patient Care* 24(7):98-101, 104, 109-10+, April 15, 1990.

"Questions and Answers about Inguinal Hernia," *Patient Care* 24(7):116, 119, April 15, 1990.

PATIENT-TEACHING AID

Recovering from hernia surgery

Dear Patient:

In most cases inguinal hernias can be repaired on an outpatient basis. This means that you'll probably leave the hospital on the same day that you have surgery.

Once you're home, follow these guidelines to minimize discomfort and speed your recovery.

The first few days
For the first 2 or 3 days, you may have a fever. Your temperature may be as high as 100° F. (37.8° C.).

Also, you may notice swelling, bruising, tenderness, or the feeling that there's a rope under the incision. Use an ice pack to help reduce swelling, bruising, and pain. Or try supporting the scrotum with a rolled towel. The doctor may also prescribe medicine to relieve any pain.

While the incision's still tender, you'll be most comfortable wearing soft, loose-fitting clothes.

Notify the doctor immediately if you experience chest pain, if you feel like throwing up, or if you have trouble breathing or difficulty urinating. These symptoms may indicate complications from the anesthetic.

Prevent and recognize infection
Keep the incision clean and covered to prevent infection.

Contact your doctor if fever, pain, swelling, and tenderness last longer than 3 days. Also contact him if you notice bleeding, redness, or drainage at the incision site or if you have chills or other flu-like symptoms. These symptoms may signal infection.

Remember to make an appointment with your doctor. He'll want to see you within a week after hernia surgery to check the wound and remove any sutures.

Take it easy
The doctor will let you know when it's safe to resume your usual activities. You'll probably be able to return to work or school within 2 or 3 days. He may advise you to avoid bathing for a couple of days and to refrain from driving for about 2 weeks. You may resume sexual activity as soon as you feel comfortable. Try to use positions that don't strain your incision.

Avoid foods that might make you constipated and cause you to strain against your incision. Don't perform any strenuous activity, such as bending, heavy lifting, or playing contact sports, until the doctor says it's okay.

If you're a parent, you may have to restrict some of your usual activities with your children. Avoid picking them up or carrying them. Explain to them why you need to take it easy, and reassure them that things will soon return to normal.

6

Endocrine Conditions

Contents

Hypoglycemia

Because this disorder requires permanent life-style changes, its management can be challenging for both you and the patient. Your first priority is teaching him to recognize hypoglycemia's telltale symptoms and to treat himself promptly so that he can prevent serious complications. But because this disorder causes fatigue, an inability to concentrate, and considerable discomfort, the patient may not always be aware of his condition or be able to start treatment immediately. As a result, you'll need to include his family in your teaching.

Besides discussing symptoms, you'll also need to teach the patient and his family about long-term treatments to control hypoglycemia, such as diet, weight reduction, medications, and surgery. In addition, you should include an explanation of the patient's particular type of hypoglycemia and tests to diagnose the disorder.

Discuss the disorder

Explain to the patient that hypoglycemia occurs when glucose, the body's major energy source, is being used too rapidly or when glucose isn't being released fast enough to meet the energy needs of vital tissues, such as brain cells. How low must blood glucose levels fall before triggering a hypoglycemic reaction? This varies greatly from patient to patient. Typically, a blood glucose level below 50 mg/dl causes hypoglycemic symptoms.

Tell the patient that the nature of his symptoms may reveal how rapidly his glucose levels are falling. For example, nervousness, diaphoresis, and an elevated heart rate can result from a rapid decline in glucose levels. Changes in mental status can result from a slow decline. (See *What happens in acute hypoglycemia,* page 280.)

Inform the patient about the three types of hypoglycemia: fasting, pharmacologic, and reactive. Then discuss his particular type. In *fasting hypoglycemia,* blood glucose levels gradually fall until, 5 hours or more after a meal, the patient has headache, dizziness, restlessness, mental status changes, and intense hunger. This rare type of hypoglycemia often occurs during the night. Untreated, it can cause severe symptoms, including seizures, unconsciousness, and coma, which resist even prompt treatment.

Tell the patient with fasting hypoglycemia that the disorder usually results from liver disease or a tumor. One type of tumor,

CHECKLIST

Teaching topics in hypoglycemia

☐ An explanation of the three types of hypoglycemia—fasting, pharmacologic, and reactive—including their causes and symptoms
☐ Importance of preventing or promptly treating hypoglycemia to avoid severe complications
☐ Preparation for diagnostic tests, such as the fasting plasma glucose test and oral glucose tolerance test
☐ Dietary modifications to prevent changes in blood glucose levels
☐ Medications and their administration
☐ Surgery for tumors
☐ Emergency treatment of a hypoglycemic episode
☐ Prevention of hypoglycemic episodes

Marlene Ciranowicz, RN, MSN, CDE, who wrote this chapter, is an independent nurse consultant from Dresher, Pa.

What happens in acute hypoglycemia

Your patient's probably reported having headaches, dizziness, or confusion during a hypoglycemic episode, but he might not realize that falling blood glucose levels produce profound changes in his body. Use the chart below to help him understand what happens in acute hypoglycemia.

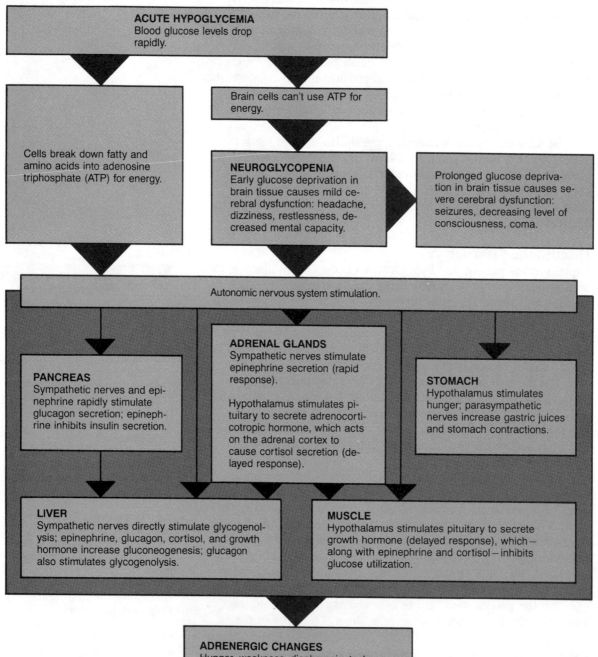

ACUTE HYPOGLYCEMIA
Blood glucose levels drop rapidly.

Brain cells can't use ATP for energy.

Cells break down fatty and amino acids into adenosine triphosphate (ATP) for energy.

NEUROGLYCOPENIA
Early glucose deprivation in brain tissue causes mild cerebral dysfunction: headache, dizziness, restlessness, decreased mental capacity.

Prolonged glucose deprivation in brain tissue causes severe cerebral dysfunction: seizures, decreasing level of consciousness, coma.

Autonomic nervous system stimulation.

PANCREAS
Sympathetic nerves and epinephrine rapidly stimulate glucagon secretion; epinephrine inhibits insulin secretion.

ADRENAL GLANDS
Sympathetic nerves stimulate epinephrine secretion (rapid response).

Hypothalamus stimulates pituitary to secrete adrenocorticotropic hormone, which acts on the adrenal cortex to cause cortisol secretion (delayed response).

STOMACH
Hypothalamus stimulates hunger; parasympathetic nerves increase gastric juices and stomach contractions.

LIVER
Sympathetic nerves directly stimulate glycogenolysis; epinephrine, glucagon, cortisol, and growth hormone increase gluconeogenesis; glucagon also stimulates glycogenolysis.

MUSCLE
Hypothalamus stimulates pituitary to secrete growth hormone (delayed response), which—along with epinephrine and cortisol—inhibits glucose utilization.

ADRENERGIC CHANGES
Hunger, weakness, diaphoresis, tachycardia, pallor, anxiety, tremors, nervousness, rebound hyperglycemia.

insulinoma, causes excessive insulin secretion. (See *Teaching about insulin-producing tumors.*) An extrapancreatic tumor can also lead to hypoglycemia, but the mechanism isn't known. Liver disease interferes with the liver's ability to raise blood glucose levels by gluconeogenesis and glycogenolysis. Other causes include adrenocortical insufficiency, growth hormone deficiency, and severe chronic renal failure.

Tell the patient with *pharmacologic hypoglycemia* that his blood glucose levels may fall slowly or rapidly in response to a drug that does one of three things: increases the amount of insulin circulating in his blood, enhances insulin action, or impairs his liver's glucose-producing capacity. If glucose levels fall slowly, he'll experience headache, dizziness, restlessness, and decreased mental capacity. If untreated, he could experience seizures, unconsciousness, or coma. If glucose levels fall rapidly, he'll have hunger, weakness, diaphoresis, tachycardia, pallor, anxiety, tremors, nervousness, and rebound hyperglycemia.

Explain that the most common causes of this type of hypoglycemia are insulin and oral sulfonylureas used to treat diabetes. Other causes include beta blockers and excessive alcohol inges-

Teaching about insulin-producing tumors

Does the doctor suspect that your patient's hypoglycemia stems from an insulinoma? If so, explain that these rare, insulin-producing tumors originate in the pancreatic beta cells. They most commonly occur in patients ages 30 to 60. Blood glucose levels decrease gradually, so the patient usually has neuroglycopenic signs and symptoms of hypoglycemia, especially in the fasting state. He also may exhibit chronic lethargy and fatigue.

Offer reassurance
Reassure the patient that about 90% of insulinomas are small, autonomously functioning, and benign. They usually produce signs and symptoms related to excess insulin secretion rather than local tumor effects.

Describe tests
Explain to the patient that these tumors produce an abnormally high insulin level but that they usually secrete excess insulin intermittently or only in slightly above-normal amounts. Therefore, the doctor must order multiple overnight fasting blood samples, prolonged fasting, or infusion of insulin secretagogues, such as tolbutamide (Orinase) or glucagon, to confirm the diagnosis. An above-normal proinsulin level also suggests these tumors.

Explain surgery
Tell the patient that the doctor will surgically remove the tumor after localizing it by angiography. A small number of these tumors are malignant, and some cancerous tumors recur after being removed. If so, hypoglycemia persists, and the doctor may order frequent high-carbohydrate feedings and oral diazoxide (Hyperstat) to maintain blood glucose levels. If these measures fail, he may use the anticancer drug streptozocin (Zanosar) as palliative therapy.

Understanding insulin-induced hypoglycemia

The patient with insulin-requiring diabetes mellitus—particularly long-standing Type I—treads a fine line between tight blood glucose control and hypoglycemia. To help him avoid insulin-induced hypoglycemia, teach him to recognize and avoid these common causes:
• chronic insulin overdose
• delayed or omitted meals
• strenuous or prolonged exercise not balanced by extra calories
• faulty insulin injection techniques (improperly mixed insulin, accidental injection into muscle rather than subcutaneous tissue, or injection into lipotrophic sites or other sites with irregular insulin absorption).

If your patient does develop insulin-induced hypoglycemia, teach him that his signs and symptoms will depend on his type of insulin:
• Short-acting insulins (regular and Semilente) cause a rapid blood glucose drop and corresponding adrenergic changes (hunger, weakness, diaphoresis, tachycardia, pallor, anxiety, tremors, nervousness, and rebound hyperglycemia).
• Intermediate- and long-acting insulins (NPH, Lente, and Ultralente) cause a gradual blood glucose drop with neuroglycopenic symptoms (headache, dizziness, restlessness, and decreased mental capacity).

tion. Signs and symptoms depend on when the patient took the particular drug. (See *Understanding insulin-induced hypoglycemia.*)

If the patient has *reactive hypoglycemia,* inform him that his blood glucose levels will fall rapidly, but they won't go drastically below normal. He'll experience hunger, weakness, diaphoresis, tachycardia, pallor, anxiety, tremors, and nervousness. These symptoms are usually mild, occurring within a few hours after a meal and resolving quickly with treatment.

Explain that three types of reactive hypoglycemia have been identified: alimentary hypoglycemia, hypoglycemia secondary to an imminent onset of Type II diabetes mellitus or impaired glucose tolerance, and idiopathic reactive hypoglycemia.

If the patient has *alimentary hypoglycemia,* tell him that it reflects digestive dysfunction, usually from extensive gastric surgery. Teach him that food passes through the stomach and enters the small intestine more rapidly than normal, causing glucose to be absorbed quickly. This first produces hyperglycemia, which stimulates the release of an excessive amount of insulin. The insulin, in turn, causes blood glucose levels to drop abruptly. Alimentary hypoglycemia usually occurs within 1 to 3 hours after eating.

Tell the patient with *reactive hypoglycemia secondary to Type II diabetes mellitus or impaired glucose tolerance* that this rare condition produces an abrupt drop in blood glucose levels 3 to 5 hours after a meal, but just why this happens remains a mystery. One theory is that delayed and excessive insulin secretion, triggered by carbohydrate ingestion, causes the drop.

Inform the patient with *idiopathic reactive hypoglycemia* that this type is the most common. Its hallmark is a rapid drop in blood glucose levels 2 to 4 hours after eating carbohydrates. The exact cause of idiopathic reactive hypoglycemia is unknown. Explain to the patient that symptoms—diaphoresis, tremors, and dizziness—will subside with appropriate therapy within 20 minutes. Reassure him that his condition doesn't predispose him to diabetes mellitus, as is commonly believed.

Complications

Emphasize the importance of preventing or promptly treating hypoglycemic episodes to avoid severe complications. Make sure your patient understands that the key danger with hypoglycemia is that once it occurs, he may quickly lose his ability to think clearly. If this should happen while he's driving a car or operating machinery, it could cause a serious accident.

Explain that brain cells can't survive long without glucose. Prolonged or severe hypoglycemia (blood glucose levels of 20 mg/dl or less) will cause permanent brain damage and could be fatal.

Describe the diagnostic workup

Explain to the patient that the types of diagnostic tests ordered will depend on whether his symptoms are related to eating or fasting. Once the doctor determines this, he'll order serial blood glucose studies, such as a plasma glucose test. He may also order an oral glucose tolerance test, an I.V. glucose tolerance test, and a C-peptide assay.

Plasma glucose test

Inform the patient that this test confirms low blood glucose levels and determines how low levels have fallen during a hypoglycemic episode. Review the symptoms of hypoglycemia with the patient, and tell him to notify you as soon as any of these symptoms occur, so that a blood sample can be drawn before treatment begins.

Instruct the patient not to eat or drink anything except water for 12 hours before a fasting plasma glucose test. Inform him that the results of this test may be inconclusive. If so, he'll need to be admitted to the hospital so that the fasting period may be extended another 24 to 72 hours. Explain that the liver can provide enough glucose to maintain adequate blood levels during a prolonged fast. But if his hypoglycemia results from an underlying pathology, such as an insulinoma, then test results will show it.

Tell the patient that a separate test will be done after a fasting plasma glucose test to measure his insulin levels and evaluate pancreatic function. If an insulinoma is present, insulin levels will be elevated.

Oral glucose tolerance test

Explain to the patient that this test helps diagnose reactive hypoglycemia. The doctor will prescribe a diet that ensures a daily intake of 150 to 300 g of carbohydrates for 3 days before the test. Then, for 12 hours before the test, the patient will need to fast. Tell him to avoid caffeine, alcohol, strenuous exercise, and smoking during the fasting and testing periods because these factors can cause misleading test results. Also discuss any medications that must be withheld during the test period.

Tell the patient that the test itself lasts 5 hours and that he'll be given a sweet solution to drink at the start of the test. Urge him to drink the entire solution, and instruct him to notify you immediately if symptoms of hypoglycemia occur. Make sure he understands that the interval between ingestion of the glucose solution and the onset of symptoms can help determine his type of reactive hypoglycemia.

I.V. glucose tolerance test

Inform the patient that this test helps detect fasting hypoglycemia caused by insulinomas and other tumors that secrete insulin or an insulin-like substance. Prepare the patient for the test in the same manner as for an oral glucose tolerance test. However, point out that instead of being given oral glucose, he'll receive an I.V. substance known to stimulate insulin secretion (such as tolbutamide, glucagon, or leucine). Here again, teach the patient the importance of reporting hypoglycemic symptoms immediately. Tell him that the test will be stopped and he'll be treated promptly if such symptoms occur.

C-peptide assay
Explain that this test helps diagnose fasting hypoglycemia. It also differentiates fasting hypoglycemia caused by an insulinoma from fasting hypoglycemia caused by insulin injections. No preparation is needed.

Teach about treatments
Treatment for hypoglycemia combines diet to prevent glucose levels from dropping rapidly and medications to control anxiety, delay gastric emptying, alleviate symptoms, and treat tumors. Surgery may also be used to remove tumors.

Diet
Emphasize to the patient the importance of carefully following the prescribed diet to prevent a rapid drop in blood glucose levels. Discuss his specific meal plan, and encourage him to comply with it. Advise him to eat small meals throughout the day, and mention that bedtime snacks also may be necessary to keep his blood glucose at an even level. Instruct him to avoid alcohol and caffeine because they may trigger severe hypoglycemic episodes.

Tell the patient with reactive hypoglycemia to avoid simple carbohydrates and other foods high in carbohydrates. Such foods load the body with glucose and may stimulate excessive insulin production, triggering a hypoglycemic episode. Help the patient plan low-carbohydrate, high-protein meals by reviewing the foods belonging to these food groups with him. Also, instruct him to add fiber to his diet because it delays the absorption of glucose from the GI tract.

If the patient is obese and has impaired glucose tolerance, suggest ways that he can restrict his caloric intake and lose weight. If necessary, help him find a weight-loss support group.

Tell the patient with fasting hypoglycemia that he'll need to increase his caloric intake because his body needs more glucose to counteract excessive insulin secretion. Warn him not to postpone or skip meals and snacks because severe and possibly prolonged hypoglycemia may develop. Tell him to call his doctor for instructions if he doesn't feel well enough to eat.

Medication
Teach the patient about prescribed drug therapy. For example, if an antianxiety drug such as diazepam (Valium) is prescribed, warn him that it may cause drowsiness. Advise him to avoid potentially hazardous activities, such as driving a car or other activities that require alertness, until this adverse reaction subsides.

If medication has been prescribed to delay gastric emptying in reactive hypoglycemia, teach the patient about possible adverse effects. Propranolol (Inderal) may also be ordered to alleviate

Hypoglycemia or hyperglycemia?

Some signs and symptoms of hypoglycemia resemble those of hyperglycemia, and patients with hypoglycemia often suffer rebound hyperglycemia.

Review the chart below with your patient and his family to help them distinguish between these two disorders and administer prompt treatment.

DISORDER	CAUSES	SIGNS AND SYMPTOMS	ACTION
Hypoglycemia	• High-carbohydrate meals • Delayed meals • Excessive amounts of certain medications • Excessive exercise • Alcohol or caffeine • Stress • Diabetes mellitus, liver disease, or tumors • Extensive gastric surgery	• Diaphoresis • Faintness • Headache • Palpitations • Trembling • Impaired vision • Hunger • Difficulty awakening • Irritability • Personality changes	• If the patient's conscious, give food or liquid containing sugar (for example, orange juice, cola, candy). • If the patient's unconscious, administer glucagon and call the doctor immediately.
Hyperglycemia	• Insufficient insulin • Failure to follow prescribed diet • Infection, fever, emotional stress	• Polydipsia and polyuria • Increased blood glucose and ketone levels • Weakness, abdominal pain, generalized aches • Deep, rapid breathing • Anorexia, nausea, vomiting	• Call the doctor immediately. • Give sugar-free fluids if the patient can swallow. • Have a diabetic patient test blood for glucose and urine for ketones every 4 hours during a hyperglycemic episode.

symptoms of a hypoglycemic episode, such as hypertension, diaphoresis, tachycardia, and palpitations.

If the patient has an inoperable insulinoma, explain that diazoxide (Hyperstat) helps treat fasting hypoglycemia by inhibiting insulin release. Together with a high-calorie diet, it helps maintain adequate blood glucose levels.

If chemotherapy has been ordered to treat inoperable tumors, explain the protocol to the patient and the possible adverse reactions to each drug.

Also advise the patient not to take nonprescription medications, such as antihistamines, without his doctor's approval. Explain that many nonprescription medications contain ingredients that mask symptoms of decreased blood glucose levels or induce hypoglycemia.

Surgery
If your patient with fasting hypoglycemia is scheduled for surgery to remove an extrapancreatic tumor or an insulinoma, you'll need to prepare him for the operation. Review standard preoperative and postoperative procedures as you would with any patient scheduled for abdominal or thoracic surgery.

After surgery, provide appropriate discharge instructions. Most important, instruct the patient to notify his doctor if symptoms of hypoglycemia recur. He should also know the symptoms of hyperglycemia, such as increased urine output and thirst. (See *Hypoglycemia or hyperglycemia?*) Hyperglycemia may occur postoperatively if more than 90% of the insulin-producing cells in the pancreas were destroyed during surgery.

Other care measures

As with diabetes mellitus, a big part of your treatment plan for a hypoglycemic patient consists of careful teaching of the patient and his family. Teach both the patient and his family the symptoms of hypoglycemia, such as tremors, palpitations, confusion, and diaphoresis. Review the treatment measures they should follow if the patient has a hypoglycemic episode, and make sure they understand the importance of *immediate* care (see *Managing a hypoglycemic episode*). Also, teach them how to administer glucagon. Advise the patient and his family to notify the doctor if hypoglycemic episodes don't respond to treatment or if they occur frequently. Help the patient and his family verbalize their feelings and concerns.

Teach the patient how to prevent hypoglycemic episodes (see *Preventing hypoglycemic episodes,* page 288). Discuss his life-style and personal habits to help him identify precipitating factors, such as poor diet, stress, or mismanagement of diabetes mellitus. Explore ways that he can change or avoid each precipitating factor you've identified. If necessary, teach him stress-reduction techniques and encourage him to join a support group. For the patient with pharmacologic hypoglycemia from insulin or oral hypoglycemic agents, review the essentials of managing diabetes mellitus, if indicated. Finally, encourage the patient to see his doctor regularly.

Further readings

Campbell, R.K. "New, Improved Glucagon Emergency Kit," *Diabetes Educator* 13(1):62, Winter 1987.

Cassmeyer, V.L. "Preventing, Recognizing, and Treating Diabetic Shock," *NursingLife* 7(1):33-40, January-February 1987.

Cerrato, P.L. "Hypoglycemia: Separating Facts from Fads," *RN* 52(4):81-83, April 1989.

"Emergency," *Clinical Diabetes* 6(1):22-23, January-February 1988.

Kitabchi, A.E., and Goodman, R.C. "Hypoglycemia: Pathophysiology and Diagnosis," *Hospital Practice* 22(11):45-56, 59-60, November 30, 1987.

Service, F.J. "Hypoglycemias: Their Etiologies and Diagnosis," *Clinical Diabetes* 7(2):25, 27-39, March-April 1989.

Wyngaarden, J., and Smith, L.H., eds. *Cecil Textbook of Medicine,* 18th ed. Philadelphia: W.B. Saunders Co., 1988.

PATIENT-TEACHING AID

Managing a hypoglycemic episode

Dear Caregiver:

A sudden hypoglycemic episode may affect the ability of the person in your care to recognize his symptoms and take appropriate action.

It will be up to you to manage the crisis for him. In such an emergency, you *must* raise his blood glucose levels immediately to prevent permanent brain damage and even death.

So be sure you have sources of glucose (sugar) available.

If the person is conscious
Give him any of the following:

Foods and fluids	Amount
Apple juice, orange juice, or ginger ale	4 to 6 oz
Regular cola or other soft drink	4 to 6 oz
Corn syrup, honey, or grape jelly	1 tablespoon
Hard candy	5 to 6 pieces
Jelly beans	6
Gumdrops	10

If the person is unconscious or has trouble swallowing
Give him a subcutaneous injection of glucagon. Be sure to check the expiration date on the glucagon kit frequently and replenish your supply as needed.

How to inject glucagon
1 Prepare the glucagon following the manufacturer's instructions included in the kit.

2 As the nurse taught you, select an appropriate injection site.

3 Pull the skin taut, then cleanse it with an alcohol swab.

4 Using your thumb and forefinger, pinch the skin at the injection site, then quickly plunge the needle into the skin fold at a 90-degree angle, up to the needle hub.

Push the plunger down to quickly inject the glucagon.

5 Withdraw the needle and rub the site with an alcohol swab.

6 Turn the person onto his side. Because glucagon may cause vomiting, this position reduces the possibility of choking.

7 If the person doesn't wake up in 5 to 20 minutes, give a second dose of glucagon and seek emergency help.

If he wakes up and can swallow, give him some sugar immediately. (See the chart at left for a selection of foods and fluids containing high amounts of sugar.) Do this because glucagon isn't effective for longer than about 90 minutes.

Then call the doctor.

Preventing hypoglycemic episodes

Dear Patient:

Although hypoglycemia can be a serious disorder, you can keep it under control and prevent most hypoglycemic episodes. Just follow these simple guidelines.

Stick to your diet
Eat all your meals and snacks at the prescribed time and in the prescribed amounts.

Also avoid alcohol and caffeine — they can cause your blood glucose level to drop.

Take your medicine
If the doctor prescribes medicine to control your hypoglycemia, strictly follow your schedule. Take the right amount of medicine at the right time.

Always check with the doctor who is treating your hypoglycemia before you take any over-the-counter medicine or any other prescribed medicine.

Also inform him about any new treatments you're having for another condition.

Control stress
Reduce stress by practicing relaxation techniques, such as deep breathing and guided imagery. Change your life-style, if possible: work less, and take more time for hobbies, traveling, and other leisure activities.

Exercise
Take some precautions when you exercise. For example, don't exercise alone, do eat extra calories to make up for those burned, and don't exercise when your blood glucose level is likely to drop.

For example, if you have *fasting hypoglycemia,* your blood glucose level is likely to drop 5 hours or more after a meal.

If you have *reactive hypoglycemia,* your blood glucose level will fall 2 to 4 hours after a meal.

If you have *pharmacologic hypoglycemia,* ask your doctor for guidelines.

If you're a *diabetic,* don't inject your insulin into a part of your body that you'll be exercising during the next few hours.

Carry carbohydrates
Carry a source of fast-acting carbohydrate, such as hard candy or sugar packets, with you at all times.

Know the warning signs
Note what symptoms you typically have before an episode of hypoglycemia. Make certain that your family, friends, and co-workers know that you have hypoglycemia, and be sure that they can also recognize the warning signs. Early recognition can prevent an acute episode.

Alert others
Wear a Medic Alert bracelet or carry a medical identification card that describes your condition and what emergency actions to take.

Renal and Urologic Conditions

Contents

Acute renal failure

When teaching about acute renal failure (ARF), you'll be dealing with a patient who is typically troubled by the disorder's initial sign—sudden onset of oliguria or, rarely, anuria. Such a patient may be frightened also by the prospect of losing renal function or becoming dependent on dialysis. To address the patient's fears, your teaching must stress that early detection and aggressive therapy can usually reverse ARF and prevent its progression to chronic renal failure.

As always, effective treatment hinges on the patient's compliance. To involve him in his care, you'll teach him to monitor his fluid balance daily by taking his blood pressure, measuring his weight, and recording his intake and output. Active self-care also means teaching him to recognize the signs and symptoms of ARF and related complications and to accept activity limits and a prescribed diet. If the patient is scheduled for dialysis, you'll review the process, including preparations and aftercare. (For more information, see the sample teaching plan, *Teaching the patient with newly diagnosed ARF*, page 292.)

Discuss the disorder

First inform the patient that ARF is the sudden inability of the kidneys to remove waste materials from the blood and to maintain proper fluid and electrolyte balance. Next, tell him whether his ARF is classified as prerenal, intrarenal, or postrenal.

Explain that *prerenal failure* results from conditions outside the kidneys that impair renal perfusion. These conditions include congestive heart failure and other cardiovascular disorders, hypovolemia, and renovascular obstruction. *Intrarenal failure* results from disorders that damage the kidneys themselves, such as acute tubular necrosis. And *postrenal failure* results from bilateral obstruction of urinary outflow caused, for example, by renal calculi or ureteral constriction.

Then explain which phase of ARF the patient is experiencing. In the *oliguric phase,* urine output usually falls to less than 500 ml/day. Advise the patient that this phase typically lasts from 7 to 21 days (a longer oliguric phase may herald chronic renal failure) and that he'll probably have to limit his fluid intake. In the *diuretic phase,* the kidneys abruptly begin producing a greater urine volume—from 3 to 7 liters/day. Because of this, many patients assume that the diuretic phase indicates improving renal function. For patients with reversible ARF, the diuretic phase often *does* in-

CHECKLIST

Teaching topics in acute renal failure

☐ Explanation of acute renal failure, including its classification (prerenal, intrarenal, or postrenal) and phase (oliguric or diuretic)
☐ Importance of treatment to prevent complications, most notably chronic renal failure
☐ Signs and symptoms of uremia, hypervolemia, hypovolemia, and hyperkalemia
☐ Preparation for diagnostic tests, such as blood and urine studies and kidney-ureter-bladder radiography, renal ultrasonography, or other imaging studies
☐ Activity limitations
☐ Dietary restrictions and, as indicated, instructions to restrict or increase fluids
☐ Medication precautions
☐ Hemodialysis or peritoneal dialysis
☐ Surgery, if appropriate
☐ How to monitor fluid balance, weight, and blood pressure

Contributors to this chapter include **Betty Dale, RN, BSN,** formerly a head operating room nurse at Abbott-Northwestern Hospital in Minneapolis; **Margery Fearing, RN, MA;** and **Carralee Sueppel, RN, BLS.** Ms. Fearing and Ms. Sueppel are clinical nursing specialists in renal medicine and urology, respectively, at the University of Iowa Hospitals and Clinics, Iowa City.

Teaching the patient with newly diagnosed ARF

If your patient is experiencing acute renal failure (ARF) for the first time, she probably knows little about this disorder. But even if she does, your teaching will still be selective. Why? Because your priority is to calm her fears and prepare her for therapy to help prevent progression to chronic renal failure.

Specifically, what will you teach your patient about ARF, and what techniques and materials will you use? Read the following account of Jane Anderson's experience to help you learn to modify a standard teaching plan to fit an individual patient's needs.

Consider Mrs. Anderson's condition
While recovering from an aortic aneurysm resection and endarterectomy of the left common iliac and femoral arteries, Jane Anderson, a 58-year-old retired teacher, develops ARF. Here is her history: Her slowly healing abdominal wound recently showed signs of infection, for which she received antibiotics. Recent angiograms revealed several arterial obstructions and significant atherosclerotic changes in the right renal artery. Mrs. Anderson has a history of hypertension and elevated serum lipid levels. She weighs 180 lb and is 5' 4" tall.

As you set diet and meal-planning goals together, you notice for the second day in a row that Mrs. Anderson is febrile. The next day she experiences a severe and prolonged drop in blood pressure, requiring fluid replacement. She also becomes acutely dyspneic. The doctor orders blood tests and chest X-rays. The test results point to a diagnosis of ARF. The doctor wants to schedule hemodialysis at once. Mrs. Anderson agrees to undergo the treatment but confides that she's scared and discouraged.

What are Mrs. Anderson's learning needs?
Using a standard teaching plan as a guide, you decide what subjects to include or adapt in your teaching about ARF. A standard plan for ARF covers:
• renal function, including anatomy and the kidneys' role in fluid and electrolyte balance
• renal failure—its causes, stages, and complications
• blood and urine tests and radiographic studies
• dialysis options (hemodialysis or peritoneal dialysis)
• other treatments, such as activity restrictions, dietary modifications, drug therapy, and surgery.

After reviewing the standard plan, you realize that Mrs. Anderson knows little about renal anatomy and function and less about renal failure. However, her acutely deteriorating condition prohibits lengthy or complex teaching. Instead, you'll give her a simple explanation of renal dysfunction and focus on teaching her about impending hemodialysis. Your goal is clear: to help her overcome her fear so she'll be better able to participate in treatment and benefit from

future teaching.

You decide to explain how hemodialysis will help her, to familiarize her with the equipment, and to introduce her to the dialysis personnel. Later, you'll teach her about activity restrictions, diet, drugs, and fluid balance (intake and output).

Setting learning outcomes
Based on Mrs. Anderson's immediate needs, together you list her learning outcomes. For example, Mrs. Anderson will be able to:

```
- describe basic kidney function and dysfunction
- relate personal symptoms to ARF
- state reason for diagnostic tests
- explain the purpose of dialysis
- describe the procedures she'll undergo before
and during dialysis
- list reportable adverse reactions to dialysis
- report signs of ARF complications
- list dietary and fluid restrictions as they
relate to her condition
- demonstrate how to measure fluids accurately
- identify life-style changes necessitated by
ARF.
```

Selecting teaching techniques and tools
What techniques and tools are available (and appropriate) for teaching Mrs. Anderson? After careful consideration, you choose *short explanations and brief discussions* of kidney function and structure, ARF causes, signs of complications, and diet, drug, and fluid restrictions. You may also use *demonstration* to teach about dialysis procedures and activity needs.

Keeping in mind Mrs. Anderson's condition and frame of mind, you choose clear and simple teaching materials. Appropriate materials may include booklets, videotapes, kidney models, diagrams, medication cards, a tour of the dialysis unit, and even household measuring devices.

Evaluating your teaching
How successful is your teaching? After teaching, what does Mrs. Anderson know about her condition? Does she know what she needs to do to prevent its progression? To find out, you'll perform an ongoing evaluation and reassessment. Perhaps you'll use *question-and-answer discussions.* You might, for instance, ask her to explain how hemodialysis removes wastes from the blood.

You can also use *return demonstration.* For instance, ask Mrs. Anderson to show you how to measure fluids accurately. Your evaluation will help you determine her progress in meeting her learning outcomes and redirect your planning and teaching.

dicate recovery. But for patients with irreversible ARF, you'll need to explain that the oliguric and diuretic phases usually form a recurrent cycle in the normal ARF progression. Mention that the diuretic phase may last from several weeks or months to a year before returning to the oliguric phase.

Complications

Emphasize that compliance with therapy may help prevent serious complications, including uremia, hypervolemia, hypovolemia, and hyperkalemia. What's more, it may prevent or delay chronic renal failure.

Define *uremia* as an accumulation of protein waste products in the blood. Explain that when these waste products reach toxic levels, such complications as uremic pericarditis and uremic pneumonitis may result. Instruct the patient to watch for and report signs and symptoms of uremia, including nausea, vomiting, headache, decreased level of consciousness, dizziness, decreased visual acuity, urinous breath odor, and elevated blood pressure.

Tell the patient that *hypervolemia* is an abnormal increase in the volume of fluid circulating in the body. This excess fluid may accumulate in the vessels or tissues. Unchecked, hypervolemia can result in such serious complications as hypertension, congestive heart failure, and pulmonary edema. Teach the patient to watch for and report signs of hypervolemia, such as sudden weight gain, swollen hands and feet, and increased blood pressure. Instruct him to go to the hospital immediately if he has difficulty breathing or can't lie down flat without breathing discomfort. Both warning symptoms suggest that hypervolemia has progressed to life-threatening congestive heart failure or pulmonary edema.

Explain that *hypovolemia,* an abnormal decrease in the volume of fluid circulating in the body, can progress to shock if it's untreated. Teach the patient to watch for and report indications of hypovolemia, such as weight loss, dry skin and mucous membranes, decreased urine output, muscle cramps, fatigue, dizziness, and decreased blood pressure.

Explain that *hyperkalemia* results when too much potassium accumulates in the blood. Mention that hyperkalemia can cause an irregular heart rate, possibly leading to cardiac arrest and death. Instruct the patient to notify the doctor if he experiences weakness, malaise, nausea, diarrhea, or abdominal cramps—all warning signs and symptoms of hyperkalemia.

Describe the diagnostic workup

Instruct the patient about the routine blood and urine tests used to evaluate renal function. Also teach about such diagnostic studies as computed tomography (CT), kidney-ureter-bladder (KUB) radiography, magnetic resonance imaging (MRI), renal angiography, renal ultrasonography, and retrograde ureteropyelography. Explain that these tests can detect abnormal kidney size or shape, fluid accumulation, and obstruction of urinary outflow. When diagnostic test results are inconclusive, the doctor may order renal biopsy to help diagnose ARF (see *Explaining renal biopsy,* page 294).

Explaining renal biopsy

When laboratory and diagnostic test results are inconclusive, the doctor may order renal biopsy to help diagnose acute renal failure, especially when oliguria lasts longer than 6 weeks.

Preparation
Teach the patient about the procedure and its purpose, explaining who will perform it, when and where it will be done, and that it takes about 15 minutes.

Then instruct the patient to restrict food and fluids for 8 hours before the test. Assure him that he'll receive a mild sedative before the test to help him relax.

Procedure
Explain that during the biopsy, he'll lie prone with a sandbag positioned under his abdomen to help stabilize the kidney. He'll feel the biopsy site being numbed with a local anesthetic. Then the doctor will ask him to hold his breath and remain still as he inserts a needle into the kidney to obtain a tissue sample for analysis. Though the needle remains in the kidney for only a few seconds, caution him that he may feel a pinching pain.

Aftercare
Inform him that after the test, he can expect pressure to be applied to stop superficial bleeding. He'll also have a pressure dressing.

Explain that for the next 12 hours, he must lie flat and motionless on his back to prevent bleeding. During that time, the nurse will closely monitor his blood pressure and heart and respiratory rates to detect any complications.

Blood and urine tests
Inform the patient that blood studies may include a complete blood count, arterial blood gas (ABG) and electrolyte analyses, and tests to determine serum protein, creatinine, uric acid, and blood urea nitrogen levels. Tell the patient what test he'll have, describing features or giving directions—for example, what happens during venipuncture or how the arterial puncture required for ABG analysis may cause momentary pain.

Mention that follow-up blood tests will be performed regularly during treatment to ensure that ARF is being managed properly.

Teach the patient having urine studies how to collect a clean-catch midstream specimen to help evaluate the kidneys' diluting and concentrating ability and to help determine the cause and degree of renal failure.

CT scan
Explain that a renal CT scan helps detect abnormalities and takes about an hour. Tell the patient that he won't have to follow any special pretest procedures. But if he's having a CT scan using an iodine-based contrast medium, he'll answer questions to detect hypersensitivity to iodine or iodine-containing foods. If the patient is sensitive to iodine, the doctor may forego the contrast medium or may prescribe antiallergenic prophylaxis.

If the patient is to receive a contrast medium, explain that when it's injected, he may feel a transient flushing, headache, metallic taste, and burning or stinging at the injection site. Then, from his position on an X-ray table, he'll hear loud clacking sounds as the scanner rotates around his body. Explain that he must lie still because motion distorts the X-ray picture.

If he received a contrast medium, instruct him to immediately report any post-test allergy signs and symptoms, such as flushing, nausea, itching, and sneezing.

KUB radiography
Inform the patient that this X-ray study shows the size and position of the urinary organs and helps detect abnormalities, such as calculi. Assure him that he doesn't need to restrict food or fluids and that the procedure takes only a few minutes.

MRI scan
Tell the patient that MRI evaluates renal structures without exposing him to X-rays. The test lasts about 1 hour.

Explain that during the test, he'll lie supine on a table that slowly moves him head first into a cylinder. He may be given earphones to muffle the scanner's loud clacking sounds as it produces images of renal structures. Advise him that the test is painless but that he may feel confined in the tunnel-like apparatus. Urge him to lie still to prevent a blurred or distorted image.

Renal angiography
Explain that renal angiography permits the doctor to visualize kidney vessels. The test takes about 1 hour.

Identify pretest preparations; for example, the patient will fast for about 8 hours before the test. Then just before the test, he may receive a narcotic analgesic, and a sedative to help him relax. Instruct him to remove all metallic objects and to void just before the procedure.

Inform him that during the test, he'll lie supine on an X-ray table, and a peripheral I.V. line will be started. He'll feel the skin over the arterial puncture site being cleansed with antiseptic solution. Then, a local anesthetic will be injected, and the femoral artery will be punctured and cannulated for instillation of a contrast medium. Warn the patient that he may experience transient discomfort (flushing, burning sensation, and nausea) as the contrast medium is injected. After this injection, a series of rapid-sequence X-ray films will be taken. Then the catheter will be removed, and pressure will be applied to the puncture site for about 15 minutes to stop bleeding.

Tell him that after the test, he'll lie flat in bed for 8 to 12 hours. He'll remain nonambulatory for 24 hours after the test. The nurse will monitor his blood pressure and heart and respiratory rates every 15 minutes for 1 hour, then every 30 minutes for 2 hours, and then once hourly until they're stable. His popliteal and dorsalis pedis pulse rates will be monitored every 4 hours.

Renal ultrasonography

Mention that this test helps detect kidney abnormalities. It takes about 30 minutes. Explain how ultrasound images are shaped by sound waves bouncing off internal structures. Reassure the patient that the test is safe and painless.

Explain that during the test, the patient will lie prone. He'll be comfortably draped, but the area to be scanned will be exposed. He'll feel the technician apply a gel (an ultrasound conductant) and pass the ultrasound transducer over the exposed area. (Some patients say that it feels like a back rub.) Inform him that he may be instructed to breathe deeply to assess kidney movement during respiration.

Retrograde ureteropyelography

Tell the patient that this test evaluates the structure and integrity of the renal collecting system. The test takes 30 to 60 minutes.

If the patient's having general anesthesia, explain that he'll have to fast for 8 hours before the test, but he'll drink plenty of fluids to ensure adequate urine flow.

Then, during the test, he'll be positioned on an X-ray table with his legs in stirrups. A contrast medium will be injected through a urethral catheter. Then X-ray films will be taken while the catheter's in place and again after it's withdrawn. Warn the patient that he may feel discomfort when the catheter and the contrast medium are inserted. Also describe the sounds made by the X-ray machine as it exposes the films.

After retrograde ureteropyelography, inform him that the nurse will frequently monitor his blood pressure and heart and respiratory rates until they're stable. She'll also check his urine color and volume. Instruct him to notify the doctor or nurse if blood continues to appear in his urine after the third voiding or if he develops chills, fever, or increased pulse or respiratory rates.

Teach about treatments

Emphasize that treatment aims to prevent progression to chronic renal failure as well as to maintain or improve the patient's quality of life. Make sure he understands any activity restrictions, diet and fluid requirements, medication directions (if any), and self-care techniques, such as blood pressure monitoring and precise intake-output measurement. If your patient will undergo dialysis or, possibly, surgery, make this a major teaching focus.

Activity

Instruct the patient with severe ARF to limit his activity to conserve energy. If the doctor orders bed rest, teach the patient early, progressive ambulation techniques, as appropriate.

Diet

Although diet alone can't treat ARF, it does play an important role in therapy. Collaborate with the doctor and the dietitian to teach the patient how to adjust his diet.

Explain that a diet high in calories and low in protein, sodium, potassium, and phosphorus can prevent further renal damage, yet maintain nutritional balance. Inform the patient that his diet is based on his renal function, so he must follow the one prescribed by the doctor or dietitian. Review the diet plan with him and discuss meal planning. Be sure to include family members in your teaching, especially those who prepare his meals.

Depending on ARF's cause, the patient may need to either restrict or increase his fluid intake. If he must restrict fluids and complains of thirst, suggest that he suck on ice chips. (Remind him to include the ice chips as part of his daily fluid intake.) Advise him to divide his fluid amounts over the day. Teach him to avoid overload by showing him how to measure fluid intake and urine output precisely. If he must increase intake, explain that the doctor will order supplemental fluids for him to drink or to receive intravenously.

Medication

Inform the patient that the doctor may recommend discontinuing the medications he normally takes, particularly if they're concentrated in the kidneys and excreted in the urine. Explain that because ARF delays urine excretion, the patient's risk for toxic drug reactions increases. Emphasize, though, that he shouldn't discontinue any medication without his doctor's approval.

If the patient's ARF is classified as prerenal, inform him that he may be given diuretics to increase his urine output—after adequate hydration has been achieved by replacing fluids.

Procedures

If ARF does not respond promptly to other treatment measures, you'll need to prepare the patient for dialysis. Explain the purpose and type the patient will receive—hemodialysis or peritoneal dialysis (see *Comparing hemodialysis and peritoneal dialysis*). And make sure he understands what to expect during and after the procedure.

Comparing hemodialysis and peritoneal dialysis

If your patient requires dialysis, use the chart below to help you explain how the treatment works. The two types of dialysis—hemodialysis and peritoneal dialysis—share a common purpose: to remove toxic wastes from the blood when renal failure prevents the kidneys from carrying out this function. But each technique—appropriate for certain situations—accomplishes this quite differently. And each technique has specific advantages and disadvantages.

HEMODIALYSIS	PERITONEAL DIALYSIS
Indications	
Hypercatabolism; hyperkalemia; severe respiratory insufficiency; a large, draining abdominal wound; intra-abdominal adhesions; a diffusely infected abdominal wall; or critical volume excess	Severe coagulopathy, cardiovascular disease, exhausted vascular access sites, religious objections to hemodialysis
Procedure	
The patient's blood circulates through an external dialyzing system. Within the dialyzer, the blood flows through a semipermeable material while a special dialysis solution is pumped around the other side under hydrostatic pressure. Because the blood contains toxic wastes and higher concentrations of hydrogen ions and other electrolytes than the solution contains, these solutes diffuse across the semipermeable material into the solution. Any solute that's more concentrated in the dialysis solution (composed of glucose or bicarbonate) diffuses into the blood.	In this technique, a hypertonic dialyzing solution is instilled through a catheter into the patient's peritoneal cavity. By osmosis, water moves from the blood, across the peritoneum, and into the dialysis solution; by diffusion, excessive concentrations of toxins also move across the peritoneal membrane. After an appropriate dwelling time, the dialysis solution (now containing the toxins) is drained.
Advantages	
• Takes only 3 to 5 hours per treatment • Requires only three treatments weekly • In an emergency, I.V. administration avoids surgical access route • After careful instruction, can be performed at home	• Can be performed immediately • Requires less complex equipment and less specialized personnel than hemodialysis; thus, costs less • Requires small amounts of heparin—or none at all—so fewer bleeding problems result • Causes no blood loss and minimal cardiovascular stress; doesn't require venipuncture • Can be performed by patient anywhere without assistance • Allows patient independence without long interruptions • Rarely causes disequilibrium syndrome • May be used for patients with unstable cardiovascular status; gives better results than hemodialysis in children and diabetic patients with renal failure • Allows for more liberal diet
Disadvantages	
• Requires surgical creation of vascular access between circulation and dialysis machine • Needs complex water treatment, expensive dialysis equipment, and highly trained personnel • Requires large heparin doses to prevent blood clotting and to maintain catheter patency • Confines patient to special treatment setup • Contraindicated in shock and hypotension; must be used cautiously in infants, small children, and patients with cardiovascular disease • May cause dysrhythmias, septicemia, air emboli, rapid fluid and electrolyte imbalance, hemolytic anemia, metastatic calcification, hepatitis, hypotension, hypertension, itching, pain (generalized or in chest), hemorrhage from heparin toxicity, leg cramps, nausea, vomiting, headache	• Requires 10 hours for significant response to treatment • May require more than three treatments weekly • Severe protein loss necessitates high-protein diet (up to 100 g/day) • Carries high risk of peritonitis; repeated bouts may cause scarring, preventing further treatments with peritoneal dialysis • Provides less urea clearance than hemodialysis • Requires abdomen free from recent surgery, adhesions, or infection • May cause dysrhythmias; hyperglycemia; bacterial or chemical peritonitis; pain (abdominal, low back, shoulder); dyspnea; atelectasis; pneumonia; severe protein loss; fluid overload or loss; constipation; catheter site inflammation, infection, or leakage

Reviewing temporary hemodialysis access sites

Inform your patient about catheter placement in hemodialysis. Two commonly used sites, the femoral and subclavian veins, allow easy access.

At both sites, the surgeon uses the Seldinger technique to insert an introducer needle into the vein. He then inserts a guide wire through the introducer needle and removes the needle. Using the guide wire, he threads a plastic or Teflon catheter (with a Y hub) into the vein. For femoral access, he may use a single catheter with a Y hub or two catheters, one for inflow and another placed about ½" distal to the first for outflow.

With femoral access, risks include infection, femoral vessel trauma, and thrombosis. Because movement could dislodge the catheter, damage the vein, or obstruct the blood flow, you'll instruct the patient to remain as immobile as possible.

With subclavian access, risks include pneumothorax on insertion and infection. You can tell the patient that this catheter site allows him more mobility.

FEMORAL VEIN CATHETERIZATION

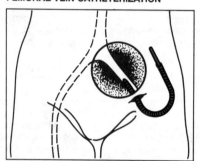

SUBCLAVIAN VEIN CATHETERIZATION

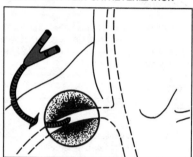

Hemodialysis. If the patient is having hemodialysis, explain that the surgeon will catheterize the subclavian or femoral veins (see *Reviewing temporary hemodialysis access sites*). Rarely, a fistula may be created to access the patient's blood. The blood leaves his body through the catheter or fistula, circulates through a dialyzer that removes waste products, and returns to his body. Tell him that the process takes 3 to 5 hours. Advise him that after hemodialysis, he may feel tired for several hours as his body adjusts to the treatment (see the patient-teaching aid *Learning about hemodialysis,* page 300).

Peritoneal dialysis. Tell the patient that this procedure may be performed manually, by an automatic or semiautomatic cycler machine, or as continuous ambulatory peritoneal dialysis. With all methods, a catheter will be inserted into the peritoneal cavity through a small incision in his abdomen. Explain that a dialysate solution will be instilled through the catheter into the peritoneal cavity, where it remains long enough to allow excess fluid, electrolytes, and accumulated wastes to move through the peritoneal membrane into the dialysate. After the prescribed dwelling time, the dialysate will be drained from the patient's peritoneal cavity, taking toxins with it. (For more information, see the patient-teaching aid *Learning about peritoneal dialysis,* page 301.)

Whether the patient is undergoing hemodialysis or peritoneal dialysis, tell him that he'll be awake and alert during the procedure. Instruct him to notify the dialysis nurse if he feels faint, dizzy, or nauseated, or if he vomits or has a headache—possible indicators of overly rapid fluid loss.

Surgery
If the patient's ARF is classified as postrenal, treatment usually includes catheterization to drain urine from the bladder and either

a surgical or nonsurgical procedure to free the obstruction. If the patient requires surgery, explain the procedure to him, including who will perform it and where, and how long it will take. For example, you may need to prepare him for removal of calculi from a ureter or the renal pelvis.

Other care measures
Prepare the patient for home care by teaching him how to monitor his fluid balance. Show him how to measure and record his daily weight, blood pressure, and intake and output (see the patient-teaching aid *How to measure fluid intake and output,* page 302).

Instruct the patient to weigh himself at the same time each day, using the same scale and wearing the same type of clothing. Tell him to notify the doctor if his weight increases or decreases by more than 5% from one day to the next. Explain the difference between weight gain from fluid accumulation and that from increased caloric intake.

Teach the patient the proper technique for taking accurate blood pressure readings. Stress that he should compare every blood pressure reading with his baseline reading. Tell him to notify the doctor if his blood pressure rises above 140/86 mm Hg or drops below 90/60 mm Hg.

Emphasize the importance of accurately recording daily fluid intake and output. When the patient totals his fluid intake, remind him to include any food that's liquid at room temperature—for example, gelatin, custard, and ice cream.

Sources of information and support
American Association of Kidney Patients
211 East 43rd Street, Suite 301, New York, N.Y. 10017
(212) 867-4486

American Kidney Foundation
6110 Executive Boulevard, Suite 1010, Rockville, Md. 20852
(800) 638-8299

National Kidney Foundation
Two Park Avenue, New York, N.Y. 10003
(212) 889-2210

Further readings
Banerjee, K., et al. "The Management of Acute Renal Failure in Intensive Care Units," *Intensive Care Nursing* 2(2):84-87, 1986.
Bihl, M.A., et al. "Comparing Stressors and Quality of Life of Dialysis Patients," *American Nephrology Nurses' Association Journal* 15(1):27-28, 33-36, February 1988.
Fuchs, J., and Schreiber, M. "Patients' Perception of CAPD and Hemodialysis Stressors," *American Nephrology Nurses' Association Journal* 15(5):282-85, 300, October 1988.
Miller, C.A., and Evans, D. "CNS Manifestations of Acute Renal Failure," *Critical Care Nurse* 7(3):94-95, May-June 1987.
Pezzarossi, H.E., et al. "High Incidence of Subclavian Dialysis Catheter-related Bacteremias," *Infection Control* 7(12):596-99, December 1986.

Learning about hemodialysis

Dear Patient:

The doctor has ordered hemodialysis for you. This procedure uses a dialyzer (pictured below) to do your kidneys' job. By filtering your blood through its internal membranes, it removes extra fluids and impurities and returns purified blood to your body.

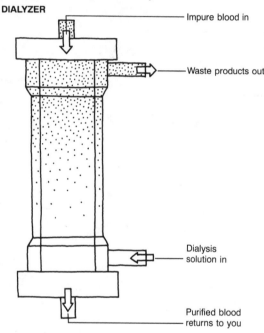

DIALYZER

Impure blood in

Waste products out

Dialysis solution in

Purified blood returns to you

Before dialysis
The nurse or dialysis technician will weigh you. She'll also take your blood pressure — once while you're lying down and once while you're standing.

Then the doctor will create an opening in your collarbone or groin area. He'll make the area numb first so that you're not uncomfortable. Into the opening he'll put a thin, hollow tube called a catheter. Stitches will keep it in place. The catheter will be used to transfer some of your blood to the dialyzer.

During dialysis
Next, the nurse will attach the dialyzer to your catheter. Then she'll turn on a machine to begin the treatment. She'll check the dialyzer and all the connections frequently.

During hemodialysis, your blood flow will gradually increase, so the nurse will check your blood pressure every half hour or so. She'll also collect blood samples every once in a while during hemodialysis and when it ends. The blood samples will be tested to see how well hemodialysis is working for you.

Be sure to tell the doctor or nurse how you feel, especially if you experience a headache, backache, nausea, vomiting, muscle twitching, difficulty breathing, or pain.

When hemodialysis is over, the nurse will disconnect the catheter from the dialyzer.

After dialysis
When you go home, remember to keep the skin around the catheter clean and dry. If the nurse has taught you how, you may cleanse it with hydrogen peroxide solution daily until healing is complete and the stitches are removed.

Call your doctor if you have pain, swelling, redness, or drainage in the catheter area.

Learning about peritoneal dialysis

Dear Patient:

Your doctor has ordered peritoneal dialysis for you. This procedure removes impurities from your blood when your kidneys aren't working properly.

Before dialysis
The nurse will take your blood pressure twice — once while you're standing and once while you're lying down. She'll also weigh you. Then she'll tell you to urinate to make you feel more comfortable and to protect your bladder.

Next, the doctor will create an opening in your peritoneal cavity, which is near your stomach. (First, he'll numb the area with an anesthetic.) He'll insert a slender tube called a catheter into the opening. (See the illustration.)

PERITONEAL CAVITY

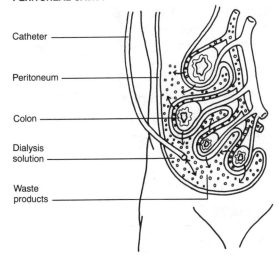

Catheter

Peritoneum

Colon

Dialysis solution

Waste products

The catheter is used to transfer a special warmed solution into your peritoneal cavity. The solution collects impurities that cross through your peritoneum (a membrane that acts like a filter). After a specified time, the solution is drained from your body.

Both you and the nurse (or the dialysis technician) will wear masks during dialysis to prevent possible infection. After the nurse connects the inflow and the drainage tubings, she'll hang the solution bag above you on a bedside pole and the drainage bag below your bed.

During dialysis
To start dialysis, the nurse will open a clamp to allow the solution to flow into your peritoneal cavity where it will remain for a prescribed time. Then it will drain into the collection bag. The procedure will be repeated until the right amount of solution has been instilled for the prescribed number of cycles.

To ensure your progress, the nurse will take your blood pressure, check your breathing, examine the tubing, and change your catheter dressing whenever it's soiled or wet.

After dialysis
The nurse will disconnect the tubing and cover the catheter with a sterile, protective cap. She'll apply ointment and bandage the catheter site.

Call your doctor if you notice any signs of infection (such as redness or swelling) or fluid imbalance (such as a sudden weight gain or swollen arms or legs). As the nurse has taught you, take your vital signs regularly and change the catheter dressing. And be sure to keep all your follow-up appointments.

How to measure fluid intake and output

Dear Patient:

Your doctor wants you to keep a daily record of your intake and output. This record can help him judge your progress and response to treatment.

What are intake and output?

Intake includes everything you drink, such as water, fruit juice, and soda. It also includes foods that become liquid at room temperature, such as gelatin, custard, and ice cream. Intake even includes fluids, liquid medicines, and solutions delivered through tubing into one of your veins (intravenously) or into your stomach.

Output includes everything that leaves your body as a fluid. It includes urine, drainage from a wound, diarrhea, and vomit.

Because your intake should balance your output, you need to keep very accurate records. Whenever possible, *measure* fluids. Don't guess.

Measuring intake

1 Measure and record the amount of fluid you have with each meal, with medicine, and between meals. Pour any liquid into a measuring cup or other graduated container before serving it in a glass or cup. Also keep in mind that labels on cans and bottles indicate exact amounts.

Don't forget to subtract any amount you don't drink. The difference, of course, is your intake amount.

2 If you're receiving medicine or nutrition intravenously or through a stomach tube, record the amounts of fluid you use.

Measuring output

1 Before throwing away any urine from a bedpan, urinal, or portable toilet, measure and record the amount (or ask your caregiver to do this). Keep a measuring container handy just for this purpose.

2 If you have a drainage bag in place, make sure you or your caregiver measures and records the amount of fluid in the bag before discarding it.

3 Measure and record any vomit or liquid bowel movements as output.

Common measures

Your doctor may want you to measure your fluid intake and output metrically. To convert your household measure, use the information below.

To convert fluid ounces (oz) to the metric equivalent of milliliters (ml), multiply by 30. To convert ml to oz, divide by 30.

APPROXIMATE EQUIVALENTS

Household	Metric
1 quart (32 oz)	1,000 ml
1 pint (16 oz)	500 ml
1 measuring cupful (8 oz)	240 ml
2 tablespoons (1 oz)	30 ml

Renal calculi

Because 90% of calculi don't exceed 5 mm in diameter, most of your patient teaching will involve explaining measures to promote their natural passage—most important, vigorous hydration and use of diuretics. However, for patients with larger calculi, your approach will differ significantly. Why? Because these sometimes excruciatingly painful calculi require removal or disintegration to avoid urinary tract obstruction. Depending on the calculi's size and location, you'll need to prepare the patient for a procedure, such as extracorporeal shock wave lithotripsy (ESWL), or for surgery.

To prevent calculi from recurring, your teaching must then stress compliance with prescribed dietary restrictions and with drug therapy, if appropriate.

Discuss the disorder

Tell the patient that calculi usually begin when tiny specks of material—normally dissolved and excreted in the urine—instead precipitate and remain in the urinary tract. As more material clings to these specks, they gradually develop into calculi. Inform him that calculi usually form in the kidneys, but can develop anywhere in the urinary tract, including the ureters and the bladder. Explain that although the exact cause of calculi is unknown, many factors have been linked to their formation (see *Calculi risk factors,* page 304).

Mention that small calculi seldom cause problems because they're easily carried through the ureter and passed in the urine. A larger calculus, however, may cause excruciating pain if it enters the ureter. It may also become lodged there. For more information, see *Where calculi form,* page 305, and *Analyzing renal calculi,* page 306.

Complications

Using an anatomic drawing of the renal and urologic system, explain how calculi too large for natural passage cause urinary tract obstruction. Point out that unless calculi are removed, urine trapped above the obstruction may set the stage for renal infection. Eventually, the kidney's collecting system may also become abnormally dilated—holding up to several liters of urine—a condition known as hydronephrosis. If untreated, hydronephrosis may lead to renal insufficiency.

June Stark, RN, BSN, and **Betty Dale, RN, BSN,** contributed to this chapter. Ms. Stark is a critical care instructor and renal nurse consultant at New England Medical Center, Boston. Ms. Dale was formerly head nurse, operating room, Abbott-Northwestern Hospital, Minneapolis.

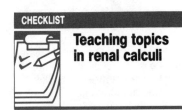

CHECKLIST

Teaching topics in renal calculi

☐ Explanation of how calculi precipitate in the urine, including factors that influence their formation
☐ Types of calculi and where they form in the urinary tract and kidneys
☐ Importance of treatment to prevent urinary tract obstruction
☐ Preparation for blood and urine tests to determine the cause and composition of calculi and for radiography or ultrasonography to pinpoint their location
☐ Importance of following prescribed dietary restrictions and adequate hydration to prevent recurrence of calculi
☐ Drugs to prevent recurrent calculi
☐ Preparation for procedures, such as extracorporeal shock wave lithotripsy, to remove calculi
☐ Home care of nephrostomy tube, if appropriate
☐ Preparation for surgery, if indicated
☐ Signs of infection
☐ Sources of information and support

Calculi risk factors

Your patient will want to know why he developed calculi. Discuss these predisposing factors.
• Metabolic disorders, including cystinuria, renal tubular acidosis, hypercalcemia, hyperoxaluria, hyperuricosuria, and hypomagnesemia.
• Familial history of calculi.
• Geography. The U.S. northwest, southeast, and southwest are known "calculi belts."
• Climate. Exposure to sunlight increases vitamin D production—and calcium absorption.
• Diet. Eating too much animal protein can raise calcium, oxalate, and uric acid levels by 50% in calculus-forming patients.
• Dehydration. Diminished water intake and reduced urine production concentrate calculus-forming substances.
• Obesity.
• Urinary tract abnormalities.
• Sedentary jobs (linked to upper urinary tract calculi).
• Infection.
• Obstruction. Urinary stasis (as in spinal cord injury) allows calculus constituents to collect.
• Drug therapy. Medications, vitamins C and D, and calcium supplements can promote calculi development. For instance, *acetazolamide* reduces urinary citrates, increases urinary uric acid levels, and raises urine pH. *Adrenocorticosteroids* elevate urine calcium levels as do *phosphate-binding nonabsorbable antacids,* which also increase urine pH.

Chemotherapeutic agents and *external radiation* may cause cellular breakdown and acute hyperuricemia. *Furosemide* may cause hyperuricemia, too, whereas *aspirin* and *probenicid* raise urine uric acid levels in hyperuricemia.

Hydrochlorothiazide may cause uric acid calculi by increasing urine uric acid levels, and *acid phosphates* may promote struvite calculus formation.

Describe the diagnostic workup

Prepare the patient for blood, urine, and imaging tests to diagnose and evaluate renal calculi.

Blood and urine tests

Inform the patient that blood will be drawn for a complete blood count and for determination of calcium, phosphorus, blood urea nitrogen, creatinine, glucose, uric acid, and electrolyte levels. Tell him who will perform the venipunctures and when. Explain that tests to measure serum calcium and phosphorus may be repeated on three different days to determine average levels; instruct him to fast for 8 hours before each test.

Teach the patient how to collect a clean-catch urine specimen for routine urinalysis and urine cultures to check for infection. If a 24-hour urine specimen is ordered—for example, to measure calcium, phosphorus, uric acid, creatinine, or magnesium levels—explain the collection technique.

KUB radiography

Prepare the patient for kidney-ureter-bladder (KUB) radiography, an X-ray of the kidneys, ureters, and bladder, to reveal calculi and other lesions. Inform him that he needn't restrict food and fluid and that the test takes only a few minutes. Explain that he'll lie supine with his arms extended over his head while a single X-ray is taken.

Excretory urography

Teach the patient that excretory urography (also known as intravenous pyelography) visualizes the kidneys and urinary tract to determine the presence of calculi. Tell him that the test takes about an hour. Instruct him to drink plenty of fluids and then to fast for 8 hours before the test. Inform him that he may receive a laxative or other bowel preparation before the test.

Explain that during the test he'll lie supine on an X-ray table. After injection of a contrast medium, X-rays will be taken at specific intervals. Mention that he'll hear loud, clacking sounds as the X-ray machine exposes the films and that a belt may be placed around his hips to keep the contrast medium in the kidneys. Warn him that he may experience a transient burning sensation and a metallic taste when the contrast medium is injected. Tell him to report these and any other sensations to the doctor. Also, instruct him to report symptoms of delayed reaction to the contrast medium, including itching, rashes, hives, and wheezing or other breathing difficulties.

Renal ultrasonography

Inform the patient that renal ultrasonography localizes urinary obstructions, such as calculi. Tell him that the test takes about 30 minutes. Reassure him that the test is safe and painless; in fact, it may feel like a back rub.

Explain that during the test he'll lie in a prone position, and the area to be scanned will be exposed. The technician will then

Where calculi form

Point out to the patient that calculi may form at various sites in the urinary tract, including the kidneys, ureters, and bladder.

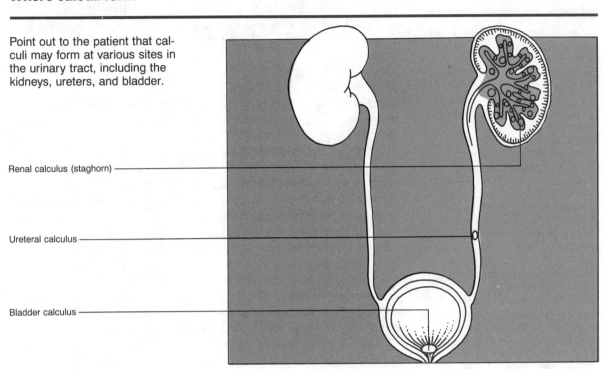

Renal calculus (staghorn)

Ureteral calculus

Bladder calculus

apply ultrasound jelly and guide a transducer over the area. During the test, the patient may be asked to breathe deeply to assess kidney movement during respiration.

Teach about treatments
Inform the patient of dietary changes and medications to prevent recurrent calculi. Warn him that about 50% of patients experience another calculus within five years of the first one, so it's vital that he practice prevention. If the patient has a calculus that's too large to pass naturally in his urine, educate him about procedures or, if appropriate, surgery to remove it.

Diet
Explain that because most calculi contain calcium he'll need to restrict this mineral. Also explain that oxalate reduction is also necessary because hypocalcemia enhances oxalate reabsorption. High urinary oxalate levels can also precipitate calculus formation. Restricting phosphorus is important, too, because phosphorus helps the body absorb calcium.

In collaboration with a dietitian, teach the patient which foods to eliminate from his diet, such as cheese for its calcium; beets, spinach, chocolate, and tea for their oxalate; and carbonated soft drinks for their phosphorus.

Tell the patient that he'll also need to restrict protein. Experts attribute 50% of the increased calcium, oxalate, and uric acid in calculus-forming patients to a diet rich in animal proteins.

Analyzing renal calculi

After the patient's calculus is removed and analyzed for its mineral content, review its distinguishing features and possible causes.

Calcium oxalate, calcium phosphate, or mixture

Inform the patient that two-thirds of calculi are formed from calcium. Such calculi are small, rough, and hard. They're gray to white and shaped like needles or a staghorn. Possible causes include hypercalciuria, hyperuricosuria, hyperoxaluria, and hyperparathyroidism.

Struvite (magnesium ammonium phosphate)

Tell the patient that struvite calculi are the second most common type. These yellow stones assume a staghorn shape and crumble easily. They're caused by microbes that split urea.

Uric acid

Explain that dye enhancement is needed for X-ray visualization of uric acid calculi. These yellow-to-red calculi are small and hard. They may be associated with gout, high uric acid levels caused by chronic diarrhea or low fluid intake, or ingestion of dietary purines.

Cystine

Inform the patient that small cystine calculi clump into smooth, waxy staghorn shapes. They may result from cystine-containing crystals in urine or diminished fluid intake.

Triamterene

Tell the patient that this recently recognized calculus type may follow ingestion of triamterene, a potassium-sparing diuretic.

Phosphate

Explain that nonopaque phosphate calculi may result from malnutrition, chronic urinary tract infection, or urine stasis.

Tell him to limit consumption of meat to once a day or less.

Instruct the patient to drink at least 12 glasses of fluid a day (to keep his urine volume at about 2 quarts daily). To prevent nocturnal dehydration, tell him to drink fluids before bedtime and to awaken at least once during the night to drink a large glass of water.

Medication

Explain that drug therapy depends on the composition of the patient's calculi and will continue indefinitely to prevent them from recurring.

To prevent calculi recurrence associated with hypercalcemia, the doctor may prescribe a thiazide, which reduces calcium reabsorption in the distal tubule. Tell the patient that thiazides lower urinary calcium excretion by about 50%. Because they work best with a low-sodium diet, instruct the patient to reduce his salt intake. Advise him to let the doctor know if he experiences extreme fatigue or sexual problems. If so, the doctor may discontinue these medications.

If the doctor prescribes a calcium-binding gel, such as sodium cellulose phosphate, to reduce the patient's calcium levels, advise him to take the drug with meals. Because this drug also binds magnesium, diminishing intestinal absorption, the patient may develop hypomagnesemia. Instruct him to take a magnesium supplement between meals.

For recurrent calcium oxalate calculi, the doctor may order cholestyramine to minimize dietary oxalate absorption by causing it to be passed in the stool. Warn the patient to avoid vitamin C—metabolism of this vitamin produces oxalate.

Other drug therapy to prevent calculi recurrence may include allopurinol for hyperuricosuria or sodium bicarbonate to alkalinize the patient's urine. For infected struvite stones, the patient requires a culture-specific antibiotic. But if antibiotics are ineffective, the doctor may prescribe acetohydroxamic acid, an inhibitor of urease-producing bacteria. Educate the patient about the purpose and administration of these drugs and about any possible adverse effects.

Procedures

Teach the patient about invasive and noninvasive procedures to remove his calculi. Such procedures include extracorporeal shock wave lithotripsy (ESWL), percutaneous nephrolithotomy, endoscopic stone manipulation, ultrasonic endoscopy, percutaneous ultrasonic lithotripsy, and laser lithotripsy. In addition, chemolysis may be used alone or in combination with these treatments.

Extracorporeal shock wave lithotripsy. Explain that this procedure successfully removes calculi in 75% of patients who have ureteral calculi; other interventions are necessary for the remaining 25%. Tell the patient that he'll sit in a large water tank or tub. The water transmits high-pressure shock waves into the body without loss of energy. Or he'll lie on a stretcher positioned over a water-filled cushion. The cushion, containing the shock electrode and reflector, is coupled to the stretcher by a layer of ultrasonic gel and placed against the patient's lower back. Inform the patient that the procedure using the water-filled cushion can be performed with a sedative-analgesic rather than a general anesthetic because improved shock generators keep shock-wave intensity high but below the patient's pain threshold.

If appropriate, teach the patient about a machine that eliminates water entirely, requiring only that the shock wave tube be positioned directly against the patient's body. Further refinements include synchronizing shock waves with the patient's respirations as well as his ECG, use of ultrasound rather than X-rays to image and localize stones, and computerized patient positioning to align the calculi with the shock waves.

Explain that ESWL can't be used for patients who can't fit in the chair (weight exceeding 300 lb); patients too large or small for the water tank; or patients with obstruction distal to the calculus, infection, abnormal kidney anatomy or calcifications, a pacemaker, or bleeding abnormalities. ESWL is also contraindicated in pregnancy, an inability to use anesthesia (if a water tank is used), most cases of hypertension, and elderly patients.

Tell the patient that ESWL is usually performed as an outpatient procedure unless a fever, hemorrhage requiring transfusion, severe pain or uncontrollable nausea, urinary obstruction from a fragmented calculus, or cardiopulmonary problems develop. Other complications include hypertension (in about 8% of patients) and decreased renal function. To prepare the patient for ESWL, give him a copy of the teaching aid *Understanding extracorporeal shock wave lithotripsy,* page 311.

Percutaneous nephrolithotomy. Inform the patient that this procedure removes renal or upper ureteral calculi. Tell him that after the doctor makes small incisions in the skin and the kidney, he uses fluoroscopy to guide the insertion of a nephroscope through the kidney. He then removes the calculus with a basket catheter.

Endoscopic stone manipulation. Explain that this procedure removes small calculi (less than 1 cm in diameter) in the lower third of the ureter. Using a cystoscope, the doctor inserts special loops or basket catheters up the ureter to capture and remove the calculus.

Inform the patient that a *ureteroscope* may allow visualization and calculi removal in the middle third of the ureter. Ureteral probes or electrohydraulic shock waves allow the doctor to fragment and remove a large calculus. If he's unable to remove the calculus, he may leave a loop or ureteral catheter in place to dilate the ureter for later manipulation. He may also leave a ureteral catheter in place after the procedure to prevent obstruction from edema. (See *Teaching about calculi removal,* page 308.)

Ultrasonic endoscopy. Tell the patient that in this procedure the doctor fragments the trapped calculus with an ultrasonic probe. He then removes the pieces by suction. A J-stent, a catheter that helps to pass the calculus and drain urine, is usually left in place until after discharge.

Teaching about calculi removal

Discuss the method chosen to remove the patient's calculi. If the surgeon chooses *percutaneous nephrolithotomy,* explain that he'll use a basket catheter to surround and then retrieve urinary stones caught in the patient's ureter. A basketing instrument housed within a flexible rod is inserted through a cystoscope or ureteroscope into the ureter and advanced to the calculus.

Once the apparatus is adjacent to the calculus,

the surgeon pushes the wire basket through the rod and beyond the calculus, allowing the flexible wires to spread out within the ureter. He slowly pulls back the wire basket to capture the calculus. Then he carefully withdraws the entire apparatus.

If the surgeon chooses *percutaneous ultrasonic lithotripsy,* inform the patient that the lithotriptor's ultrasonic probe breaks up calculi by vibration and continuously suctions the fragments from the kidney.

EXTRACTOR IN PLACE

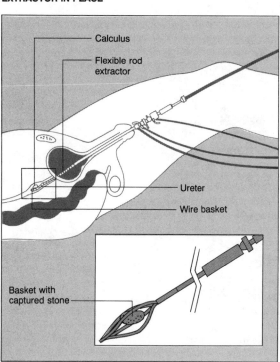

Calculus

Flexible rod extractor

Ureter

Wire basket

Basket with captured stone

PROBE IN PLACE

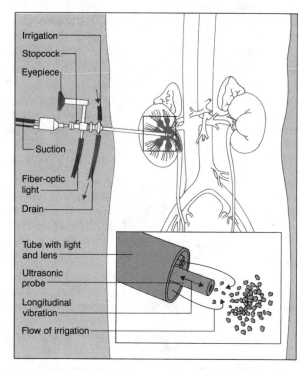

Irrigation

Stopcock

Eyepiece

Suction

Fiber-optic light

Drain

Tube with light and lens

Ultrasonic probe

Longitudinal vibration

Flow of irrigation

Percutaneous ultrasonic lithotripsy. Inform the patient that this procedure (also called percutaneous nephrolithotripsy) removes kidney or upper ureteral calculi. Explain that the doctor uses electrohydraulic or ultrasonic probes to fragment larger calculi with electrical or ultrasonic energy. He removes larger fragments with a basket catheter and smaller pieces with continuous suction through a nephroscope. Afterward, he places a catheter in the tract to drain the kidney and control bleeding, a possible major complication. The external lumen of the large nephrostomy catheter and its inflated balloon (if the doctor uses a balloon catheter) applies direct pressure to bleeding areas.

Laser lithotripsy. Explain that this procedure involves direction of laser light through a ureteroscope to the calculus, where strobe-light pulsations create tiny shock waves. These pulsations fragment calculi but don't damage the ureteral wall.

Chemolysis. Explain that this procedure uses drugs to break up calculi. Drugs can be delivered through a nephrostomy tube to renal calculi or through a catheter to bladder and ureteral calculi. Hemiacidrin is used for struvite dissolution; sodium bicarbonate for uric acid dissolution.

Surgery

If the patient requires surgery to remove calculi, reinforce the doctor's explanations, and answer any questions. Tell the patient what type of anesthetic he'll receive—local, spinal, or general—and advise him of any preoperative food and fluid restrictions or bowel preparation.

Pyelolithotomy, ureterolithotomy, or nephrolithotomy. If the patient is scheduled for surgery to remove calculi from the kidney (pyelolithotomy) or the ureter (ureterolithotomy), inform him that he'll be positioned on his side and that the doctor will remove the calculi through an incision in his flank. Nephrolithotomy involves incising the kidney to remove staghorn calculi and calculi embedded too tightly for removal by pyelolithotomy. Or it may be used for calculi that don't fragment well, such as calcium oxalate or phosphate calculi.

Tell the patient that he'll receive fluids through an I.V. line for 1 or 2 days after surgery. If a drainage tube will be inserted during surgery, tell him that it will be removed before he goes home. If the ureter will be opened during surgery, explain that he'll have a catheter until the ureter heals (usually 4 to 6 days after surgery). Full recovery will take 6 to 8 weeks.

Percutaneous nephrostomy. When calculi are in the renal pelvis or upper ureter, you may need to prepare the patient for percutaneous nephrostomy. Explain that the doctor will insert a catheter and guide wire through a puncture in the patient's flank. Guided by fluoroscopy or ultrasonography, he'll move the catheter to the renal pelvis or upper ureter and inject a contrast medium to visualize the collecting system and to locate the calculi. Then he'll either grasp and remove the calculi or shatter them with ultrasound waves and flush away the fragments.

Tell the patient that he'll return from surgery with a urinary drainage tube in place. If the patient has a permanent drainage tube, such as a nephrostomy tube, teach him how to care for it at home. (See *Caring for your nephrostomy tube,* page 312.)

If the drainage tube is temporary, tell the patient that it will be removed 1 to 3 days after surgery, when X-rays reveal that the kidney is healing properly and no calculi remain. Inform the patient that he can return to work immediately if he has a sedentary job or in 2 weeks if his job requires any lifting.

Nephrectomy. If the calculi are embedded in one of the renal calyces (staghorn calculi) and the kidney is severely damaged or not working, the doctor may order a nephrectomy. Emphasize that the body can adapt well to one healthy kidney.

Explain that nephrectomy is the removal of part or all of a kidney. Show the patient where the incision will be made—in the flank over the affected kidney. Tell him that the surgery takes 2 to 3 hours.

Discuss that with a partial nephrectomy, the doctor removes

a portion of the kidney, usually the lower pole, in a patient with severe obstruction and permanent kidney damage. Unless removed, the damaged region may produce more calculi.

Inform the patient that he'll have a catheter in his bladder after nephrectomy to carefully monitor his urine volumes. Mention that he may also have a Penrose or Hemovac drain in place to remove fluid from the surgical site, thereby preventing infection. Both the catheter and drain will be removed before the patient goes home. Tell him that full recovery takes 6 to 8 weeks.

Teach the patient about complications of surgery, including bleeding, wound infection, emboli, periureteral abscess, chronic fistula, or ureteral obstruction. Instruct him to report the following signs and symptoms to the doctor immediately: bleeding, difficulty breathing, diminished urine output, foul-smelling dressings, chills, fever, and pain, especially between the ribs and ileum (known as flank pain).

Other care measures

After most calculi removals, instruct the patient to strain his urine after voiding and to save any solid material for analysis. Explain that knowing the composition of calculi will help the doctor pinpoint what's causing them to form. Advise him to report continuing passage of bloody urine to the doctor right away.

Finally, tell the patient to watch for and report signs of infection, such as increased pain, inability to void, change in the color or odor of his urine, or fever exceeding 101° F.

Sources of information and support

American Urological Association Allied
P.O. Box 9397, 6845 Lake Shore Drive, Raytown, Mo. 64133
(816) 358-3317

National Kidney and Urologic Diseases Information Clearinghouse
P.O. Box NKUDIC, Bethesda, Md. 20892
(301) 468-6345

Further readings

Brennan, C. "Lithotriptor Treatment of Kidney Stones in Outpatient Surgery," *Journal of Post Anesthetic Nursing* 4(3):170-71, June 1989.
Coe, F.L., et al. "Pathophysiology of Kidney Stones and Strategies for Treatment," *Hospital Practice* 23(3):185-89, 193-95, 199-200, March 15, 1988.
Conner, P.A., et al. "Nursing Implications of Renal Pelvis Irrigations for Chemolysis," *Journal of Urologic Nursing* 7(1):350-56, January-March 1988.
Ghiotto, D.L. "A Full Range of Care for Nephrostomy Patients," *RN* 51(4):72-74, 76-77, April 1988.
Mactariane, F.J. "Getting Ready for Certification...Urinary Tract Calculi," *American Urologic Association Allied Journal* 23-24, 28, January-March 1988.
Parker-Cohen, P.D. "Extracorporeal Shock-Wave Lithotripsy Treatment for Kidney Stones," *Nurse Practice* 13(3):32, 37-38, 40-42, March 1988.
Reid-Czarapata, B.J. "Post ESWL Positioning... Extra-Corporeal Shock Wave Lithotripsy," *Urologic Nursing* 9(2):14-15, October-December 1988.

Understanding extracorporeal shock wave lithotripsy

Dear Patient:

Your doctor will perform a special procedure called extracorporeal shock wave lithotripsy to get rid of your stone.

During this procedure, a machine will direct shock waves through water or a water-filled cushion and send them into your body, where they will crush the stone.

Keep in mind that the energy from these shock waves is targeted at the stone and shouldn't damage your body tissues. Here's what to expect.

Before the procedure
On the night before the procedure, don't eat or drink anything after midnight. The next day when you arrive at the hospital at your scheduled time, a nurse will take blood and urine samples. She may also perform an electrocardiogram to evaluate your heart function.

Then a nurse will start an I.V. line in your arm or hand so you can receive fluids and drugs. A doctor will give you an anesthetic to prevent pain and help you stay still during the procedure. And a technician will X-ray your kidneys, ureters, and bladder to find out the size and location of your stone.

During the procedure
You'll sit in a special chair, and be secured with a belt. A thin catheter, called a J-stent, may be placed in your urinary tract to help remove the stone fragments after the stone has been crushed. The J-stent will remain in place for several days afterward.

Next you'll be lowered into a tub of water that reaches to your shoulders. If necessary, you'll be shifted in the chair so you're in the best position for your treatment. Or you may lie on a stretcher that's positioned over a water-filled cushion to receive your treatment.

Throughout the procedure, you'll be asleep or feel drowsy.

After the procedure
You're usually allowed to go home right after the procedure unless a fever or other complications develop. Expect the doctor to give you prescriptions for medication to relieve pain and prevent possible infection.

Because internal bleeding is possible, don't take any aspirin or other anti-inflammatory medicines for 7 to 10 days after the procedure. These drugs could worsen any bleeding.

Expect blood-tinged urine and bruising, especially on your back for several days. If these signs continue longer or if you experience fever or excessive pain, call the doctor immediately.

For several days afterward, strain all your urine and save the stone fragments for your doctor to look at. If you have a J-stent catheter in place, make an appointment for the doctor to remove it. Also, make an appointment for follow-up X-rays and blood studies.

Caring for your nephrostomy tube

Dear Patient:

A nephrostomy tube allows urine to drain from your kidney into a drainage bag. This bag is attached to the tube's free end with a length of tubing.

Because the nephrostomy tube goes directly into your kidney, you'll need to take proper care of the tubing and bag each day to prevent infection.

How to change the tubing and drainage bag

1 Gather your equipment: a clean drainage bag and connecting tube and alcohol swabs. Wash your hands.

Important: Always keep the drainage bag lower than the nephrostomy tube.

2 Disconnect the nephrostomy tube from the used tubing and drainage bag. Don't use your fingernails to disconnect the tubing. Clean the end of the nephrostomy tube with an alcohol swab. Also clean the end of the tubing that connects the new drainage bag to the nephrostomy tube.

3 Now attach the ends of the nephrostomy tube and the connecting tube securely. Don't touch the end of either tube. Check the tubing periodically for kinks.

How to clean the bag and tubing

1 Wash the used bag and tubing with a weak detergent solution daily. Avoid a biodegradable or chlorine product because it may erode the bag.

2 Twice weekly, wash the bag and tubing with a weak vinegar solution (one part vinegar and three parts water) to prevent crystalline buildup. Rinse with plain water and hang them on a clothes hanger to air dry.

How to change the dressing
Change the dressing daily, as your doctor orders.

1 Gather the necessary equipment: Desitin powder, sterile gauze pads, and adhesive tape. Then wash your hands and remove the old dressing.

2 Gently wash around the tube with soap and water. Inspect the skin around the tube. Is any redness present? If so, apply Desitin powder.

If you notice white, yellow, or green drainage, with or without odor, suspect infection, and report it to the doctor. If you see drainage that looks or smells like urine, the tube may be displaced. Report this to the doctor.

3 Next, fold several sterile gauze pads in half and place them around the base of the tube. Cover with an unfolded gauze pad. Apply adhesive tape to secure the gauze pads to your skin.

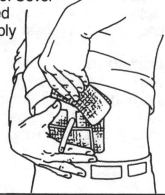

Benign prostatic hyperplasia

Because benign prostatic hyperplasia (BPH) progresses slowly, a patient may not recognize its symptoms right away. Eventually, though, he'll notice a frequent urge to urinate, difficulty starting his urine stream, and waking throughout the night to urinate.

Besides helping your patient identify these and other warning symptoms of BPH, your teaching must explain why prostatic enlargement causes these symptoms. You'll need to discuss what will happen if the patient doesn't have BPH corrected, which tests he'll have to evaluate it, and which treatments he'll undergo, such as surgery to remove prostatic tissue and relieve pressure on the urethra.

Your teaching may be complicated because BPH most commonly affects elderly men. With this in mind, be prepared to overcome age-related learning barriers, such as impaired vision and memory, hearing loss, and other physical limitations.

Discuss the disorder

Using an anatomic drawing of the male genitourinary system, explain normal structure and function. Point out the prostate gland at the base of the bladder surrounding the urethra. Tell the patient that BPH is a nonmalignant overgrowth of prostatic tissue. As the gland size increases, it presses inward, compressing the urethra and obstructing urine flow. (See *How BPH obstructs urine flow,* page 314.) Eventually, he'll notice symptoms of obstruction. (See *Recognizing BPH signs and symptoms,* page 315.) Inform him that BPH is related to aging and that by age 70 most men have some degree of prostate enlargement. Explain that the cause of BPH is unknown, but researchers suspect a hormonal or metabolic etiology.

Complications

Caution the patient that BPH may lead to serious complications if it remains untreated. For instance, the patient may notice a decreasing ability to empty his bladder as the enlargement causes resistance to urine flow. This residual urine can cause urinary tract infection. Warn him that ultimately, he may be unable to void. Then he'll experience acute urine retention and increased bladder pressure, which can result in renal damage if untreated.

Describe the diagnostic workup

Explain the physical examination that the patient will have to evaluate BPH. Tell him that the doctor will examine the prostate

CHECKLIST

Teaching topics in BPH

☐ Explanation of nonmalignant tissue overgrowth in the prostate
☐ Signs and symptoms of benign prostatic hyperplasia
☐ Importance of treatment to prevent complications, such as renal damage
☐ Preparation for diagnostic evaluation, including physical examination, laboratory studies, and radiologic and endoscopic tests
☐ Experimental drug treatments and balloon dilatation
☐ Explanation of transurethral resection of the prostate or open prostatectomy
☐ At-home catheter care, if appropriate
☐ Referral for sexual counseling, if indicated
☐ Sources of information and support

Contributors to this chapter include **Betty Dale, RN, BSN,** and **Gloria Perry, RN.** Ms. Dale was formerly head nurse, operating room, Abbott Northwestern Hospital, Minneapolis. Ms. Perry is a urology nurse clinician at Duke University Hospital, Durham, N.C.

How BPH obstructs urine flow

Explain normal prostate structure and function to the patient. Then show him how benign prostatic hyperplasia (BPH) constricts the urethra, interfering with urine flow. This may result in urine retention and eventually cause renal damage.

NORMAL PROSTATE GLAND

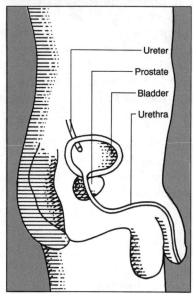

Ureter
Prostate
Bladder
Urethra

BENIGN PROSTATIC HYPERPLASIA

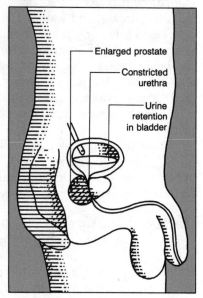

Enlarged prostate
Constricted urethra
Urine retention in bladder

gland by inserting a gloved finger into the patient's rectum. He'll also evaluate the rectal sphincter, which indirectly reflects bladder innervation. Inform the patient that the doctor will observe him as he voids to determine the size and force of his urine stream. He'll be catheterized immediately after urination to measure postvoiding residual volume. Reassure him that he'll be given complete privacy during these often embarrassing procedures.

Next, explain the blood and urine tests that evaluate BPH. Also prepare him for radiologic tests, such as excretory urography, and endoscopic tests, such as cystourethroscopy.

Blood and urine tests
Inform the patient that blood samples will be drawn to measure blood urea nitrogen, serum creatinine, and acid phosphatase levels. Urine specimens will also be collected for urinalysis and to check for infection.

Excretory urography
If the patient is scheduled to undergo excretory urography (intravenous pyelography), tell him that this test evaluates the structure and excretory function of the kidneys, ureters, and bladder. Tell

him who will perform the test and where and that it takes about 1 hour.

Ask the patient about allergies. If he's allergic to shellfish or the iodine they contain, tell him to notify the doctor because the contrast medium contains iodine. Instruct the patient to drink plenty of fluids and then to fast for 8 hours before the test. Inform him that he may receive a laxative or other bowel preparation.

Explain that during the test the patient will lie in a supine position on an X-ray table. After injection of a contrast medium, X-rays will be taken at specific intervals. Describe the X-ray machine's loud, clacking sounds as it exposes films. Mention that a belt may be placed around his hips to keep the contrast medium at a certain level. Warn him that he may experience a transient burning sensation and metallic taste when the contrast medium is injected. Tell him to report these and any other sensations to the doctor, including delayed reaction to the contrast medium.

Cystourethroscopy
Explain that this test allows visualization of the bladder and urethra, permitting evaluation of bladder neck construction, the degree of prostatic enlargement, and urinary obstruction.

Tell the patient who will perform the test and where and that it takes about 20 minutes. If a general anesthetic has been ordered, instruct the patient to fast for 8 hours before the test. If a local anesthetic has been ordered, he may receive a sedative before the test to help him relax.

Describe what happens during the test. Explain that the patient will lie supine on an X-ray table with his hips and knees flexed. His genitalia will be cleaned with an antiseptic solution, and he'll be draped.

Then the doctor will administer a local anesthetic, if appropriate, and introduce the cystourethroscope through the urethra into the bladder. Next, he'll fill the bladder with irrigating solution and rotate the scope to inspect the entire bladder wall surface. If the patient receives a local anesthetic, warn him that he may feel a burning sensation when the cystourethroscope passes through the urethra. He may also feel an urgent need to urinate as the bladder fills with irrigating solution.

If the patient receives a general anesthetic, inform him that for the first hour after the test his blood pressure, heart rate, and respirations will be monitored every 15 minutes; then they'll be monitored hourly until stable. Instruct him to drink plenty of fluids and to take the prescribed analgesics. However, he should avoid alcohol for 48 hours after the test. Reassure him that urinary burning and frequency will soon subside. Instruct him to take antibiotics, as ordered, to prevent bacterial infection.

Tell the patient to report flank or abdominal pain, chills, fever, or decreased urine output to the doctor immediately. In addition, tell him to notify the doctor if he doesn't void within 8

Recognizing BPH signs and symptoms

Help your patient recognize the signs and symptoms of benign prostatic hyperplasia (BPH). Inform him that he may experience some of the following:
- urgent desire to void
- frequent urination (day and night)
- difficulty starting his urinary stream
- decreased size and force of his urinary stream
- dribbling of urine
- incontinence
- incomplete bladder emptying
- urinary tract infection
- acute urine retention.

Dilating the urethra

To preserve function and avoid infection in men with benign prostatic hyperplasia (BPH), more and more doctors are trying noninvasive treatments. One such treatment uses a balloon to dilate the urethra, compressing the prostate gland. This expands the urinary passageway.

If the doctor offers this experimental option, tell the patient that this outpatient procedure takes about 30 minutes. Inform him that he'll receive either a local or a general anesthetic.

Then the doctor inserts a guide wire into the urethra and passes a balloon-tipped tube over the wire into the prostate and bladder area.

Next, he'll inflate the balloon with a saline solution. The inflation widens the urethra and compresses the enlarged prostate gland to allow urine flow. This accomplished, the doctor will remove the balloon apparatus.

Explain that preliminary results offer promise, but more procedures must be done to assess the technique's full value.

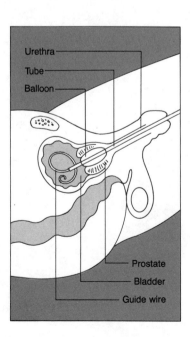

hours after the test or if bright red blood continues to appear after three voidings.

Teach about treatments

Tell the patient that surgery is currently the primary treatment for BPH; however, researchers are investigating certain drugs and procedures to provide long-term relief.

Medication

Discuss two investigational drugs, leuprolide acetate (Lupron) and nafarelin acetate. Both hold promise for patients who aren't candidates for surgery. If your patient will become part of these investigational studies, explain the advantages and disadvantages of participation. Make sure he understands the guidelines for his participation.

Explain that leuprolide acetate reduces prostate volume and improves such signs and symptoms as urinary frequency and urgency and diminished urine stream. Inform the patient that researchers believe nafarelin acetate helps BPH by blocking testosterone production. Warn him that this drug causes impotence, which persists until therapy is discontinued.

Procedures

If appropriate, teach the patient about balloon dilatation to treat BPH. This procedure relieves obstruction by using a balloon to dilate the part of the urethra that passes through the prostate. For more information, see *Dilating the urethra*.

Surgery

Describe two types of surgery—transurethral resection (TUR) and open prostatectomy—to remove some or all prostatic tissue. (See *Teaching about surgical correction of BPH*.)

For either type of surgery, explain that the patient may be placed on a low-residue diet before surgery. Tell him that the night before surgery he may receive a cleansing enema. The doctor will also prescribe antibiotics, usually erythromycin 500 mg and neomycin 1 g every 4 hours for 24 hours before surgery.

If the patient is having a *transurethral resection,* tell him that the surgeon passes a small tubular instrument into the urethra, enabling him to visualize the obstructing prostatic tissue. Then he passes an electric cutting loop through the instrument to trim away the tissue. Explain that TUR typically takes less time, requires a shorter hospital stay, and produces less postoperative pain than an open prostatectomy. If the prostate gland is extremely large, however, a TUR isn't feasible and an open procedure is usually necessary.

During an *open prostatectomy,* the surgeon makes one of three incisions to expose and remove the obstructing prostatic tissue: suprapubic, retropubic, or perineal. Regardless of the incision type, the patient will have an indwelling catheter for several days after surgery. The catheter will be connected to a continuous fluid irrigation system to facilitate the passage of blood clots. Tell him

Teaching about surgical correction of BPH

Inform the patient facing surgery for benign prostatic hyperplasia (BPH) that the operation he'll have depends on several factors, including the extent of prostatic enlargement and the doctor's preferred technique. Describe which operation the surgeon will perform: a transurethral resection or a suprapubic, retropubic, or perineal prostatectomy. Note that the arrows indicate the direction for surgical removal.

Transurethral resection of the prostate
Explain that transurethral resection is the most commonly used surgical procedure for BPH. After the surgeon inserts a transurethral rectoscope, he excises prostatic tissue under direct visualization. He uses cautery to control any bleeding during the surgery. Tell the patient that he'll probably have a spinal anesthetic because it achieves better relaxation than a general anesthetic and prevents postoperative nausea and vomiting.

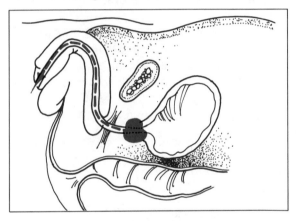

Suprapubic prostatectomy
If the prostate is too large for transurethral removal, inform the patient that the surgeon may perform a suprapubic prostatectomy. In this procedure, the doctor incises the bladder to reach the prostate; then he enucleates the enlarged gland by blunt dissection.

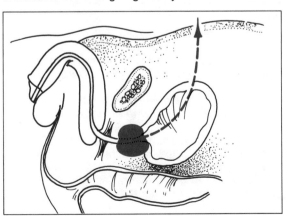

Retropubic prostatectomy
Like the suprapubic approach, a retropubic prostatectomy removes a prostate that's too large for transurethral removal. The surgeon incises the abdomen below the bladder, allowing him to see the prostatic bed and control bleeding.

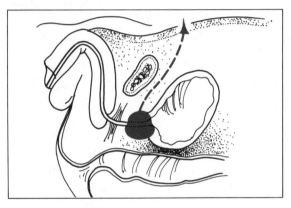

Perineal prostatectomy
Inform the patient that in perineal prostatectomy the surgeon makes a curved incision behind the scrotum and in front of the anus. This perineal approach permits removal of extensive intraurethral lateral lobe hyperplasia. However, because this method may damage nerves that stimulate erection, it may cause sexual dysfunction. The surgeon probably won't use it if the patient has severe arthritis or chronic obstructive pulmonary disease that prevents the required exaggerated lithotomy position.

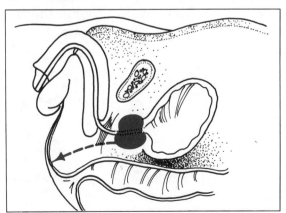

to expect blood in his urine for several days afterward.

Inform the patient that when the bleeding has subsided, the catheter will be removed. Warn him that bladder spasms may occur while the catheter is in place, but that medication can be given to provide relief. For a time following catheter removal, he may experience a sensation of heaviness in the pelvic region, urinary urgency, burning during urination, difficulty controlling urination, and the reappearance of some blood in the urine. Tell him that these effects will improve with time, and explain measures to help control them. (See *Speeding your recovery after prostate surgery.*)

Other care measures

If the patient will be going home with an indwelling (Foley) catheter in place, teach him how to care for the catheter. Reinforce your instruction by providing a copy of the patient-teaching aid *How to care for your urinary catheter,* page 320. Tell him when to return to the hospital for the catheter's removal.

Rarely, a patient will experience temporary or permanent impotence after surgery. More commonly, a patient may still be able to have an erection but will become sterile because his semen is expelled backward into the bladder instead of being ejaculated. Reassure the patient that seminal fluid in the bladder does no harm; it's simply eliminated in the urine. If the patient has problems adjusting sexually, refer him and his partner to a reputable counselor.

Sources of information and support

Impotents Anonymous (I-Anon)
Impotence Institute of America
5119 Bradley Boulevard, Chevy Chase, Md. 20815
(301) 656-3649

Resolve, Inc.
P.O. Box 474, Belmont, Mass. 02178
(617) 484-2424

Further readings

Azar, I. "The Transurethral Prostatectomy Syndrome," *Current Reviews for Post Anesthesia Care Nurses* 9(9):71-76, 1987.

Libman E., et al. "Determining What Patients Should Know About Transurethral Prostatectomy," *Patient Education and Counselling* 9(2):145-53, April 1987.

Reddy, P.K., et al: "Balloon Dilatation of the Prostate for Treatment of Benign Hyperplasia," *The Urologic Clinics of North America* 15(3):529-35, August 1988.

Roberts, A. "Senior Systems: The Aging Urinary System: Part 34," *Nursing Times* 85(10):Systems of Life 169; 59-62, March 8-14, 1989.

Schlegel, P.N., and Brendler, C.B. "Management of Urinary Retention Due to Benign Prostatic Hyperplasia Using Luteinizing Hormone-Releasing Hormone Agonist," *Urology* 34(2):69-72, August 1989.

Speeding your recovery after prostate surgery

Dear Patient:

Here's what you can expect after prostate surgery, along with directions for caring for yourself.

Expect trouble urinating

At first, you may have a feeling of heaviness in the pelvic area, burning during urination, a frequent need to urinate, and loss of some control over urination. Don't worry. These symptoms will disappear with time.

If you notice blood in your urine during the first 2 weeks after surgery, drink some fluids and lie down to rest. The next time you urinate, the bleeding should decrease.

Let your doctor know right away if you continue to see blood in your urine or if you can't urinate at all.

Also let him know immediately if you develop a fever.

Prevent constipation

Eat a well-balanced diet and drink 12 glasses of fluid a day unless the doctor prescribes otherwise. Don't strain to have a bowel movement. If you do become constipated, take a mild laxative.

Don't use an enema or place anything, such as a suppository, into your rectum for at least 4 weeks after surgery.

Cut back on activities

Take only short walks, and avoid climbing stairs as much as possible. Don't lift heavy objects. Also, don't exercise strenuously for at least 3 weeks.

Strengthen your perineal muscles

Perform this simple exercise to strengthen your perineal muscles after surgery: Press your buttocks together, hold this position for a few seconds, and then relax. Repeat 10 times.

Perform this exercise as many times daily as your doctor orders.

Don't have sex just yet

Don't have sex for at least 4 weeks after surgery because sexual activity can cause bleeding.

When you do have sex, most of the semen (the fluid that contains sperm) will pass into your bladder rather than out through your urethra. This won't affect your ability to have an erection or an orgasm. However, it will decrease your fertility.

Don't be alarmed if the semen in your bladder causes cloudy urine the first time you urinate after intercourse.

Ask about work

At your next doctor's appointment, ask when you can return to work. The timing will vary, depending on the type of surgery you had, the kind of work you do, and your general health.

Schedule an annual checkup

Continue to have an annual examination so your doctor can check the prostate area that wasn't removed during surgery.

PATIENT-TEACHING AID

How to care for your urinary catheter

Dear Patient:

Your catheter is a tube that will continually drain urine from your bladder, so you won't need to urinate. To care for your catheter, follow these guidelines.

Empty the drainage bag
How often? Usually, every 8 hours will do. First, unclamp the drainage tube and remove it from its sleeve, without touching the tip.

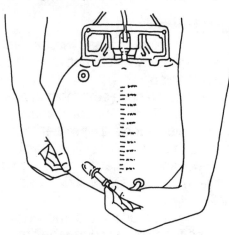

Then let the urine drain into the toilet or into a measuring container, if required. When the bag's completely empty, swab the end of the drainage tube with povidone-iodine solution.

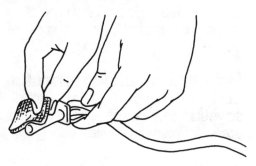

Reclamp the tube and reinsert it into the sleeve of the drainage bag.
   To maintain good drainage from the catheter, frequently check the drainage tubing for kinks and loops. Never disconnect the catheter from the drainage tubing, for any reason. Also, keep the drainage bag below your bladder level, whether you're lying down, sitting, or standing.

Care for your skin
Use soap and water to wash the area around your catheter twice each day.

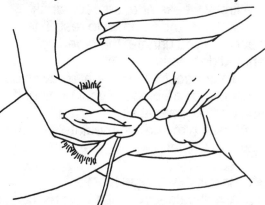

Also wash your rectal area twice each day and after each bowel movement. Periodically check the skin around the catheter for signs of irritation, such as redness, tenderness, or swelling.

Report problems early
Contact the doctor immediately if you have any problems, such as urine leakage around the catheter, pain and fullness in your abdomen, scanty urine flow, or blood in your urine.
   Above all, never pull on your catheter or try to remove it yourself.

Hydronephrosis

Beginning insidiously, without signs or symptoms, hydronephrosis may eventually cause pain severe enough to require hospitalization. In fact, the patient who experiences acute pain from this disorder may be hunched over, clutching his abdomen in distress. Or he may pace the floor or begin to vomit. But whatever his symptoms, you'll need to explain—to the extent his condition permits—that his pain results from a urinary tract obstruction and will cease when the obstruction is relieved.

Review the tests the patient will have to locate the obstruction, assess any renal damage, and determine its cause. Inform him about medication to relieve his discomfort and, if necessary, about catheterization or nephrostomy tube insertion to promote urine drainage. Finally, teach him how to recognize the signs and symptoms that signal another obstruction.

Discuss the disorder

Inform the patient that hydronephrosis is characterized by dilation of the renal pelvis and calyces with urine. Dilation is more common in one kidney, although it can affect both. Describe normal renal anatomy and physiology to help explain how dilation disrupts renal function (for more information, see *Understanding renal structures and functions,* page 322).

Point out that dilation results from an obstruction in the patient's urinary tract, which may be caused by a calculus, a tumor, a kink in the ureter, an infection or inflammation, or scar tissue. (In older men, obstruction may develop secondary to prostatic hyperplasia.) Even though muscles in the affected area contract to force the urine around the obstruction, urine eventually backs up into the kidney, filling the organ beyond its capacity and exerting pressure on the renal wall. This results in renal dilation and loss of function.

Whereas obstruction in the lower urinary tract causes bladder distention, obstruction in the upper urinary tract leads quickly to hydronephrosis because the ureters and renal pelves are small. Increased pressure produces partial ischemia of the arteries between the renal cortex and the medulla and dilation of the renal tubules, leading to tubular damage. Then, compensatory mechanisms cause urine to flow from the renal tubules back into the veins and the lymphatic system. This prompts increased activity by the unaffected kidney. With prolonged obstruction, the unaffected kidney hypertrophies and may function as effectively alone as both kidneys did before the obstruction. If kidney function remains ade-

Diane Kaschak Newman, RN, MSN, CRNP, who wrote this chapter, is a nurse practitioner with Golden Horizons, Inc., Newtown Square, Pa.

CHECKLIST

Teaching topics in hydronephrosis

☐ Normal renal structures and functions
☐ How hydronephrosis affects the kidneys
☐ Signs and symptoms of hydronephosis, especially pain
☐ Complications, including infection
☐ Diagnostic studies, including antegrade pyelography, cystoscopy, retrograde cystography, renal ultrasonography, and excretory urography
☐ Medications to minimize pain, control nausea and vomiting, and combat infection
☐ Urinary bladder catheterization to promote urine flow
☐ Nephrostomy tube care
☐ Surgery to remove a urinary tract obstruction
☐ Other care measures, such as increasing fluid to counterbalance postobstructive diuresis and recognizing signs and symptoms of infection and additional obstruction
☐ Source of information and support

Understanding renal structures and functions

To help your patient understand his condition, explain the structure and function of the kidneys. Inform him that the bean-shaped kidneys lie near and on either side of the spine, at the small of the back. They have a dual function: extracting waste products from the blood and forming urine from waste products and other fluids.

Explain that the kidneys receive waste-filled blood from the renal artery. This blood filters through a complicated network of smaller blood vessels and nephrons (the kidney's basic functioning units). Purified by this process, the blood returns to the circulation via the renal vein.

Explain that waste products and other fluids that form urine take a different route. They move from the renal pyramids, through the renal calyces, into the renal pelvis, and out into the ureters, where peristalsis forces the urine forward into the urinary bladder. The bladder stores the urine briefly and then expels it through the urethra.

INSIDE THE KIDNEY

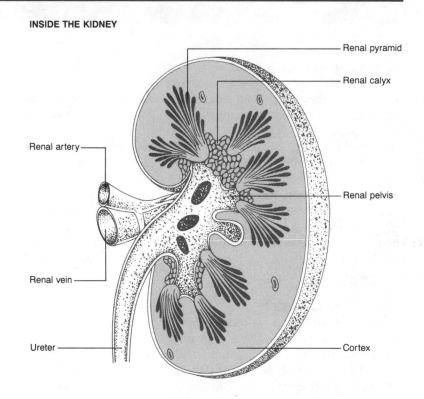

quate and urine can drain, the onset of signs and symptoms of hydronephrosis will be delayed.

Emphasize that the damaging effects of hydronephrosis depend on the obstruction's duration, extent, and location. As hydronephrosis progresses, tissue expansion and muscle spasms around the obstructed area produce pain. Usually localized, pain may occur during activity or urination. Dull flank pain suggests slowly developing hydronephrosis. Pain that radiates to the genitalia and the flank occurs when ureteral smooth muscle increases peristaltic motion to dislodge the obstruction or to force urine around it (for more information, refer to *How signs and symptoms characterize obstruction*).

Complications
Explain that pooled urine in the dilated renal pelvis provides a culture medium for bacteria, so the patient faces a high risk of infection. Furthermore, such an infection exacerbates renal damage and, left untreated, can lead to life-threatening illness.

What's more, calculi may form in the dilated renal pelvis, adding to renal damage. Over time, pressure from backed-up urine in the kidney may cause irreversible nephron destruction and renal failure.

If the patient with a lower urinary tract obstruction experiences prolonged bladder distention, muscle fibers may hypertrophy, and diverticula (herniated sacs of bladder mucosa) may develop. Then, pooled urine stagnating in the diverticula may harbor infection and promote the formation of bladder calculi.

Describe the diagnostic workup

Prepare the patient for an in-depth examination of the urinary tract, including such diagnostic tests as antegrade pyelography, computed tomography (CT), cytoscopy, retrograde cystography, renal ultrasonography, and excretory urography. Tell him that these tests can confirm the diagnosis, locate the obstruction, and assess the damage. As needed, provide the teaching aids *Preparing for renal ultrasonography,* page 327, and *Preparing for excretory urography,* page 328.

Antegrade pyelography

Inform the patient that this radiographic test allows examination of the kidney and evaluates the extent of hydronephrosis detected during excretory urography or renal ultrasonography. Performed in the radiology department, the test lasts about 1 hour.

Advise the patient that during the test he'll be positioned prone on an X-ray table and given a sedative to help him relax. Next, the skin over his kidney will be cleaned with a cold antiseptic solution and numbed with a local anesthetic. Then the doctor will insert a needle into the kidney to inject contrast medium (a dyelike substance that highlights kidney structures during X-ray studies). Explain that urine also may be collected for testing. After the X-ray studies are done, a nephrostomy tube may be inserted in the kidney for urine drainage.

Warn the patient that he may feel mild discomfort from the injection and transient burning and flushing from the contrast medium. Also describe the loud, clacking sounds made by the X-ray machine.

After the test, tell the patient to expect a nurse to monitor his blood pressure and heart and respiratory rates every 15 minutes for the first hour, every 30 minutes for the second hour, and every 2 hours for the next 24 hours. She'll also check his dressing for blood or urine leakage and monitor his fluid intake and urine output for 24 hours. If the doctor inserted a nephrostomy tube, explain that the nurse will inspect it for patency and adequate drainage.

Advise the patient to report posttest chills, fever, and irregular or unusually rapid heartbeats or breathing to the doctor immediately. Also tell him to report any abdominal or flank pain, sudden chest pain, or dyspnea.

CT scan

Inform the patient that a CT scan uses three-dimensional X-ray images to detect calculi and soft tissue obstructions in and around the renal collecting system and ureters.

Instruct the patient to avoid eating or drinking anything after midnight before the test but to continue taking medication as or-

How signs and symptoms characterize obstruction

Help your patient understand that signs and symptoms of hydronephrosis differ because they commonly reflect the duration and extent (partial or complete) of a urinary tract obstruction. What's more, they provide a clue to its location.

Signs and symptoms of lower urinary tract obstruction
• Lower abdominal pain
• An urge to void but an inability to do so
• Increasing urinary frequency or nocturia, suggesting a partial obstruction (common in benign prostatic hyperplasia). The bladder fails to empty completely at each voiding and therefore refills more quickly.

Signs and symptoms of upper urinary tract obstruction
• Pain associated with stretching of tissue and hyperperistalsis. Dull flank pain suggests slowly developing hydronephrosis. Severe, colicky pain in the flank or abdomen indicates a ureteral blockage. If pain radiates to the genitalia and thigh, the patient may become immobilized. Pain on one side results from a unilateral obstruction.
• Nausea and vomiting (a reflex reaction to pain) associated with acute ureteral obstruction and usually relieved when pain subsides. GI symptoms may continue if a markedly dilated kidney presses on the stomach. Ongoing nausea and vomiting may signal uremia (which suggests severely impaired renal function). The patient may also experience a loss of appetite, leading to nutritional and electrolyte imbalance.
• Local tenderness
• Abdominal muscle spasms
• A mass in the kidney region

dered. Explain that during the test he'll lie on a hard X-ray table that will slide into the tunnel-like CT scanner. Advise him to lie still, relax, breathe normally, and remain quiet because movement will blur the images and prolong the test.

If the doctor orders an I.V. contrast medium, inform the patient that he may experience discomfort from the needle puncture and a localized feeling of warmth when the doctor injects the dye-like substance. Tell him to report any discomfort or rare hypersensitivity reactions, such as dizziness, headache, hives, nausea, or vomiting. Inform him that he may resume eating after the test.

Cystoscopy

Tell the patient that this 20-minute test usually is performed in the doctor's office. It allows the doctor to visualize internal bladder structures. If the patient is a man, he may receive a general anesthetic. Instruct him not to eat for 8 hours before the test. If he'll have a local anesthetic, tell him that he may receive a sedative to help him relax before the test. (If the patient is a woman, she will not receive any anesthetic.)

Describe how the patient will lie supine (with his hips and knees flexed) on an X-ray table. Then, his genitalia will be cleaned with an antiseptic solution, and he'll be covered with a sterile drape. Next, the doctor will administer a local anesthetic, if appropriate, and introduce the cystoscope (a tubular optical instrument) through the urethra into the bladder. He'll fill the bladder with irrigating solution and rotate the cystoscope to inspect the bladder wall's surface.

If the patient will receive a local anesthetic, warn him that he may feel a burning sensation as the cytoscope advances through the urethra. He may also feel an urgent need to void as the bladder fills with the irrigating solution.

If the doctor plans to take bladder X-rays, tell the patient that he may receive a preparation to clean his bowels to ensure sharper, clearer X-ray images.

Retrograde cystography

Point out that this test evaluates the structure and integrity of the bladder and the renal collecting system. Performed in the radiology department, the procedure may take up to 1 hour.

Advise the patient that he'll lie on his back on an X-ray table so that preliminary X-rays can be taken and a catheter can be inserted into his bladder. Then a contrast medium will be instilled through the catheter. After the catheter is clamped shut, he'll assume various positions as more X-ray films are taken.

After the test, tell the patient to expect a nurse to monitor his vital signs until they're stable and also to check urine color and volume. Instruct him to notify the doctor or nurse if blood continues to appear in his urine after the third voiding or if he develops chills, fever, or increased pulse or respiratory rates.

Teach about treatments

Clarify treatment goals, such as pain relief, infection control, and relief from urinary tract obstruction. Then discuss drug therapy options and surgery, if appropriate.

Medication

Advise the patient who has severe, colicky pain that the doctor may prescribe pain relievers, such as the narcotic analgesics morphine or meperidine (Demerol); antispasmodics, such as propantheline bromide (Pro-Banthine) and belladonna preparations; and antiemetics, such as prochlorperazine (Compazine). He may also prescribe antibiotics to control infection.

Instruct the patient receiving *narcotic analgesics* to take these drugs as directed. Advise him to seek medical attention if he experiences an abnormally slow heartbeat (bradycardia), abnormally slow breathing (bradypnea), shortness of breath (dyspnea), lightheadedness or fainting (hypotension), confusion, severe dizziness, restlessness, or weakness. He should also watch for dry mouth, nausea, and vomiting. Emphasize that drug tolerance may develop with long-term use. However, drug dependence seldom occurs in patients who require narcotic analgesics for pain relief.

Inform the patient taking *antispasmodics* that adverse effects of these drugs include constipation, decreased sweating, dizziness, drowsiness, and dry mucous membranes.

If the patient receives *antiemetics* to control nausea and vomiting, warn him about possible adverse effects, such as dizziness, dry mouth, and sedation.

Advise the patient taking any of these drugs not to participate in activities requiring mental or physical alertness, such as driving a car or operating heavy machinery, until he knows the full effects of the medication. Recommend that he use ice chips or sugarless hard candy or gum to relieve dry mouth.

The doctor may prescribe *antibiotics* to prevent or treat infection. Instruct the patient to complete the full course of medication. Advise him to watch for and report adverse effects, such as hematuria, difficulty breathing or swallowing, hives, itching, numbness and tingling, sore throat, fever, unusual fatigue and weakness, and other reactions associated with the specific drug.

Procedures

If urine retention and bladder distention accompany hydronephrosis, tell the patient that he may need to catheterize himself intermittently or have an indwelling catheter to promote continuous urine flow and prevent recurrent obstruction. Demonstrate how to care for the catheter and the drainage bag, and show him how to care for surrounding skin to prevent breakdown and infection. Give him the patient-teaching aid *How to care for your urinary catheter* on page 320.

Surgery

Explain that the doctor may recommend using a nephrostomy tube to drain urine from the renal pelvis, or he may suggest surgery (depending on the obstruction) to relieve the blockage that causes hydronephrosis.

Nephrostomy tube. Inserted through the patient's flank and into the kidney, a nephrostomy tube allows urine to drain from the kidney, preventing renal damage from the increased pressure associated with continuous urine formation without adequate urine flow. Teach the patient how to care for the nephrostomy tube. Demonstrate the technique for cleaning and changing the tubing and drainage bag. Tell him to change the dressing daily and show him how to do so. Provide the patient-teaching aid *Caring for your nephrostomy tube* on page 312.

Urinary tract surgery. To relieve a urinary tract obstruction, the surgeon may perform ureterolithotomy (removal of a calculus from the ureter), cystoscopy with prostatic resection, or removal of a bladder tumor. Explain that a nephrectomy may be done to remove an irreparably damaged kidney.

Before surgery, reinforce and clarify the doctor's explanations. Allow time to answer the patient's questions and listen to his concerns. If possible, tell him which type of anesthetic he'll receive, and advise him of any preoperative food or fluid restrictions or bowel preparation. Outline what the patient can expect after surgery by discussing pain relief, breathing and coughing techniques, and ambulation.

Other care measures

Remember to inform your patient about postobstructive diuresis. Removal of a urinary tract obstruction relieves the pressure on the renal parenchyma, and untrapped urine begins to flow freely. Caution him that this reflexive diuresis can lead to fluid depletion. Encourage him to increase his fluid intake to maintain a safe fluid balance. Advise him to drink at least 2,000 ml (68 oz) of fluid daily. (Note, if appropriate, that increased fluid intake may also help him to pass a kidney stone.) Reassure him that postobstructive diuresis normally ceases as the kidneys readjust.

Finally, instruct the patient to contact the doctor for signs and symptoms of infection that suggest another obstruction and further hydronephrosis. These include chills, fever, pain, anorexia, and general malaise.

Source of information and support

National Kidney and Urologic Diseases Information Clearinghouse
P.O. Box NKUDIC, Bethesda, Md. 20892
(301) 468-6345

Further readings

Baille, M.D. "The Total Costs of Ultrasonography," *Pediatrics* 86(2):323, August 1990.

DuBose, T.J. "Standards for Color Doppler Imaging," *American Journal of Roentgenology* 154(6):1348-49, June 1990.

Goldberg, B.B., et al. "Getting the Most Out of Ultrasound," *Patient Care* 24(16):22-26, 35-36, 38, October 15, 1990.

PATIENT-TEACHING AID

Preparing for renal ultrasonography

Dear Patient:

The doctor wants you to undergo renal ultrasonography to determine how healthy your kidneys are.

How the test works
During the test, a transducer will be passed over your abdomen. This small instrument projects high-frequency sound waves. As these sound waves meet your kidneys and surrounding structures, they bounce back (like echoes). A microphone on the transducer picks up these reflected sound waves, and a computer converts them into electrical impulses that are displayed visually on a TV screen.

These ultrasound images help the doctor to evaluate the size, shape, position, and internal structure of the kidneys and the tissues that surround them. The test also helps the doctor to locate and evaluate a urinary tract obstruction.

How to get ready
This safe, painless test may take about 30 minutes. Before the test, you may drink and eat as usual.

What to expect
The test can be done in the hospital's ultrasound lab or in an office. During the test, you'll lie flat on your back on an X-ray table. The technician will spread a water-soluble gel on your abdomen to improve sound wave transmission. The gel may feel cold and slippery.

Next, the technician will pass the transducer over the exposed area of your skin. You may feel a light pressure as she moves the instrument. Try to remain as still as possible.

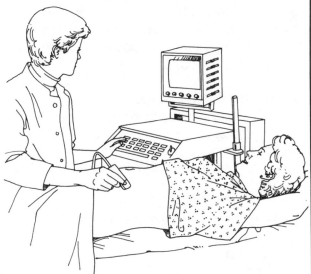

You may be instructed to breathe deeply. This will allow the doctor to assess how your kidney moves when you inhale and exhale. As the scan progresses, the technician may use a marking pen to trace an outline of your kidney on your abdomen. She may ask you to change positions so additional scans can be made.

Afterward
Upon completing the test, the technician will wipe off the ultrasound gel. If you're a patient in the hospital, the nurse may remove the gel when you return to your room.

Preparing for excretory urography

Dear Patient:

The doctor wants you to have a test called excretory urography. (Some doctors call this test intravenous pyelography, or IVP.) The test uses X-rays to create images of the kidneys, ureters, and bladder. This lets the doctor evaluate kidney function and locate urinary tract obstruction.

How the test works
An iodine-containing contrast medium, which shows up on X-rays, will be injected into your bloodstream. Circulating blood carries the medium to the kidneys and distributes it throughout the urinary tract. Then a series of X-ray images will be taken to show these structures.

How to get ready
You'll be asked to name any allergies you have and to say if you're allergic to shellfish or the iodine they contain.

Most likely, you'll be asked to drink six to eight glasses of water the day before the test and not to eat any food for 8 hours before the test. You'll also need to take a laxative the night before the test to rid your system of waste and gas.

In the radiology department or the radiologist's office, you'll undress and put on a hospital gown. Remove any jewelry or metal objects that may interfere with the X-rays.

What to expect
Performed by a radiologist and an X-ray technician, the test takes about 1 hour.

You'll be asked to urinate immediately beforehand so that the urine in the bladder won't interfere with the contrast medium.

During the test, you'll lie on your back on an X-ray table while a preliminary film is taken to identify landmarks in the test area. This film will be developed and viewed before the test continues.

Next, a needle will be inserted into a vein (usually the one on the inside of your arm). The contrast medium will be injected here. You may experience a temporary burning sensation and metallic taste in your mouth during the injection. Also, you have a slight risk for hypersensitivity reactions, such as flushing, nausea, vomiting, hives, or wheezing. Report these and any other sensations to the doctor.

Then X-ray films will be taken at 5-minute intervals. Try to hold still for each film. You may hear loud, clacking noises made by the X-ray machine.

You may have a compression belt placed around your hips to confine the contrast medium to your urinary tract. If the belt hurts or feels too tight, tell the technician.

Afterward
When the test ends, you may be asked to urinate. Then an X-ray will be taken to assess how well your bladder empties. Remember to drink lots of fluids to flush the contrast medium from your system.

Check the injection site periodically. If you notice swelling or redness, apply warm compresses and notify the doctor.

Urinary tract infection

Among the most common urologic disorders, urinary tract infections (UTIs) affect people of all ages and women about 10 times more often than men. UTIs may occur without causing signs and symptoms, so your teaching must emphasize prevention as well as treatment.

Establishing a good rapport with your patient is especially important because you'll need to discuss preventive measures that may require the patient to adopt new dietary and personal hygiene habits and new voiding patterns. Your teaching will also include the pathophysiology and risks of UTI, test procedures, and drug therapy. (See *Teaching the patient with recurrent UTIs,* page 330, for additional information.)

Discuss the disorder

Inform the patient that the naturally sterile urinary tract can harbor infection when bacteria enter the nonsterile area near the urethra. Explain that lower UTIs, such as *urethritis* and *cystitis,* involve the urethra or bladder or both. Upper UTIs, called *pyelonephritis,* affect the kidneys (see *Explaining UTIs,* page 331).

Tell her that symptoms may develop rapidly (if they occur at all) over a few hours or a few days. And although symptoms may resolve without treatment, residual infection is common, and symptoms are likely to recur.

Explain that lower UTIs usually produce urinary urgency and frequency, dysuria, bladder cramps or spasms, itching, a feeling of warmth during urination, and nocturia. Male patients may complain of urethral discharge. If the bladder wall's inflamed, the patient may also have fever and hematuria. Other common symptoms include abdominal pain or tenderness over the bladder, chills, flank pain, low back pain, malaise, nausea, and vomiting.

Explain that upper UTIs cause similar symptoms, including urinary urgency and frequency, burning during urination, dysuria, nocturia, and hematuria (usually discovered microscopically but sometimes apparent to the eye). What's more, the patient's urine may appear cloudy and have an ammonia or fishlike odor. Other typical signs and symptoms include a fever of 102° F. (38.9° C.) or higher, chills, flank pain, anorexia, and fatigue.

Identify common UTI risk factors. This will help your patient understand why prevention ranks high in self-care. Use illustrations to supplement your teaching (see *Reviewing UTI risk factors,* page 332).

Sarah J. Griesbach, RN, BSN, who works at Dakota Hospital, Fargo, N.D., wrote this chapter.

CHECKLIST

Teaching topics in UTI

☐ Types of urinary tract infections (UTIs), including their signs and symptoms
☐ Risk factors for UTIs
☐ Complications, such as renal disease
☐ Explanation of diagnostic tests, such as urinalysis and radiography
☐ Activity and diet guidelines
☐ Prescribed medications, such as antibiotics
☐ Explanation of surgery, if necessary
☐ Preventive measures, including healthful hygiene practices and urination patterns

Teaching the patient with recurrent UTIs

When you're teaching a patient with recurrent urinary tract infections (UTIs), you'll need to pare down a standard teaching plan to target specific needs. Here's an example of how to do this.

Gather assessment data
Jane Hart, a 24-year-old part-time office worker and law student sits before you in the hospital's outpatient clinic. She has a 103° F. fever and complains of burning and frequent urination, nausea, and abdominal pain. She tells you that she was sick a month ago with a UTI. She took her medication until she felt better, then she threw away the pills. She adds that she resumed her daily routine at the health club, where she works out, rides an exercise bike, and relaxes in the whirlpool before she gulps a cola and heads for classes or her part-time job.

You smile and acknowledge that she seems busy. She sighs, agreeing that with job, school, and trying to stay fit she hardly has time to go to the bathroom, let alone eat. Usually, she grabs a cup or two of coffee and keeps a full pot nearby when she studies.

Identify learning needs
Starting with a standard teaching plan, decide which topics to feature for Ms. Hart. A standard teaching plan for UTI includes:
• types of UTIs and where they occur
• signs, symptoms, and risk factors
• complications
• diagnostic tests and how to collect a urine specimen
• treatments, including activity and diet, medications, surgery (if needed), and preventive measures.

You eliminate from the standard teaching plan what Ms. Hart already knows. She's been sick before, so she can identify UTI signs and symptoms. She's familiar with tests that she'll have and she's provided a clean-catch urine specimen. What's more, she knows where her infection occurs.

That leaves you with complications, treatments, and prevention. Most important, Ms. Hart needs to understand the serious, long-term consequences of recurrent UTIs. From your interview with Ms. Hart, you conclude that she's so busy attending to daily details that she's overlooking her future needs. Specifically, she needs first to learn to take her medicine exactly as directed (not discard it when she thinks she doesn't need it). And second, she needs to identify and change behaviors that promote recurrent infection.

The next time you talk with Ms. Hart, you relate your thoughts about her learning needs. You add that assuming she learns and applies what she learns, you won't expect to see her with a UTI again.

Set learning outcomes
Together you and Ms. Hart review learning needs and set learning outcomes. You agree that she'll be able to:

```
-explain the long-term complications of UTIs
-list the side effects of prescribed drugs
-tell why she should finish her prescribed medicine
 and state the consequences of not doing so
-discuss how prolonged bicycle riding and coffee
 drinking increase her susceptibility to a UTI
-develop a menu plan that incorporates high-acid
 foods and the suggested amount of daily fluid
-state why showers are more healthful than baths
-name the type of outerwear and underwear she'll
 choose to avoid recurrent UTIs
-explain the purpose of emptying her bladder fre-
 quently throughout the day.
```

Select teaching techniques and tools
Begin with *discussion* to involve Ms. Hart in finding solutions as she asks and answers questions. First talk about UTI as it relates to kidney disease. Then discuss how adequate drug treatment can cure UTIs and thereby eliminate the threat of long-term illness.

Consider using *simulation* to initiate life-style modifications, such as planning frequent rather than delayed urination. For example, ask Ms. Hart to imagine that she's an attorney preparing to defend a client. It's morning. She dresses and fixes breakfast before leaving for court. What will she wear? What will she eat and drink? Arriving at court early, will she pour a cup of coffee or use the bathroom?

She leaves court and goes to the health club. Will she ride the exercise bike or work on the treadmill? Will she use the whirlpool or take a shower? Suggest that she make a mental list of moments when she can take a break and exercise healthful choices.

Introduce Ms. Hart to *self-monitoring* to help her initiate diet changes. Ask her to keep a written record of how much fluid she drinks daily. Suggest that she keep and use a checklist of high-acid foods and healthful beverages.

For teaching tools, select *printed medication and diet guidelines* and *printed teaching aids.* If you can, offer *videotape* and *audiocassette* reinforcements.

Evaluate your teaching
How can you tell if your teaching was effective? Ask Ms. Hart to perform a *return demonstration* by acting out a typical day at school and the health club and showing how she'll plan time to use the bathroom and drink liquids without caffeine. Ask *open-ended questions,* such as "What did you eat and drink yesterday?" Her responses will tell you if she grasps what you've taught and if she practices it.

Explaining UTIs

Use a simple illustration like this one to enhance your teaching on urinary tract infections (UTIs). Then identify the patient's specific infection and the affected area. If appropriate, name the organism causing the patient's UTI.

Lower UTI
If your patient has urethritis (an infection of the urethra) or cystitis (an infection of the urethra and the bladder), point out the urethra and the bladder. Explain that lower UTIs result from infection by bacteria, such as *Escherichia coli, Klebsiella, Proteus, Enterobacter, Pseudomonas,* or *Serratia* species.

Upper UTI
If your patient has pyelonephritis (an infection of the kidneys and renal pelvis), show her where the kidneys lie. Explain that infectious bacteria usually are normal intestinal and fecal flora that grow readily in urine. Mention that the most common causative organism is *E. coli.* Other disease-causing organisms include *Proteus, Pseudomonas, Staphylococcus aureus,* and *Streptococcus faecalis.*

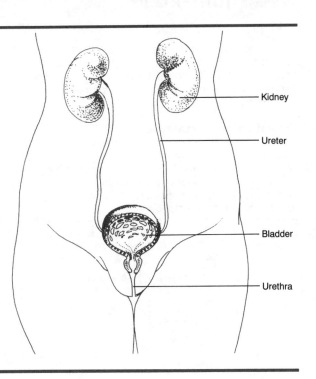

Kidney
Ureter
Bladder
Urethra

Complications
Warn the patient that complications, such as chronic pyelonephritis—a leading cause of end-stage renal disease—may result from failure to observe treatment guidelines. And without vigilance and treatment, other kidney damage may occur from chronic UTIs—especially if the patient has a neurogenic bladder, which permits urine retention and consequent infection. Caution the pregnant patient that careful compliance with treatment is necessary because her UTI can progress to pyelonephritis. This can pass on to the fetus and cause hypertension, eye infections, and decreased motor activity.

Describe the diagnostic workup
Discuss scheduled tests, beginning with laboratory tests, such as urinalysis and culture, smear and stain of urethral discharge, and a complete blood count (CBC). Then, if appropriate, discuss radiographic tests, such as kidney-ureter-bladder (KUB) radiography, excretory urography, and voiding cystourethrography.

Laboratory tests
Explain that *urinalysis* involves examination of a urine specimen for signs of infection, such as a cloudy appearance and a foul odor; bacteria, pus, and proteins; red and white blood cells; and alkaline pH. A *urine culture* can identify the disease-causing agent.

Inform the patient that the test requires a urine specimen. Then provide a copy of the patient-teaching aid *How to collect a*

Reviewing UTI risk factors

Inform your patient that certain factors increase the risk for a urinary tract infection (UTI). They include natural anatomic variations, trauma or invasive procedures, urinary tract obstruction, urine reflux, and other conditions.

Natural anatomic variations
Explain that women are more prone to UTI than men because the female urethra is shorter (about 1" to 2" [2.5 to 5 cm] compared with about 7" to 8" [18 to 20 cm] in men) and closer to the anus than the male urethra. Naturally, bacteria survive longer by traveling shorter distances to colonize.

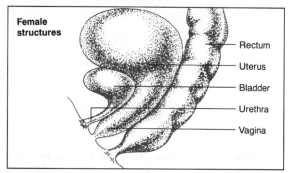

Female structures — Rectum, Uterus, Bladder, Urethra, Vagina

Pregnant patients are especially prone to UTIs—first because of hormonal changes and second because the enlarged uterus exerts greater pressure on the ureters. This restricts urine flow, allowing bacteria to linger in the urinary tract.

In men, the release of prostatic fluid serves as an antibacterial shield. However, men lose this protection after about age 50, when the prostate gland begins to enlarge. In turn, this enlargement may promote urine retention.

Trauma or invasion
Explain that fecal matter, sexual intercourse, and instruments—for example, catheters and cystoscopes—can introduce bacteria into the urinary tract to trigger infection.

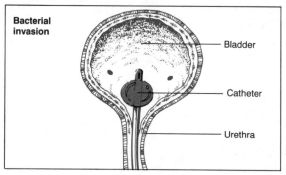

Bacterial invasion — Bladder, Catheter, Urethra

Obstruction
Tell the patient that a narrowed ureter or calculi (stones) lodged in the ureters or the bladder can obstruct urine flow. Slowed urine flow allows bacteria to remain and multiply—risking damage to the kidneys.

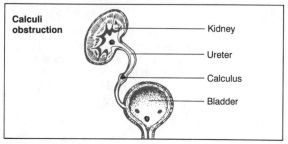

Calculi obstruction — Kidney, Ureter, Calculus, Bladder

Reflux
Inform the patient that vesicourethral reflux results when pressure inside the bladder (caused by coughing or sneezing) pushes a small amount of urine from the bladder into the urethra. When the pressure returns to normal, the urine flows back into the bladder, bringing bacteria from the urethra with it.

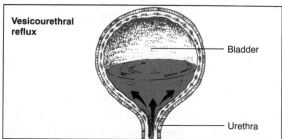

Vesicourethral reflux — Bladder, Urethra

In vesicoureteral reflux, urine may flow back from the bladder to one or both ureters. Normally, the vesicoureteral valve shuts off reflux. Damage, however, can prevent the valve from doing its job.

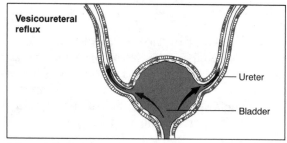

Vesicoureteral reflux — Ureter, Bladder

Other risk factors
Caution your patient that stasis of urine in the bladder can promote infection, which, if undetected, can spread to the entire urinary system. And because urinary tract bacteria thrive on sugars, diabetes is also a risk factor.

urine specimen: For males, page 338, or *How to collect a urine specimen: For females,* page 339. If the patient collects the specimen at home, advise her to store it in the refrigerator to keep bacteria from multiplying. Instruct her to take it to the laboratory within 1 hour to ensure accurate results.

If the doctor suspects urethritis, explain that he'll order a *smear and stain* of the patient's urethral discharge to help identify the causative organism.

Tell the patient that typical *blood tests* include a CBC to measure white blood cell (WBC) and neutrophil levels and to determine the erythrocyte sedimentation rate (ESR). Explain that in simple cystitis the WBC level remains within the normal range. With complicated cystitis or pyelonephritis, however, it may rise. An increased ESR may also occur in pyelonephritis.

Radiographic tests

Tell the patient that a *KUB,* an abdominal X-ray study, identifies the position of the kidneys, ureters, and bladder and helps detect any abnormalities. Depending on KUB findings, the patient will usually have other studies, too. Tell her that she won't have to restrict foods or fluids. Mention who will perform the test and where and that the test takes only a few minutes. For more information, see *What happens in a KUB study,* page 334.

If the doctor orders *excretory urography* (also called intravenous pyelography), inform the patient that this test evaluates the structure and excretory function of the kidneys and urinary tract. Tell her who will perform the test and where and that it takes about 1 hour. Advise her to drink plenty of fluids and then to fast for 8 hours before the test. Inform her that she may receive a laxative or other bowel preparation before the test.

Tell the patient that she'll lie supine on an X-ray table. After contrast medium injection, a technician will take X-ray films at specific intervals. Mention that the technician may place a belt around the patient's hips to keep the contrast medium at a certain level. Also warn her that she may experience a transient burning sensation and a metallic taste from the contrast medium. Advise her to report these and any other sensations to the technician or the doctor. Explain that the X-ray machine will make loud, clacking sounds as it exposes films. Instruct her to report symptoms of delayed reaction to the contrast medium, such as itching and hives or difficulty breathing.

If the doctor orders a *voiding cystourethrography,* explain that this test assesses the bladder and urethra and detects abnormalities, such as vesicoureteral reflux, neurogenic bladder, prostatic hyperplasia, and urethral strictures or diverticula. Tell the patient who will perform the test and where. Add that it takes 30 to 45 minutes.

Tell the patient that she'll lie supine while a nurse inserts a bladder catheter and then instills a contrast medium through the catheter. She may have a full sensation and feel an urge to void. Explain that she'll be asked to assume various positions for X-ray films of her bladder and urethra.

What happens in a KUB study

Inform the patient that the kidney-ureter-bladder (KUB) study uses X-rays to find abnormalities that may contribute to urinary tract infections.

Precise positioning
Explain that only one X-ray picture will be made, so the technician must position the patient precisely. Prepare the patient to lie supine on an X-ray table with his arms extended over and behind his head. This will help align his body. Inform him that the technician will check his iliac crests — again to ensure symmetrical positioning.

Tell the patient that he must lie perfectly still to ensure a quality image. If he's obese, suggest that he exhale and hold his breath.

Special considerations
If the patient's male, reassure him that his sexual organs will be shielded to protect them from radiation. If the patient's female, however, her sexual organs cannot be shielded because they're too close to the kidneys, ureters, and bladder.

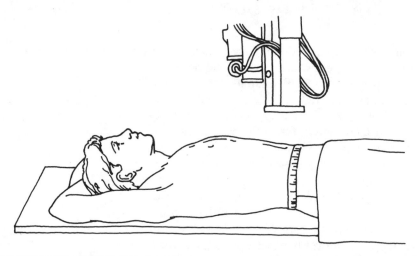

Inform the patient that after the test the nurse will observe and record the time, color, and amount of each voiding. The patient should drink plenty of fluids to reduce burning on urination and to flush away any residual contrast medium. Tell her to report chills or fever; these may be symptoms of infection.

Teach about treatments
Discuss the primary treatment for UTI—medication. (Refer to *Teaching about drugs for urinary tract infections,* for more information.) Then discuss life-style changes to prevent recurrent UTIs, mild activity restrictions, dietary measures, and surgery (if indicated). Provide a copy of the patient-teaching aid *Self-care tips in urinary tract infections,* page 340.

Activity
Tell the patient that she needn't restrict most activities. She should, however, avoid prolonged bicycling, motorcycling, and horseback riding. These activities may promote urine reflux and may damage the urinary tract.

Teaching about drugs for urinary tract infections

DRUG	ADVERSE REACTIONS	TEACHING POINTS
Antibiotics		
amoxicillin (Amoxil, Trimox)	• Watch for bloody urine, difficulty breathing, face and ankle swelling, hives, itching, large amounts of pale urine, rash, unusual tiredness, and weakness. • Other reactions include abdominal cramps, diarrhea, fever, increased thirst, nausea, seizures, unusual bleeding or bruising, vomiting, and weight loss.	• Explain that the drug can be taken on a full or an empty stomach. • Inform the patient that the liquid form may be taken straight or mixed with juice or water. If the patient mixes the drug, advise her to drink it immediately. Remind her to drink all of the liquid to ensure a full dose. • Remind her to finish the entire prescription even if she begins to feel better after a few days. • Advise her to take a missed dose as soon as possible, but warn her not to overdose. Tell her to call the doctor, pharmacist, or nurse as questions arise.
co-trimoxazole (Bactrim) **sulfamethoxazole** (Gantanol) **sulfamethoxazole and phenazopyridine** (Azo-Gantanol) **sulfisoxazole** (Gantrisin) **sulfisoxazole and phenazopyridine** (Azo-Gantrisin)	• Watch for aching joints and muscles; bloody urine; difficulty swallowing; itching; pale skin; rash; redness; skin blistering, peeling, or loosening; sore throat and fever; unusual bleeding or bruising; unusual tiredness or weakness; and yellow eyes or skin. • Other reactions include appetite loss, diarrhea, dizziness, headache, nausea, photosensitivity, and vomiting.	• Instruct the patient to take the drug with 8 oz of water and to drink an additional 8 to 10 glasses of water daily to prevent unwanted effects, such as renal calculi. • Teach her to take the drug at evenly spaced times around the clock to keep constant levels of the medicine in her blood or urine. If this schedule interferes with sleep and other activities, tell her to consult with her doctor, pharmacist, or nurse. • Remind her to continue the medication even after symptoms subside. • Caution her not to drive or operate equipment requiring mental alertness until the drug's effect is known. • Advise her to avoid the sun while taking this drug to prevent a reaction. • Tell her to take care brushing her teeth and using dental floss because this drug can cause bleeding. Suggest that she delay dental work until her blood counts are normal. • Warn the patient taking drugs with phenazopyridine that it causes urine to turn reddish orange.
nitrofurantoin (Furadantin, Nitrofan)	• Watch for chest pain, chills, difficulty breathing, dizziness, drowsiness, face or mouth burning, fever, numbness or tingling, pallor, unusual tiredness or weakness, and yellow eyes or skin. • Other reactions include abdominal pain, appetite loss, diarrhea, itching, nausea, rash, and vomiting.	• Suggest that the patient take the drug with food or milk to lessen GI upset and improve absorption of the medicine. • Caution her not to drive or operate equipment requiring mental alertness until the drug effects are known. • Alert her that the drug may turn her urine a rust-yellow to brown color. • Warn her that the oral suspension drug form may temporarily discolor or stain teeth. To avoid this, suggest that she rinse her mouth with water after swallowing the medication. • Tell her to notify the doctor if symptoms don't improve within a few days or if they become worse. • Instruct her not to store the drug in pillboxes made of stainless steel or aluminum.

continued

Teaching about drugs for urinary tract infections — *continued*

DRUG	ADVERSE REACTIONS	TEACHING POINTS
Antibiotics — *continued*		
norfloxacin (Noroxin)	• Watch for dizziness; headache; lightheadedness; depression; and vision problems, including blurred or decreased vision, double vision, halos around lights, increased eye sensitivity to light, and overbright appearance of lights. • Other reactions include abdominal pain, appetite loss, bloody urine, burning or pain while urinating, constipation, diarrhea, dry mouth, GI upset, insomnia, itching, lower back pain, nausea, rash, redness, swollen or inflamed joints or tendons, and vomiting.	• Instruct the patient to take the drug with at least 8 oz of water on an empty stomach, either 1 hour before or 2 hours after meals, and to drink additional water (6 to 8 glasses a day) to maintain adequate urine output. • Teach her to take the drug at evenly spaced intervals around the clock to keep a constant level of the medicine in her blood or urine. If this schedule interferes with sleep and other activities, tell her to consult her doctor, pharmacist, or nurse. • Remind her to continue taking the drug even after symptoms subside. • Caution her not to drive or operate equipment requiring mental alertness until the drug effects are known. • Advise her to wear sunglasses and, if possible, avoid exposure to bright light. • Suggest that she use sugarless candy or gum to relieve mouth dryness. • Suggest that she take antacids at least 2 hours after taking the drug.
Nonnarcotic analgesic		
phenazopyridine (Pyridium)	• Watch for blue or bluish purple skin, difficulty breathing, rash, yellow eyes or skin, and unusual tiredness or weakness. • Other reactions include dizziness, headache, indigestion, and stomach cramps or pain.	• Inform the patient that this drug treats pain associated with urinary tract infections. • Advise her to take this drug with food or immediately after eating to minimize GI upset. • Instruct her to take a missed dose as soon as possible. If she's scheduled to take the next dose within 2 hours, however, she should skip the missed dose and continue with the usual dosage schedule. Caution her not to double-dose. • Warn her that the drug will turn her urine reddish orange, and urine that permeates clothing may stain it. • Advise her to notify the doctor if symptoms worsen or don't improve.

Diet

When you talk about diet, include the patient's family if possible—especially if the patient doesn't do the grocery shopping or cooking. Essentially, encourage additional fluids—up to 14 glasses of water daily—and increased acid intake—especially meats, nuts, fruit juices, and other high-acid foods.

Medication

When culture results identify the causative microorganism, explain to the patient that the doctor will prescribe the single-dose or short-term drugs most likely to kill or control the infection. Advise her that an effective drug should rapidly sterilize the urine and relieve her symptoms. Urge her to have her urine reanalyzed 1 to 3 days after treatment starts to judge the drug's effectiveness.

If the patient has frequent UTIs, tell her that she may require long-term, low-dose antibiotic prophylaxis.

Explain that other antibiotics, such as sulfonamides and urinary tract antiseptics, may also be used to treat UTIs. Mention that the doctor may prescribe a nonnarcotic analgesic to treat infection-related pain.

Surgery

If appropriate, inform the patient that the doctor may recommend surgery to correct an obstruction causing recurrent UTIs. Explain that common obstructive disorders include calculi, tumors, and benign prostatic hyperplasia.

Other care measures

Suggest life-style changes to help the patient fight recurrent UTIs. Such changes include improved hygiene habits—for example, wiping from front to back after going to the bathroom to prevent fecal contamination and avoiding tight or synthetic underpants. Also recommend taking showers instead of baths and avoiding any products that can irritate the perineum, and advise the patient to urinate more frequently and to urinate after sexual intercourse.

Further readings

Cameron, G.L., and Brenner, D.A. "Low Urinary Bacterial Counts in Symptomatic Patients," *New Zealand Journal of Medical Laboratory Technology* 43(1):10-11, March 1989.

Conway, J. "Taking a Look at Lower UTIs...Urinary Tract Infection," *Journal of Urology Nursing* 8(2):641-43, April-June 1989.

Fekety, R., et al. "Does Antibiotic Prophylaxis Help?" *Patient Care* 23(9):76-80, 89, 93+, May 15, 1989.

Fiorelli, R.L. "Recurrent Urinary Tract Infections in Women: Pathogenesis and Treatment," *Journal of Urology Nursing* 7(4):510-14, October-December 1988.

Hanno, P.M. "Cystitis: A Management Guide to Recurrent Cases," *Physician Assistant* 13(2):25-28, 31-32, 137-40+, February 1989.

Lewis, S. "Nursing Management of Urinary Tract Infection," *Infection Control* 3(3):18-19, September-October 1988.

Lohr, J.A. "The Foreskin and Urinary Tract Infections," *Journal of Pediatrics* 114(3):502-04, March 1989.

Millette-Petit, J.M. "Urinary Tract Infections in Older Adults," *Nursing Practice* 13(12):21-24, 29, December 1988.

Pitt, M. "Fluid Intake and Urinary Tract Infection," *Nursing Times* 85(1):36-38, January 4-10, 1989.

Smaill, F. "Diagnosis of Urinary Tract Infections," *Infection Control Canada* 4(1):20-21, 23, March-April 1989.

PATIENT-TEACHING AID

How to collect a urine specimen: For males

Dear Patient:

Your doctor wants you to have your urine tested. A urine test can tell whether you have a infection, or it can tell whether you have too much or too little of certain substances in your body. To make sure that the test results are accurate, your urine shouldn't contain "outside germs" from your hands or your penis.

Follow these directions carefully. Read them through to the end before collecting your specimen.

1 Wash your hands thoroughly. Open the package of disposable wipes that the nurse gave you, and place it on a clean, dry, nearby surface.

2 Remove the lid from the specimen cup and place it flat side down. *Do not* touch the inside of the cup or lid.

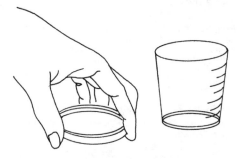

3 Prepare to urinate (if you're uncircumcised, first pull back your foreskin). Using a disposable wipe, clean the head of your penis from the urethral opening toward you, as shown at the top of the next column. Then discard the used wipe.

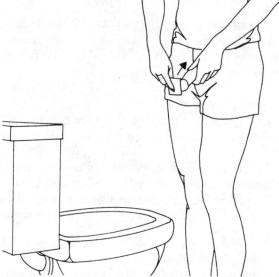

4 Urinate a small amount into the toilet. After 1 or 2 seconds, catch about 1 ounce (30 ml) of urine in the specimen cup.

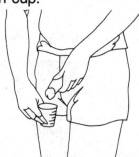

The nurse will tell you how far to fill the cup. As a rule, you'll fill it about one-fourth or more full.

Don't allow the cup to touch your penis at any time. When you're done, place the lid on the cup and return it to the nurse.

Note: Don't drink a lot of water before the test. This could affect the accuracy of test results.

How to collect a urine specimen: For females

Dear Patient:

Your doctor has asked you to provide a urine specimen for testing. It can tell whether you have an infection, or it can tell whether you have too much or too little of certain substances in your body.

To make sure that the test results are accurate, your urine shouldn't contain "outside germs" from your hands, your labia, or your urethral opening.

Follow the instructions below carefully. Read them through to the end before collecting your specimen.

1 Wash your hands thoroughly. Open the package of disposable wipes that the nurse gave you, and place it on a clean, dry, nearby surface.

2 Remove the lid from the specimen cup and place it flat side down. *Do not* touch the inside of the cup or lid.

3 Sit as far back on the toilet as possible. Spread your labia apart with one hand, keeping the folds separated for the rest of the procedure.

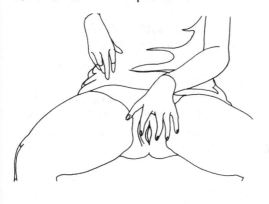

4 Using the disposable wipes, clean the area between the labia and around the urethra thoroughly from front to back. Use a new wipe for each stroke.

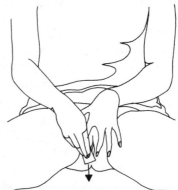

5 Urinate a small amount into the toilet. After 1 or 2 seconds, hold the specimen cup below your urine stream and catch about 1 ounce (30 ml) of urine in the cup. Don't allow the cup to touch your skin at any time.

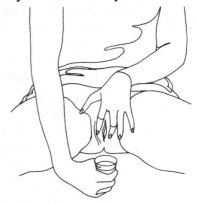

6 Place the lid on the cup and return it to the nurse.

Note: Don't drink large amounts of water before the test. This could affect the accuracy of test results.

PATIENT-TEACHING AID

Self-care tips in urinary tract infections

Dear Patient:

Here's some advice to help you treat your urinary tract infection (UTI) and prevent it from occurring again.

Treatment guidelines
• Take your prescribed medicine exactly as your doctor directs. *Do not* stop taking your medicine just because you feel better. Finish the prescription to kill all infection-causing germs. Otherwise, you run the risk of the infection coming back.
• Lay a warm heating pad on your abdomen and sides to soothe any pain and burning sensations you may have. Try a warm sitz bath, or ask your doctor to prescribe a pain reliever.

Diet tips
• Drink 10 to 14 glasses of fluid a day to increase urine flow and flush out germs.
• Eat foods and drink fluids with a high acid content. This will acidify your urine. Acid urine inhibits urinary tract germs.

High-acid foods include meats, nuts, plums, prunes, and whole-grain breads and cereals. High-acid drinks include cranberry and other fruit juices.

Here's a note of caution: If you're taking a sulfonamide drug (such as Gantrisin or Gantanol) to treat your infection, *avoid* cranberry juice because its high acid content can interfere with the action of the drug.
• Limit your intake of milk and other products with a high calcium content.
• Avoid caffeine, carbonated beverages, and alcohol because these substances irritate the bladder.

Prevention tips
• Practice sensible hygiene. For example, wipe from front to back each time you go to the bathroom. This reduces the chance that germs from bowel movements will enter your urinary tract.
• Change your underpants daily.
• Wear cotton undergarments because cotton "breathes." This enhances ventilation, which deters germ growth.
• Avoid tight slacks that prevent air circulation. Inadequate ventilation encourages germs to multiply and grow.
• Take showers instead of baths because germs in the bath water can enter your urinary tract.
• Avoid bubble baths, bath oils, perfumed vaginal sprays, and strong bleaches and cleansing powders in the laundry. These products can irritate crotch skin, which may trigger germ growth and infection.
• Urinate frequently (every 3 hours) to completely empty your bladder.
• Use the bathroom as soon as you sense you need to. Delayed urination is a major cause of UTIs.
• Urinate after sexual relations. This will help rid your urinary tract of any germs.

When to call the doctor
• Call your doctor right away if you suspect you have a new or repeated UTI.
• Also call the doctor if you notice such symptoms as an increased urge to urinate, increased urination (especially at night), pain when you urinate, or bloody or cloudy urine.

Epididymitis

Most common in men ages 18 to 40, this infection of the epididymis is usually unilateral. Bilateral infection or testicular involvement, however, may lead to sterility.

Because of the risk of sterility, you'll emphasize the early signs and symptoms of epididymitis, so the patient can learn to recognize them and seek immediate care if he suspects a recurrence. You'll also stress compliance with antibiotic therapy to combat the infection, and you'll help him cope with the discomfort caused by this disorder.

Furthermore, you'll identify the causes of epididymitis and review male reproductive anatomy to help the patient understand how this disorder occurs. You'll also cover how it's diagnosed. If drug therapy fails, you'll teach him about surgery—epididymectomy or bilateral vasectomy. If sterility is already present, you'll provide emotional support and refer him for counseling if needed.

Discuss the disorder

Explain that epididymitis is an infection of the epididymis, the testicle's tubular excretory duct. The epididymis carries sperm from the testicle to the urethra. Show the patient a diagram of the male reproductive system to point out the infection site and explain how this disorder can decrease sperm development. (See *How epididymitis can affect fertility,* page 342.)

Inform the patient that epididymitis most commonly results from pyogenic organisms, such as staphylococci, *Escherichia coli,* or streptococci. Usually, these organisms spread from an established urinary tract infection or prostatitis through the lumen of the vas deferens to the epididymis. The disorder may also result from gonorrhea, syphilis, or *Chlamydia* infection. Or it may follow prostate surgery or urinary catheterization. Rarely, it's caused by a distant bacterial infection, such as tonsillitis or tuberculosis. In this case, bacteria travel through the lymphatic system or, less commonly, through the bloodstream to reach the epididymis.

Chemical epididymitis (from nonbacterial causes) results from traumatic injury to the epididymis or irritation from urine reflux into the vas deferens. This form of epididymitis is common in military recruits (during basic training) who exercise with a full bladder, which causes urine reflux.

Tell the patient that signs and symptoms of epididymitis include sudden scrotal pain; redness, swelling, and extreme tender-

---

Gloria Perry, RN, who wrote this chapter, is a urology nurse clinician at Duke University Medical Center, Durham, N.C.

CHECKLIST

Teaching topics in epididymitis

☐ How epididymitis occurs
☐ Causes of epididymitis, primarily pyogenic bacteria
☐ Key signs and symptoms, such as sudden onset of acute pain, tenderness, and swelling in the groin and scrotum
☐ Complications, including sterility and orchitis
☐ Diagnosis by history and physical examination, blood and urine tests, and cultures
☐ Activity restrictions
☐ Use of antibiotics and analgesics
☐ Pain control measures, including scrotal elevation and ice packs
☐ Importance of increasing fluids
☐ Explanation of epididymectomy and vasectomy
☐ Counseling for sterilized patients and those whose epididymitis results from a sexually transmitted disease
☐ Sources of information and support

How epididymitis can affect fertility

Use the diagram below to help the patient understand how sperm normally develop and what can go wrong if he has epididymitis.

Inform the patient that the male reproductive cells, called spermatozoa (sperm), are produced in the testicles—a complex system of coiled tubules. The immature sperm swim out of the testicles into a long, coiled duct, called the epididymis, where the maturing process continues. From here, they pass into the vas deferens, where they become fully mature. The vas deferens terminates in the prostatic urethra. Finally, the sperm leave the body through the urethra when ejaculation occurs.

Tell the patient that in epididymitis bacteria from other parts of the urogenital system, such as the urethra, can travel backward through the reproductive tract to invade the epididymis. Here, these infecting organisms can interfere with sperm development, decreasing the patient's fertility.

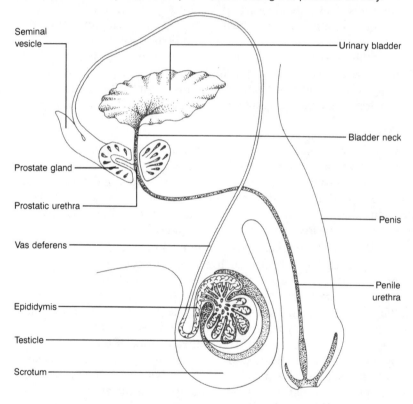

ness of the scrotum and groin (from enlarged lymph nodes in the spermatic cord); fever; chills; and malaise. The patient also exhibits a characteristic waddle—an attempt to protect the groin area when walking.

Complications
Warn the patient that untreated epididymitis can result in sterility. To help him understand what happens, explain that an infection

What is orchitis?

If your patient has orchitis, explain that this infection of the testicles is a severe complication of epididymitis that can cause permanent sterility.

Signs and symptoms include tenderness, redness, and warmth in one or both testicles, swelling of the scrotum and testicles, gradual onset of pain, and nausea and vomiting. Warn the patient that if the pain suddenly stops he may have testicular ischemia, which can permanently damage one or both testicles.

Tell the patient that antibiotics are given immediately to treat orchitis. Corticosteroids have also been tried, but their use is still experimental. Explain that in severe cases surgery may be needed to incise and drain the hydrocele and to improve circulation in the testicles. Otherwise, treatment is similar to that for epididymitis without orchitis.

that spreads to one or both testicles can cause orchitis, resulting in atrophy of the testes and decreased sperm production, which can lead to sterility (see *What is orchitis?*). Mention that bilateral epididymitis also causes sterility.

Another complication, fibrosis of the epididymal tissue, can occur if the infection occludes the epididymis. Untreated epididymitis can also rapidly lead to necrosis of testicular tissue and life-threatening septicemia.

Describe the diagnostic workup

Inform the patient that the doctor may tentatively diagnose epididymitis from the patient's medical history and a physical examination. Then the doctor will order tests to confirm the diagnosis, including a white blood cell (WBC) count, a urinalysis, a urine culture and sensitivity test, urethral discharge and prostatic secretion cultures, and, possibly, segmented bacteriologic localization cultures.

History and physical examination

Tell the patient that the doctor will ask him to describe his signs and symptoms and his general health. Explain that he'll examine the patient's scrotum and testicles for redness, swelling, and warmth. Then he'll gently palpate the scrotum, checking for enlargement and induration (hardness) of the epididymis. He'll also palpate the testicles, checking for tenderness and other symptoms of orchitis. Reassure the patient that the doctor will be careful not to hurt him.

WBC count

Explain to the patient that he'll have a blood sample drawn to determine the presence of infection. Tell him who will perform the venipuncture, when and where it will be done, and that no test preparations are necessary. Inform him that an increased WBC count indicates an infection.

Urinalysis

Tell the patient that he'll be asked to give a urine sample and that he needs no test preparation. Explain that WBCs in the urine are a sign of infection.

Urine culture and sensitivity test

Inform the patient that this test can identify the specific bacteria causing the infection so that the doctor can choose the best treatment. Show him how to collect the specimen without contaminating it. Then, give him a copy of the patient-teaching aid *How to collect a urine specimen: For males,* page 338.

Urethral discharge culture

Tell the patient that this test helps identify the bacteria causing the infection. If any urethral discharge is present, the doctor will swab the end of the penis to obtain a specimen for culture.

Prostatic secretion culture

Explain that this test also helps identify the bacteria causing the patient's infection. The doctor gently massages the prostate gland to stimulate the discharge of any secretions. He performs this procedure by inserting his gloved index finger into the patient's rectum and palpating the anterior rectal wall above the prostate gland. Reassure the patient that this is painless.

Segmented bacteriologic localization cultures

Tell the patient that these tests can help pinpoint the infection site. Explain that the test procedure involves collecting specimens all at once for a urinalysis, urine culture and sensitivity test, and prostatic secretion culture.

To prepare for the test, instruct the patient to drink several glasses of water. Then he'll provide four specimens, each in a different collection tube. Three of the tubes will be used for urine specimens. For the fourth specimen tube, the doctor will massage the prostate gland to stimulate prostatic secretion.

Teach about treatments

Teach the patient that treatment for epididymitis aims to combat the infection and relieve signs and symptoms. Treatment must begin immediately (particularly if the patient has bilateral epididymitis) because sterility is always a threat. Treatment includes antibiotics and analgesics; bed rest with scrotal elevation and ice packs; increased fluids; and occasionally, surgery (epididymectomy or bilateral vasectomy).

Activity

Tell the patient that during the acute phase of this illness he must remain on bed rest to reduce swelling and relieve pain. Advise him to start walking when his pain and swelling subside and to wear an athletic supporter. Caution him to avoid vigorous activity until all his signs and symptoms resolve.

Medication

Explain that the doctor will prescribe antibiotics to treat the infection (unless the patient has chemical epididymitis) and analgesics to relieve the pain. The choice of antibiotic depends on the results of culture and sensitivity tests. However, for severe illness the doctor may prescribe a broad-spectrum antibiotic immediately. Stress the importance of taking the antibiotic exactly as prescribed and for as long as ordered, even if the patient feels better; otherwise, the infection may recur.

A mild analgesic, such as aspirin (Ecotrin) or acetaminophen (Panadol), will usually relieve the patient's pain. If the patient has acute epididymitis, tell him that the doctor may inject the spermatic cord just above the testicle with an anesthetic, such as lidocaine (Xylocaine), to alleviate pain. If the patient has a fever, suggest that he consult his doctor before taking aspirin or acetaminophen.

Procedures

Inform the patient that elevating his scrotum will help relieve pain and reduce swelling while he's confined to bed. He can simply fold a soft towel and place it under the scrotum. Suggest applying an ice pack to the scrotum to help reduce swelling. Instruct him to fill an ice bag one-third to one-half full, expel the air, and close the top. He should wrap the ice pack in a towel and apply it to his scrotum, refilling it as needed. Advise him to remove the ice pack for several minutes every hour to prevent burns. Warn him not to take sitz baths or apply heat to his scrotum because heat destroys sperm cells.

Surgery

Two surgical procedures are used to treat epididymitis. An epididymectomy is performed when antibiotic therapy fails, and a bilateral vasectomy is occasionally performed in patients with chronic epididymitis or in elderly patients undergoing open prostatectomy.

Epididymectomy. In an epididymectomy, the surgeon makes a small incision in the scrotum and removes the inflamed portion of the epididymis. Tell the patient that he'll undergo this procedure on an outpatient basis and that he'll receive a local anesthetic. Make sure he understands that an epididymectomy results in sterility.

Outline postoperative care. Instruct the patient to apply an ice pack to his scrotum and take sitz baths for minor pain and swelling. Advise him to rest and wear an athletic supporter for 48 hours after surgery. He should abstain from sexual intercourse until his doctor directs otherwise. Emphasize the importance of avoiding strenuous activity or heavy lifting for a week or until his doctor directs. Also warn him to notify the doctor if fever, persistent abdominal or scrotal pain, or incisional bleeding develops.

Vasectomy. In a vasectomy, the surgeon makes a small incision in the scrotum and ties off the vas deferens so that fluid and organisms can no longer pass to the epididymis. Explain that the patient will have this surgery on an outpatient basis. He'll have a local anesthetic before undergoing the surgery. Inform the patient that afterward he'll be sterile.

Review postoperative care. For minor pain and swelling, direct the patient to apply an ice pack to his scrotum and take sitz baths. He'll need to rest and wear an athletic supporter for 48 hours after surgery. Tell him to avoid strenuous activity or heavy lifting for a week or until his doctor directs. Advise him to ask the doctor when he can resume sexual intercourse. Warn him to notify the doctor if he experiences fever, persistent abdominal or scrotal pain, or incisional bleeding.

Other care measures

Tell the patient to increase fluid intake to help fight the infection. Advise him to drink at least 2 to 3 liters of fluid a day.

If the patient's epididymitis stems from a sexually transmitted disease, recommend that his sexual partner seek treatment to prevent reinfection. If the patient is sterile as a result of bilateral epididymitis or surgery (epididymectomy or vasectomy), refer him to a counselor.

Sources of information and support

American Urological Association
11512 Allecingie Parkway, Richmond, Va. 23235
(804) 379-5513

National Kidney and Urologic Diseases Information Clearinghouse
P.O. Box NKUDIC, Bethesda, Md. 20892
(301) 468-6345

Further readings

Bips, M. "Investigating Male Infertility," *Journal of American Academy of Physician Assistants* 2(2):85-94, March-April 1989.

Conti, M.T., and Eutropius, L. "Preventing UTI's: What Works?" *American Journal of Nursing* 87(3):307-9, March 1987.

Kaler, S.R. "Epididymitis in the Young Adult Male," *Nurse Practitioner* 15(5):10, 12, 14, May 1990.

Nero, F.A. "When Couples Ask About Infertility," *RN* 51(11):26-33, November 1988.

Oates, R.D. "Male Infertility: Actual or Potential," *Hospital Practice* 24(9A):20, 22, 25, September 30, 1989.

Roberts, A. "Senior Systems: The Aging Urinary System," Part 34. *Nursing Times* 85(10):59-62, March 8-14, 1989.

Tonetti, J.A. "Testicular Torsion or Acute Epididymitis? Diagnosis and Treatment," *Journal of Emergency Nursing* 16(2):96-98, March-April 1990.

8

Obstetric and Gynecologic Conditions

Contents

Dysfunctional uterine bleeding

Dysfunctional uterine bleeding can be frightening and puzzling for a patient. Her first questions, "What's happening to my body?" and "Do I have cancer?" will challenge you to provide not only information but also emotional support. You'll need to review the disorder's many causes, explain how the menstrual cycle works, and discuss appropriate tests and treatments. Most importantly, you'll need to reassure her that dysfunctional uterine bleeding is common and treatable. And if treatment includes a hysterectomy, you'll need to help her accept her altered body image and cope with possible depression or moodiness.

Discuss the disorder

Explain to the patient that dysfunctional uterine bleeding is characterized by excessive and irregular uterine bleeding for which no organic cause can be found. Inform her that bleeding is judged abnormal based on its amount, time of occurrence, and duration (see *When is uterine bleeding abnormal?* page 350).

Tell the patient that the disorder can be classified as true dysfunctional or pseudodysfunctional uterine bleeding. *True dysfunctional uterine bleeding* results from a disruption in the hormones that regulate the menstrual cycle and estrogen-progesterone secretion, which, in turn, causes endometrial abnormalities and abnormal bleeding. Explain that this hormonal disruption has several variations. Either the body produces no progesterone (resulting in nonovulatory dysfunctional uterine bleeding); too little progesterone (resulting in irregular endometrial ripening); too much progesterone or slow withdrawal of progesterone (resulting in irregular endometrial shedding); or too little estrogen and no progesterone (resulting in endometrial atrophy).

Pseudodysfunctional uterine bleeding, on the other hand, results from local disorders, endocrine disorders or systemic diseases or both, and certain drugs. Local disorders include uterine fibroids, cervicitis, pelvic inflammatory disease (PID), and ovarian tumors. Endocrine disorders and systemic diseases include adrenal dysfunction, diabetes mellitus, hypothalamic or pituitary disorders, thyroid dysfunction, idiopathic thrombocytopenic purpura, leukemia, systemic lupus erythematosus, renal or hepatic disease, and obesity. Anticoagulants, oral contraceptives, and possibly digitalis can also cause abnormal uterine bleeding.

Pamela Klauer Triolo, RN, PhD, ARNP, CNM, wrote this chapter. She is associate director of nursing at the University of Iowa Hospitals and Clinics, Iowa City.

CHECKLIST

Teaching topics in dysfunctional uterine bleeding

☐ Explanation of dysfunctional uterine bleeding
☐ Description of a normal menstrual cycle
☐ Classifications and causes of dysfunctional uterine bleeding
☐ Diagnostic procedures and tests, including D & C, endometrial biopsy, and laparoscopy
☐ Hormonal therapy and adverse reactions
☐ Hysterectomy, if appropriate
☐ Home care after surgery, if appropriate
☐ Source of information and support

When is uterine bleeding abnormal?

Is your patient uncertain about whether her uterine bleeding episodes signify a temporary upset in her menstrual cycle or an ongoing disorder requiring treatment?

If so, explain that when, how long, and how much bleeding occurs determines whether it's abnormal. For example, the patient should seek medical attention when her bleeding episodes occur:
• between menstrual periods
• as a *consistently* heavy or prolonged period (more than 8 days)
• as a *consistently* short menstrual cycle (fewer than 18 days)
• more than 1 year after the last menstrual period
• after sexual intercourse
• as consistent bloody discharge
• as hemorrhaging.

Complications

Emphasize that untreated dysfunctional uterine bleeding can cause anemia. Urge the patient to report changes in breathing rate, dizziness, faintness, fatigue, and sweating to her doctor. Point out that hemorrhage from dysfunctional uterine bleeding can be life-threatening.

Describe the diagnostic workup

Tell the patient to expect a thorough physical and gynecological examination. Forewarn her that because dysfunctional uterine bleeding can stem from many causes, the doctor may order several diagnostic tests. Tell the patient who will perform each test and when and where it will be done.

Blood and urine tests

Inform the patient that these tests may provide clues about her health. For instance, they can tell whether she has anemia or abnormal follicle stimulating hormone, luteinizing hormone, prolactin, or testosterone levels. Thyroid function and glucose tolerance tests can determine whether a systemic disease is causing the bleeding.

Other tests may include a complete blood count, platelet count, prothrombin time, activated partial thromboplastin time, LE preparation (to rule out systemic lupus erythematosus), and an antinuclear antibody test (to rule out a connective tissue disease). An SMA-12 and a urinalysis may be done to rule out renal and hepatic disease.

Diagnostic procedures

Besides dilatation and curettage (D & C) and endometrial biopsy, the doctor may perform hysterosalpingography, hysteroscopy, laparoscopy, or pelvic ultrasonography.

D & C. Inform the patient that this procedure takes about 1 hour and serves as both a test and a treatment. Explain that the doctor will obtain tissue samples from the uterus, cervix, endometrium and other sites for laboratory analysis to determine the cause of bleeding. Also explain that a D & C alone may correct abnormal bleeding.

Reassure the patient that she'll receive either a local or a general anesthetic. If she'll be an outpatient, caution her to arrange for transportation home because she'll be groggy afterward. Then describe the procedure, pointing out steps to take before and after surgery. Allow time to answer her questions and give her a copy of the patient-teaching aid *What to expect with a D & C,* page 358.

Endometrial biopsy. If the doctor suspects cancer, he may perform an endometrial biopsy without a D & C. Explain that the biopsy can be done only during a bleeding episode. Describe it as being similar to a D & C. Mention that a local anesthetic will prevent pain during the biopsy, but that she may feel mild to moderate cramping afterward.

Hysterosalpingography. Inform the patient that this 15-minute test can help identify uterine and fallopian tube abnormalities. No special test preparations are needed.

Tell her that during the test, she'll lie on her back with her legs in stirrups. The doctor will insert a speculum into her vagina and swab the cervix to remove any mucus that could obscure the area he needs to see. Then he'll insert a cannula into the uterus and slowly inject a radiopaque contrast agent. If this dyelike substance triggers cramping, he'll stop the injection until the cramps subside. Then he'll view the uterus and fallopian tubes with a fluoroscope and take X-ray films.

Caution the patient to watch for signs of infection after the test and to report them to the doctor. Also warn her that this test may increase her chances of becoming pregnant because as the contrast agent flows through the fallopian tubes, it may break up adhesions, stimulate cilia that promote passage of the ovum, or make cervical mucus more receptive to sperm.

Hysteroscopy. Explain that hysteroscopy allows the doctor to see abnormalities inside the uterine cavity. The test takes about 10 minutes and no special preparations are needed.

Describe the lithotomy position that the patient will assume and explain that the doctor will insert a speculum into her vagina and swab the cervix to remove any mucus. Next he'll insert a hysteroscope (an optical instrument resembling a periscope) and look for abnormalities.

After the test, caution her to report any signs of infection, including fever, pelvic pain, increased pulse rate, and malaise.

Laparoscopy. Tell the patient that like a D & C, laparoscopy can be both a test and a treatment. Describe how this procedure allows the doctor to view the pelvic organs through a tubelike apparatus. The procedure may be done with either local or general anesthetics and takes about 1 hour.

Inform the patient that during the test, the doctor makes a small abdominal incision and then inserts the laparoscope through it. If minor surgery is necessary—such as removal of an endometrioma or small fibroid tumors—he'll perform it by passing instruments through the laparoscope.

Explain that the doctor may inject air into the abdominal cavity to help him see the internal structures better. If this occurs, warn the patient that after the test, she might have some shoulder pain from air irritating her diaphragm. Suggest that lying in a prone position with a pillow under her abdomen may help. Also caution her to watch for signs of infection, such as redness, warmth, or increased tenderness at the incision site. As appropriate, remind her to follow the doctor's orders regarding douching and resuming sexual intercourse.

Pelvic ultrasonography. Inform the patient that this test detects foreign bodies in the uterus and distinguishes between cysts (containing liquid or semisolid material) and tumors (containing solid material). It takes about 30 minutes and requires no anesthetic.

Tell her that she must drink 6 to 8 glasses of clear fluid, such as water, ginger ale or apple juice, 1½ to 2 hours before the test. Warn her not to void until afterward—a full bladder helps to position other pelvic organs. Reassure the pregnant patient that the test won't harm the fetus.

Explain that she'll lie on her back during the test and that her abdomen will be coated with a conductant, such as mineral oil. The technician will guide a transducer over her abdomen, revealing images of the uterus, vagina, and adjoining structures.

Tell the patient that she can empty her bladder after the test.

Teach about treatments

Explain that once the doctor determines the cause of uterine bleeding, appropriate treatment can start. For true or PID-induced dysfunctional uterine bleeding, drug therapy is customarily used, unless the patient has cancer or is pregnant. For bleeding caused by fibroids, uterine cancer, or uterine prolapse, a hysterectomy may be performed.

Medication

If your patient has true dysfunctional uterine bleeding, explain that the doctor will probably prescribe hormonal therapy. See *Teaching about drugs for dysfunctional uterine bleeding,* pages 354 and 355. If your patient has pseudodysfunctional uterine bleeding from a disorder such as PID, the doctor may prescribe other drug therapy.

Hormonal therapy. Various hormonal combinations and amounts are used depending on the underlying disorder. *For nonovulation or irregular ovulation,* estrogen and progesterone may help the endometrium develop normally and stimulate ovulation. Estrogen supplements "prime" the endometrium during the menstrual cycle's proliferative phase. Progesterone supplements, such as medroxyprogesterone (Provera) or norethindrone (Micronor), promote secretory development of the endometrium. If the doctor orders medroxyprogesterone, tell the patient to take it for 10 days, beginning on day 16 of her menstrual cycle. If he prescribes norethindrone, tell her to start the drug on day 5 of her cycle and discontinue it on day 25. She should expect bleeding 3 to 7 days after discontinuing either drug.

For irregular endometrial ripening, the doctor may prescribe progesterone cautiously, because if the patient's in the first 4 months of pregnancy, fetal abnormalities may result.

For irregular endometrial shedding, the doctor may prescribe a monophasic, a biphasic, or a triphasic oral contraceptive. Explain that a monophasic drug supplies the same hormonal formula for 21 days, that a biphasic drug supplies two different formulas for 21 days, and that a triphasic drug supplies three different formulas for 21 days.

For endometrial atrophy, indicating both estrogen and progesterone deficiencies, the doctor usually prescribes an oral contraceptive, such as estrogen with progestin (Enovid, Ovulen). Tell

Questions patients ask about hysterectomy

I hear so much about hysterectomies being done unnecessarily—and now my doctor says I need one. How do I know it's really necessary?
One way to ease your mind and help form your decision is to get a second opinion. The second doctor will review your records and give you a physical examination, which will either support the first doctor's judgment or conflict with it. If the second doctor doesn't think that you need surgery, get a third opinion. Then consider all three judgments before making your decision—because it is your decision, after all.

Will I gain weight after a hysterectomy?
Not usually—unless you eat more and exercise less.

However, if the doctor removes your ovaries along with your uterus, you'll experience menopause unless you have supplemental hormonal therapy. Because postmenopausal women require one-third fewer calories, you could gain weight if you continue eating the same amount of food you did before your hysterectomy.

Will a hysterectomy ruin my sex life?
No. Many women find that sexual interest and enjoyment increases when pregnancy isn't an issue. If your ovaries are removed along with your uterus, however, your vagina may be drier. Using a water-soluble lubricating jelly or taking supplemental estrogen may help with this problem.

---

the patient to start taking the drug on day 5 of her menstrual cycle, taking one color tablet for 10 days and the next color tablet for 11 days. Explain that withdrawal bleeding similar to a normal menstrual period should follow the last tablet.

Other drugs. If your patient has PID-induced bleeding, explain that the doctor may prescribe antimicrobial therapy.

Surgery
Explain that the surgery involves removing the uterus either abdominally or vaginally, depending on the causative disorder. (See *What happens in abdominal hysterectomy,* page 356.)

Preoperative teaching. Tell the patient that she won't be allowed any food or fluids after midnight the night before surgery. That night, she'll need to shower with an antibacterial soap, and she may have to douche. She may also be given a cleansing enema. The morning of surgery, she'll have an indwelling urinary catheter inserted, which will stay in place 24 hours, and an I.V. line started. Shortly before surgery, she'll receive a sedative.

Postoperative teaching. Tell the patient that she'll return from surgery with a perineal pad in place. Inform her that she can expect some abdominal pain, and advise her not to wait until the pain is intense to ask for medication. Besides showing her how to do leg exercises to prevent thromboembolism, explain that she'll need to get out of bed and walk several times a day. Let her know that she will still have an I.V. line in place and will be allowed nothing by mouth until she has bowel sounds and is passing flatus—then her diet will progress from clear liquids to solid foods, as tolerated.

continued on page 357

Teaching about drugs for dysfunctional uterine bleeding

DRUG	ADVERSE REACTIONS	TEACHING POINTS
Progestins		
medroxyprogesterone acetate (Provera) **norethindrone** (Micronor)	• Be alert for abdominal pain; amenorrhea; arm or leg weakness or pain; breakthrough bleeding; breast discharge, enlargement, or tenderness; chest pain; depression; dizziness; dysmenorrhea; headache; jaundice; melasma; shortness of breath; slurred speech; rash; and visual disturbances. • Other reactions include ankle and foot swelling, appetite changes, lethargy, nausea, vomiting, and weight changes.	• Warn the patient to discontinue the drug immediately if she suspects that she's pregnant and to have a pregnancy test. • If she misses a dose, advise her to take the next dose as soon as she remembers it, but not to double-dose. • Teach her to take the drug at the same time each day at 24-hour intervals (nighttime dosing may reduce nausea and headaches), to keep the tablets in their original container, and to take them in correct (color-coded) sequence. • If she misses one menstrual period and has taken the tablets on schedule, instruct her to continue taking them. If she misses two consecutive periods, tell her to discontinue the drug and to have a pregnancy test. Progestins may cause birth defects if taken early in pregnancy. • Stress the importance of having a yearly Pap test and gynecologic examination while taking progestin combinations. • Warn the patient of a possible delay in achieving conception when the drug is discontinued. Advise her to check with her doctor about how soon conception can be safely attempted. • Warn her of the risks associated with simultaneous use of cigarettes and oral contraceptives—for example, thrombophlebitis and cerebrovascular accident. • Instruct her to weigh herself at least twice a week and to report any sudden weight gain or edema to the doctor. • Inform her that this drug decreases cervical mucus viscosity and heightens susceptibility to vaginal infections, so good hygienic practices are essential.
Combination oral contraceptives		
norethynodrel with mestranol (Enovid)	• Be alert for breathing difficulty, chest pain, hypertension, leg pain or tenderness, severe headache, tachycardia, and yellow skin or sclera. • Other reactions include ankle swelling; breast discharge, enlargement, or tenderness; dizziness; mild headache; nausea; and spotting or breakthrough bleeding.	• Explain to the patient that this drug helps treat excessive uterine bleeding. • Advise her to take the tablets at the same time each day for greatest effectiveness. • Warn the patient that mild headache, nausea, dizziness, breast tenderness, spotting, and breakthrough bleeding are common at first. Spotting and breakthrough bleeding may diminish between 1 and 3 months of therapy but should be reported to the doctor. • If she misses one menstrual period and has taken the tablets on schedule, instruct her to continue taking them. If she misses two consecutive periods, tell her to discontinue the drug and have a pregnancy test. Progestogens may cause birth defects if taken early in pregnancy. • If she has nausea or headache, tell her to take the tablets at night. Taking them with food may also help reduce nausea. • Stress the importance of having a yearly Pap test and gynecologic examination while taking this drug. • Warn her of a possible delay in conceiving when she discontinues the drug. Advise her to check with her doctor about how soon conception can be safely attempted. • Warn her of the risks associated with simultaneous use of cigarettes and oral contraceptives. • Instruct her to weigh herself at least twice a week and to report any sudden weight gain or edema to the doctor. • Caution her to avoid exposure to ultraviolet light or prolonged exposure to sunlight—it aggravates chloasma. If she expects such exposure, advise taking the drug at bedtime. This may lower daytime levels of circulating hormone. • Inform her that this drug decreases cervical mucus viscosity and heightens susceptibility to vaginal infections, so good hygienic practices are essential.

continued

Teaching about drugs for dysfunctional uterine bleeding — *continued*

Oral contraceptives

Monophasic type:
mestranol and norethynodrel

Biphasic type:
ethinyl estradiol and norethindrone
(Ortho-Novum 10/11)

Triphasic type:
ethinyl estradiol and norethindrone
(Tri-Norinyl 28-Day)

• Be alert for abdominal pain, hypertension, leg pain or tenderness, and yellow skin or sclera.
• Other reactions include breast discharge, enlargement, or tenderness; dizziness; mild headache; intolerance of contact lenses; rash or acne; spotting or breakthrough bleeding; and vision loss.

• Inform the patient that the prescribed drug helps to control excessive uterine bleeding.
• Teach the patient to take the drug at the same time each day at 24-hour intervals, to keep the tablets in their original container, and to take them in correct (color-coded) sequence. Tablets are colored differently to indicate different strengths, and they may be less effective if taken in random order.
• Suggest that the patient use an additional birth control method for the first drug cycle (or 3 weeks) to provide further protection from pregnancy.
• Warn the patient that mild headache, nausea, dizziness, breast tenderness, spotting, and breakthrough bleeding are common initially. Spotting and breakthrough bleeding may diminish after 1 to 3 months of therapy but should be reported to the doctor.
• If the patient misses one menstrual period and has taken the tablets on schedule, instruct her to continue taking them. If she misses two consecutive periods, tell her to discontinue the drug and to have a pregnancy test. Progestins may cause birth defects if taken early in pregnancy.
• If the patient has nausea or headache, tell her to take the tablets at night. Taking them with food may also help reduce nausea.
• Urge the patient to keep monophasic, biphasic, or triphasic tablets in their original containers, which are marked to help her keep track of her dosage schedule.
• Stress the importance of having a yearly Pap test and gynecologic examination while taking estrogen-progestin combinations.
• Advise the patient to schedule medical checkups every 6 to 12 months, depending on her condition. Some doctors may require more frequent visits.
• Warn the patient that this drug may cause a possible delay in conception when it's discontinued. Advise her to check with her doctor about how soon she can safely attempt conception.
• Warn her of the risks associated with simultaneous use of cigarettes and oral contraceptives.
• Instruct the patient to weigh herself at least twice a week and to report any sudden weight gain or edema to the doctor.
• Caution the patient to avoid exposure to ultraviolet light or prolonged exposure to sunlight—it aggravates chloasma. If she expects such exposure, advise her to take the drug at bedtime. This may help reduce daytime levels of circulating hormone.
• Inform her that this drug decreases cervical mucus viscosity and heightens susceptibility to vaginal infections, so good hygienic practices are essential.
• Instruct her to tell her doctor or dentist that she is taking this drug before undergoing any surgical procedure or emergency treatment because this drug may cause clotting, stroke, or heart attack.
• Tell the patient to check with her doctor if she is wearing contact lenses and notices any change in vision or is unable to wear them.

What happens in abdominal hysterectomy

The patient facing an abdominal hysterectomy will have many questions about the surgery and its aftermath. To answer her questions, review the surgery with her. Begin by describing, as appropriate, the three types of hysterectomies: total (the surgeon removes the entire uterus); subtotal (the surgeon removes part of the uterus, leaving the cervical stump intact); and radical (the surgeon removes the uterus, upper vagina, cervix, and parametrial tissue).

Depending on the surgeon and the operation, the patient may have a midline (vertical) incision, from the umbilicus to the symphysis pubis, or a Pfannenstiel (horizontal, or bikini line) incision.

Once the surgeon makes the incision, he identifies major organs and structures, carefully removes the diseased portions, then closes the incision and applies a pad or dressing. Reassure the patient that the incision usually heals rapidly and the scar fades over time.

REPRODUCTIVE ORGANS

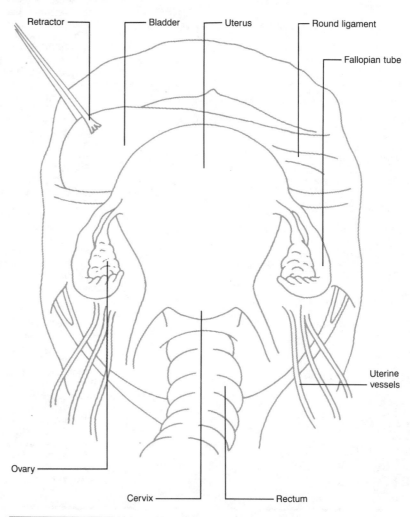

Home care instructions. Before the patient leaves the hospital, review home care measures with her. Discuss signs of complications she should report to her doctor, and how to clean her wound to prevent infection. Instruct her to check vaginal discharge daily, explaining that small spots of blood or brownish staining are normal and may last about a week. Warn her to report bleeding that resembles a menstrual period, severe cramping, or hot flashes. Emphasize that she shouldn't use a tampon, douche, or insert anything into her vagina for 6 weeks. To prevent constipation, suggest a diet high in fiber and tell her to drink plenty of fluids.

Caution her not to exercise vigorously, lift any heavy objects, or have sexual intercourse for 6 weeks. Urge her, however, to walk or exercise regularly and as tolerable.

Other care measures

The patient may feel depressed or discouraged, especially if the cause of her bleeding has been difficult to diagnose. If she needs a hysterectomy, she might feel even more depressed after surgery because of abrupt hormonal fluctuations. Reassure her that depression and irritability are common and are only temporary. Encourage her to express her feelings about her altered body image and to feel free to ask you and the doctor questions. Counsel her family about possible mood swings, encouraging them to respond calmly and with understanding. As appropriate, refer the patient and her family to support and information groups.

Source of information and support

Endometriosis Association
P.O. Box 9187
Milwaukee, Wisc. 53202
(414) 962-8972

Further readings

Haslett, S. "Hysterectomy," *Nursing* (London) 3(25):962-65, January 1988.
Mechcatie, E. "When Is Hysterectomy Really Needed?" *Patient Care* 21(1):62-66, 68, 73, January 15, 1987.
Modica, M.M., et al. "Transvaginal Sonography Provides a Sharper View into the Pelvis," *Journal of Obstetric, Gynecologic, and Neonatal Nursing* 17(2):89-95, March-April 1988.
Pinsonneault, O., et al. "Dysfunctional Uterine Bleeding and Breast Masses in Adolescents," *Physician Assistant* 11(4):77-78, 82-85, April 1987.
Rubin, D. "Gynecologic Cancer: Uterine and Ovarian Malignancies," *RN* 50(6):52-57, June 1987.

What to expect with a D & C

Dear Patient:

Dilatation and curettage (a D & C for short) is a surgical procedure designed to control abnormal uterine bleeding and to determine its cause.

Before the procedure

Before you enter the hospital, you'll describe your health history and the doctor will give you a physical and gynecological examination. You'll have a Pap test and blood and urine tests to make sure you're ready for surgery.

You may be asked to shower with an antibacterial soap the night before the procedure; you may also be given an enema to cleanse your bowel — a precaution against infection. You'll probably be told not to eat or drink anything after midnight.

In the hospital, you'll be given a mild tranquilizer before surgery, and an I.V. line will be started to give you fluids or medicine that you may need during the procedure.

During the procedure

If you have a general anesthetic to let you sleep through the procedure, you'll wake up in about an hour in the recovery room, where a nurse will check your progress. If you have a local anesthetic, you'll be awake during the procedure. Here's what to expect:

The surgical team will help you lie on your back on the operating table. You'll see stirrups for your legs.

The doctor will examine you internally.

As he does, he may remove polyps (growths that can cause bleeding) and take tissue samples from your cervix and uterus. (The tissue will be studied to find out the reason for your bleeding.) Then he'll do the D & C using surgical instruments to stretch (dilate) your cervix and to gently scrape the surface lining of the uterus (the endometrium).

If you feel temporary cramping, nausea, or light-headedness, breathe deeply and try to relax. It's unlikely you'll feel discomfort. However, if you do, tell the doctor. He can give you medicine.

After the procedure

When your anesthetic wears off, you'll feel mild to severe cramping, similar to a menstrual period. You may also have some lower back pain for 1 or 2 days. Here are some tips for your recovery:
- Ask your doctor or nurse to recommend a pain medicine.
- Use a sanitary napkin, *not a tampon,* for mild spotting or staining that may last a few days or more.
- Resume your normal activities, but ask your doctor about vigorous execise.
- Don't have sexual intercourse until healing is complete — about 2 weeks.
- Report any of the following to your doctor: vaginal bleeding that resembles a menstrual period; fever; sharp, constant pelvic pain; increased pulse rate; or foul-smelling vaginal drainage. Also call him if you just don't feel right.
- Be sure to make and keep your appointment for a checkup.

Abortion

Abortion refers to the expulsion of the products of conception from the uterus before the fetus is viable. It may be spontaneous (also called miscarriage) or induced (also called therapeutic abortion). Although the result remains the same, the two types of abortion may trigger very different responses and feelings in your patient, so plan to personalize your instruction.

Because most women have intense, mixed feelings about abortion, you may spend as much time offering emotional support as you will offering instruction. If your patient's hospitalized for spontaneous abortion—either threatened or actual—you'll discuss causes, signs and symptoms, complications, and tests and treatments. As appropriate, you'll cover activity restrictions, drug therapy, surgery, and other care.

If your patient's having an induced abortion, teach her about preabortion testing, describe the surgical procedure, and discuss possible complications. Sum up with postoperative and home care.

Discuss the disorder

Tailor this information to the patient's needs. If she's just had a spontaneous abortion, or if she's trying to prevent one, explain that a miscarriage occurs when the fertilized ovum can't grow in the uterus. Tell her that at least 15% of all pregnancies end in spontaneous abortion, usually before 13 weeks of gestation. Then, if appropriate, explain the types of spontaneous abortion (see *Reviewing types of spontaneous abortion,* page 360).

Inform the patient that certain fetal, placental, and maternal factors may cause spontaneous abortions. Possible fetal causes include embryologic defects, faulty implantation of the fertilized ovum, and failure of the endometrium to accept the fertilized ovum. Possible placental causes include premature separation of the placenta, abnormal placental implantation, and platelet dysfunction. Possible maternal causes include infection, reproductive abnormalities, endocrine dysfunction, trauma, blood group incompatibility, and drug ingestion—especially cocaine and alcohol. In most cases, the abortion's cause will remain unknown (unless the patient obviously abused drugs). Spend extra time, if necessary, to reassure the patient that she wasn't at fault.

If the patient has a threatened abortion, describe the signs and symptoms of spontaneous abortion. Tell her that the first sign may be brown spotting, lasting for several weeks, or a pink discharge, lasting for several days. If her condition progresses, she'll notice old, dark blood or fresh, bright red blood. She'll begin to

Linda Byers, RN,C, BSN, MS, who wrote this chapter, is director of clinic services for Community Action, Family Planning Program, San Marcos, Texas.

CHECKLIST

Teaching topics in abortion

☐ Causes, signs, and symptoms of spontaneous abortion
☐ Types of spontaneous abortion
☐ Complications of untreated incomplete abortion
☐ Diagnostic tests, including those that confirm pregnancy and spontaneous abortion and those that test for anemia and infection
☐ Activity restrictions after abortion
☐ Medications to relieve pain, prevent infection, reduce blood loss, and cause uterine contractions
☐ Preparation and surgical procedure for incomplete or induced abortion
☐ Rationale for contraception
☐ Pregnancy after abortion
☐ Sources of information and support

Reviewing types of spontaneous abortion

Your patient may not know that a spontaneous (or threatened) abortion takes many forms. Use the information below to help her differentiate among the various types.

Impending abortion
Bloody vaginal discharge during the first half of pregnancy signals an impending miscarriage. About 20% of pregnant women have vaginal spotting or actual bleeding early in pregnancy; of these, about 50% abort. Instruct the patient to contact her doctor if she has this sign of threatened abortion.

Inevitable abortion
In this condition, membranes rupture and the cervix dilates. Contractions and bleeding accompany labor as the uterus expels the products of conception.

Complete abortion
The uterus passes all the products of conception. Usually, minimal bleeding occurs. That's because the uterus contracts normally to compress or seal the maternal vessels that supplied blood to the placenta.

Incomplete abortion
In incomplete abortion, the uterus retains part or all of the placenta. Before 10 weeks of gestation, the uterus usually expels the fetus and placenta together; after 10 weeks, separately. Because some placenta may still adhere to the uterine wall, bleeding continues. Hemorrhage can result because the uterus doesn't contract to compress or seal the large vessels that supplied blood to the placenta.

Missed abortion
In this type of abortion, the uterus retains the fetus for 2 months or more after the fetus dies. Uterine growth ceases. In some cases, uterine size appears to decrease. Prolonged retention of the fetus may cause coagulation defects (such as disseminated intravascular coagulation) and infection.

Habitual abortion
Spontaneous loss of three or more consecutive pregnancies constitutes habitual abortion.

Septic abortion
When accompanied by infection, an abortion is called septic. The condition typically results from a nonsterile procedure performed by untrained personnel. It may also accompany a spontaneous abortion if the patient has a uterine infection.

---

have cramps. The cramps will intensify over a few hours as the cervix dilates to expel the uterine contents—blood clots or fetal tissue.

If the patient is having an induced abortion, explain that this procedure surgically removes the products of conception. It's usually performed between 8 and 17 weeks of pregnancy, preferably in the first trimester (before 13 weeks). Reassure her that a first-trimester abortion is a simple procedure with few risks. Also, although a second-trimester abortion (between 14 and 26 weeks) may be a more complex procedure, it carries fewer risks than childbirth.

Complications
Tell the patient with a threatened or actual spontaneous abortion that few complications occur if the products of conception are completely expelled. However, if any tissue remains in the uterus, she'll need surgery. Without treatment, cramping and bleeding will continue. Hemorrhage or infection may follow.

Describe the diagnostic workup
Inform the patient that certain tests along with her health history and physical examination will confirm pregnancy or spontaneous abortion. Tell her that she may also have tests to detect whether anemia, infection, Rh factor or, possibly, sexually transmitted diseases (STDs) contributed to the abortion.

Pregnancy tests
Inform the patient that she can expect to have blood or urine tests (or both) to confirm pregnancy, even if a home pregnancy test already gave her positive results. Tell her that human chorionic gonadotropin (HCG) in the blood or urine confirms pregnancy, whereas decreased HCG levels suggest spontaneous abortion.

Pelvic ultrasonography
Inform the patient that pelvic ultrasonography may be done to detect a gestational sac and to date the pregnancy. Tell her that the test takes about 30 minutes, and discuss any necessary preparations. Explain that during the test she'll lie on her back and her abdomen will be coated with a conductant, such as mineral oil. Then the technician will guide a transducer over her abdomen to visualize the uterus.

Blood tests
If the patient with a threatened abortion has heavy bleeding, explain that a complete blood count will be done to check for anemia and infection. Her blood will also be tested for Rh factor. If she's Rh negative, she'll be given Rh-immune globulin to prevent incompatibility problems in future pregnancies.

Tests to confirm spontaneous abortion
If the patient's already had a spontaneous abortion, tell her that the doctor will confirm this by performing a pelvic examination, inspecting tissue expelled from the uterus (if available), and ordering tissue studies.

Other tests
Inform the patient that many hospitals and clinics also test for STDs, such as gonorrhea, syphilis, or chlamydia, possible causes of spontaneous abortion.

Teach about treatments
After a complete spontaneous abortion, treatment includes bed rest and medication. For an incomplete, missed, or induced abortion, treatment will also involve surgery. All patients will need contraceptive information.

Activity
Explain honestly to the patient with a threatened abortion that the only treatment is complete bed rest and even that may fail. If she's already had a spontaneous abortion, with or without subsequent surgery, tell her that avoiding vigorous activity for a few days will decrease the risk of hemorrhage. But advise her to resume activity later as tolerated. If she's having a therapeutic abortion, the same instructions apply.

Medication
Teach the patient about medications she may receive to prevent infection, reduce bleeding, and relieve pain. Explain that she'll probably take an antibiotic—ampicillin, tetracycline, or erythro-

mycin, for example—to prevent a uterine infection.

Tell the patient to take the entire drug dose exactly as prescribed. Warn that she may experience GI upset, especially if she has or had morning sickness. Reassure her, though, that few patients have severe hypersensitivity reactions, such as breathing disorders or hives and rashes.

Inform the patient that she may receive ergonovine maleate and methylergonovine maleate to reduce blood loss after a spontaneous or induced abortion and to help the uterus contract to normal size. Forewarn her that contractions begin within minutes of taking these drugs and may continue for several hours. Adverse reactions include dizziness, headache, nausea, and vomiting.

Tell the patient that an over-the-counter, nonaspirin analgesic, such as acetaminophen, or a nonsteroidal anti-inflammatory drug, such as ibuprofen, may relieve the cramping that follows a spontaneous or an induced abortion. Caution her not to take products containing aspirin, which can increase bleeding.

Surgery

Discuss the types of surgery used to remove uterine contents: suction curettage, dilatation and curettage (D&C), and dilatation and evacuation (D&E). Suction curettage, used at about 4 to 6 gestational weeks, requires little or no cervical dilation. In this procedure, the doctor inserts a cannula, which is attached to a vacuum source, through the cervix and gently curettes the uterus. After about 7 weeks, a D&C or D&E is usually required.

Explain the D&C or D&E. Inform the patient having surgery for an *incomplete abortion* that she'll receive a general anesthetic, a regional paracervical block, or a local anesthetic. Afterward, she'll lie in the dorsal lithotomy position. The doctor will perform a preliminary bimanual pelvic examination. He'll expose the cervix and check the depth and direction of the uterine cavity. Then he'll dilate the cervical canal. If he performs a D&C, he'll examine the uterine cavity and perform standard curettage to scrape away the superficial endometrial layer. Then he'll remove the remaining products of conception. If he performs a D&E, he'll use a suction curette to extract the uterine contents.

Explain to the patient having a first-trimester *induced abortion* that she'll usually receive a local anesthetic instilled into the cervix. And she may be asked to self-administer nitrous oxide. Then the doctor performs a D&E. The full procedure may take fewer than 10 minutes.

If the patient's pregnancy is advanced past 11 weeks, explain that the procedure may be done in two stages on two consecutive days. On the first day, the doctor inserts one or more laminaria (compressed natural or synthetic materials) into the cervical os. Laminaria expand with moisture, inducing cervical dilation slowly. On the second day, the patient has the abortion either with a suction catheter or by curettage.

Outline preoperative measures. Whether the patient's being treated for a spontaneous abortion or having an induced abortion, your instructions will be similar. Tell her who will perform the surgery and describe where it will be done. If appropriate, explain that because she'll be admitted as an outpatient, she'll be unlikely to stay in the hospital.

Explain to the patient that she'll have preliminary tests, including a urinalysis, hematocrit, and hemoglobin measurements. She may have a Pap smear. If she's scheduled for an induced abortion, inform her that she'll receive counseling before the procedure. Tell her not to eat or drink anything after midnight before surgery and, if ordered, to give herself an enema in the morning. Remind her that she'll be groggy after the procedure, so she should plan to have someone transport her home.

Explain that she may receive preoperative medications, such as diazepam (Valium). She'll also have an I.V. line inserted for administering fluids and, possibly, anesthesia. If she's bleeding heavily from an incomplete abortion, the doctor may administer I.V. oxytocin (Pitocin) to promote uterine contractions and thereby decrease blood loss.

Discuss postoperative procedures. Inform the patient that she'll have a perineal pad in place after surgery and that she'll probably have spotting and discharge for at least a week. Advise her that she can expect to feel abdominal cramping and pelvic and low back pain after the procedure. These aftereffects are temporary. If she feels any continuous, sharp abdominal pain that doesn't diminish with analgesics, however, she should contact her doctor. This symptom may signal a rare complication—a perforated uterus, for instance. She should also contact her doctor if she has any signs of infection (such as purulent, foul-smelling vaginal drainage) or hemorrhage (such as bright red blood or bleeding that lasts more than 8 days).

Caution the patient that she may experience mood swings resulting from hormonal changes. Add that these should subside in a few days. Also warn her that she may continue to have symptoms of pregnancy, such as morning sickness and breast engorgement or leakage for 2 to 7 days after surgery (or after spontaneous abortion). If these symptoms last longer after an induced abortion, suggest that she notify her doctor.

Mention that in about 1% of patients, the procedure fails and the pregnancy continues (this occurs mostly in induced abortions performed before 8 weeks of pregnancy).

Other care measures

Advise the patient to prevent infection by avoiding intercourse, douching, and tampons for at least 2 weeks after abortion. If she wants to get pregnant again, advise her to wait about 3 to 6 months. This gives the placental site time to heal and her body time to readjust. For more information, see *Questions women ask about pregnancy after miscarriage*.

Discuss contraception with the patient, covering the use, reliability, and possible adverse effects of various methods. Then inform her that though she may not have a menstrual period for 4 to 8 weeks, she can still become pregnant. If she expresses interest, help her choose a method of contraception that's compatible

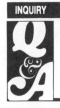

INQUIRY

Questions women ask about pregnancy after miscarriage

I just had a miscarriage. What are my chances of having another one?
If this was your first miscarriage, your chances of having another one are no greater than any other woman's. If you've had two or more, or a late miscarriage (after 13 weeks of pregnancy), you may be more likely to have another one. Make sure to discuss your concerns with your doctor before becoming pregnant again.

Should I have any tests before getting pregnant again?
Unfortunately, no test can predict whether you'll have another miscarriage. If possible, your doctor may test the tissues expelled during your past miscarriage. What he finds may pinpoint why you miscarried.

You can increase your chances of a healthy pregnancy by having a Pap smear and a gynecologic checkup annually.

How soon can I try to get pregnant again?
Most experts advise waiting between 3 and 6 months. Your body needs some time to heal and get back to normal. Consider practicing birth control briefly. And watch for your first menstrual period. It may be a little late. Your second period may be a little late also. If you don't have a period for 8 weeks, consult your doctor and schedule a checkup.

with her life-style. And refer her to Planned Parenthood or another family planning agency if desired.

Throughout your contact with the patient, offer emotional support. If she had a spontaneous abortion, she may crave a sympathetic ear. She may blame herself, and if she felt ambivalent about the pregnancy, she may feel guilty after the abortion. Help her to express her feelings, and encourage her to find a trusted friend or family member to talk to. Be sure to include the patient's partner in your counseling. If she and her partner voice interest, refer them to an appropriate support group. If the patient's had several spontaneous abortions, refer her to a fertility specialist.

A patient who's undergone an induced abortion needs emotional support as well. Help her through this time by encouraging her to express her feelings to you or to share them with a relative or close friend. Support her efforts to seek more information from her local Planned Parenthood organization, family planning agency, or public health service.

Sources of information and support

Center for Population Options
1012 14th Street, NW, Suite 1200, Washington, D.C. 20005
(202) 347-5700

Compassionate Friends (National Office)
P.O. Box 3696, Oak Brook, Ill. 60522
(708) 990-0010

National Abortion Federation
900 Pennsylvania Avenue, SE, Washington, D.C. 20003
(202) 546-9060; Abortion Hotline: 1-800-772-9100

National Abortion Rights Action League
1101 14th Street, NW, 5th Floor, Washington, D.C. 20005
(202) 371-0779

Planned Parenthood Federation of America
810 Seventh Avenue, New York, N.Y. 10019
(212) 541-7800

Pregnancy and Infant Loss Center
1421 E. Wayzata Boulevard, Suite 40, Wayzata, Minn. 55391
(612) 473-9372

Further readings

Hatcher, R.A., et al. *Contraceptive Technology 1988-1989,* 14th rev. ed. New York: Irvington Publishers, 1988.
Hern, W.M., and Stubbefield, P. *Abortion Practice.* Philadelphia: J.B. Lippincott Co., 1984.
National Abortion Federation. *Celebrating Roe v. Wade: Dramatic Improvements in American Health.* Washington, D.C.: National Abortion Federation, 1989.

Pregnancy-induced hypertension

Also called preeclampsia or eclampsia, pregnancy-induced hypertension (PIH) accounts for more than 30,000 stillbirths and neonatal deaths in North America each year. That means when you teach about PIH, you'll be dealing with parents who are understandably concerned about their neonate's survival. This concern frequently translates into high patient compliance; for example, a patient with mild PIH may be eager to learn how to monitor her condition at home. For such a patient, you'll teach her how to accurately measure her daily weight, blood pressure, and urine protein level, and you'll emphasize the importance of reporting any symptoms of worsening PIH immediately. You may also need to teach about medications, a high-protein diet, and the importance of bed rest. Your teaching here can help ensure a healthy pregnancy and a normal delivery.

A patient with severe PIH requires immediate hospitalization and, possibly, emergency delivery. If emergency delivery is necessary, you'll teach the patient and her partner about induced labor or cesarean section. And if the infant's life can't be saved, you'll need to help them cope with stillbirth or neonatal death.

Discuss the disorder

Inform the patient that PIH is a disorder of late pregnancy in which the mother's blood pressure rises, her body retains excess fluid, and her urine contains excess protein. Explain that blood pressure is the force exerted by the heart as it pumps blood through the arteries to all body parts. Blood pressure is partly determined by the size of the arteries: the narrower they are, the harder the heart must work. It can also be affected by the amount of blood moving through the arteries. Because a woman's blood supply normally increases during pregnancy, her heart must pump harder to circulate blood. This can cause hypertension in susceptible women.

Explain that PIH causes spasms in the blood vessels that diminish cardiac output and decrease blood flow to all body organs—including the placenta, which provides the fetus with nutrients and oxygen. This may result in fetal malnutrition and growth retardation.

Discuss three categories of PIH: gestational hypertension alone, preeclampsia (mild, moderate, or severe), and eclampsia. Eclampsia is always severe, including symptoms of preeclampsia as well as seizures. (See *Classifying PIH*, page 366.)

Miriam Horwitz, RN, MS, and **Darlene Whenry, RN, BSN,** contributed to this chapter. Ms. Horwitz is president of Executive Search Consultants, Westwood, Mass. Ms. Whenry is nurse manager of the outpatient department at Chester County Hospital, West Chester, Pa.

CHECKLIST

Teaching topics in PIH

☐ Explanation of how pregnancy-induced hypertension (PIH) compromises maternal and fetal blood flow
☐ Categories of PIH: gestational hypertension, preeclampsia, and eclampsia
☐ Predisposing factors
☐ Complications of uncontrolled PIH, such as heart failure, pulmonary edema, and renal failure
☐ Description of diagnostic tests, including laboratory tests, pelvic ultrasonography, amniocentesis, and antepartal external fetal monitoring
☐ Activity restrictions, including how to deal with bed rest
☐ Importance of a nutritious, high-protein diet
☐ Drug administration and adverse effects
☐ Home monitoring of PIH by measuring daily weight, blood pressure, and urine protein level
☐ Preparation for emergency delivery by induced labor or cesarean section
☐ Symptoms of worsening PIH
☐ Sources of information and support

Classifying PIH

Explain that pregnancy-induced hypertension (PIH) can be classified by its severity. Then use the following information to discuss the patient's form of PIH.

Gestational hypertension
Blood pressure of 140/90 or above occurs after 20 weeks of pregnancy and disappears within 6 weeks after delivery.

Preeclampsia
Hypertension and proteinuria occur with or without generalized edema. This form develops in primigravidas, usually after 20 weeks of pregnancy.

In *mild preeclampsia,* blood pressure is less than 140/90, with a rise of 15 mm Hg or greater above the patient's normal diastolic pressure, measured on two occasions, 6 hours apart, while the patient is at rest. Proteinuria and edema may both be present.

Moderate preeclampsia is defined as blood pressure greater than 140/90 and less than 160/110, or a rise of 30 mm Hg or greater above the patient's normal systolic pressure or 15 mm Hg or greater above the patient's normal diastolic pressure. Appreciable proteinuria and, usually, edema of the lower extremities are also present.

Severe preeclampsia refers to blood pressure greater than 160/110 on at least two occasions, 6 hours apart, while the patient is resting, along with proteinuria of 5 g/24 hours or more. Headaches and blurred vision usually occur, along with right upper quadrant or epigastric pain, oliguria, pulmonary edema, visual or cerebral disturbances, and edema of the face, hands, and lower extremities.

Eclampsia
Patients have hypertension, proteinuria, and seizures. The initial seizure may occur up to 24 hours postpartum.

Tell the patient that the cause of PIH is unknown; however, it's most common in primigravidas who are under age 20 or over age 35, because pregnant teenagers are often too embarrassed or uninformed to seek medical attention until the disease is severe. Older pregnant women are at increased risk for chronic hypertension. Other predisposing factors include multiple fetuses, hydatidiform mole, malnutrition, coexisting renal disease, immunologic disorders, diabetes mellitus, and possibly, a familial tendency to PIH.

Complications
Explain that inadequate treatment and uncontrolled PIH can have devastating effects on both the expectant mother and her fetus. In the mother, PIH can cause heart failure from increased cardiac work load; pulmonary edema from heart failure; renal failure from decreased renal perfusion; hepatic rupture from subcapsular liver hematomas; and seizures or cerebrovascular accident from cerebral vasospasm or cerebral hemorrhage.

PIH can also reduce uteroplacental perfusion, resulting in microscopic placental lesions, large placental infarcts, markedly small placental size, and abruptio placentae. At its worst, it can lead to fetal or neonatal death.

Describe the diagnostic workup
Prepare the patient for diagnostic tests to evaluate maternal and fetal health. These may include laboratory tests, such as a complete blood count and a 24-hour urine collection, pelvic ultrasonography, amniocentesis, and antepartal fetal monitoring.

Laboratory tests
Outline blood and urine tests to assess the patient's overall health. Such tests include a complete blood count, liver enzyme and uric acid tests, coagulation studies, blood urea nitrogen and serum creatinine tests, and a 24-hour urine collection for total protein and creatinine clearance. If appropriate, teach the patient how to collect a clean-catch midstream urine specimen or a 24-hour urine specimen.

Pelvic ultrasonography
Tell the patient that pelvic ultrasonography is performed to evaluate fetal viability, position, and gestational age. The test determines the fetal biparietal diameter, detects early evidence of fetal growth retardation, locates the placenta, identifies placental infarcts, measures the fetal head-to-abdomen ratio, and rules out oligohydramnios. It also detects multiple fetuses, erythroblastosis, and hydatidiform mole. In addition, the test helps to guide amniocentesis by determining the location of the placenta and fetus.

Reassure the patient that the test is painless and won't harm the fetus. Tell her that it takes about ½ hour. Explain that 1½ to 2 hours before the test she should start drinking 6 to 8 glasses of fluid. A full bladder serves as a landmark to define other pelvic organs, so she shouldn't urinate before the test.

Explain that the patient will lie on her back with her legs extended. The technician will coat her abdomen with a conductant, such as mineral oil, then guide a transducer over her abdomen to visualize the uterus, vagina, and adjoining organs. She can empty her bladder after the test.

Amniocentesis

Explain that amniocentesis evaluates fetal health and maturity and can also identify the sex of the fetus. The doctor usually performs this test if the mother's PIH worsens or if he suspects fetal growth retardation. If the test shows an L/S ratio greater than 2.0 (mature), the doctor usually delivers the fetus, regardless of its size. (The L/S ratio refers to measurement of chemicals, such as lecithin and sphingomyelin, which can predict lung maturity.) Reassure the patient that complications, such as infection, miscarriage, and fetal damage, are rare.

Tell the patient that the test usually takes about ½ hour. Instruct her to urinate just before the test to minimize the risk of a punctured bladder or of aspirating urine instead of amniotic fluid. Explain that the doctor will use ultrasonography to locate the placenta and the fetus, allowing him to select the safest position to insert the needle without injuring either.

Inform the patient that she'll lie on her back with her upper body slightly elevated (to relax the abdominal muscles) and her legs extended. The doctor will examine the abdomen to reconfirm the position of the fetus and to assess its heartbeat. Then he'll clean the abdominal area with an antiseptic and inject a local anesthetic. He'll gently insert a special needle through the abdominal wall into the uterus and aspirate an amniotic fluid specimen. After removing the needle, he'll apply a sterile dressing over the puncture site.

Explain that afterward the nurse will monitor the patient's heart rate, blood pressure, and respirations for about ½ hour. Caution the patient to report any discomfort, fever, leakage of fluid, or change in fetal activity after the test.

Antepartal external fetal monitoring

Inform the patient that antepartal external fetal monitoring assesses placental function during stressful and nonstressful situations, measures fetal heart rate as an indicator of fetal health, and measures fetal ability to withstand the stress of contractions induced before actual labor begins. Tell her the test takes about 2 hours. Reassure her that the test is painless and that it won't harm the fetus or interfere with the normal progress of labor. Mention that the test can also be performed without stimulated contractions to assess fetal health.

Unless otherwise ordered, instruct the patient to eat a meal just before the test to reduce bowel sounds and to increase fetal activity. Also tell her to empty her bladder. Then explain that she'll lie in a semi-Fowler's or left-lateral position with her abdomen exposed. An ultrasound transducer will be attached over the area with the most distinct fetal heart sounds. For the *nonstress*

INQUIRY

Questions patients ask about PIH treatments

I've always been active, but now my doctor says I can't exercise. Why not?
Because exercise increases your heart rate, causing it to pump more and more blood into your arteries and circulatory system. This increased force causes your blood pressure to rise even higher. Most women with PIH are advised to restrict activities; some are even ordered to stay in bed.

Why do I have to cut back on salty foods?
Large amounts of salt absorbed into your blood can cause your kidneys to retain water. When this happens, the blood exerts more force against the artery walls and your blood pressure increases. Besides reducing your salt intake, try to eat a well-balanced diet that's high in protein (including meat, fish, poultry, eggs, milk, cheese, and nuts).

I've been resting at home, but now my doctor says I have to go to the hospital. Why?
Your doctor has obviously decided that conservative treatment isn't working and that your PIH is progressing to a more serious stage. This can affect your health and your baby's life. By admitting you to the hospital, the doctor can monitor your baby's health and your blood pressure, diet, and activity much more closely.

He can also give you medication to help you relax, help lower your blood pressure, and reduce the likelihood of seizures.

test, she'll hold a pressure transducer in her hand and push it each time she feels the fetus move. For the *stress test,* she'll receive a low-dose infusion of oxytocin (Pitocin) until she has three or four uterine contractions within 10 minutes, each contraction lasting longer than 30 seconds.

Teach about treatments
Explain that therapy for PIH is designed to halt the disorder's progress—specifically, the early effects of eclampsia, such as seizures, residual hypertension, and renal shutdown—and to ensure fetal survival. Inform the patient that mild PIH requires bed rest, dietary restrictions, home monitoring of blood pressure, weight, and urine protein level, and reporting the signs and symptoms of worsening PIH. Treatment for more severe cases includes medication and emergency delivery, either by inducing labor or performing a cesarean section.

Activity
If the patient has mild PIH, the doctor may recommend bed rest at home. (See *Making the most of bed rest,* page 372.)

Diet
In collaboration with the dietitian, stress to the patient the importance of eating a well-balanced, nutritious diet that's high in protein. (See *Questions patients ask about PIH treatments.*)

Medication
If the doctor has prescribed drugs for PIH, teach the patient about their purpose, how to take them, and what adverse effects to watch for. Explain that beta-adrenergic blockers (atenolol, propranolol) decrease cardiac output to lower blood pressure, and vasodilators (minoxidil) and centrally acting antihypertensive drugs (clonidine) directly or indirectly dilate the arteries, decreasing the resistance against which the heart has to pump. If appropriate, teach the patient about other drugs, such as phenobarbital (Luminal), which promotes relaxation, helps lower blood pressure, and reduces the likelihood of seizures. Drug therapy for severe preeclampsia may include magnesium sulfate for increased muscle tonicity and diazepam I.V. (maximum 10 mg I.V.) for seizures. Drug therapy does not include diuretics except for patients unresponsive to other drugs. (For more information, see *Teaching about drugs for PIH.*)

Procedures
If appropriate, teach the patient how to monitor PIH at home by measuring and recording her daily weight, blood pressure, and urine protein level. Instruct her to weigh herself at the same time each day, using the same scale and wearing the same type of clothing. Tell her to notify the doctor if she gains more than 2½ lb per week after the 34th week of pregnancy.

Teach her how to take her blood pressure accurately, and emphasize that she should compare each reading against her baseline

Teaching about drugs for PIH

DRUG	ADVERSE REACTIONS	TEACHING POINTS
Beta-adrenergic blockers		
atenolol (Tenormin) **labetalol** (Trandate) **propranolol** (Inderal)	• Watch for depression, dizziness, dyspnea, rash, very slow heart rate, and wheezing. • Other reactions include decreased libido, diarrhea, fatigue, headache, insomnia, nasal stuffiness, nausea, nightmares, vivid dreams, and vomiting.	• If the patient takes one dose daily, instruct her to take a missed dose within 8 hours. If she takes two or more doses daily, tell her to take a missed dose as soon as possible. Make sure to caution her never to take a double-dose. • Warn against suddenly discontinuing the drug. To avoid serious complications, the doctor will gradually decrease, or taper, the dosage. • Teach the patient to check her pulse rate before taking the drug and to notify the doctor if it falls below 60 beats/minute. • To help prevent insomnia, advise her to take the drug no later than 2 hours before bedtime. • Suggest she take the drug with food to increase its absorption.
Centrally acting antihypertensives		
clonidine (Catapres)	• Watch for ankle edema, nightmares, skin pallor, and vivid dreams. • Other reactions include constipation, drowsiness, dry mouth, insomnia, and slow heart rate.	• Advise the patient to take one dose just before bedtime to take advantage of the drug's tendency to cause drowsiness. • To avoid constipation, tell her to increase her fluid and fiber intake and to use bulk laxatives. • To relieve dry mouth, suggest she use sugarless gum, hard candy, or mouth rinses. • Instruct her to limit alcohol intake. • Warn her against stopping the drug even if she feels better.
methyldopa (Aldomet)	• Watch for chest pain, depression, edema, fever, syncope, very slow heart rate, weakness, and weight gain. • Other reactions include decreased libido, diarrhea, dizziness, drowsiness, dry mouth, nausea, slightly slow heart rate, stuffy nose, and vomiting.	• Tell the patient to take a missed dose as soon as she remembers. Caution her, however, never to take a double-dose. • Suggest that she take one of her scheduled daily doses at bedtime to take advantage of the drug's tendency to cause drowsiness. • Reassure her that drowsiness is usually transient, but tell her to notify her doctor if it persists. • Tell her to rise slowly from a sitting or lying position to minimize postural hypotension. • Advise her to chew gum, suck on hard candy, or use mouth rinses to relieve dry mouth. • Advise her to limit her alcohol intake.
prazosin (Minipress)	• Watch for chest pain, dyspnea, edema, rapid heart rate, and syncope. • Other reactions include drowsiness, gastric upset, headache, and slight dizziness.	• Tell the patient to take a missed dose as soon as possible, but warn her not to double-dose. • Advise her to take the initial dose at bedtime because dizziness is most pronounced after this dose. • To reduce dizziness during therapy, instruct her to take the drug with food. • Instruct her to limit her alcohol intake. • Caution her not to operate heavy machinery or drive a motor vehicle during the first week of therapy, in case syncope occurs. • Tell her to rise slowly from a sitting or lying position to minimize postural hypotension.

continued

Teaching about drugs for PIH — *continued*

DRUG	ADVERSE REACTIONS	TEACHING POINTS
Vasodilators		
hydralazine (Apresoline)	• Watch for chest pain, numbness, palpitations, rapid heart rate, systemic lupus erythematosus-like syndrome (fever, joint pain, malaise, skin rash), and tingling. • Other reactions include anorexia, diarrhea, headache, nasal congestion, and nausea.	• If a q.i.d. schedule is prescribed, tell the patient to take a missed dose only up to 2 hours before her next scheduled dose, but not to double-dose. Help her work out a regular medication schedule. • To prevent GI distress, advise her to take the drug on an empty stomach, 1 hour before or 3 hours after meals.
minoxidil (Loniten)	• Watch for distended neck veins, dyspnea, edema, rapid heart rate, and weight gain. • Other reactions include lengthening and darkening of fine body hair.	• Tell the patient to take a missed daily dose within 8 hours of the scheduled time, but no later. Warn her not to double-dose. • Suggest that she remove unwanted hair by shaving or using a depilatory. • Instruct her to weigh herself at least every other day and to report any sudden weight gain.
Miscellaneous		
phenobarbital (Luminal)	• Watch for ataxia, bradycardia, bradypnea, confusion, depression, easy bleeding or bruising, fever, hives, hyperexcitability, insomnia, jaundice, joint or muscle pain, rash, severe drowsiness or weakness, shortness of breath, slurred speech, and sore throat. • Other reactions include anxiety, dizziness, drowsiness, headache, irritability, nausea, nightmares, and vomiting.	• Tell the patient that this drug helps control seizures. • Tell her to take a missed dose as soon as possible, unless it's almost time for the next dose. Warn her not to double-dose. • Warn her not to crush, chew, or break extended-release capsules. • Tell her to operate machinery cautiously and to avoid driving if she feels dizzy or drowsy. • Tell her to avoid alcohol as well as hay fever, allergy, cold, and sleeping medications that contain central nervous system depressants, such as antihistamines. • Warn her to take the drug as ordered to prevent possible dependence. • Caution her never to stop the drug abruptly because withdrawal seizures could occur. • Tell her that she should inform her doctor or dentist that she's taking this drug before they perform any surgery.

reading. She should notify the doctor immediately if her systolic pressure rises 30 mm Hg above baseline or her diastolic pressure rises 15 mm Hg above baseline. Also teach the patient how to measure protein in her urine.

First, instruct her to collect a clean-catch midstream urine specimen—preferably in the morning, when urine is most concentrated and yields the most reliable information. Tell her to dip the reagent strip into the urine and to remove excess urine by tapping the strip against a clean surface or the edge of the container. Next, have her hold the strip in a horizontal position, place it close to the color block on the bottle, and carefully compare colors. Explain that the color block corresponds to levels of protein in the urine. Tell her to notify the doctor immediately if she detects protein levels of 300 mg/dl or more.

Surgery

If the patient doesn't respond to conservative treatment, or if PIH is severe, the doctor may attempt emergency delivery—either by inducing labor or by performing a cesarean section. Stress that delivery is necessary to preserve the health and possibly the life of the infant, the mother, or both. Reinforce the doctor's explanation of the procedure and answer any questions. Encourage parent-infant bonding after delivery.

Unfortunately, it's not always possible to save the infant's life through emergency delivery. Besides providing emotional support for the parents, you'll need to help them cope with stillbirth or neonatal death by describing the grieving process.

Other care measures

Teach the patient with mild PIH to watch for and report symptoms of a worsening condition. Symptoms include apprehension, dizziness, epigastric or right upper quadrant pain, excitability, frontal or occipital headaches resistant to ordinary analgesics, nausea, visual disturbances ranging from slight blurring to blindness, and vomiting.

Sources of information and support

American Heart Association
7320 Greenville Avenue, Dallas, Texas 75231
(214) 373-6300

Heart, Blood, and Lung Program Information Center
4733 Bethesda Avenue, Suite 530, Bethesda, Md. 20814
(301) 951-3260

National Hypertension Association
324 East 30th Street, New York, N.Y. 10016
(212) 889-3557

Further readings

Burke, M.E. "Hypertensive Crisis and the Perinatal Period," *Journal of Perinatal and Neonatal Nursing* 3(2):33-47, October 1989.
Ferris, T.F. "Caring for the Hypertensive Pregnant Patient," *Consultant* 29(2): 27-30, 33, February 1989.
Lao-Nario, B.T. "Nursing Care of Patients with Pregnancy-Induced Hypertension," *Philippine Journal of Nursing* 58(4):14-25, October-December 1988.
Poole, J.H. "Getting Perspective on HELLP Syndrome," *Maternal Child Nursing* 13(6):432-37, November-December 1988.
Remich, M.C., and Youngkin, E.Q. "Factors Associated with Pregnancy-Induced Hypertension," *Nurse Practitioner* 14(1):20, 22, 24, January 1989.
Simpson, D. "The Epidemiology and Aetiology of Pre-eclampsia," *Midwife Health Visitor and Community Nurse* 25(3):62, 64, 66-67, March 1989.

Making the most of bed rest

Dear Patient:

Your doctor has prescribed bed rest to help control your blood pressure. Bed rest may prevent your heart from beating faster. If your heart rate slows down, less blood will be pumped into your arteries. This may keep your blood pressure stable.

If you don't get better in 3 or 4 days, your doctor will probably admit you to the hospital. That way, you'll be sure to get the proper rest and care.

As long as your high blood pressure remains mild, you can manage it at home. But because your condition can quickly get worse, you must follow your doctor's instructions precisely. The following suggestions will help.

Most important: stay in bed
Bed rest means lying quietly in a darkened room with as little stimulation as possible. You should lie on your left side to help increase the blood flow to your baby. Leave your bed only to go to the bathroom.

Get help
Ask your family and friends to help by preparing meals, doing the laundry, shopping, and cleaning. If no help is available, ask the doctor or nurse to help you arrange for a home health care aide or volunteer.

If you have young children, ask a family member or friend to babysit, or better yet, to keep them for several days. This can be an exciting experience for children if it's viewed as a "vacation."

Do what you can
Remaining in bed doesn't mean that you can't do anything. You can still plan meals, balance your checkbook, pay bills, read, watch television, or give yourself a manicure. Any activity is fine—as long as you lie in bed, and the activity doesn't cause excitement or stress.

The bottom line
Staying in bed is hard when you're used to being active and when you have a house and family who need attention. But it's worth it. Following your doctor's orders will help you deliver a healthy baby and keep you healthy, too.

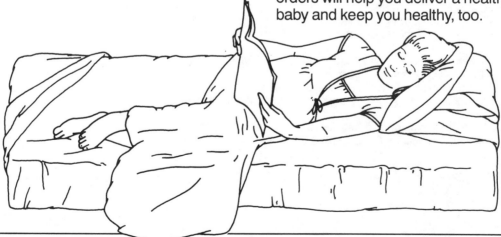

Mastitis

Effective patient teaching and successful breast-feeding go hand in hand—especially in preventing a disruptive development, such as mastitis. In this era of early postpartum discharge, you'll need to ensure that the new mother learns how to recognize and prevent mastitis before she leaves the hospital. Mastitis occurs most often in the first weeks after initiating breast-feeding.

Your teaching's equally important for the patient who already has mastitis. By helping her understand the disorder, you'll promote her compliance with treatment and help her prevent a recurrence. To do this, you'll discuss the cause of mastitis and how it's diagnosed. You'll also explain treatment measures, including rest, proper nutrition, and medication. Above all, you'll reassure the breast-feeding patient that she can continue to breast-feed her infant, if she chooses, despite having mastitis (for more information, see *Teaching the new mother with mastitis,* page 374).

Discuss the disorder

Inform the patient that mastitis is a breast infection that causes localized tenderness, redness, and warmth. The infection may also produce flulike symptoms, such as chills, muscle aches, and fever.

If your patient is breast-feeding an infant, inform her that mastitis typically occurs 3 to 4 weeks after breast-feeding starts. Explain that the most common cause is bacteria (staphylococcus or streptococcus) from the infant's skin or nasopharyngeal area. Describe factors that contribute to mastitis—a crack or a fissure in the nipple; blockage of a milk duct, resulting from inadequate or infrequent breast emptying; and fatigue, stress, poor nutrition, and insufficient fluid intake. For more information, see *How mastitis develops,* page 375.

Dispel the myth that mastitis causes permanent breast damage. Also reassure the patient that it doesn't increase her risk for breast cancer or other breast diseases. Assure her that she'll be able to breast-feed other infants in the future if she wishes, probably without developing mastitis again.

If your patient isn't breast-feeding, explain that fibrocystic breast disease or a recurrent subareolar abscess may also cause mastitis. Inform her that the infection usually results from a ruptured breast cyst or subareolar abscess.

Complications

Advise your patient that prompt treatment may help her to avoid a

Mary R. Wood, BSN, MSN, CNM, wrote this chapter. She's a certified nurse-midwife with the Austin-Travis County Health Department in Austin, Texas.

CHECKLIST

Teaching topics in mastitis

☐ How lactation relates to mastitis
☐ Cause of mastitis and predisposing factors, such as nipple cracks, fatigue, and blocked milk ducts
☐ Mastitis signs and symptoms, such as fever, localized tenderness, and redness; and complications, including breast abscess
☐ Importance of rest, proper diet, and adequate fluid intake
☐ Analgesic and antibiotic therapy
☐ Maintaining breast-feeding despite mastitis
☐ Comfort measures, including warm or ice packs and a well-fitting bra
☐ Preventing a recurrence
☐ Source of information and support

Teaching the new mother with mastitis

Teaching a new mother with mastitis can be challenging—especially if she's breast-feeding and wants to continue. She may be poorly informed about the disorder, and she may be too busy meeting her infant's needs to consider her own health. Mastitis may make her reconsider breast-feeding, especially if she feels discouraged by sore nipples, fatigue, or criticism from family or friends who may try to convince her that breast-feeding isn't worth the trouble. Discuss her concerns, correct any misinformation, and assist her to succeed with breast-feeding if she chooses to continue.

Assess the patient's condition
Suppose your patient is Susan Taylor, a 28-year-old office manager who's breast-feeding her first infant, born 24 days ago. This morning the doctor advised her to come to the clinic when she called to report that her right breast was very sore, red, and warm and that she had a fever of 103° F. (39.4° C.).

Talking with Mrs. Taylor, you learn that she has pain and flulike symptoms and breast-feeding problems too. "My nipples feel sore, the baby cries a lot—mostly at night—and he nurses fitfully. Could my cracked nipple affect how he nurses?" She reports that her nipple cracked about a week ago.

When you ask how often she breast-feeds, you learn that she waits at least 4 hours between feedings—because her mother said to. By then her breasts are usually so engorged that it's difficult for the infant to hold her nipple in his mouth.

As she talks, you notice how tired Mrs. Taylor looks. You ask how much rest she gets. She volunteers, "Not much since my mother left 2 weeks ago."

The doctor examines Mrs. Taylor, diagnoses mastitis, and prescribes antibiotic therapy. He asks if she has any questions, and she asks, "Can I continue breast-feeding?" He sees no reason not to and tells her that you'll give her pointers. He adds that you'll tell her how to prevent a recurrence too.

Outline the patient's learning needs
Exactly what will you teach Mrs. Taylor? Begin by comparing what she already knows about mastitis with the standard teaching plan, which includes:
• a description of breast anatomy and the physiology of lactation, including how regular milk expression promotes continued lactation
• an explanation of mastitis
• treatment measures, including drugs, rest, and diet, to promote cure and prevent recurrent infection or a breast abscess
• comfort measures, for example, supporting the breast with a well-fitting bra.

From your conversation with Mrs. Taylor, you realize that she knows little about mastitis, that she wants to continue breast-feeding, and that she needs rest. You decide that you'll need to cover all of the standard teaching plan topics. Your initial goals are clear: to expedite Mrs. Taylor's recovery and to support her decision to continue breast-feeding. Next you'll focus on steps to prevent a recurrence.

Set learning outcomes
You and Mrs. Taylor work together on learning outcomes. You agree that she'll be able to:

```
-identify the cause of mastitis and explain
how mastitis and a breast abscess develop
-describe treatment she'll carry out at home,
including a plan for getting adequate rest
-name her medicine and explain her dosage
-demonstrate proper breast-feeding and breast
massage techniques
-specify ways to enlist the support of her
husband and friends to help her obtain rest
-continue to breast-feed successfully if she
desires.
```

Choose teaching tools and techniques
Because Mrs. Taylor's in pain and is uncomfortable from the fever, her attention span is short. So you'll keep today's teaching session short, using *discussion* and *explanation* to explain mastitis and to describe treatment and prevention plans. You select *visual aids*—a diagram showing how mastitis develops and a pamphlet depicting breast-feeding techniques—to enhance comprehension and retention. Then you reinforce the instruction with a *patient-teaching aid* on breast-feeding and mastitis for home review.

In a few days, you'll call Mrs. Taylor to support her progress and review what you taught today.

Evaluate your teaching
Does Mrs. Taylor understand mastitis and its treatment? Does she know how to prevent a recurrence? To find out, evaluate your teaching. If needed, revise your plan. During your follow-up phone contact, use *questions and answers* to decide whether Mrs. Taylor understands how to avoid a recurrence. Ask her to review with you why breast emptying's important. Adapt a *demonstration* technique by asking her to describe the breast-feeding positions she uses to reduce stress on the infected breast. And use *discussion* to evaluate her current feelings about breast-feeding and to help you identify additional learning needs.

How mastitis develops

Explain mastitis in the context of breast-feeding physiology. Doing so can help a patient realize the importance of proper feeding technique in preventing and treating this disorder. Use these diagrams to illustrate the breast-feeding process and how predisposing factors, such as a blocked mammary duct and a cracked nipple, contribute to the development of mastitis.

Breast structures
Start by describing breast structures, which include lobules containing milk-secreting cell clusters called alveoli. Each alveolus empties into a secondary tubule that leads into a mammary duct. Near the nipple these ducts widen into an ampulla—or sinus—that stores milk.

Let-down reflex
Explain that the infant's sucking on the breast signals the posterior pituitary to release oxytocin. This hormone prompts the alveoli to eject milk into the sinuses. From the sinuses, the milk flows through mammary ducts into the nipple and out of the breast.

Portal of infection
Inform the patient that a cracked nipple provides a route through which bacteria from the infant's skin or nasopharyngeal area can enter the breast. There the milk stored in the sinuses provides an excellent medium for bacterial growth. If a duct becomes blocked, even more milk remains in the sinuses to support bacterial growth.

Preventive measures
Stress that frequent breast-milk expression (by the infant or manually by the mother) reduces the reservoir of milk in the sinuses and ducts, helping to prevent mastitis.

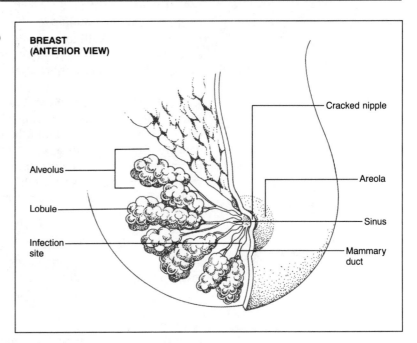

BREAST (ANTERIOR VIEW)

Alveolus

Lobule

Infection site

Cracked nipple

Areola

Sinus

Mammary duct

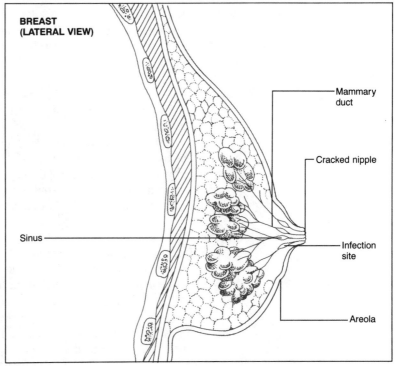

BREAST (LATERAL VIEW)

Sinus

Mammary duct

Cracked nipple

Infection site

Areola

breast abscess. This condition, which develops in fewer than 10% of mastitis patients, causes increased localized pain, swelling, and redness, sometimes with purulent discharge from the nipple.

If your patient's breast-feeding, stress that compliance with treatment can also minimize disrupted breast-feeding and mother-infant bonding. Antibiotic therapy should quickly reduce her discomfort. What's more, continued breast emptying will sustain milk production and remove the milk in which bacteria can grow.

Describe the diagnostic workup

Inform the patient that her clinical symptoms form the basis for a diagnosis of mastitis. Explain, however, that sometimes the exudate from the nipple or abscess may be cultured to identify the infecting organism. The culture may be followed by antibiotic sensitivity testing to permit selection of a maximally effective antibiotic. Mention that she needn't make special preparations for these tests.

Teach about treatments

Tell the patient that treatment for mastitis consists of antibiotics, rest, and increased fluid intake. If an abscess is present, explain that the doctor may open and drain it.

Activity

Urge the patient to stay in bed and rest as much as possible until the infection begins to resolve. Remind her that fatigue and stress contribute to mastitis. If necessary, encourage her to recruit family members, friends, or others to share in family care and household chores.

Diet

Stress the importance of good nutrition to promote recovery. If the patient's breast-feeding and wishes to continue, tell her to eat a balanced diet and to increase her caloric intake. Also instruct her to drink plenty of water, juice, and milk, especially if she's dehydrated from fever. Advise her to limit her intake of coffee, tea, and other caffeine-containing beverages. Explain that caffeine can contribute to dehydration and can also disturb her sleep.

Medication

Inform the patient that medications for mastitis include analgesics to reduce pain and antibiotics to kill bacteria.

Analgesics. Explain that pain inhibits the let-down reflex, making breast-feeding difficult and uncomfortable. By reducing pain, an analgesic will permit the patient to express milk from the breast more frequently and completely. See *Safe analgesics for breast-feeding patients*.

Antibiotics. Inform the patient that the doctor may prescribe antibiotic therapy for 10 days. Reassure her that she'll probably begin to feel better within 24 to 48 hours of starting therapy. In-

Safe analgesics for breast-feeding patients

Many drugs ingested by the mother pass through breast milk to the infant, making them unsafe to take while breast-feeding. Inform your patient that the analgesics listed below, however, can be taken safely during breast-feeding to relieve mastitis pain:
- acetaminophen (Datril, Tylenol)
- aspirin (Bufferin, Ecotrin, Empirin) after the first postpartum week
- ibuprofen (Advil, Motrin)
- propoxyphene (Darvon)

Teaching points
Forewarn the patient that any of these drugs may cause GI upset. Advise her that taking them with food or milk may prevent this reaction. Then explain that hypersensitivity reactions are rare, but she should contact her doctor if she has such signs and symptoms as itching, hives, rash, and wheezing or other breathing problems.

If the patient takes ibuprofen, advise her to avoid activities that require alertness until she knows how the drug affects her.

Caution her to take propoxyphene (and all medicines) only as directed. Explain that it may cause drowsiness, constipation, and nausea or vomiting as well as general GI upset. Tell her to watch for drowsiness and slowed breathing in her infant. She should stop taking the drug if this happens.

---

struct her to take the medication for the full 10 days to prevent recurrent infection. (Refer to *Teaching about antibiotic therapy for mastitis,* page 378, for information about specific antibiotics.)

Procedures
Tell the patient with a breast abscess that the doctor will drain the abscess. Explain that drainage procedures vary, depending on the abscess's severity and location. If the abscess is superficial and unilocular, the doctor may perform needle aspiration of the contents. Reassure the patient that she'll receive a local anesthetic for this procedure.

If the patient has several deep abscesses, however, inform her that the doctor may admit her to the hospital to incise and drain the abscesses. Explain that the doctor may use a curvilinear incision, which produces less noticeable scarring. Or if necessary, he may make a radial incision to promote proper drainage.

After evacuating the pus from the abscess, the doctor will leave a drain in place for several days. Until the breast heals, the lactating patient won't be able to breast-feed her infant. Suggest that she sustain milk production by manually expressing milk. After the abscess heals, she should be able to resume breast-feeding.

If the patient has chronic recurrent subareolar abscesses, inform her that a cure involves surgical removal of the fistulous tract or duct.

Teaching about antibiotic therapy for mastitis

DRUG	ADVERSE REACTIONS	TEACHING POINTS
Cephalosporins		
cefadroxil (Duricef, Ultracef) **cephalexin** (Keflex)	• Watch for abdominal pain and distention; diarrhea (severe, watery, perhaps bloody); fever; hives; itching; nausea; rash; unusual fatigue, thirst, weakness, or weight loss; vomiting; and wheezing. • Other reactions include mild diarrhea, mild GI upset, or sore mouth or tongue.	• Suggest the patient take the drug with food or milk to decrease GI upset. • Tell her to complete the prescribed course of therapy by taking every dose. • Instruct her to store the reconstituted suspension form in the refrigerator and to shake the liquid well before using. Inform her that the suspension form remains stable for 14 days if refrigerated. • Tell the patient to contact her doctor before taking an antidiarrheal medicine if diarrhea develops after taking this antibiotic. • Caution the diabetic patient that this drug may cause false-positive results on some urine glucose tests. Also advise her to check with her doctor before changing her diet or her drug dosage.
Erythromycin		
erythromycin (E-Mycin, Erythrocin, Ilosone)	• Watch for dark or amber urine, fever, pale stools, severe abdominal pain, unusual fatigue or weakness, and yellowing of eyes or skin (more common with Ilosone). • Other reactions include abdominal cramps, diarrhea, nausea, sore mouth or tongue, and vomiting.	• Advise taking this drug 1 hour before or 2 hours after meals. If prescribed, the patient can take enteric-coated, estolate, or ethylsuccinate forms without regard to meals. • Advise her to take the drug with a full glass of water. • Tell her not to swallow chewable tablets whole. • Instruct her to complete the prescribed course of therapy by taking every dose.
Penicillinase-resistant penicillins		
cloxacillin (Cloxapen, Tegopen) **dicloxacillin** (Dycill, Dynapen) **methicillin** (Staphcillin) **nafcillin** (Unipen) **oxacillin** (Bactocill)	• Watch for breathing problems, hematuria, hives, itching, jaundice, rash, unusual tiredness or weakness, and wheezing. • Other reactions include diarrhea, dizziness, muscle weakness, and nausea or vomiting.	• Review signs and symptoms of penicillin hypersensitivity. Emphasize that the patient should contact the doctor immediately if these occur. Urge her to report any unusual reactions. • Review drug dosage directions. Instruct her to complete the prescribed therapeutic course by taking every dose. • Caution her to discard expired or unused medication and not to give it to family members or friends.

Other care measures

Encourage the patient to wear a supportive, well-fitting but non-binding bra. Explain that a too-tight bra can contribute to a blocked milk duct, which can then predispose her to recurrent mastitis.

Offer tips to reduce discomfort. For example, when the patient lies on the affected side, advise her to use pillows to support her breast. If she's lactating, instruct her to breast-feed her infant frequently to ensure adequate breast emptying. Suggest that she apply a warm or ice pack before breast-feeding to decrease pain, and tell her to start the feeding on the affected breast. Teach the patient how to massage her breasts to promote complete emptying of the ducts as the infant feeds. Also give her a copy of the patient-teaching aid *Breast-feeding tips for the mother with mastitis,* page 380, to review at home.

To prevent recurring mastitis, review general breast-feeding guidelines. For example, to distribute stress evenly on the nipple, encourage the patient to rotate feeding positions. Instruct her to massage any tender or firm areas while the infant feeds. Is the infant sucking correctly? Remind her to check that the infant is sucking with the areola well back into his mouth. Explain that this helps prevent cracked nipples.

Advise the patient to air-dry her nipples carefully after each feeding. Air-drying her nipples helps toughen them and prevents them from remaining damp for long periods of time. In addition, suggest she apply a vitamin-based skin ointment—for example, A and D Ointment— to her nipples if they develop any dryness or cracking.

Stress that the patient should wash her hands and her nipples gently before breast-feeding. This will help prevent transmitting another infection. If she expresses interest, refer her to a support group for nursing mothers, such as a local chapter of La Leche League.

Source of information and support

La Leche League International
9616 Minneapolis Avenue, P.O. Box 1209, Franklin Park, Ill. 60131
(708) 455-7730

Further readings

Briggs, K.D. "Recurring Mastitis, Increased Sodium and Chloride Levels and Unilateral Breast Refusal: A Case Study," *Breastfeeding Review* 12(5):32-34, May 1988.
Cantlie, H.B. "Treatment of Acute Puerperal Mastitis and Breast Abscess," *Canadian Family Physician* 34(10):101-04, October 1988.
Ellerhorst-Ryan, J.M., et al. "Evaluating Benign Breast Disease," *Nurse Practitioner* 13(9):13, 16, 18, September 1988.
Ogle, K.S., and Davis, S. "Mastitis in Lactating Women," *Journal of Family Practice* 26(2):139-44, February 1988.

Breast-feeding tips for the mother with mastitis

Dear Patient:

Although mastitis makes breast-feeding uncomfortable, it doesn't mean you have to stop breast-feeding your baby. In fact, continuing to breast-feed can speed your recovery.

Feed your baby as often as he's hungry. Frequent emptying of the affected breast prevents milk from accumulating there and allowing bacteria to grow.

Here are some tips to help you and your baby continue to benefit from breast-feeding.

Condition yourself
• Get plenty of rest. If possible, stay in bed for a few days.
• Eat a balanced diet, and drink plenty of juice, milk, and water.
• Avoid caffeine-containing drinks, such as coffee, tea, and colas, which tend to be dehydrating.
• Take your prescribed antibiotic exactly as directed. If you don't feel better in 48 hours, call the doctor. Make sure to finish taking all of the medicine. Why? This will help prevent your infection from recurring.

Relieve discomfort
• Take pain-relieving medicine that's safe to use while breast-feeding—Advil or Tylenol, for example.
• Wear a comfortable bra that provides good support, and make sure that it isn't too tight.
• Apply heat or cold to your breast to reduce pain. Try a warm, moist wash-cloth, take a warm shower, or use a cold, moist washcloth or an ice pack.

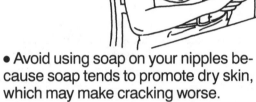

• Avoid using soap on your nipples because soap tends to promote dry skin, which may make cracking worse.
• Soften sore or cracked nipples with A and D Ointment or a breast cream with lanolin.

When you breast-feed
• Offer the sore breast first to promote complete emptying.
• Be sure that the baby takes most of the areola in his mouth.
• Massage the breast while your baby nurses. This will also help to empty it.
• Reposition your baby at each feeding so that stress on the affected breast's nipple will be distributed evenly.
• Allow your nipples to air-dry after breast-feeding—and after showering.

Watch for warning signs
If an abscess forms despite your care and precautions, an area of the breast may become hard and increasingly painful, or pus may drain from the nipple. Call your doctor at once if you have these signs.

Vulvovaginitis and cervicitis

The incidence of vulvovaginitis and cervicitis is rising—possibly because of increased sexual activity and decreased use of barrier-type contraceptives by heterosexual partners. Clearly, patients with these disorders require information to help limit contagion as well as to avoid the complications of cervicitis. But you may need to overcome emotional obstacles before you can teach effectively. After all, the patient may feel hesitant about describing her symptoms to the doctor. Or she may be too embarrassed to discuss treatment and preventive measures.

Once you establish a rapport with a patient, your teaching will focus on promoting compliance with treatment. You'll also need to encourage regular gynecologic checkups, especially if the patient is sexually active, and prompt treatment for new or recurring symptoms of infection.

Discuss the disorder

Tell the patient that vulvovaginitis and cervicitis are inflammations of the vulva, vagina, and cervix that cause vaginal discharge. Discuss the patient's type of vulvovaginitis: candidiasis, trichomoniasis, nonspecific vaginitis, or atrophic vaginitis. In these disorders, discharge originates in the vagina. If appropriate, explain that two major types of cervicitis are chlamydia and gonorrhea. In these disorders, discharge originates from the cervix.

Caused by various microorganisms or conditions, the disorders may be episodic and easily treated or chronic, requiring recurrent treatment. Except for candidiasis, nonspecific vaginitis, and atrophic vaginitis, the inflammations may be sexually transmitted. (For more information, see *Distinguishing among types of vulvovaginitis and cervicitis,* page 382.) As appropriate, discuss sexually transmitted diseases (STDs) that may coexist with or mimic these infections (see *Learning about sexually transmitted diseases,* pages 384 and 385).

Complications

Stress that strict compliance with treatment is the best way to avoid complications. Although vulvovaginitis rarely causes complications, fissures and adhesions may develop from inflammation and scarring in chronic atrophic vaginitis.

Inform the patient that cervicitis complications are more severe because of the infection's type and the proximity to the upper

Sandra Ludwig Nettina, RN,C, MSN, CRNP, formerly of Temple University Hospital, Philadelphia, wrote this chapter. She is an adult nurse practitioner at the Student Health Center, LaSalle University, Philadelphia.

CHECKLIST

Teaching topics in vulvovaginitis and cervicitis

☐ Types of vulvovaginitis and cervicitis
☐ Predisposing factors and signs and symptoms
☐ Sexually transmitted diseases resembling vulvovaginitis and cervicitis
☐ Complications, such as pelvic inflammatory disease
☐ Discussion of the diagnostic workup, including blood tests, pelvic examination, and smears
☐ Medications, such as antifungals, antiprotozoals, antibiotics, and conjugated estrogen
☐ How to administer an intravaginal medication
☐ Importance of sexual abstinence or modification of sexual activity during treatment
☐ Treatment for sexual partners
☐ Hygiene and comfort measures
☐ Sources of information and support

Distinguishing among types of vulvovaginitis and cervicitis

TYPE	PREDISPOSING FACTORS	SIGNS AND SYMPTOMS
Vulvovaginitis		
Candidiasis (moniliasis or yeast vaginitis) A change in the vaginal environment permits an overgrowth of *Candida albicans,* a common inhabitant of the vagina.	Pregnancy, oral contraceptives, antibiotic use, obesity, douching, diabetes, excessive carbohydrate intake, and constrictive clothing with poor ventilation—girdles, for example	Tell the patient that she may have a thick, white, curdlike vaginal discharge and vaginal itching, slight burning, and erythema.
Trichomoniasis (Trichomonas vaginitis) *Trichomonas vaginalis* bacteria are sexually transmitted to the vagina.	Multiple male sexual partners	Inform the patient that she may have profuse, thin, foul yellow and possibly frothy vaginal discharge; vaginal spotting; vaginal and vulvar erythema; hemorrhagic spots on the cervix; and vaginal burning. Additional symptoms may include perineal irritation, dysuria, and urinary frequency.
Nonspecific vaginitis (Gardnerella vaginitis or Haemophilus vaginitis) By an unclear mechanism, vaginal microorganisms, predominantly *Gardnerella vaginalis,* multiply, creating bacterial overgrowth.	Vaginal tissue trauma, sexual intercourse	Tell the patient that she may have moderately increased, thin, grey-white, fishy-scented vaginal discharge.
Atrophic vaginitis Decreased estrogen levels in menopause cause atrophy of the vaginal mucosa. Because the vagina can't maintain a correct acid pH, the vagina becomes thin and fragile.	Menopause	Inform the patient that she may have scant, thin vaginal discharge; vaginal spotting; dryness on sexual intercourse; vaginal burning; pruritus; thin labia or less pubic hair; fissuring of the vulva; or smooth, red, shiny vaginal walls.
Cervicitis		
Gonorrhea *Neisseria gonorrhoeae* bacteria are sexually transmitted to the vagina.	Multiple male sexual partners	Tell the patient that she may or may not have symptoms, including profuse, yellow, purulent vaginal discharge; dysuria; cervical erythema; and cervical edema and tenderness. Add that other possible symptoms include vulvovaginal irritation; and (possibly) pharyngitis, proctitis, or pelvic involvement. Mention that her male sexual partners may have urethritis.
Chlamydia cervicitis *Chlamydia trachomatis* bacteria are sexually transmitted to the vagina.	Multiple male sexual partners	Explain to the patient that she may or may not have symptoms. For example, she may have mild, mucoid, clear to creamy vaginal discharge; dysuria; and cervical erythema and edema. Add that her male sexual partners may experience urethritis.

reproductive tract. Both chlamydia and gonorrhea can cause pelvic inflammatory disease, which can lead to infertility.

What's more, chlamydia can be passed from a mother to a neonate during birth. Inclusion conjunctivitis will result if the bacteria come in contact with the neonate's eyes; pneumonia, if bacteria infect the upper airways.

In the same way, gonorrhea can be transmitted to the neonate, causing ophthalmic infection and rare disseminated infection—if the pregnancy reaches term. Explain that patients who are pregnant and who have gonorrhea have a higher incidence of spontaneous abortion and premature births.

Additional complications of untreated gonorrhea include arthritis-dermatitis syndrome and—rarely—meningitis, endocarditis, or pericarditis. Adult conjunctivitis may occur from autoinoculation with purulent discharge. Even more serious are the epidemic complications caused by disease spread. For example, the microorganisms *Chlamydia trachomatis* and *Neisseria gonorrhoeae* are transmitted sexually from partner to partner. Untreated chlamydia may cause urethritis and epididymitis. And untreated gonorrhea in men may cause urethritis, epididymitis, urethral stricture, or disseminated gonococcal infection.

Describe the diagnostic workup
Inform the patient that the doctor will perform a pelvic examination to assess vaginal discharge and to obtain vaginal and cervical smears for analysis. He may also order blood tests to help diagnose the disorder.

Blood tests
Prepare the patient for venipuncture, and explain that she'll have a complete blood count to detect infection.

Pelvic examination
Because many patients feel apprehensive about a pelvic examination, take extra time to allay your patient's anxiety—especially if this is her first examination. Show her the examination table, and briefly explain the equipment the doctor will use. Encourage her to express her feelings and to let the doctor know if she experiences discomfort during the examination. Aided by a diagram or a model, show her how the doctor will use a speculum to examine the vulva, vagina, and cervix and use his hands to examine the uterus, fallopian tubes, and ovaries. Mention that the doctor may or may not perform a rectal examination. Give her a copy of the patient-teaching aid *Preparing for a pelvic exam,* page 392, and answer any questions.

Explain that the vaginal smear obtained during the examination will be studied with a microscope to identify the type of vulvovaginitis (fungal hyphae point to a candidiasis diagnosis; motile, flagellated protozoa confirm trichomoniasis; and bacteria-stipled "clue" cells indicate nonspecific vaginitis; smear findings appear

Learning about sexually transmitted diseases

Inform your patient that some sexually transmitted diseases (STDs) may be identified at the same time that vulvovaginitis, cervicitis, or both are diagnosed. Like vulvovaginitis and cervicitis, these diseases may cause vaginal discharge and genital lesions, pain, itching, irritation, and other symptoms as well. As appropriate, use the chart below when you discuss STDs with your patient.

STD AND CAUSE	SIGNS AND SYMPTOMS	TEACHING POINTS
Chancroid Caused by *Haemophilus ducreyi,* a gram-negative bacillus	Erosion of a genital vesiculopustule leaves a tender, shallow, or deep ulcer with purulent drainage. Enlarged, tender lymph nodes called buboes may also develop.	• Explain that the doctor may suspect this rare disease if the patient's traveled to a tropical climate or had multiple sexual partners. • Inform the patient that the doctor will order a Gram stain of drainage and a culture to confirm the diagnosis. • Tell her that treatment includes oral erythromycin or trimethroprim-sulfamethoxazole or ceftriaxone I.M. • Advise her to relieve buboes with warm soaks. Buboes should not be incised.
Condylomata acuminatum (genital warts) Caused by human papilloma virus types 6 and 11	Single or multiple soft, fleshy vegetating growths appear on the genital organs.	• Explain that the doctor will perform a Pap smear and obtain a tissue sample for biopsy. • Tell the patient that treatment includes local podophyllin or trichloroacetic acid therapy, scalpel excision, cryotherapy, or CO_2 laser therapy. • Warn her that this disease, which has a long incubation period, increases her risk for cervical cancer. • Add that the disease can be intraurethral, cervical, or rectal, as well as external. • Tell the pregnant patient that podophyllin is teratogenic. Large doses have been associated with fetal death. Also mention that vaginal delivery may be impossible if warts grow large.
Genital herpes Caused by herpes genitalis, a virus	Vesicles clustered on an erythematous base rupture, ulcerate, or crust. Other symptoms include paresthesias, pain, fever, and headache.	• Tell the patient that the doctor will order a Tzanck smear and tissue culture to confirm the diagnosis. • Inform her that treatment includes acyclovir (an antiviral agent) and pain medication. • Explain that recurrent disease may occur with systemic infection, fever, stress, menses, and pregnancy. • Inform her that she can transmit the disease even when she has no symptoms. • Warn the pregnant patient that the disease may cause neonatal infection.
Granuloma inguinale Caused by *Calymnatobacterium granulomatis,* a gram-negative bacillus	A painless, indurated genital ulcer with friable base develops, possibly with inguinal induration (pseudobuboes).	• Explain that the doctor may suspect this rare disease if the patient's traveled to Africa or Southeast Asia or has had multiple sexual partners. • Inform the patient that the doctor will order a Gram stain of the affected tissue to diagnose the disorder. • Treatment includes oral tetracycline, doxycycline, erythromycin, or ampicillin. • Suggest using warm soaks to relieve pseudobuboes.
Lymphogranuloma venerum Caused by *Chlamydia trachomatis* types L1, L2, and L3 of subgroup A, an intracellular bacillus	Development of a small, nontender, transient papule or genital ulcer may be followed by buboes.	• Explain that the doctor may suspect this rare disease if the patient's traveled to Africa or Southeast Asia or has had multiple sexual partners. • Inform the patient that the doctor will diagnose the disorder by microimmuno-fluorescence or complement fixation testing and treat it with oral tetracycline, doxycycline, or erythromycin. • Advise her to relieve buboes with warm soaks. Buboes should not be incised.

continued

Learning about sexually transmitted diseases — *continued*

STD AND CAUSE	SIGNS AND SYMPTOMS	TEACHING POINTS
Syphilis Caused by *Treponema pallidum,* a spirochete	Initially, a transient, shallow, non-tender genital ulcer appears, possibly followed by generalized rash, soft genital warts, or lymphadenopathy.	• Explain that the doctor will order blood tests, either the RPR (rapid plasma reagin) or the VDRL (Venereal Disease Research Laboratory) test to diagnose syphilis. • Tell her that she'll receive an injection of benzathine penicillin for primary, secondary, and early latent syphilis. Add that for late latent syphilis, she'll receive three injections over 3 weeks. • Stress that she may be asymptomatic for long periods (between the primary and secondary stages and in the latent stage) but that the disease is still transmittable. • Explain that untreated syphilis may result in tertiary syphilis many years later with severe cardiac, neurologic, and dermatologic complications. • Warn the pregnant patient that syphilis may cause neonatal infection.

normal in atrophic vaginitis). Once the doctor knows the patient's type of vulvovaginitis, he can target appropriate drug therapy.

If the doctor suspects cervicitis, inform the patient that he'll send the smear to the laboratory for culture and sensitivity studies and a Gram stain to detect gonorrhea or for other analysis to detect chlamydia. Mention that test results will be available within 48 hours.

Mention that vulvovaginitis or cervicitis may be detected if routine Pap smear results indicate inflammation—white blood cells but no malignant cells. Inform the patient that the infectious organism may or may not be identified on the Pap smear but that treatment is necessary, and that the Pap smear should be repeated in 3 months.

Teach about treatments
Inform your patient that medication is the primary treatment for vulvovaginitis and cervicitis. Emphasize that she and her partner require concurrent treatment to avoid reinfection and recurrent cervicitis. The doctor will also advise sexual abstinence during treatment and may recommend sitz baths to soothe perineal irritation and to minimize odor.

Medication
Explain that the doctor may prescribe medication based on his initial clinical impression. However, he may change the medication, depending on diagnostic test results. Remind the patient that effective drug therapy kills or controls the causative microorganism (see *Teaching about drugs for vulvovaginitis and cervicitis,* pages 386 and 387). The doctor will prescribe antifungal agents to treat candidiasis, antiprotozoal agents for trichomoniasis, other antimicrobial agents for nonspecific vaginitis and both kinds of cervici-

continued on page 388

Teaching about drugs for vulvovaginitis and cervicitis

DRUG	ADVERSE REACTIONS	TEACHING POINTS
Antimicrobials		
butoconazole nitrate (Femstat) **clotrimazole** (Gyne-Lotrimin, **miconazole nitrate** (Monistat 3) **nystatin** (Mycostatin, Nilstat) **terconazole** (Terazol 3, Terazol 7) **tioconazole** (Vagistat)	• Watch for hives; itching; skin blisters, burning, peeling, rash, redness or swelling; and vaginal burning (with vaginal use). • Other reactions include abdominal cramps, diarrhea, nausea, and vomiting.	• Instruct the patient to complete the prescribed course of therapy. Remind her to take every dose. • If she's using a topical cream, show her how to apply it on the affected area and surrounding skin. Warn her *not* to cover the area with an occlusive wrapping or dressing. • If she's using a vaginal drug form, advise her to wear clean cotton panties or pantyhose with cotton crotches. • If she has vaginal discharge while using this drug, advise her to wear a sanitary napkin to protect her clothing. • Instruct her to continue therapy during menstruation and to wash the vaginal applicator thoroughly after each use. • Tell her to store the drug away from heat and light and according to manufacturer's directions.
Antiparasitic agent		
metronidazole (Flagyl)	• Watch for new dryness or discharge, hives, paresthesias in the hands or feet, rash, seizures, and vaginal irritation. • Other reactions include abdominal pain, anorexia, constipation, darkened urine, diarrhea, dizziness, dry mouth, headache, nausea, metallic taste, and vomiting.	• Suggest taking this drug with meals to minimize GI upset. • Instruct her to take every dose of medicine. • Warn her not to perform tasks requiring mental alertness if the drug causes dizziness. • Tell her to avoid alcohol and alcohol-containing products for the first 48 hours after taking this drug. • Tell the pregnant patient that the drug's safety during pregnancy hasn't been established. • Tell the patient with trichomoniasis that sexual partners should be treated simultaneously to avoid reinfection.
Estrogens		
dienestrol (DV Cream) **estradiol** (Estrace) **estradiol valerate** (Estradiol LA) **estrogen, conjugated** (Premarin) **estrogen, esterified** (Estratab) **estropipate** (Ogen) **ethinyl estradiol** (Estinyl, Feminone) **quinestrol** (Estrovia)	• Watch for abdominal pain, acne, altered menstrual flow, amenorrhea, arm or leg weakness, breakthrough bleeding, breast lumps, curdlike vaginal discharge, depression, dysmenorrhea, dysuria, jaundice, lethargy, rash, severe headache, shortness of breath, slurred speech, sudden chest pain, urinary frequency, and visual disturbances. • Other reactions include anorexia, bloating, breast tenderness, dizziness, edema, hair loss, headache, leg cramps, nausea, photosensitivity, and vomiting.	• Explain that this drug corrects estrogen deficiency and should help atrophic vulvovaginitis. Instruct the patient to read the package insert information carefully and to ask her doctor or pharmacist to clear up any questions. • Discourage smoking when taking this drug to reduce the risk of myocardial infarction, cerebrovascular accident, pulmonary emboli, and thrombophlebitis. • Teach the patient how to perform breast self-examination. • Suggest using a sunscreen when outdoors because estrogens can cause photosensitivity reactions. • If appropriate, review instructions on vaginal administration of the drug. • Advise taking the drug with meals to minimize GI upset. • If the patient suspects that she's pregnant, tell her to discontinue the drug and notify her doctor. Using this drug during pregnancy may cause birth defects.
Penicillins		
amoxicillin (Amoxil) **ampicillin** (Omnipen, Polycillin) **penicillin G procaine** (Crysticillin, Duracillin, Uticillin VK)	• Watch for abdominal cramps, seizures, severe diarrhea, signs of hypersensitivity (hives, itching, rash, wheezing), unusual thirst, and weight loss. • Other reactions include leukopenia, mild diarrhea, nausea, sore mouth or tongue, and vomiting.	• If the patient's using ampicillin, instruct her to take the drug on an empty stomach. She can take amoxicillin, however, without regard to mealtimes unless the drug causes GI upset; then advise taking the drug with meals. • Tell her to take every dose to complete the therapy. • Advise the patient taking oral contraceptives to use a back-up birth control method, because these drugs may reduce the oral contraceptive's effectiveness. • If the patient's taking a suspension form of drug, remind her to check the drug label for storage directions.

continued

Teaching about drugs for vulvovaginitis and cervicitis – *continued*

DRUG	ADVERSE REACTIONS	TEACHING POINTS
Penicillinase-resistant agents		
ceftriaxone (Rocephin)	• Watch for abdominal pain, easy bruising, infections, severe diarrhea, and seizures. • Other reactions include anemia, diarrhea, dizziness, dyspnea, fever, flushing, genital pruritus, hair loss, hives, increased gouty arthritis attacks, pain at injection site, rash, renal pain, sweating, and urinary frequency.	• Caution the patient that if she's allergic to penicillin, she may be allergic to this drug, too. Advise her to contact her doctor immediately if she has signs and symptoms of hypersensitivity. • Tell her that this drug contains sodium (3.6 mEq/g of the drug). She should advise her doctor of any fluid retention. • Suggest that consuming yogurt or buttermilk may help prevent a secondary intestinal infection from developing. • Instruct her to notify her doctor if she suspects a secondary bacterial or fungal infection, such as candidiasis. • If the patient has diabetes, caution her to use a glucose monitoring test other than Clinitest, because the drug may alter test results.
spectinomycin (Trobicin)	• Reactions include chills and fever; decreased urine output; dizziness; hives, itching, or rash; insomnia; nausea or vomiting; and pain at injection site.	• Warn the patient that the injection site may be painful. • Inform the patient that because this drug's ineffective against syphilis, she should take care to seek medical attention for any genital lesions that develop.
Renal tubular blocking agent		
probenecid (Benemid, Probalan)	• Watch for easy bruising, infections, and excessive weakness. • Other reactions include dizziness, GI distress, fever, flushing, hair loss, headache, hematuria, hypotension, increased gouty arthritis attacks, leukopenia, renal pain, sore gums, sweating, and urinary frequency.	• Tell the patient that this drug will delay urinary excretion of antibiotic drugs, thereby ensuring more effective blood-antibiotic levels to fight infection. • Advise the patient to increase fluid intake to prevent kidney stone formation. • Advise taking drug with food or milk to avoid GI upset. • If the patient has diabetes, caution her to use a glucose monitoring test other than Clinitest, because the drug may alter test results.
Tetracyclines		
demeclocycline (Declomycin) **doxycycline** (Doxy-Caps, Vibramycin) **minocycline** (Minocin) **tetracycline** (Achromycin, Tetracyn)	• Watch for diarrhea; increased pigmentation of skin or mucous membranes; unusual thirst, fatigue, or weakness; and urinary frequency or increased urine volume. • Other reactions include abdominal cramps or burning, discolored tongue, dizziness, genital or rectal itching, light-headedness, nausea, photosensitivity, sore mouth or tongue, and vomiting.	• Instruct the patient to take tetracycline on an empty stomach – 1 hour before or 2 hours after meals. • Tell her to take the drug with plenty of water at least 1 hour before bedtime to prevent esophageal irritation. • Advise against taking tetracycline with milk. • Tell her to avoid taking antacids or other calcium- or magnesium-containing preparations within 2 hours of taking tetracycline. • Instruct her to avoid taking iron preparations within 3 hours of taking tetracycline. • Remind her to take every dose to complete therapy. • Teach the patient good oral hygiene. And show her how to check her tongue for signs of candidal infection. If superinfection occurs, instruct her to notify the doctor. • Warn her to avoid direct sunlight and ultraviolet light and to use a sunscreen if she can't avoid exposure. Explain that photosensitivity may continue after she finishes therapy. • Explain that these drugs shouldn't be used by a child under age 8 or by a pregnant patient because the drugs may permanently damage teeth and retard bone growth. • Instruct the patient to store reconstituted solutions in the refrigerator. Tell her that they're stable for 48 hours. • Advise her not to use medication that has changed color, taste, or appearance.

Tips for relieving vulvovaginal irritation

If your patient has vulvovaginal irritation, offer the following tips for soothing irritation and avoiding recurrent infection.

- Shower daily, washing between showers with soap and water if discharge or odor seems excessive. Rinse soap away thoroughly to avoid increasing irritation.
- Avoid tub baths, especially with bubbles or oils.
- Change underwear daily.
- Avoid using feminine hygiene deodorant sprays, douches, perfumes, creams, or chemicals around the perineum.
- Use unscented, white toilet tissue and sanitary napkins.

- Wear white cotton underwear.
- Stay away from nylon pantyhose without a cotton crotch and tight panties made of synthetic fabrics that inhibit ventilation.
- Change a wet bathing suit promptly rather than wear it until it dries.
- Avoid contamination by remembering to wipe the perineal area from front to back each time you use the bathroom.
- Take antibiotics cautiously because some can cause candidiasis.
- Consider using alternative birth control methods if oral contraceptives cause recurrent candidiasis.

tis, and conjugated estrogen for atrophic vaginitis. Add that the drugs may be administered orally or intravaginally.

Then review dosages, possible adverse effects, and precautions for the patient's medication. If the doctor prescribes intravaginal medication, give the patient a copy of the teaching aid *How to administer a vaginal medication,* pages 390 and 391. Stress that she complete the prescribed medication regimen, cautioning her that absence of symptoms doesn't necessarily mean absence of infection.

Other care measures

Discuss specific hygiene measures and sexual abstinence that accompany drug treatment.

Personal hygiene. Teach the patient about personal hygiene practices that minimize perineal irritation and odor (see *Tips for relieving vulvovaginal irritation*). Instruct her to irrigate the perineum with warm water or normal saline solution. This rinses away discharge from an irritated vulva.

Sexual abstinence. Inform the patient that sexual abstinence is essential in cervicitis and in some forms of vulvovaginitis. Tell her that her partner also must be treated for and cured of STDs before he can resume sex. If appropriate, direct her to advise her sexual partners to be examined and treated by their own doctors, a public health clinic, or an STD clinic.

Caution the patient and her infected sexual partner to wait 48 hours to 1 week or longer after completing treatment before resuming sexual relations. Explain that the doctor may need to perform a follow-up examination, and that cultures may be necessary before he approves resumed sexual activity. Point out that some patients have intercourse using condoms during treatment. However, they still risk infecting each other.

Tell the patient with gonorrhea that her name will be reported to the local public health department. Explain that she'll be asked to identify her sexual partner or partners to ensure that they receive treatment.

Inform her that the law requires her doctor to report gonorrhea to the public health department.

Advise the patient with a nonsexually transmitted vulvovaginitis (candidiasis, nonspecific vaginitis, and atrophic vaginitis) that sexual abstinence may minimize vulvovaginal irritation. Add that her partners don't need treatment unless she has recurrent infection.

For the patient with atrophic vaginitis, suggest using a lubricant during intercourse to enhance her comfort.

Finally, urge the patient to seek prompt evaluation and treatment for recurrent vaginal discharge or irritation.

Explain that because infection—especially cervicitis—can recur with or without symptoms, she should schedule regular gynecologic checkups.

Sources of information and support

American Foundation for the Prevention of Venereal Disease (Sexually Transmitted Disease)
799 Broadway, Suite 638, New York, N.Y. 10003
(212) 759-2069

American Social Health Association (Sexually Transmitted Diseases)
P.O. Box 13827, Research Triangle Park, N.C. 27709
(919) 361-2742

Further readings

Hammerschlag, M.R., et al. "When to Suspect Chlamydia," *Patient Care* 21(18):64-70, 75-76, 78, November 15, 1987.

McCauley, K.M., and Oi, R.H. "Evaluating the Papanicolaou Smear, Part 1," *Consultant* 28(12):31-34, 37, 40, December 1988.

McCauley, K.M., and Oi, R.H. "Evaluating the Papanicolaou Smear: Four Possible Colposcopic Findings and Corresponding Management Strategies, Part 2," *Consultant* 29(1):36-38, 41-42, January 1989.

Nettina, S. "Diagnosis and Management of Sexually Transmitted Genital Lesions," *Nurse Practitioner* 15(1):20, 22, 24, 26, 31, 34-36, 38, 39, January 1990.

Secor, R.M.C. "Bacterial Vaginosis: A Comprehensive Review," *Nursing Clinics of North America* 23(4):865-75, December 1988.

Simon, W. "Feminine Hygiene," *Nursing (London)* 3(35):31-34, March 1989.

Wordell, D.W. "Chronic Exposure to Sexually Transmitted Diseases," *Nursing Clinics of North America* 23(4):947-57, December 1988.

How to administer a vaginal medication

Dear Patient:

Your doctor has prescribed a vaginal medication for you. To insert the medication, follow these instructions:

1 Plan to insert the vaginal medication after bathing and just before bedtime to ensure that it will stay in the vagina for an appropriate amount of time.
   Collect the equipment you'll need: the prescribed medication (suppository, cream, ointment, tablet, or jelly), an applicator, water-soluble lubricating jelly (such as K-Y Jelly), a towel, a hand mirror, paper towels, and a sanitary pad.

2 Next, empty your bladder, wash your hands, and place the towel on the bed. Sit on the towel, and open the medication wrapper or container.

3 Using the hand mirror, carefully inspect your perineum. If you see

signs of increased irritation, don't insert the medication. Notify the doctor. He may change your medication.

4 Place a vaginal suppository or tablet in the applicator, or fill the applicator with cream, ointment, or jelly.

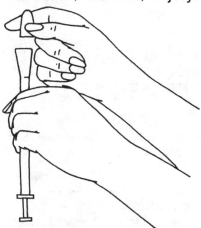

5 To make insertion easier, lubricate the suppository or applicator tip with water or water-soluble lubricating jelly.

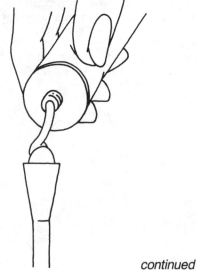

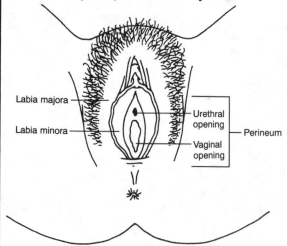

Labia majora —
Labia minora —
Urethral opening —
Vaginal opening —
Perineum

continued

How to administer a vaginal medication — *continued*

Now, lie down on the bed with your knees flexed and legs spread apart.

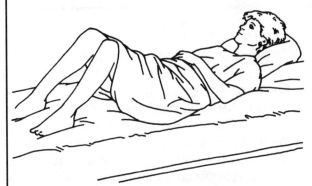

Spread apart your labia with one hand, and insert the applicator tip into the vagina with the other hand. Advance the applicator about 2 inches (5 cm), angling it slightly toward your tailbone.

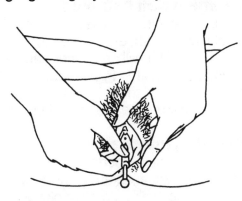

6 Push the plunger to insert the medication. Be aware that the medication may feel cold.

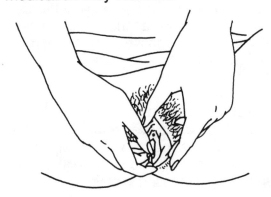

7 Remove the applicator and discard it—if it's disposable. If it's reusable, thoroughly wash it with soap and water, dry it with a paper towel, and return it to its container.

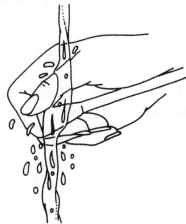

8 If your doctor prescribes it, apply a thin layer of cream, ointment, or jelly to the vulva (the area including the vagina, labia majora, and labia minora).

9 Remain lying down for about 30 minutes so the medicine won't run out of your vagina. Apply the sanitary pad to avoid staining your clothes or bed linens.

Then check your vagina for signs of an allergic reaction. If the area seems unusually red or swollen, contact the doctor.

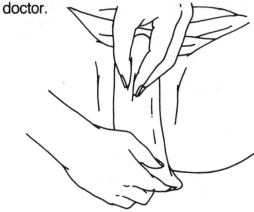

PATIENT-TEACHING AID

Preparing for a pelvic exam

Dear Patient:

If just thinking about a pelvic exam makes you feel uncomfortable, remember this: The exam won't hurt, and it could save your life. How? During the exam, you'll have a Pap test, which is a simple, painless, cervical smear that can detect cancer cells.

The pelvic exam can also check that your reproductive organs are healthy. And it can help detect sexually transmitted diseases and other infections while they're treatable. Another plus—the exam takes only about 5 minutes.

Before the exam
First, the nurse will ask about your health history, take your blood pressure, and request a urine specimen.

Next you'll enter an examination room, remove your clothes, and put on a front-opening examination gown. Then you'll sit on an examining table, and the nurse will give you a sheet to drape across your legs.

A brief physical
The doctor may check your throat, neck, heart, lungs, and breasts. (Ask how to perform a breast self-examination if you don't already know how.)

Positioning
Then you'll need to position yourself so that your buttocks are at the table's edge, and your heels are in the table's stirrups. Once a sheet is draped over your legs, you'll be instructed to spread your knees apart.

Inspection
The doctor will inspect your external genitals (called the perineum) for irritation or other abnormalities.

Next, he'll insert a speculum into your vagina. This instrument enables him to inspect your vagina and cervix. It may feel cool. But usually it will be warmed and lubricated so that it slides easily and causes little sensation.

If you resist the speculum, however, you may feel uncomfortable. So take a deep breath and relax.

Obtaining cell samples
Now, using a thin wooden or plastic spatula, tiny brush, and cotton-tipped swab, the doctor will obtain cell samples for tests, such as the Pap smear—most women don't feel this at all. Once that's done, he will remove the speculum.

Checking internal organs
Next, the doctor will perform a two-handed (bimanual) exam to feel your internal organs. He'll insert two gloved and lubricated fingers into your vagina up to the cervix. Then with his other hand on your abdomen, he'll feel the size, shape, and location of your uterus, ovaries, and fallopian tubes and check for tenderness, masses, or other abnormalities. If you tense up, take a deep breath to relax.

After the exam
When the exam's over, remember to ask any questions you have. Then wipe the lubricant from your perineum with a tissue and get dressed in private.

Musculoskeletal Conditions

Contents

Herniated nucleus pulposus

In North America, low back pain rivals the common cold as one of the most prevalent health problems. One cause of low back pain, herniated nucleus pulposus (HNP), requires your command of a wide range of teaching topics. You'll need to convey the importance of strict activity restrictions—for example, bed rest—and pain-control techniques, including medication, which are typically the first treatment measures selected. You'll also need to routinely emphasize proper body mechanics to help prevent further or recurrent back injury. Your teaching here can often mean the difference between successful home care and necessary hospitalization.

For some patients, hospitalization is the only alternative, forcing difficult career and life-style changes. So you may need to teach the patient about surgery and about care measures during convalescence. Other teaching topics include an explanation of how HNP develops in a disk, the signs and symptoms of nerve root compression, and various diagnostic tests for HNP. And because severe, debilitating pain can lead to frustration and depression, you'll also need to offer patients strong emotional support.

Discuss the disorder

Inform the patient that HNP is commonly called a ruptured or herniated disk, or by the misnomer, a "slipped" disk. Explain how HNP occurs by first reviewing the anatomy of a normal disk, then describing the three stages of herniation. (See *How HNP develops*, page 396.)

What causes HNP? Tell the patient that it may occur suddenly—from heavy lifting, twisting, or direct injury. Or it may arise gradually from degenerative changes related to aging. The most common site for herniation is the L4-L5 disk space, but the problem also occurs at L5-S1, L2-L3, L3-L4, C6-C7, and C5-C6. Lumbar herniation usually develops in people ages 20 to 45; cervical herniation in those 45 or older. More men than women suffer from HNP.

Explain that pain is the most common symptom. It typically worsens with activity, coughing, and sneezing, and subsides with rest. It may be unilateral or bilateral. If the sciatic nerve root in the spine is compressed, pain will radiate down the leg (the sciatic nerve runs along the hip, buttocks, and leg). Other signs and symptoms include muscle spasms, muscle weakness, and sensory and motor loss in the area innervated by the compressed spinal nerve root.

Marilyn A. Folcik, RN, BA, MPH, ONC, and **Marianne K. Ostrow, RN, BSN,** contributed to this chapter. Ms. Folcik is a staff development instructor in orthopedics, neurosurgery, and rehabilitation nursing at Hartford Hospital, Hartford, Conn. Ms. Ostrow is a clinical nurse at Thomas Jefferson University Hospital, Philadelphia.

CHECKLIST

Teaching topics in HNP

☐ An explanation of herniated nucleus pulposus (HNP), including how it causes back and leg pain
☐ Warning signs and symptoms of nerve root compression
☐ Procedures to confirm sciatica
☐ Preparation for X-rays, myelography, computed tomography scan, magnetic resonance imaging, and electromyography
☐ Initial treatments, such as bed rest, back-strengthening exercises, proper body mechanics, and weight reduction
☐ Medications and their administration, including epidural steroid injections
☐ Other pain-control measures, such as heat and cold, positioning, and transcutaneous electrical nerve stimulation
☐ Procedures, such as pelvic traction and chemonucleolysis
☐ Preparation for and explanation of surgery (laminectomy, diskectomy, or spinal fusion)
☐ Postoperative instructions, including wound care and activity guidelines
☐ Sources of information and support

396 Herniated nucleus pulposus

How HNP develops

Before describing to the patient how a disk herniates, review the normal anatomy of an intervertebral disk.

A disk consists of two parts—a semigelatinous center called the nucleus pulposus and a tough, surrounding fibrous ring called the anulus fibrosus. The nucleus pulposus acts as a shock absorber, distributing the mechanical stress applied to the spine when the body moves.

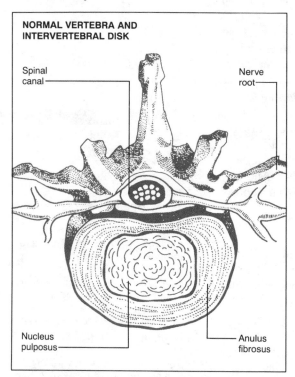

NORMAL VERTEBRA AND INTERVERTEBRAL DISK

Spinal canal

Nerve root

Nucleus pulposus

Anulus fibrosus

Inform the patient that physical stress—usually a twisting motion—can cause the anulus fibrosus to tear or rupture, allowing the nucleus pulposus to push through (herniate) into the spinal canal. This process causes the vertebrae to move closer together as the disk compresses, resulting in pain and possible sensory and motor loss as pressure is placed on the nerve roots as they exit between the vertebrae.

A herniated disk also may be related to intervertebral joint degeneration. If the disk has begun to degenerate, minor trauma may cause herniation.

Herniation occurs in three stages: protrusion, extrusion, and sequestration.

Stage I: Protrusion
The nucleus pulposus presses against the anulus fibrosus.

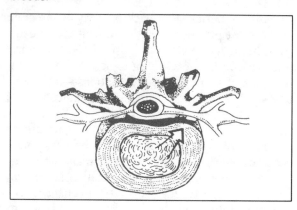

Stage II: Extrusion
The nucleus pulposus bulges forcefully through the anulus fibrosus, pushing against the nerve root.

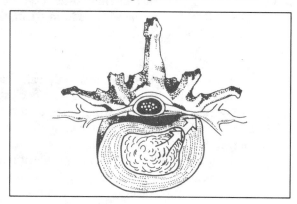

Stage III: Sequestration
The anulus fibrosus gives way, and the inner core bursts through to press against the nerve root.

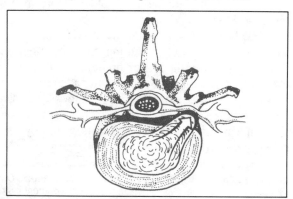

Complications
Although symptoms occasionally abate spontaneously, HNP may cause persistent sciatica without treatment. It may also cause permanent motor or sensory loss, such as weakness in one or both legs, and bowel or bladder problems.

Describe the diagnostic workup
Tell the patient that several tests are used to confirm HNP, including a physical examination, X-rays, myelography, computed tomography (CT) scan, magnetic resonance imaging (MRI), and electromyography (EMG).

Physical examination
Explain that the doctor may perform some tests to confirm sciatica. In the first test, the straight leg raise, the patient lies on his back. The doctor lifts the patient's leg, supporting the heel and keeping the knee straight. A person without sciatica won't feel pain until his leg's lifted to an 80-degree angle. If the patient feels pain at a lesser angle, the doctor will lower the leg slightly and dorsiflex the foot. If this also elicits pain, the patient has sciatica.

Explain that in the second test, the sitting root test, the patient sits on the examination table with his legs dangling and his chin touching his chest. The doctor holds the patient's thigh against the table and tries to straighten the leg. If the patient feels pain before his leg is completely extended, he has sciatica.

X-rays
Tell the patient that X-rays will be ordered to detect bone abnormalities but that X-rays alone won't confirm the presence of HNP.

Myelography
Explain that myelography may be performed to pinpoint the level of the herniation. Tell the patient that the test is done in the X-ray department and takes about 1 hour. Inform him that he'll lie prone on a tilting X-ray table. After cleansing the skin on the patient's lower back, the doctor injects an anesthetic.

Warn the patient that he may feel a stinging sensation. Next, the doctor inserts a needle between two vertebrae of the patient's spinal cord and injects an oil- or water-based contrast medium.

Warn the patient that he may feel a transient burning sensation during injection. He may also feel flushed and warm and experience a headache, a salty taste, or nausea and vomiting.

Explain that the doctor takes a series of X-rays as the table tilts vertically and then horizontally to allow the contrast medium to flow through the spinal canal. After the test is finished, the doctor withdraws the oil-based medium or allows the water-based medium to absorb. He then places an adhesive bandage over the puncture site.

Describe what will occur after the test: If an oil-based medium was used, the patient should lie flat in bed for 6 to 8 hours and avoid abrupt movement. He should drink plenty of fluids and resume his normal diet, as tolerated. If nausea prevents this, he may require I.V. fluids or an antiemetic. If a water-based medium was used, advise him to lie with the head of the bed elevated 30 degrees for 6 to 8 hours, then to remain on bed rest for an additional 6 to 8 hours. He should drink plenty of fluids and resume his normal diet, as tolerated. If he's on phenothiazine therapy, tell him to temporarily discontinue the drug, as ordered by the doctor.

In any case, warn him to notify the doctor if he has a headache for more than 24 hours after the test or if he develops weakness, numbness, or tingling in his legs.

CT scan

Teach the patient that a CT scan uses X-ray images to detect bone and soft-tissue abnormalities. It can also visualize spinal canal compression, resulting from herniation. Tell him that the test takes from 30 to 60 minutes. Explain that he won't be allowed food or fluids for 4 hours before the scan if a contrast medium will be used. Also explain that the room will be chilly because the equipment requires a cool environment, and that he must wear a hospital gown, remove all his jewelry, and void before the test.

Inform the patient that the technician positions him on an X-ray table and places a strap across the part of his body to be scanned, to restrict any movement. The table then slides into the scanner. If a contrast medium is ordered, the infusion takes about 5 minutes. Instruct the patient to report any discomfort, such as burning, warmth, or itching, immediately. (The technician can see and hear him from an adjacent room.) Tell him that the table will move a small distance every few seconds and that the scanner will rotate around him and may make a clicking or buzzing noise. He should remain still during the test. If he receives a contrast medium, tell him to drink plenty of fluids after the test.

MRI test

Instruct the patient that MRI uses a magnetic field to produce images of areas where bones usually obscure visualization. The test takes about 1 hour. Tell him to alert the doctor if he has any metal objects in his body such as aneurysm clips, a metal prosthesis, an implanted infusion pump, a pacemaker, or bullet fragments, so the machine can be adjusted. Warn him that he'll be in an enclosure, so he should alert the doctor if he's claustrophobic.

Inform the patient that he'll lie on a table while his head, chest, and arms are restrained to help him remain still and ensure sharp images. The table slides into a large cylinder housing the MRI magnets. Describe the loud, knocking sound the machine makes, and tell him to ask for earplugs or pads if the noise bothers him. Reassure him that the technician will be able to see and communicate with him from an adjacent room.

Electromyography

Teach the patient that EMG can confirm nerve involvement by measuring the electrical activity of muscles innervated by the herniated disk. Tell him the test takes about 1 hour.

Tell the patient that he'll lie on his abdomen on a bed or table. The technician cleanses the skin over the muscle to be tested, then he inserts a needle attached to an electrode into the muscle.

Warn the patient that he may experience some discomfort as the needle's inserted. The technician places another electrode, which delivers a mild electrical charge, on the patient's limb. This may also cause discomfort as each muscle is stimulated to test its response at rest and during voluntary contraction. Tell the patient to remain still, except when asked to contract or relax a muscle.

Teach about treatments
Inform the patient that treatment for HNP initially includes bed rest (sometimes with traction), medication, application of heat or cold, proper body positioning, back-strengthening exercises, and if necessary, weight reduction. If these measures fail, epidural steroid injections, chemonucleolysis, and surgery may be necessary.

Activity
Tell the patient that for acute HNP the doctor may order 2 weeks of bed rest. Explain that bed rest reduces pressure on the spine, allowing the herniated disk to subside. This, in turn, relieves pressure on the irritated nerve root. Suggest that the patient lie in a semi-Fowler's or side-lying position with his knees flexed, to reduce tension on his spine. Recommend that he use a bedpan or a bedside commode, as ordered.

Explain that when his acute pain eases, the physical therapist will give him an exercise program to strengthen his back and abdominal muscles and to promote good posture. Include the family in your teaching to give the patient extra encouragement and support.

Emphasize the use of proper body mechanics. Advise the patient not to lift heavy objects or to bend at the waist. Suggest assistive devices, such as reachers. The patient may have to change his life-style to avoid aggravating his back problem.

Diet
Explain to the overweight patient that excess body weight aggravates the strain on his spine. If the doctor prescribes a weight-reduction diet, make sure the patient has a written copy of it. When teaching about meal planning, include other family members—especially the one who does most of the cooking.

Medication
Tell the patient that for acute HNP the doctor may order narcotic analgesics, muscle relaxants, and nonsteroidal anti-inflammatory agents to relieve pain and steroids to reduce inflammation. Because narcotic analgesics can cause constipation, he may also suggest concomitant use of a laxative. Teach the patient that a high-fiber diet and adequate fluid intake also help to prevent constipation. (For more information, see *Teaching about drugs for HNP symptoms*, pages 400 and 401.)

If the patient's pain results from nerve root irritation and conservative medication regimens fail, explain that the doctor may

continued on page 402

Teaching about drugs for HNP symptoms

DRUG	ADVERSE REACTIONS	TEACHING POINTS
Narcotic analgesics		
codeine sulfate **hydromorphone** (Dilaudid) **methadone** (Dolophine) **morphine sulfate** **oxycodone** (Percocet, Percodan, Tylox) **propoxyphene** (Darvon)	• Watch for confusion, unusually slow breathing, and unusually slow, fast, or pounding heartbeat. • Other reactions include constipation, diaphoresis, dizziness, drowsiness, headache, and unusual tiredness or weakness.	• For maximum effectiveness, advise the patient to take this drug before pain becomes intense. Regularly scheduled doses often provide more consistent pain relief than doses ordered "as needed." • Remind him to use this drug only for severe pain; when pain decreases, he should use a less potent pain reliever to avoid drug dependency and tolerance. • Tell him to avoid central nervous system (CNS) depressants, such as antihistamines and alcohol, when taking this drug. • Caution him to avoid activities requiring concentration, balance, and coordination because this drug can impair these functions. • Advise him to rise slowly from a sitting or lying position to minimize dizziness and fainting resulting from lowered blood pressure. • Discuss measures to prevent constipation, such as adding dietary fiber to his diet or increasing fluids and activity.
Nonsteroidal anti-inflammatory agents		
diflunisal (Dolobid) **ibuprofen** (Advil, Motrin, Nuprin) **indomethacin** (Indocin, Indocin SR) **meclofenamate** (Meclomen) **naproxen** (Anaprox, Naprosyn) **piroxicam** (Feldene) **sulindac** (Clinoril) **tolmetin** (Tolectin)	• Watch for bloody or tarry stools, bloody urine, bruises, decreased urine output, fever, skin rash, sore throat, unusual bleeding, wheezing, and yellowing of skin and eyes. • Other reactions include diarrhea, dizziness, heartburn, indigestion, nausea, and vomiting.	• Tell the patient to take a missed dose as soon as he remembers. If it's almost time for the next dose, tell him to skip the missed dose. Warn him not to double-dose. • If gastric upset occurs, tell him to take this drug with an antacid. • Caution him not to drive a car or operate machinery if he becomes drowsy. • Warn him not to take this drug along with aspirin, acetaminophen, or alcohol. • For best absorption, advise him to take this drug on an empty stomach 1 hour before or 3 hours after meals. • Teach him signs of GI bleeding: bloody or coffee ground-like vomit or bloody or black, tarry stools.
Skeletal muscle relaxants		
carisoprodol (Rela, Soma)	• Watch for blurred or double vision; fever; itching; hives; shortness of breath; skin rash; swollen lips, tongue, and face; unusually fast, slow, or pounding heartbeat; and wheezing. • Other reactions include dizziness, drowsiness, hiccups, nausea, stomach cramps, and vomiting.	• Tell the patient to take a missed dose if he remembers within an hour; otherwise, he should skip the missed dose. Warn him not to double-dose. • Because this drug may cause dizziness or drowsiness, caution him to get out of bed and to change positions slowly, and to lie down whenever he feels dizzy. Warn him not to drive a car or operate machinery when he feels this way. • Instruct him to check with the doctor or pharmacist before taking over-the-counter CNS depressants, such as antihistamines or sleeping pills, along with this drug. • Advise him against drinking alcohol.

continued

Teaching about drugs for HNP symptoms — *continued*

DRUG	ADVERSE REACTIONS	TEACHING POINTS
Skeletal muscle relaxants — *(continued)*		
chlorzoxazone (Paraflex, Parafon Forte DSC, Strifon Forte DSC)	• Watch for itching, hives, skin rash, and yellow skin and mucous membranes. • Other reactions include agitation, constipation, depression, diarrhea, dizziness, drowsiness, epigastric distress, headache, insomnia, irritability, nausea, tremor, and vomiting.	• Tell the patient to take a missed dose if he remembers within an hour; otherwise, he should skip the missed dose. Warn him not to double-dose. • Caution him to avoid hazardous activities that require alertness or physical coordination until CNS depression is determined. • Instruct him to avoid alcohol and use caution when taking cough and cold preparations because they may contain alcohol or other CNS depressants. • Advise him to store this drug away from direct heat or light (not in the bathroom medicine chest). • Warn him not to stop taking this drug without first consulting the doctor. • Tell him that his urine may turn orange or reddish purple but that this is a harmless effect.
cyclobenzaprine (Flexeril)	• Watch for breathing difficulty, buzzing in ears, confusion, fainting, fever or decreased temperature, hallucinations, hives, muscle stiffness, severe drowsiness, severe vomiting, and unusually fast or irregular heartbeat. • Other reactions include dizziness, dry mouth, and slight drowsiness.	• Tell the patient to take a missed dose if he remembers within an hour; otherwise, he should skip the missed dose. Warn him not to double-dose. • Instruct him to check with the doctor or pharmacist before drinking alcoholic beverages or taking over-the-counter CNS depressants, such as antihistamines or sleeping pills, along with this drug. • Because this drug may cause dizziness or drowsiness, advise him to get out of bed and change positions slowly and to lie down when he feels dizzy. Warn him not to drive a car or operate machinery when he feels this way. • Suggest sucking on ice chips or sugarless hard candy or chewing gum to relieve a dry mouth.
diazepam (Valium)	• Watch for confusion, hallucinations, hostility, insomnia, restlessness, severe drowsiness, severe weakness, slurred speech, and staggering. • Other reactions include constipation, dry mouth, nausea, transient drowsiness, vomiting, and weakness.	• Advise the patient to take this drug with food or a full glass of water. He should swallow capsules whole and not chew or crush them. • Tell him to take a missed dose if he remembers within an hour; otherwise, he should skip the missed dose. Warn him not to double-dose. • Instruct him not to drive a car or operate machinery while taking this drug. • Warn him that this drug may be habit-forming. • Tell him not to take this drug with alcohol or any over-the-counter CNS depressants, such as antihistamines or sleeping pills. • Warn him not to discontinue this drug abruptly, especially after long-term use.
methocarbamol (Robaxin)	• Watch for fever, hives, itching, and skin rash. • Other reactions include blurred vision, dizziness, drowsiness, headache, lightheadedness, nausea, nervousness, unsteadiness, and vomiting.	• Explain that this drug can be taken by mouth or injection. To take by mouth, the patient can crush the tablets and mix them with food or liquid. • Tell him to take a missed dose as soon as he remembers, unless it's almost time for the next dose. Warn him not to double-dose. • Instruct him not to drive a car or operate machinery if the drug makes him drowsy. • Tell him not to take the drug with other CNS depressants, such as antihistamines or sleeping pills, or with alcohol.

perform an epidural steroid injection. Tell the patient that this procedure is performed in the hospital, usually by an anesthesiologist, who injects a steroid around the nerve where it exits between the facet joints. The procedure is usually done in three stages, 2 weeks apart. Warn the patient that pain relief may not occur after the first injection. Add that indications for the procedure are limited, and research is still being conducted on its long-term effects.

Procedures

Discuss adjunctive measures for pain relief: Applying local heat or cold helps to reduce muscle spasms, and using pillows, a bed board, or a firm mattress helps to ensure comfortable positioning. If the patient has decreased sensation, advise frequent skin checks for safety during heat or cold therapy. If necessary, describe how transcutaneous electrical nerve stimulation (TENS) works to manage pain and muscle spasms.

The doctor may order traction to enhance the effects of bed rest. If the patient will be in traction at home, teach him and his caregiver what devices will be used, how traction works, and how long he'll be in traction. Give him a copy of the patient-teaching aid *Learning about pelvic traction*, page 404.

If these methods fail to relieve the patient's pain, one alternative to surgery still exists—chemonucleolysis. Explain that this procedure may be done in a hospital X-ray department or operating room, under local or general anesthesia, and that it takes about 45 minutes. Tell the patient that he'll receive an injection of the enzyme chymopapain, which shrinks the nucleus pulposus, thereby relieving his pain. (Mention that diagnostic tests can't always reveal how far the nucleus pulposus has pushed into the spinal canal. Sometimes, the enzyme can't reach this herniated tissue, especially if it's fragmented.) Explain that most patients experience immediate relief, but total relief may not occur for 3 to 6 weeks. After the procedure, he'll probably be on bed rest for 24 hours. Reinforce any prescribed exercise program.

Surgery

When conservative measures fail, you'll need to prepare the patient for surgery—most commonly, laminectomy—to relieve back pain. Tell him that laminectomy involves the removal of a flat, bony section of the vertebra known as the lamina. Once the surgeon removes the lamina, he can remove the protruding fragments of the disk or the entire disk (diskectomy) to relieve nerve root compression. Occasionally, the surgeon may perform spinal fusion to enhance vertebral stability. Explain that this surgery involves placing bone chips from the patient's iliac crest or a bone bank over the unstable area of his spine.

Emphasize that laminectomy and spinal fusion won't immediately relieve back pain and neurologic symptoms. That's because irritation and swelling from chronic nerve root compression will take some time to subside. In fact, warn the patient that he may temporarily have more back pain, stiffness, or muscle spasms after surgery. Assure him that analgesics and muscle relaxants will be available. If the doctor also orders a back brace or corset to support the spine, teach the patient how to apply it. Also teach him to logroll when he gets in and out of bed, to prevent back strain and twisting.

Discharge instructions. Before discharge (usually 6 to 10 days after surgery), make sure the patient understands the importance of resuming *activity* gradually. Have him start with a few short walks inside his home, then progress to longer walks outdoors. He should rest between activities to avoid overdoing it. He may prefer to lie down—rather than sit—to rest, because sitting adds stress on the spine. For the same reason, advise him to avoid long car trips at first. When sitting, he should prop his feet on a low stool so that his knees are higher than his hips—this keeps his lower back flat against the back of a chair. When standing, he should alternately place one foot on a low stool to straighten his lower back and relieve strain. Advise him to wear supportive shoes with a moderate heel, to avoid bending over or lifting heavy objects, and to use a firm mattress or bed board.

Tell him that he can resume *sexual activity* whenever he feels comfortable doing so, but suggest a side-lying or supine position to reduce back strain. Also, discuss any exercises the doctor will prescribe, such as the pelvic tilt, leg lifts, and toe pointing. Explain that he'll probably begin them about 2 months after surgery.

Instruct the patient or his caregiver about *daily care of the posterior surgical incision.* Advise him to shower facing the stream of water and not to soak his wound in the bath until the stitches have been removed (usually 1 to 2 weeks after surgery). Describe signs of infection to report to the doctor: redness, swelling, increased pain or tenderness, fever exceeding 102° F. (38.9° C.), or changes in drainage color or odor.

Sources of information and support

International Association for the Study of Pain
909 N.E. 43rd Street, Suite 306, Seattle, Wash. 98105-6020
(206) 547-6409

National Committee on the Treatment of Intractable Pain
P.O. Box 9553, Friendship Station, Washington, D.C. 20016-6717
(202) 965-7617

Further readings

Brooks, B.J. "Percutaneous Lumbar Discectomy: An Alternative to Lumbar Laminectomy," *Association of Operating Room Nursing* 49(5):1332, 1334-38, 1340-41, May 1989.
Brown, M.D., and Tompkins, J.S. "Pain Response Post-Chemonucleolysis or Disc Excision," *Spine* 14(3):321-26, March 1989.
Schretlen, E., and Spring, M. "Acute Disc: Trends in Treatment," *Canadian Nurse* 85(7):31-32, August 1989.

Learning about pelvic traction

Dear Patient:

The doctor has ordered pelvic traction for you. For about 2 weeks, you'll be spending most of your time in this device. You'll be allowed out of traction for about 4 hours a day to eat meals, use the bathroom, and perform other necessary activities.

Here's what to expect:

The traction setup
A beltlike device will be placed around your hipbones over the iliac crests. Make sure that you have the correct size belt. It should fit snugly.

Straps on each side of the belt attach to pulleys, which are attached to weights (8 to 10 pounds each). Each strap has its own pulley system. Your body weight provides countertraction.

How traction works
By exerting a pulling force on your body, traction aligns the lower spine and reduces pressure on the spinal nerve roots. This helps ease back pain and muscle spasms.

Proper positioning
The head of your bed will be raised 20 to 30 degrees. The traction will hold your lower legs parallel to the floor. Make sure to lie with your hips and knees flexed 30 degrees, so your back stays flat against the mattress. However, avoid lying totally flat. This hyperflexes the lumbar spine and may increase your pain.

Some cautions
Most patients feel comfortable in pelvic-belt traction. However, if your pain increases, contact the doctor. He may stop the traction or have you use it intermittently.

Because the traction device is attached directly to the skin, skin breakdown can occur. Remember to check your skin at least twice a day for signs of inflammation, such as redness and swelling.

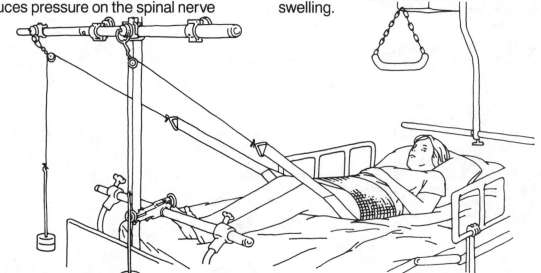

Congenital hip dysplasia

When teaching about congenital hip dysplasia (CHD), your biggest challenge may be dealing with anxious, perplexed parents. They may ask, "Why did this happen to our child?" "What did we do to cause it?" or "What did we neglect to do?" Besides explaining CHD and helping to assuage their feelings of guilt, your teaching must help them understand the importance of early treatment. In neonates, conservative measures like splinting can usually correct CHD. Older infants and children may require traction or surgery along with a hip spica cast.

Many parents may be bewildered by orthopedic devices and techniques such as traction. Reassure them that these devices won't cause their child pain or impede his growth and development.

Whatever technique is used, expect treatment to be long-term. Because children may face 2 to 6 months of hospitalization, you'll need to address parental feelings about separation from their child and the psychological effects of hospitalization. Parents will need patience and strength to cope with this. But long-term hospitalization can provide one teaching advantage: It may motivate parents to learn about home care. After all, the sooner they can master skills like cast care, the quicker their child will return home. To help develop confidence and competence, combine written instruction with return demonstration and allow ample time for asking questions.

Discuss the disorder

Describe CHD to parents as a common hip joint abnormality that's present at birth. Hip dislocation usually occurs at birth or shortly thereafter; occasionally, it occurs during fetal development. Explain the type of hip dysplasia their child has: unstable hip dysplasia, subluxation, or frank dislocation. In unstable hip dysplasia, the ligaments around the hip are lax, making the hip prone to dislocation. In subluxation, the head of the femur is partially displaced out of the acetabulum, whereas in frank dislocation, it's totally displaced (see *Comparing degrees of dysplasia*, page 406).

If parents ask about the cause of CHD, explain that this question has yet to be answered for certain. According to one theory, hormones that relax maternal ligaments in preparation for labor may also cause laxity of infant ligaments around the capsule

Madeline T. Albanese, RN, MSN, Marianne K. Ostrow, RN, BSN, and **Teresa A. Pellino, BSN, MS,** contributed to this chapter. Ms. Albanese, manager of patient education, and Ms. Ostrow, clinical nurse III, work at Thomas Jefferson University Hospital, Philadelphia. Ms. Pellino is a staff nurse in orthopedics at Meriter Hospital, Madison, Wis.

CHECKLIST

Teaching topics in CHD

☐ Explanation of the type of dysplasia: unstable hip dysplasia, subluxation, or frank dislocation
☐ Screening tests
☐ Importance of treatment to ensure a normal gait and to avoid degenerative joint disease later in life
☐ Explanation of selected treatment: external splinting, application of traction, or surgery (open or closed reduction)
☐ Child care in a hip spica cast or Pavlik harness
☐ Home traction
☐ Car seat safety

Comparing degrees of dysplasia

When teaching the parents of a child with congenital hip dysplasia (CHD), you'll need to clarify the extent of dysplasia. Begin by explaining how the head of the femur normally fits snugly into the acetabulum, allowing the hip to move properly. In CHD, flattening of the acetabulum prevents the head of the femur from rotating adequately. The hip may be unstable, subluxated (partially dislocated), or completely dislocated. Explain that the degree of dysplasia and the child's age determine the doctor's treatment choice.

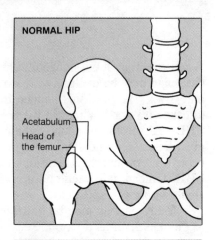

NORMAL HIP

Acetabulum

Head of the femur

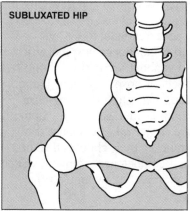

SUBLUXATED HIP

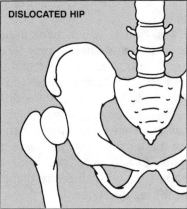

DISLOCATED HIP

of the hip joint. The disorder is 10 times more common after breech delivery than after cephalic delivery.

Complications

Emphasize to the parents that without treatment, a child with CHD will develop an abnormal gait and restricted mobility of the hip joint. The femur and acetabulum must fit together correctly to continue growing normally. Otherwise, the hip joint will lose the ability to move correctly. A unilateral dislocation will also shorten one of the child's legs, which may cause functional scoliosis. Bony abnormalities of the femur and acetabulum may also develop, possibly causing painful degenerative joint disease later in life.

Describe the diagnostic workup

Explain the clinical tests that the doctor may perform to detect CHD, including Ortolani's, Barlow's, and Trendelenburg's tests. Explain to the parents that during these tests, the doctor manipulates the child's hip to see if the femur fits snugly into the hip joint or if it slips out, which may indicate subluxation or dislocation (see *Ortolani's test*).

Also prepare parents for X-ray studies to evaluate the extent of dislocation and any bony abnormalities or soft-tissue contraction around the hip. Assure parents that the small amount of radiation used in these studies won't harm their child; X-ray shields are used to protect the genital area. During treatment, inform them that follow-up X-rays will be taken to ensure that the hip is healing properly.

Teach about treatments
Inform the parents that the earlier the infant receives treatment, the better his chance for normal development. Depending on his age, the patient may undergo external splinting, traction, or closed or open reduction.

Procedures
Typically, *external splinting* corrects CHD in neonates. Available devices include the Frejka pillow splint and the Pavlik harness. Usually the doctor will allow parents to apply and remove a splint if the hip is unstable but not dislocated. If so, teach them to do this, and review the schedule for wearing the splint. If the neonate has a harness, stress that parents mustn't remove it without the doctor's approval (see *Caring for your child in a Pavlik harness,* page 409).

If treatment is postponed until the infant is several months old, or if splinting proves unsuccessful, the patient may require *traction* to correct soft-tissue contraction around the hip joint. Explain to the parents that traction pulls down on the femur, stretching the muscles and soft tissues around the hip. This allows the femoral head to be reduced into the acetabulum. Traction may take several weeks or more, until X-rays show that the soft tissues have been stretched enough.

Assess the parents' ability to maintain traction at home, taking into account such factors as employment demands and the people available to help. If skin traction is to be used at home, teach the parents how to apply and maintain it. Tell them the hospital or home care agency will help them acquire equipment and show them how to set it up. Also teach them how to check neurovascular status. To prevent pooling of secretions in the pharyngeal cavity, which leads to otitis media, have them keep the child's head and trunk elevated whenever possible. (See the patient-teaching aids *How to set up traction using the Bradford frame,* page 410, and *Caring for your child in traction,* page 411.)

Surgery
To replace the head of the femur into the acetabulum, the doctor may perform closed or open reduction. Carried out in the operating room, both interventions require anesthesia. Explain to the parents that open reduction involves an incision (whereas closed reduction does not) and is usually necessary when soft tissue lies between the head of the femur and the acetabulum.

After reduction, the doctor may place the child in a series of

Ortolani's test

A technique for assessing congenital hip dysplasia (CHD), Ortolani's test may cause some discomfort. Warn parents that the child may fuss or cry.

To perform this test, place the infant supine with his hips and knees flexed at right angles. Abduct the thighs until the lateral aspects of the knees are almost touching the table. In CHD, the femoral head moving over the acetabular rim may produce a click or jerk. In an infant under 1 month old, this sound indicates subluxation. In an older infant, it may indicate subluxation or complete dislocation.

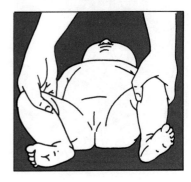

Car seat safety

Advise parents on car safety for a child wearing a Pavlik harness or a spica cast. Modifications may be needed for a commercially manufactured car seat. In this illustration, the plastic bucket of the car seat has been cut to accommodate a child with a hip spica cast. To ensure safety, though, a reputable testing organization should evaluate crashworthiness.

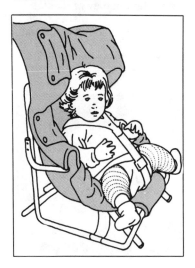

spica casts so that the hip joint can remodel. You'll need to teach the parents the basics of cast care (see *Caring for your child in a hip spica cast,* page 412). Their most challenging task will be keeping the cast clean. If the child has been toilet-trained, instruct them to tuck plastic wrap around the cast's edges to prevent soiling. If the child hasn't been toilet-trained, teach them how to diaper around the cast or describe available devices, such as the split Bradford frame, that help prevent soiling. Inform the parents that the child may need to wear a splint at night after cast removal. If so, teach them to apply it correctly.

Other care measures
If a child wears a Pavlik harness or a spica cast, inform the parents that modifications may have to be made to a commercially manufactured car seat to ensure the child's safety when riding in an automobile (see *Car seat safety*). The hospital or the doctor may be able to suggest modifications. For further information, refer parents to the organizations listed below.

Sources of information and support
American Academy of Pediatrics
Division of Public Education
141 Northwest Point Boulevard, P.O. Box 927, Elk Grove Village, Ill. 60007
(312) 228-5005

Automotive Safety for Children Program
James Whitcomb Riley Hospital for Children
Indiana University School of Medicine
702 Barnhill Drive, P-121, Indianapolis, Ind. 46223
(317) 264-2977

Evenflo Juvenile Furniture Company (Safe Passage Program)
1801 Commerce Drive, Piqua, Ohio 45356
(513) 773-3971

E-Z On Products, Inc. of Florida (safety vests and restraints)
500 Commerce Way, West, Jupiter, Fla. 33458
(312) 537-0066, (800) 323-6598

National Passenger Safety Association
1705 DeSales Street, N.W., Suite 300, Washington, D.C. 20036
(202) 429-0515

Further readings
Corbett, D. "Information Needs of Parents of a Child in a Pavlik Harness," *Orthopaedic Nursing* 7(2):20-23, March-April 1988.
Cuddy, C.M. "Caring for the Child in a Spica Cast: A Parent's Perspective," *Orthopaedic Nursing* 5(3):17-21, May-June 1986.
Feller, N., et al. "A Multidisciplinary Approach to Developing Safe Transportation for Children with Special Needs," *Orthopaedic Nursing* 5(5):25-27, September-October 1986.
Shesser, L.K., and Kling, T.F., Jr. "Practical Considerations in Caring for a Child in a Hip Spica Cast: An Evaluation Using Parental Input," *Orthopaedic Nursing* 5(3):11-15, May-June 1986.

PATIENT-TEACHING AID

Caring for your child in a Pavlik harness

Dear Parent:

The doctor has applied a Pavlik harness to correct your baby's hip problem. Carefully follow these guidelines at home.

An important caution
Never remove the harness without the doctor's approval. He probably won't let you remove it for any reason because removal may cause the baby's hip to dislocate again. However, if the hip is partially dislocated, he may let you remove the harness just for bathing.

Checking the harness
Several times a day check the straps to see if they've loosened. You can tell by checking the black lines that the doctor marked on the harness to show where the straps should pass through the buckles. Adjust as necessary.

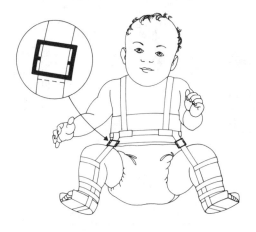

If the harness becomes fully unbuckled, call the doctor.

Bathing your baby
Give your baby a daily sponge bath and check his skin, especially under the straps, for irritation. Also gently massage the skin to stimulate circulation. Avoid using powder or lotion, which may become caked and irritate the skin.

Dressing and diapering your baby
With the doctor's approval, you can undo the shoulder straps to change your baby's shirt. Carefully adjusting these straps, as instructed, shouldn't affect the baby's hip position.

When changing your baby, fasten diaper ends *under* the straps so that the diaper doesn't pull on them. Use plastic pants with side snaps to keep the harness clean. Or choose disposable diapers with elastic legs.

Dress your baby in undershirts and one-piece stretch suits with a snap crotch under the harness, and put on high socks under the leg pieces to decrease skin irritation. Clothe your baby in baggy pants, sweatsuits, dresses, and buntings placed over the harness.

Cleaning the harness
If the harness becomes soiled, simply sponge it clean with a mild soap. If your baby has a subluxated hip, the doctor may let you remove the harness to wash it. But he'll give you another for the baby to wear in the meantime.

How to set up traction using the Bradford frame

Dear Parent:

The nurse will show you how to apply traction and allow you to practice so you'll feel more comfortable when doing it on your own. Use the following guidelines to reinforce the nurse's teaching when applying traction at home.

1 Attach the footboards and rope to moleskin strips. Place the moleskin strips (foam side against the skin) on your child's legs.

2 Apply the jacket restraint to your child, and secure it to the Bradford frame.

3 Now wrap the elastic bandage around the moleskin strips from your child's ankle to his groin in a diagonal, circular motion, keeping a small amount of tension on the bandage as you wrap.

4 Thread the cords attached to the footboards through the pulleys, and attach the weights.

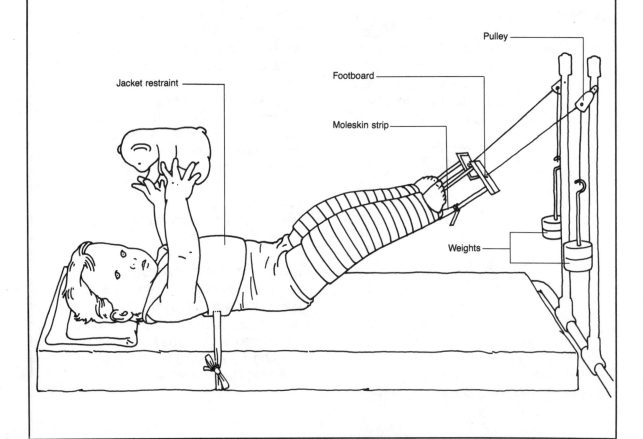

Jacket restraint

Pulley

Footboard

Moleskin strip

Weights

Caring for your child in traction

Dear Parent:

When your child arrives home, he'll be spending most of the time in traction. Use the following guidelines to help you care for him during this time.

Check circulation
Make sure you haven't wrapped the elastic bandage too tightly around your child's legs. To do this, check your child's toes by briefly pressing on his large toenail. Release when the skin under the toenail turns white.

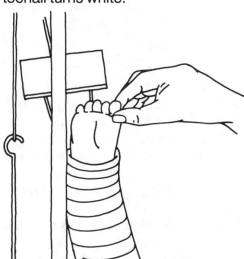

If normal pink color doesn't return quickly, remove the traction and keep pressing and releasing the toes. Reconnect your child to traction after normal color has returned. To avoid decreasing the circulation, wrap the elastic bandage less tightly this time. Also check your child's feet for color, warmth, and movement.

Check equipment
Rewrap traction at least every 4 hours. Make sure the traction weights hang freely, and inspect the cord to be sure it's moving properly over the pulleys. Replace a frayed cord.

Provide skin care
Check your child's skin pressure points, such as his buttocks and elbows, for irritation and redness. Place pieces of sheepskin beneath areas vulnerable to irritation.

Examine the back of your child's head for baldness. You may use a satin pillowcase to keep his hair from breaking and matting.

Show your emotions
Be sure to cuddle and touch your child when he's in traction. Your child needs stimulation and emotional support whether he's in or out of traction. Also provide books and toys to play with during this time.

Monitor free time
Your doctor will tell you how long (usually around 4 hours) your child is allowed out of traction. You may have to divide this time into several short periods, including bath time and mealtime. Be sure your child doesn't put weight on his legs during these periods. Elevate the head of your child's bed if he returns to traction after mealtime.

Caring for your child in a hip spica cast

Dear Parent:

To help your child's hip heal correctly, follow these instructions.

Check circulation
At least three times a day check your child's circulation by pressing on his large toenail until the skin under the nail turns white. Release pressure. If pink color doesn't return quickly, call the doctor. Also call him if the skin above or below the cast looks blue or mottled or if your child's toes feel cold and don't warm up when you cover them.

Check sensation
Several times a day squeeze your child's toes. If he pulls away or seems in pain or does not seem to feel you touching him, call the doctor. Also call him if your child seems unusually irritable or uncomfortable or keeps his feet and legs increasingly still.

Cleanse the skin
Every day wash the skin along the cast's edges using water and mild soap. Be sure to first cover the edges with plastic wrap. Also cleanse the skin you can reach under the cast, but don't wet the cast itself. Remove the wrap when you're finished. Finally, massage the skin under and along the cast's edges.

Check the skin
Every day inspect as far under the cast as possible. Look for possible irritants and redness. Place tape over any rough cast edges. To "petal" the cast with tape, put one end of the tape under the inside edge of the cast and secure to the lining. Pull the free end over the edge of the cast and secure it on the cast surface.

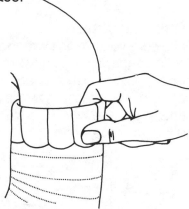

Call the doctor if you notice any object stuck in the cast, any change in the cast's fit, or a foul smell or fresh stain.

Don't let your child put anything inside the cast. To relieve any itching, try using a hair dryer set on "cool." Never apply lotion or powder in or around the cast.

Keep the cast dry and clean
If your child isn't toilet-trained, tuck a folded disposable diaper under the perineal edges of the cast (around the crotch area). To hold the diaper in place, fasten a second diaper around the cast.

If your child is toilet-trained, insert plastic wrap under the edges of the cast's perineal area before placing him on a bedpan. Be sure to remove the plastic after cleaning the child.

When the cast becomes dirty, clean it with a damp cloth and mild soap.

Fractures

Because fractures are relatively common, your patient may not regard the injury as serious. To help correct this misconception, you'll need to emphasize the reasons for complying with therapy and reporting signs of possible complications. Poor compliance, after all, can lead to permanent deformity or disability. Worse yet, it can lead to life-threatening complications, such as fat embolism and compartment syndrome.

Begin by explaining what happens when a bone fractures, so that your patient can understand his injury. Then teach him about treatments, such as those performed to realign displaced bone fragments and immobilize the injury. To promote recovery, teach him appropriate self-care measures. For example, he may need instruction on how to care for his cast, walk with crutches, and recognize possible complications. Finally, discuss ways to prevent common accidents, because most fractures result from them.

Discuss the disorder

Explain that a fracture is a partial or complete break in bone continuity. Typically, it results from major trauma, such as a fall or a skiing accident. A less common injury, called a fatigue fracture, occurs when normal bone is subjected to repeated stress. This type of fracture may result from prolonged standing, walking, or running. If the patient has a bone-weakening disease, such as osteoporosis or bone tumors, minor trauma or even normal activities may produce a pathologic fracture. (See *How bones break,* page 416.)

Fractures are classified by several criteria, such as their location, the direction of the fracture line, and the position of bony fragments. (See *Classifying fractures,* pages 414 and 415.) Tell the patient that healing begins almost immediately after a fracture occurs. Unlike other tissues, which heal by scar formation, bone heals through the regeneration of bone cells. For more information, give him a copy of the patient-teaching aid *How broken bones heal,* page 422.

Explain that the rate of healing depends on the type of fracture, although most heal within 6 months. Typically, arm bones heal quicker than leg bones. An impacted fracture, in which bone fragment ends are pushed into each other, may heal in several weeks. A displaced fracture, in which the fragments must be realigned to normal anatomic position, may take months or years to heal fully (see *Average healing times for fractures,* page 417)

Madeline P. Albanese, RN, MSN, ONC, who wrote this chapter, is manager of patient education at Thomas Jefferson University Hospital, Philadelphia.

CHECKLIST
Teaching topics in fractures

□ Explanation of the types of fractures and how bones heal
□ Possible complications, such as compartment syndrome and fat embolism
□ Diagnostic tests, such as X-rays and CT scan, if necessary
□ Limitations on activity and weight-bearing
□ Instructions for cast care, exercises for casted limbs, and crutch walking, if necessary
□ Importance of nutritious diet for bone healing
□ Analgesics and their possible adverse reactions
□ Procedures and surgery to align displaced bone fragments and immobilize the injury
□ Tips for preventing accidental fractures
□ Sources of information and support

Classifying fractures

To help your patient understand his injury and its treatment, teach him about his type of fracture. A fracture may be classified as:
- open—a fracture in which bone fragments penetrate the skin
- closed—a fracture that doesn't penetrate the skin
- complete—an interruption in bone continuity
- incomplete—an incomplete interruption in bone continuity

Then describe the fracture in terms of location. For example, in long bones, fractures are described as distal, proximal, or midshaft. Near a joint, fractures are called intracapsular or extracapsular. Within a joint, they're called intra-articular.

As described below, fractures are further classified by the direction of the fracture line and the position of bony fragments. Keep in mind that your patient's fracture may combine several types.

FRACTURE LINE DIRECTION

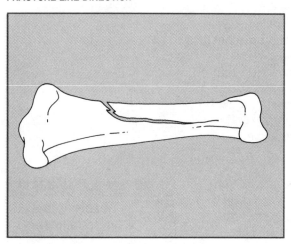

Longitudinal
Fracture line runs parallel to the bone axis

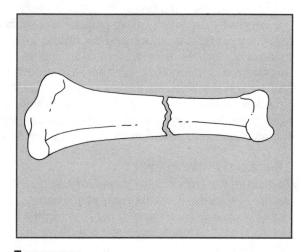

Transverse
Fracture line crosses the bone at a right angle to its axis

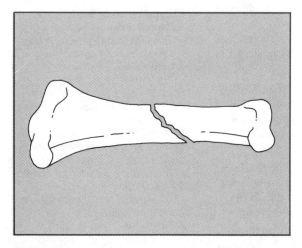

Oblique
Fracture line breaks the bone at a slanted angle to the bone's axis

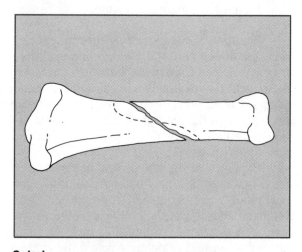

Spiral
Fracture line runs through the bone in a coil-like manner or twists around the bone, usually caused by torsion or a twisting force

continued

Classifying fractures— *continued*

BONY FRAGMENT POSITION

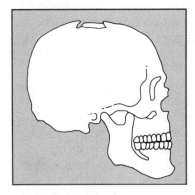

Depressed
Broken bone is driven inward

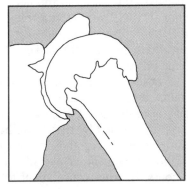

Impacted
One fragment is forced into or
onto another fragment

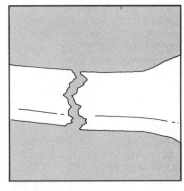

Nondisplaced
Fragments maintain
essentially normal alignment

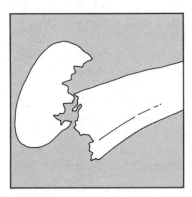

Displaced
Disrupted anatomic bone
relationships occur with deformity

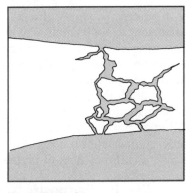

Comminuted
Three or more fragments

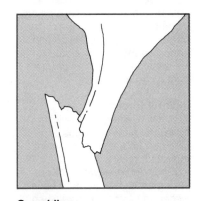

Overriding
Fragments overlap and
shorten total bone length

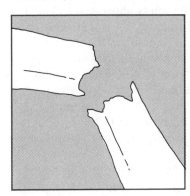

Angulated
Fragments deviate from their
normal linear alignment so that
they're at angles to each other

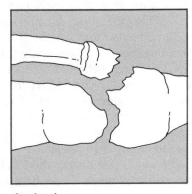

Avulsed
Fragments are pulled from their
normal position by forceful
muscle contractions or ligamen-
tous resistance

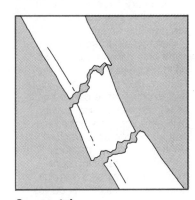

Segmental
Fractures occur in two adjacent
areas with an isolated central
segment

How bones break

Your patient may be surprised to learn he has a broken bone, especially if his fracture was caused by a low-energy force, such as a sudden twist to his leg. Explain that bones can absorb considerable force before breaking and that fractures can be caused by both direct and indirect forces.

Direct forces
A high-energy, violent force can cause serious fractures. Direct forces include:
• *wedging force,* which fractures the bone and propels a fragment into another fragment or into a joint
• *compression force,* which propels bones together, causing an incomplete fracture in which the cortex breaks on one side and bends on the opposite side
• *crushing force,* which splinters bones into fragments.

Indirect forces
This lower-energy, less-violent force can fracture bones at a distance from the impact point. Indirect forces include:
• *torsion force,* a twisting force strong enough to fracture bone
• *shearing force,* exerted when part of the bone is fixed, fracturing the part above or below
• *angulatory force,* exerted on an angle so that the bone fractures at that angle.

Sometimes a fracture will occur if only *minimal force* is applied. For example, a stress fracture may occur when fatigue and exercise have caused a small crack in a bone. Later, minimal force may extend the crack to a complete fracture.

After a fracture, the force that caused it (or resulting bone fragments) may also damage adjacent soft tissue, blood vessels, nerves, ligaments, muscles, and tendons, with subsequent edema, bleeding, and hematoma formation.

Complications
Inform the patient that complications may arise shortly after his injury or may develop later. Help him understand how he will be monitored for possible problems. Explain that bleeding normally occurs with a fracture, so his blood pressure will be routinely checked. Tell him that the neurovascular status of his involved limb also will be checked frequently, because fractures may be associated with vascular and nerve damage. To minimize such complications, remind him to keep his fractured limb elevated and immobilized.

Discuss compartment syndrome—a serious complication that, if untreated, may cause permanent dysfunction and deformity. It may arise suddenly, right after injury, or gradually, over several days. It's caused by tissue swelling within muscle groups, which compresses nerves and arteries, resulting in muscle ischemia. Without treatment, irreversible muscle damage may occur within 6 hours. Instruct your patient to immediately report early signs and symptoms of compartment syndrome: worsening pain that's unrelieved by analgesics, increased swelling, and numbness and tingling in the affected limb.

If the patient has a long-bone fracture, inform him that he'll be monitored for signs of a fat embolism. This potentially life-threatening complication may occur after the injury as the bone marrow releases fat into the veins. The fat can lodge in the lungs, obstructing breathing, or pass into the arteries, eventually affecting the central nervous system.

Caution the patient that failure to comply with treatment may cause malunion (fracture fragments that unite in an angulated or deformed position), delayed union (slow healing), or nonunion (absence of healing). Stress that these complications will delay his recovery and may lead to permanent deformity or disability.

Describe the diagnostic workup
Inform the patient that X-rays can diagnose most fractures. The diagnosis is confirmed by X-rays of the suspected fracture from two angles, as well as by X-rays of the joints above and below it.

If the patient has a complicated fracture, the doctor may order a computed tomography (CT) scan to confirm the diagnosis or plan treatment. Explain that a CT scan produces cross-sectional views of bone, helping to pinpoint abnormalities. Mention who will perform the test and where, and that it takes 30 to 90 minutes. If the patient's scheduled to receive a contrast medium, tell him not to eat or drink for 4 hours before the test. Tell him to wear a hospital gown, to remove all jewelry, and just before the test, to empty his bladder.

Explain that during the test he'll lie on a table within a large tunnel-like scanner. Then, he may be given a contrast medium. The table will move a small distance every few seconds during the test. Tell him that the scanner will rotate around him and may make a clicking or buzzing sound. Instruct him to remain still during the test. Although he'll be alone in the room, assure him that he can talk to the technician through an intercom. If the patient received a contrast medium, encourage him to drink plenty of fluids afterward to help expel it.

Teach about treatments

Explain that treatment aims to restore function and motion to the injured part. Stress the importance of limiting activity and weight-bearing to allow the fracture to mend properly. Encourage the patient to eat a well-balanced diet to obtain essential nutrients for bone healing. Depending on the treatment plan, teach him about procedures to heal the fracture and how to care for his cast and use crutches.

Activity

Inform the patient that he may need to curtail his activities to give his fracture time to heal. Initially, he may be in traction or confined to bed. Tell him that the doctor will decide when he should begin a program of passive and active range-of-motion exercises, as well as start to use his injured body part. If he's wearing a cast, give him a copy of the patient-teaching aid, *Exercises for casted limbs,* pages 428 and 429.

Instruct him to reduce or eliminate weight-bearing on his injured limb, as his doctor recommends. Teach him how to use crutches or other assistive devices for ambulation. To help him review your instructions, give him a copy of the patient-teaching aids, *Choosing crutches,* page 430, *Learning to walk with crutches,* pages 431 and 432, and *Using crutches on stairs and with chairs,* pages 433 and 434.

Diet

Stress the importance of following a nutritious diet to promote bone healing. Encourage the patient to eat foods rich in vitamin C (such as citrus fruits and tomatoes) and calcium (such as dairy products, salmon, and broccoli). Tell him that these nutrients are necessary for bone repair. Also advise him to get adequate vitamin D (found in fortified milk and produced by sun-exposed skin), because this vitamin promotes calcium absorption and bone remodeling. Tell him to eat adequate protein and vitamin A (found in carrots, sweet potatoes, and other yellow or orange fruits and vegetables) for proper wound healing. If his diet lacks these nutrients, mention that the doctor may prescribe calcium and vitamin D supplements.

Medication

Inform the patient that the doctor may prescribe narcotic or non-narcotic analgesics to reduce pain. The nonnarcotic analgesics of choice are acetaminophen and nonsteroidal anti-inflammatory drugs (NSAIDs).

If the patient is taking a narcotic analgesic, such as codeine, advise him to avoid activities that require alertness. Tell him to report a rash, itching, or GI upset. If the drug causes constipation, instruct him to check with his doctor about using a stool softener.

Tell the patient taking an NSAID that the drug may cause GI upset and bleeding. Instruct him to report loss of appetite, nausea, vomiting, diarrhea, or other GI symptoms. Urge him to call his doctor immediately if he has black, tarry stools or bloody vomit—signs of GI bleeding.

Average healing times for fractures

"How long will it be until my broken bone is healed?" Expect to hear that question often from patients with fractures. Using the chart below, give your patient an estimate of the healing time for his fracture. Remind him, though, that his own fracture may require more or less time to mend than average. Emphasize that he can speed recovery by complying with his prescribed treatment and rehabilitation.

BONE	WEEKS OF HEALING TIME
Collar bone	6
Upper arm	
Neck	6
Shaft	12
Forearm	
Both bones	12
One bone	6
Hand	6-10
Finger	3
Hip	12
Upper leg	16-24
Lower leg (tibia)	
Plateau	8
Shaft	16-24
Ankle	8-12
Lower leg (fibula)	
Shaft	8
Ankle	8
Heel	8-12
Foot	8
Toe	3

If the patient has an open fracture or is undergoing surgery, explain that the doctor will prescribe antibiotics to prevent infection.

Procedures

Inform the patient that the first step in healing his fracture is to correct the alignment of bone fragments—a procedure called reduction. The next step is to immobilize the injury with a cast, splint, or other support to prevent dislocation of the bone fragments and to aid healing.

Closed reduction. For most fractures, closed reduction is the treatment of choice. Explain that the doctor manipulates the limb to lock the ends of the bone fragments together and restore normal alignment. In some patients, traction may be used to achieve closed reduction. (See *Comparing traction techniques.*)

If the patient is undergoing closed reduction by manipulation, assure him that he will receive a sedative, an I.V. muscle relaxant, or local anesthetic to relieve pain. If the fracture is severe, he may receive a general anesthetic.

Immobilization. After the fracture has been reduced, specify the patient's type of immobilization—sling, splint, cast, brace, or other external support. If the limb is markedly swollen, inform the patient that he may have a temporary splint. If he needs a cast, give him a copy of the patient-teaching aids, *How to care for your cast,* pages 423 to 425, and *Troubleshooting your casted limb,* pages 426 and 427.

Cast bracing or a molded orthosis also may be prescribed for immobilization. These devices help support the fracture, preventing further displacement of the bone fragment ends. Explain that hinges in these supports permit some exercise and use of joints around the fracture. Emphasize that wearing a brace or molded orthosis will speed the patient's recovery.

Surgery

If closed reduction isn't possible or advisable, tell the patient that open reduction will be necessary to restore normal alignment of bone fragments. Open reduction may be achieved by internal or external fixation.

Open reduction with internal fixation. This surgery involves inserting internal fixation devices—pins, screws, nails, wires, rods, or plates—into the affected bones to maintain positioning during healing.

Tell the patient that internal fixation has several benefits, such as earlier return of function than with external fixation or skeletal traction. The patient also may not need to wear a cast or other immobilizing device. On the other hand, internal fixation increases the risk of infection, because the fracture site is surgically opened.

Prepare the patient for surgery, and instruct him on any postoperative activity restrictions. Advise him to report signs and symptoms of possible complications, such as redness, tenderness, swelling, drainage, or increasing pain in the affected limb. Assure the patient that the body tolerates internal fixation devices well.

Comparing traction techniques

Mention the word "traction," and your patient may picture himself helpless, imprisoned in a cast with his limbs suspended in mid-air. If your patient is undergoing traction, clear up any misconceptions he may have. Start by explaining that traction can reduce muscle spasms and restore broken bone ends to their normal alignment. Traction also can be a definitive treatment to reduce and immobilize a fracture.

Inform the patient about the several types of traction. Depending on his treatment plan, the patient may be confined to bed for an extended period, and movement of his affected limb or body part will be restricted. If so, reassure him that he can continue to exercise his unaffected body parts during treatment. If traction is being used to reduce a fracture, tell him that X-rays will be taken periodically to check if the bone ends are correctly aligned.

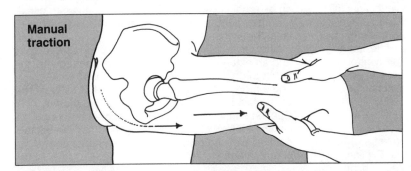

Manual traction

This traction technique temporarily immobilizes an injured area through hands pulling on the injured body part. It can be used before more permanent traction and while applying a cast.

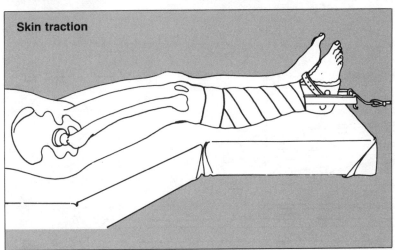

Skin traction

This technique immobilizes a body part intermittently over an extended period by directly applying a pulling force on the patient's skin. The force may be applied using adhesive or nonadhesive traction tape or other skin traction devices, such as a boot, belt, or halter. Adhesive attachment allows more continuous traction, whereas nonadhesive attachment allows easier removal for daily care. Skin traction is commonly used to decrease muscle spasms preoperatively in the hip fracture patient.

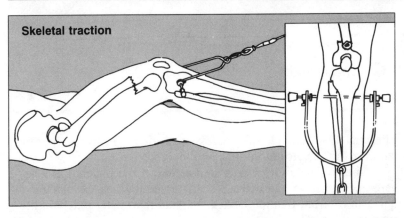

Skeletal traction

Skeletal traction immobilizes a body part for prolonged periods by attaching weighted equipment directly to the patient's bones with pins, screws, wires, or tongs. It allows more prolonged traction with heavier weight than do the other two techniques. Skeletal traction is commonly used in femoral fractures and cervical spine fractures. It may also be used to reduce some fractures.

Mending fractures with motion and stimulation

Your patient may require additional treatment to speed bone healing and restore mobility. In particular, you may need to teach the patient about two advanced treatments—continuous passive motion (CPM) and electrical bone growth stimulation.

Continuous passive motion
This treatment employs an electrically or manually powered machine (shown below) to move a joint through its normal range of motion for an extended period. CPM is used to minimize or prevent joint stiffness during recovery from internal fixation of knee or ankle fractures. It also may be used with traction.

Set the machine's speed and degree of flexion as ordered. Teach the patient how to use the control cord to stop and start the machine as prescribed. Explain that the duration of treatment depends on his injury and rehabilitation plan.

Electrical stimulation
This treatment is usually reserved for patients whose fractures fail to heal within 6 to 9 months. Explain that a mild electric current will be directed at bone fracture fragments to help stimulate new bone growth and speed healing.

Three types of stimulators are currently used. The *invasive stimulator* consists of electrodes and a power source implanted under the skin. Instruct the patient to follow his doctor's advice on weight-bearing and activity restrictions. Tell him treatment usually lasts 5 to 6 months.

The *semi-invasive stimulator* involves the insertion of electrodes under the skin at the fracture site, with an external power source. Teach the patient to avoid weight-bearing during this treatment, which typically lasts 3 months.

The *noninvasive stimulator* uses external wire coils and an external power source at the fracture site. Instruct the patient to use the device for 10 to 12 hours a day, or as ordered. Suggest that he wear the coils while sleeping to avoid interrupting therapy. Caution him to avoid weight-bearing as ordered. Teach him how to test the unit and to call the doctor if it isn't working properly or if the external power source alarm signals.

CONTINUOUS PASSIVE MOTION MACHINE

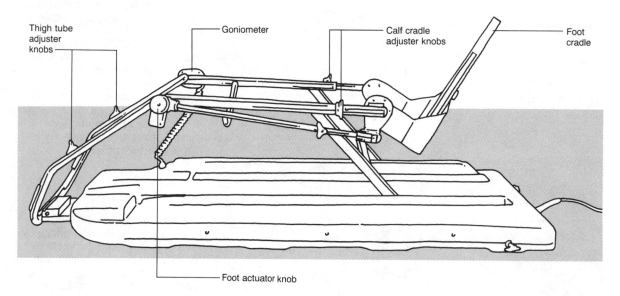

Thigh tube adjuster knobs — Goniometer — Calf cradle adjuster knobs — Foot cradle — Foot actuator knob

The implants are made of stainless steel, titanium, or Vitallium (an alloy of cobalt, chromium, and molybdenum).

Open reduction with external fixation. If the patient has a severe open fracture and extensive soft tissue injuries, he may require an external fixation device. Explain that metal pins will be surgically inserted above and below the fracture to hold bones and bone fragments together, then the pins will be securely attached to the device's frame.

Assure the patient that an external fixation device, once in place, won't hurt. Teach him to clean his external pins daily with alcohol, soap and water, or a half-strength solution of saline and peroxide. Instruct him on proper wound care. Advise him to watch for and report signs and symptoms of complications, such as redness, tenderness, swelling, drainage at the surgical site, or loose pins.

Other care measures

Encourage the patient to participate in his rehabilitation program, which may include physical and occupational therapy. If appropriate, explain that he may be treated with continuous passive motion to regain movement of joints near the fracture site, or electric bone growth stimulation to speed healing. (See *Mending fractures with motion and stimulation*.)

Because most fractures result from trauma, address safety issues. For example, teach an elderly patient how to prevent falls at home, such as by installing safety rails around the shower or bath. If the patient needs crutches or other ambulatory devices, make sure he knows how to use this equipment safely. Suggest that he wear nonskid, flat-soled supportive shoes. Advise him to remove throw rugs and avoid walking on slippery, wet, or waxed floors.

Sources of information and support

American Association of Orthopedic Medicine
926 East McDowell Road, #202, Phoenix, Ariz. 85006
(602) 254-5315

American Fracture Association
P.O. Box 668, Bloomingham, Ill. 61701
(309) 663-6272

Further readings

Cruwys, A. "Ankle Fracture," *Nursing Times* 84(1):52-55, January 6-12, 1988.
Dubrovskis, V., and Wells, D. "Hip Fracture in the Elderly: Program Planning Puts These Patients on Their Feet Again," *Canadian Nurse* 84(5):20-22, May 1988.
Hansell, M.J. "Fractures and the Healing Process," *Orthopedic Nursing* 7(1):43-50, January-February 1988.
Hughes, J.H. "Critical Decisions in Managing Fractured Ribs," *Hospital Medicine* 23(12):25, 29-30, 31-33, December 1987.
"Internal Fixation for Open Fractures," *Patient Care* 21(14):25, September 15, 1988.
Mullin, W.J. "A Patient's-eye View," *Canadian Orthopaedic Nurses Association Journal* 9(4):13, December 1987.
Pryor, G.A., et al. "Team Management of the Elderly Patient with Hip Fracture," *Lancet* 1(8582): 401-03, February 20, 1988.
Tomford, W. "Basics of Broken Bones for the Nonorthopedist," *Emergency Medicine* 19(15):24-28, 30-32, 43, September 15, 1987.

How broken bones heal

Dear Patient:

A broken bone starts to heal the moment the break occurs. But rigid bone tissue fragments take a long time to reestablish a firm union. That's why you should continue your rehabilitation program, even after your injured bone seems normal again.

Here are the stages your broken bone goes through when it heals.

Blood collects at the site

First, blood collects around the broken bone ends, forming a sticky, jellylike mass called a clot. Within 24 hours, a meshlike network forms from the clot. This becomes the framework for growing new bone tissue.

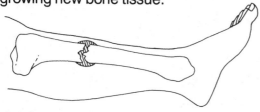

Cells start bone healing

Soon, osteoclasts and osteoblasts—the cells that do the bone healing—invade this clot. *Osteoclasts* start smoothing the jagged edges of bone. Meanwhile, *osteoblasts* start bridging the gap between the bone ends. Within a few

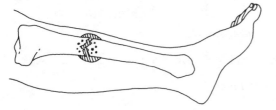

days, these cells form a granular bridge, linking the bone ends.

Callus forms

Six to ten days after the injury, the granular bridge of cells becomes a bony mass called a callus, which eventually hardens into solid bone.

But for now, the callus is fragile, and abrupt motion can split it. That's why keeping a broken bone from moving while it's healing is so important.

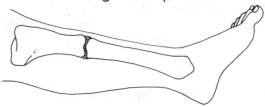

Bone hardens

Three to ten weeks after the injury, new blood vessels start bringing calcium to the area to harden the new bone tissue. This process is called ossification, in which the ends of the bones "knit" together.

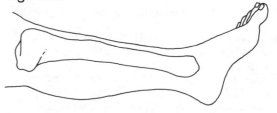

After ossification, the bone becomes solid and is considered healed. Although the cast may be removed, up to a year may pass before the healed bone is as strong as it was before the break.

How to care for your cast

Dear Patient:

Think of your new cast as a temporary body part—one that needs the same attentive care as the rest of you. While you wear your cast, follow these guidelines.

Speeding up drying time
The doctor may apply a cast made of plaster, fiberglass, or a synthetic material. The wet material must dry thoroughly and evenly for the cast to support your broken bone properly. At first, your wet cast will feel heavy and warm. But don't worry—it will get lighter as it dries.

To speed drying, keep the cast exposed to the air. Fiberglass and synthetic casts dry soon after application, but plaster casts don't (a plaster arm or leg cast dries in about 24 to 48 hours). Obviously, drying a plaster cast in less time makes it more comfortable sooner.

When you raise the cast with pillows, make sure the pillows have rubber or plastic covers under the linen case. Use a thin towel placed between the cast and the pillows to absorb moisture. Never place a wet cast directly onto plastic.

Drying evenly
To make sure the cast dries evenly, change its position on the pillows every 2 hours—using your palms, not your

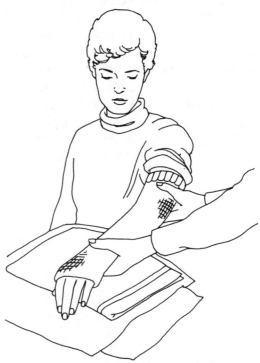

fingertips. (You can have someone else move the cast for you, if necessary.) To avoid creating bumps *inside the cast*—bumps that could cause skin irritation or sores—don't poke at the cast with your fingers while it's wet. Also, be careful not to dent the cast while it's still wet.

Keeping your cast clean
After your cast dries, you can remove dirt and stains with a damp cloth and powdered kitchen cleaner. Use as little water as possible, and wipe off any moisture that remains when you're done.

continued

PATIENT-TEACHING AID

How to care for your cast — *continued*

Protecting your cast

Avoid knocking your cast against any hard surface. To protect the foot of a leg cast from breakage, scrapes, and dirt, place a piece of used carpet (or a carpet square) over the bottom of the cast. Slash or cut a V-shape at the back, so the carpet fits around the heel when you bring it up toward the ankle. Hold the carpet in place with a large sock or slipper sock. Extending the carpet out beyond the toes a little also will help prevent bumped or stubbed toes.

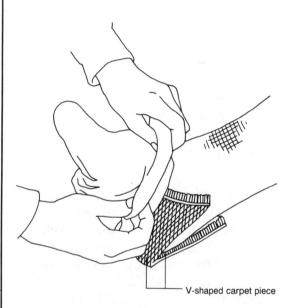

V-shaped carpet piece

Preventing snags

To keep an arm cast from snagging clothing and furniture, make a cast cover from an old nylon stocking. Cut the stocking's toe off, and cut a hole in the heel. Then, pull the stocking over the cast to cover it. Extend your fingers through the cut-off toe end, and poke your thumb through the hole you cut in the heel. Trim the other end of the stocking to about 1½ inches longer than the cast, and tuck the ends of the stocking under the cast's edges.

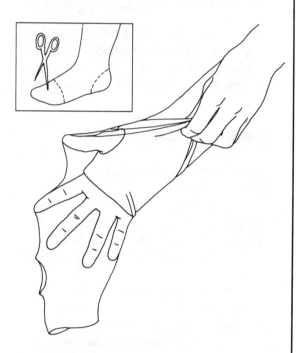

Caring for your skin

Wash the skin along the cast's edges every day, using a mild soap. Before you begin, protect the cast's edges with plastic wrap. Then, use a washcloth wrung out in soapy water to clean the skin at the cast's edges and as far as you can reach inside the cast. (Avoid getting the cast wet.) Afterward, dry the skin thoroughly with a towel, then massage the skin at and beneath the cast's edges with a towel or pad saturated with rubbing alcohol. (This helps toughen the skin.) To help prevent skin irritation, remove any loose plaster particles you can reach inside the cast.

continued

How to care for your cast — *continued*

Relieving itching

No matter how itchy the skin under your cast may feel, *never* try to relieve the itch by inserting a sharp or pointed object into the cast. This could damage your skin and lead to infection. Don't put powder or lotion in your cast, either, or stuff cotton or toilet tissue under the cast's edges (this may cut down on your circulation).

Here's a safe technique to relieve itching: Set a hand-held blow-dryer on "cool" and aim it at the problem area.

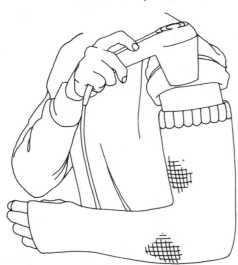

Staying dry

If you have a plaster cast, you'll need to cover it with a plastic bag before you shower, swim, or go out in wet weather. You can use a garbage bag or a cast shower bag, which you can buy at a drug store or medical supply store. *Above all, don't get a plaster cast wet.* Moisture will weaken or even destroy it. If the cast gets a little wet, let it dry naturally, such as by sitting in the sun. Don't cover the cast until it's all dry.

If you have a fiberglass or synthetic cast, check with your doctor to find out if you may bathe, shower, or swim. If he does allow you to swim, he'll probably tell you to flush the cast with cool tap water after swimming in a chlorinated pool or a lake. (Make sure that no foreign material remains trapped inside the cast.)

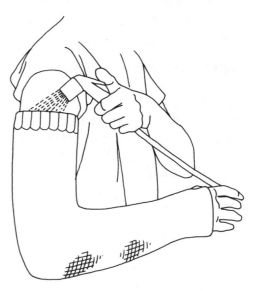

To dry a fiberglass or synthetic cast, first wrap the cast in a towel. Then, prop it on a pad of towels to absorb any remaining water. The cast will air-dry in 3 to 4 hours; to speed drying, use a hand-held blow-dryer.

Signing the cast

Family members and friends may want to sign their names or draw pictures on the cast. That's okay, but don't let them paint over large cast areas. Why? Because this could make those areas nonporous and damage the skin beneath them.

Troubleshooting your casted limb

Dear Patient:

After you leave the hospital, you'll need to check for possible problems with your casted limb, such as wound drainage or excessive swelling. Get in the habit of checking your cast every day.

Watch for wound drainage

When a cast also covers a wound, you can expect some red or reddish-brown drainage during the first 48 hours after the cast is applied. Drainage may stain the cast or, if it leaks from the cast's ends, the bed linens. If drainage occurs, use a felt-tipped pen to outline it on the cast. Jot down the date and time, too.

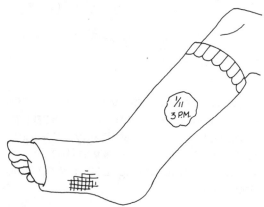

Drainage may signal a problem that requires the doctor's attention. *Notify the doctor* if the drainage:
• stains the cast or bed linens bright red.
• occurs even though the cast wasn't applied over a wound (pressure from the cast may have caused a sore).
• changes in odor or color (this may indicate infection).
• spreads.

Test sensation and movement

Several times a day, check for changes in sensation by touching the area above and below the cast. Do you feel any numbness, tingling, or pain?

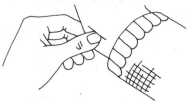

Wiggle your fingers or toes on the casted arm or leg. If you can't move your fingers or toes, or if you have more pain than usual when you move them, contact the doctor.

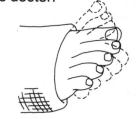

Check circulation

Press a fingernail or large toenail of the casted limb until the color fades. Then let go.

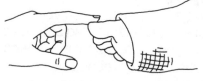

If normal flesh color doesn't return quickly (within 3 seconds), contact the doctor at once. Repeat this check at least three times a day.

If your fingers or toes are cold, first try covering them. If that doesn't warm them, contact the doctor.

continued

PATIENT-TEACHING AID

Troubleshooting your casted limb — *continued*

Look for swelling

A little swelling of a casted limb is normal, but a lot isn't. To help prevent excessive swelling, keep the cast raised above heart level, as much as possible, on two regular-size pillows. Apply ice as directed by your doctor. If your leg's in a cast, sit or lie down and raise the leg on pillows.

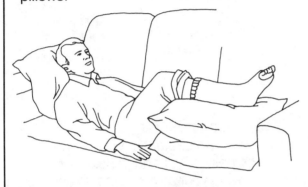

If your arm's in a cast, prop the arm so that your hand and elbow are higher than your heart. (Call your doctor if raising the cast *doesn't* reduce the swelling.)

Check for severe swelling above and below the cast several times daily. To do this, compare the casted limb with the healthy one.

Relieve skin irritation

After the cast dries completely, rough edges may cause skin irritation. To smooth them, try these techniques.

If the cast is fiberglass, remove rough edges by filing with a nail file. If the cast is plaster, "petal" rough edges using adhesive tape or moleskin. This prevents catching the material on clothing or peeling it off accidentally.

To petal a plaster cast, first cut several 4-inch by 2-inch strips of tape or

moleskin and trim the ends that will be outside the cast so they're rounded, like toenails.

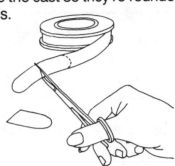

Next, place the first strip, rounded end down, on the outside of the cast.

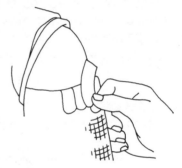

Then tuck the straight end just inside the cast edge.

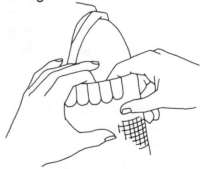

Smooth the tape or moleskin with your finger to remove any creases, which can also irritate your skin.

Now apply the remaining strips. Overlap them, as needed, until you've covered all the cast's rough edges.

Exercises for casted limbs

Dear Patient:

Depending on which of your limbs has a cast, the doctor may recommend exercises for any of its joints not covered by the cast. Exercising a joint will help keep the entire limb strong and help to reduce or prevent swelling.

Your doctor will give you instructions for which exercises you should do. As he directs, do your exercises at least three times a day, several times each. If you feel pain when you do any exercise or have trouble moving any of the joints, call the doctor.

Finger exercise

Hold up your hand and separate the fingers; then, close them up.

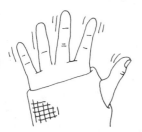 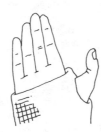

Next, hold up your hand and touch the little finger and thumb together. Repeat with the other three fingers.

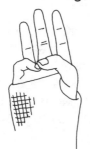

Finally, bend all the fingers on your hand up and down, as though waving goodbye.

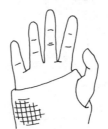 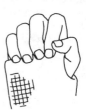

Shoulder exercise

With your arm straight down at your side and the palm of your hand next to your body, swing your arm out and up until it's even with your shoulder. Now bring your arm back to your side, then swing it across your chest toward your other arm. If necessary, use your unaffected arm to help lift the injured arm up to shoulder level. Then bring the casted arm back to your side.

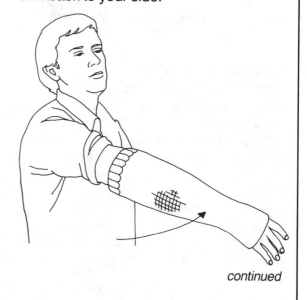

continued

Exercises for casted limbs — *continued*

Wrist exercise

Rest your forearm on the arm of a chair. Extend your hand straight out with your palm down. Slowly bend your wrist up and down to raise and lower your hand.

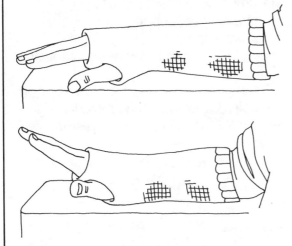

Ankle exercise

Make a circle with your foot, first moving it clockwise, then counterclockwise.

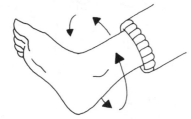

Next, stretch your foot so your toes reach back toward you. Then reverse this position, so your toes stretch away from you.

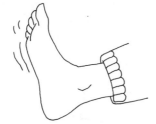

Toe exercise

Flex and wiggle your toes.

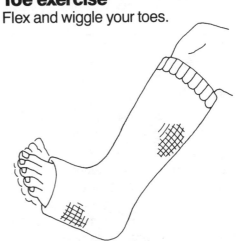

Hip exercise

Sit in the middle of your bed with both legs extended directly in front of you. Move the casted leg slowly out to the side, as far as it will comfortably go. Then, move it slowly back to its original position.

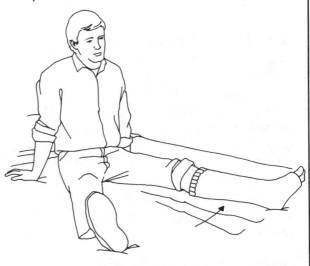

Next, lie flat on your back and bend your casted leg at the knee. Move it to your chest and then back to the bed.

Choosing crutches

Dear Patient:

Your doctor wants you to use crutches to reduce or eliminate the amount of weight you put on your casted leg or foot. Using crutches helps to speed the healing process by taking pressure off your injured bone as you stand or walk.

Before you select a pair of crutches, put them to the test. Ask yourself these questions to determine if you've found the right ones.

Are the crutches in good condition?

Make sure that your crutches have rubber tips, to prevent sliding. Also make sure they have padded underarm pieces for comfort.

Are they the right size?

Stand with your crutches, and place their tips about 6 inches from the sides of your feet. Check to see if the underarm pieces come to about 1 to 1½ inches (roughly 2 finger widths) below your armpits. If the underarm pieces touch your armpits, the crutches are too long. Ask the doctor to shorten them. Remember, you should support your weight with the handgrips, not the crutch tops.

Do they cause problems?

Support yourself by distributing your weight on your hands, wrists, and arms.

If you feel any tingling or numbness in the side of your chest below your armpits or in your upper arms, you're probably using the crutches improperly — or you may need to adjust their size or fit.

It's important to use your crutches correctly. Otherwise, they may damage the nerves in your armpits or palms.

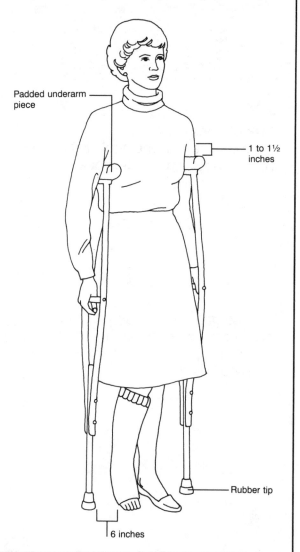

Padded underarm piece

1 to 1½ inches

Rubber tip

6 inches

Learning to walk with crutches

Dear Patient:

Learning to walk with crutches requires time and patience. You'll use one of the techniques described below.

Crutch-walking with *partial* weight on your injured leg

The doctor may allow you to place some of your weight on the injured leg. To do this, look over the diagrams below. They show how to walk with crutches if your right leg is injured. (If your left leg is the injured one, place most of your weight on your right leg, and adapt the instructions. You may want to draw the step patterns for yourself.)

1 Stand straight, with your shoulders relaxed and your arms slightly bent. Lean your body slightly forward, distributing your weight between the crutches and your uninjured leg. You can put some weight on your injured leg (shown as the patterned foot).

2 Move the crutches forward. Then move your *injured* leg up to meet them.

3 Put some weight on your injured leg as you move your *uninjured* leg *ahead* of the crutches.

Now repeat these steps to keep walking.

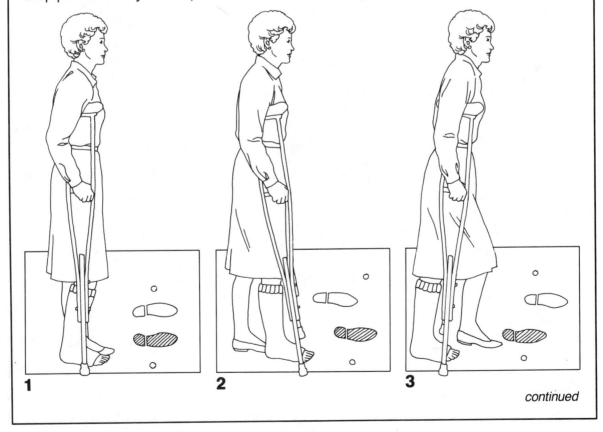

1

2

3

continued

Learning to walk with crutches — *continued*

Crutch-walking with *no* weight on your injured leg

If the doctor says you shouldn't put any weight on your injured leg while walking with crutches, use the method below.

The step patterns below show how to walk with crutches if your left leg is injured. (If your right leg is injured, rest your weight on your left leg, and adapt the instructions. You may want to draw the step patterns for yourself.)

1 Stand straight, with all your weight on your *uninjured* leg. Relax your shoulders. Hold the foot of your *injured* leg off the floor, flexing your knee slightly.

Balancing all your weight on the crutches, position the uninjured leg's foot so it's even with the crutch tips, slightly in front of you. Use the uninjured leg and the crutches to support your weight as you lean your body slightly forward.

2 Shift *all* your weight to the uninjured leg and move the crutches forward together, swinging the injured leg along with them. *Don't put any weight on your injured leg!*

3 Now shift all your weight back to the crutches via your hands and wrists, swing your uninjured leg forward, and again place all your weight on this leg — using the crutches to keep your balance.

To keep walking, repeat steps 2 and 3.

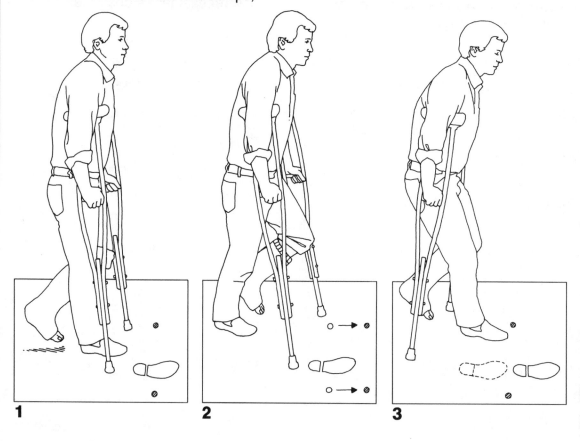

Using crutches on stairs and with chairs

Dear Patient:

Climbing stairs and getting into and out of a chair with your crutches may seem hard. Put yourself at ease, and do these maneuvers slowly at first. The following guidelines will help.

How to climb stairs

If the banister is on your left side and your right leg is injured, follow the directions below.

1 Standing at the bottom of the stairs, shift both crutches to your right hand. Then grasp the banister firmly with your left hand. Using your right hand, carefully support your weight on the crutches.

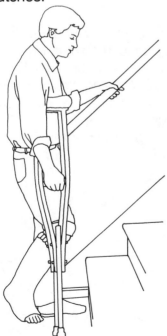

2 Next, push down on your crutches and hop onto the first step, using just your uninjured leg. Lift your injured leg as you go.

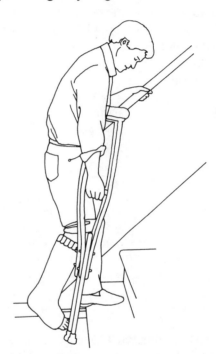

Support your weight on that leg as you continue to grasp the banister tightly. Then swing the crutches up onto the first step. Now hop onto the second step, using your uninjured leg. Repeat this procedure, but go slowly.

To get down the stairs, reverse these maneuvers. But always advance the crutches and your injured leg *first.* Remember: Your strong leg goes up first and comes down last.

continued

PATIENT-TEACHING AID

Using crutches on stairs and with chairs — *continued*

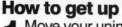

How to sit down

1 Using your crutches, walk over to the chair. Turn around, and step backward until the back of your uninjured leg touches the chair's front edge.

2 Keeping your weight on your uninjured leg, transfer both crutches to the hand on the same side as your injured leg. Support most of your weight on your crutches. Next, reach back with your other hand and grasp the chair arm.

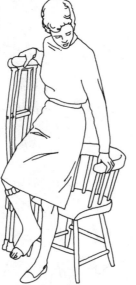

3 Carefully sit down, making sure to keep your weight off your injured leg. Keep your crutches next to the chair.

How to get up

1 Move your uninjured leg backward until it touches the back of the chair's front edge. While you're still sitting, take the crutches and stand them upright.

2 Using the hand on the same side as your injured leg, hold onto the handgrips. With your other hand, hold onto the chair arm.

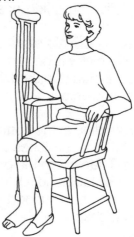

3 Slide forward, with your uninjured leg slightly under the chair. Push yourself up onto your uninjured leg. Once you're standing, transfer a crutch to your uninjured side. Or push yourself up while grasping the hand grip of a crutch in each hand.

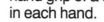

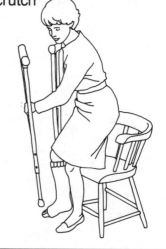

Carpal tunnel syndrome

A serious occupational health problem, carpal tunnel syndrome affects people who repetitively and strenuously use their hands. It's most common in women between ages 30 and 60. Occupations of affected people range from homemakers and computer operators to assembly line workers, meat cutters, machinists, mechanics, and carpenters.

Your teaching will emphasize that recovery depends almost entirely on compliance with treatment. You'll pinpoint activities that trigger or aggravate the disorder and suggest ways to avoid or modify them. For instance, you could suggest how the patient can modify her hand motions at home and at work. You'll also describe medications for pain and inflammation, immobilization devices, surgery, and strengthening exercises. Of course, your teaching will cover related topics, such as the pathophysiology of carpal tunnel syndrome, the physical examination, and electrophysiologic tests.

Discuss the disorder

Explore the patient's symptoms. Carpal tunnel syndrome causes weakness, pain, burning, numbness, or tingling in one or both hands. Sometimes these symptoms extend to the forearm (or the shoulder in severe cases). Other signs and symptoms include paresthesia of the thumb, index, and middle fingers, and half of the ring finger; inability to make a fist; atrophy of the fingernails; and dry, shiny skin on the hands and fingers. Vasodilation and venous stasis may cause some symptoms to intensify at night and in the morning. Usually, the patient can relieve the discomfort by vigorously shaking her hands or dangling her arms at her sides.

One of the most common entrapment neuropathies, carpal tunnel syndrome occurs when the median nerve is compressed where it passes through the carpal tunnel (for more information, see *Locating the carpal tunnel,* page 436). Explain that the median nerve controls many types of movement in the forearm, wrist, and hand, such as turning the wrist toward the body, flexing the index and middle fingers, and many thumb movements. It also supplies sensation to the index, middle, and ring fingers. Compression of this nerve causes loss of movement and sensation in the wrist, hand, and fingers.

Inform the patient that the exact cause of carpal tunnel syndrome remains unknown. However, some edema-causing conditions, such as diabetes, rheumatoid arthritis, pregnancy,

Julie Tackenberg, RN, MA, CNRN, who wrote this chapter, is a clinical specialist at the University Medical Center in Tucson, Ariz.

CHECKLIST

Teaching topics in carpal tunnel syndrome

☐ Anatomy and function of the median nerve and carpal tunnel
☐ Relationship between repetitive wrist activity and carpal tunnel syndrome
☐ Diagnostic tests, including the physical examination and electrophysiologic studies
☐ Modifying work habits and the workplace to reduce symptoms
☐ Using protective gloves and splints
☐ Strengthening and stretching exercises for the wrist, hand, and fingers
☐ Medications, including corticosteroids, nonsteroidal anti-inflammatory drugs, and pyridoxine
☐ Surgery to relieve carpal tunnel syndrome
☐ Discharge instructions, including incision site care and reportable signs
☐ Care tips for patients with contributing systemic disorders

Locating the carpal tunnel

Give your patient a short anatomy lesson by showing her the tunnel made by the transverse carpal ligament in this cross section and palmar view of a right hand.

Also show her where the median nerve and the flexor tendons pass through the tunnel at the wrist to innervate the fingers and the hand. In this way, she can visualize how inflammation and swelling compress the nerve to produce the symptoms known as carpal tunnel syndrome.

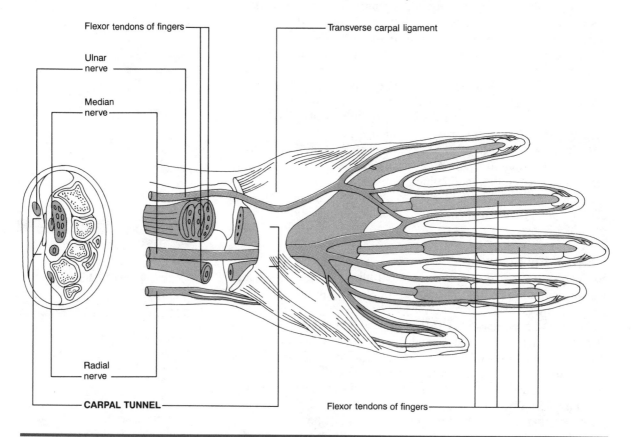

Flexor tendons of fingers — Transverse carpal ligament

Ulnar nerve

Median nerve

Radial nerve

CARPAL TUNNEL

Flexor tendons of fingers

premenstrual fluid retention, renal failure, and congestive heart failure, may be predisposing factors. Add that rapid, repetitive wrist motions involving excessive wrist flexion or extension also cause the carpal tunnel structures—for example, tendons—to swell and press the median nerve against the transverse carpal ligament. Furthermore, some experts think that a vitamin B_6 deficiency may contribute to carpal tunnel syndrome.

Complications
Warn that continued overuse of the affected wrist will increase tendon inflammation, compression, and neural ischemia. Wrist function will decrease. Stress that untreated carpal tunnel syndrome can produce permanent nerve damage with movement and sensation losses.

Describe the diagnostic workup

Tell the patient that a physical examination and health history are necessary to diagnose carpal tunnel syndrome. During the physical examination, the doctor may perform tests for Tinel's and Phalen's signs, which gauge sensation when she moves her wrist in certain directions (for more information, see *Two signs of carpal tunnel syndrome*). She may also undergo electrophysiologic studies to confirm the condition.

Electrophysiologic tests

Explain that before the tests a technician may ask about the patient's symptoms and reassure her that these nerve stimulation procedures aren't painful, although they may feel uncomfortable or strange. Mention that these tests use electrical current in amounts too small to be harmful.

Two signs of carpal tunnel syndrome

Tell the patient that two simple tests—for Tinel's sign and for Phalen's sign—may confirm carpal tunnel syndrome. The tests elicit symptoms confirming that certain wrist movements compress the median nerve, causing pain, burning, numbness, or tingling in the hand and fingers.

Tinel's sign

Tell the patient that the doctor will lightly percuss (or tap) the transverse carpal ligament lying over the median nerve where the patient's palm and wrist meet. If the patient feels discomfort, such as numbness or tingling, shooting into her palm and fingers, she has Tinel's sign—or positive confirmation of carpal tunnel syndrome.

Phalen's sign

The doctor or nurse flexes the patient's wrist for about 30 seconds. If the patient feels subsequent pain or numbness in her hands or fingers, she has Phalen's sign—positive evidence of carpal tunnel syndrome.

The more severe the carpal tunnel syndrome, the more rapidly the symptoms develop.

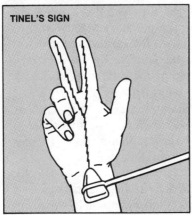

TINEL'S SIGN

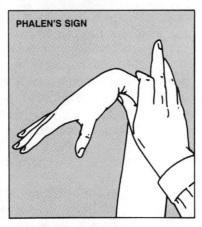

PHALEN'S SIGN

If the patient is having a *digital electrical stimulation test,* inform her that the technician will place ringlike electrodes around the index and middle fingers to stimulate the fingers electrically. Also, he'll attach an electrode over the median nerve in the wrist to record the nerve stimulation. If the median nerve's compressed, the stimulating current will take longer than usual to travel from the fingers to the wrist. Or the stimulation may be weak, depending on the degree of compression.

In a *motor function test* of the median nerve, the technician places stimulating electrodes over the median nerve at the wrist and recording electrodes over the thumb and directly below it on the inside of the hand. Then he watches for thumb movement. Delayed movement usually signals median nerve compression and carpal tunnel syndrome.

For electromyography, the technician inserts very fine needles into the wrist and thumb to check for irritability (spontaneous electrical activity) of the hand muscles innervated by the median nerve. Warn the patient that the needles may hurt—but only briefly because the test takes just a few minutes.

Teach about treatments

Inform the patient that her treatment plan will be designed to accommodate her life-style and the changes she's willing to make. If she's had symptoms only a short time, if her symptoms suggest mild carpal tunnel syndrome, or if they're expected to subside on their own (for example, after pregnancy), treatment may begin with conservative measures, such as rest, splinting, and medication. However, if symptoms affect both wrists or provoke severe discomfort and disability, treatment may involve surgery.

Activity

Teach the patient that resting the affected wrist or wrists can relieve the symptoms induced by nerve compression. Can she stop the repetitive activity that produces her symptoms? This is the ideal solution. If this isn't feasible, suggest she try slowing her pace and decreasing the activity. If a work task aggravates her symptoms, explore ways to decrease or eliminate this activity. Emphasize that rest can relieve only the immediate symptoms; it can't cure the underlying problem. Stress that resuming the activity will cause continued symptoms and damage. Reinforce your instruction by providing a copy of the patient-teaching aid *Relieving symptoms of carpal tunnel syndrome,* page 442.

If the doctor prescribes a restraining device, such as a glove or a splint, show the patient how to wear it. Explain that these devices limit motion and thereby decrease inflammation, compression, and discomfort. Acknowledge that the device may feel uncomfortable at first. Even so, encourage her to wear it as directed, especially when she's performing the activity that aggravates symptoms. If the device remains too cumbersome, help her to find ways to work with it. Remind her to wear the device whenever she has symptoms—even at night, if necessary.

Finally, if the patient has a splint, review the exercise program that complements splinting therapy. Emphasize that certain exercises maintain joint motion, prevent wrist stiffness, and preserve function and strength of muscles not affected by the wrist movement. Then give her the patient-teaching aids *Selecting a splint or a glove,* page 443, and *Exercises for patients with carpal tunnel syndrome,* page 444.

Medication

Inform the patient that the drugs most commonly prescribed for carpal tunnel syndrome include corticosteroids given by injection and nonsteroidal anti-inflammatory drugs (NSAIDs) taken orally. These drugs may be prescribed alone or in combination. If the doctor suspects that a vitamin B_6 deficiency contributes to symptoms, he may also prescribe pyridoxine.

Corticosteroids. Explain that a steroid injection, which reduces inflammation, will relieve the patient's symptoms almost immediately—but only temporarily. Inform her that the doctor may desensitize the area with a local anesthetic and then use a medium-sized needle to inject the drug into the carpal tunnel tendons. Caution her to report any burning sensations or loss of feeling or movement in the treated area.

NSAIDs. Explain that these drugs typically accompany corticosteroid and splinting therapy. They help control pain and reduce inflammation.

Instruct the patient to take the drug exactly as prescribed. Caution her that the drug may take 2 to 4 weeks to reach maximum effectiveness. If her drug regimen includes indomethacin (Indocin), mefenamic acid (Ponstel), phenylbutazone (Butazolidin), or piroxicam (Feldene), advise her to take the drug with food or antacids to avoid GI upset. Suggest she take other NSAIDs 30 minutes before or 2 hours after a meal to speed their effect (especially in the first few days of therapy). However, she may also take them with food or antacids if GI upset occurs.

Tell the patient to take all tablets or capsules with an 8-oz glass of water. Then warn her not to lie down for 15 to 30 minutes after taking the tablet to prevent it from lodging in the esophagus. Does she have trouble swallowing pills? If so, advise her to ask the doctor or pharmacist if the drug is available in liquid or suspension form. Or she can ask whether she can crush the solid drug and mix it with food or fluids.

Caution the patient to avoid hazardous activities or those that require alertness, such as driving a car, until she knows how the drug affects her central nervous system. Advise her to avoid alcohol, which may increase the risk of GI irritation and bleeding. Instruct her to report GI bleeding signs to her doctor at once. They include severe abdominal pain or cramping; bloody or black, tarry stools; and vomit that contains blood or looks like coffee grounds. Other reactions to report at once include a sudden decrease in urine output, shortness of breath, a rash, and swollen hands, face, or neck.

Surgical incision for carpal tunnel syndrome

If your patient's scheduled for carpal tunnel surgery, describe the 1- to 1½-inch incision the surgeon will use to transect the transverse carpal ligament.

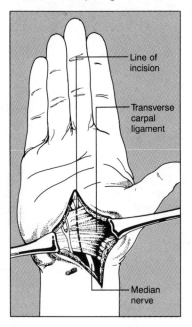

Line of incision

Transverse carpal ligament

Median nerve

If the patient is pregnant, advise her to avoid NSAIDs—even nonprescription NSAIDS—for example, ibuprofen (Advil, Nuprin). Caution her that NSAIDs are associated with dystocia and bleeding complications during delivery.

Pyridoxine. Explain to the patient with vitamin B_6 deficiency that she'll take this drug daily for at least 3 weeks; then the doctor will reevaluate her status. Instruct her to keep the drug in a dark bottle protected from light. If the doctor prescribes maintenance therapy to prevent vitamin B_6 deficiency from recurring, urge the patient to comply with the medication regimen and follow a nutritious diet. Food sources of vitamin B_6 include yeast, wheat germ, liver, whole-grain breads and cereals, bananas, and legumes.

Surgery

If conservative measures fail to improve carpal tunnel syndrome after about 6 months of treatment or if objective neurologic changes occur in the hand, the doctor will probably recommend surgical decompression of the median nerve at the carpal tunnel. Explain that the surgery involves transecting the ligaments that bridge the median nerve in the wrist.

Discuss preoperative care. If the patient will receive a general anesthetic, inform her that she won't be allowed food or fluids after midnight before the operation. If she's having a local anesthetic, tell her that she'll be admitted as an outpatient and will probably leave the hospital about 6 hours after surgery. Before surgery, the affected arm will be shaved and cleansed.

Describe the operation. Tell the patient that the doctor will apply a tourniquet-like Esmarch's bandage to her arm near the wrist to prevent blood from circulating in her hand. This provides a clear, visible surgical field. With the patient's hand positioned palm up and immobilized, the doctor can make an incision over the wrist (for more information, see *Surgical incision for carpal tunnel syndrome*). Then he'll perform the transection, suture the incision closed, and apply a pressure dressing. After surgery, the nurse will assess the patient's vital signs regularly and check the circulation in the affected hand. Reassure the patient that she'll receive pain relievers as needed.

Review postoperative care. If the patient has a pressure dressing, instruct her to leave it in place until the doctor approves its removal—usually between 6 and 24 hours after surgery. Direct her to elevate her hand for the first 24 hours and to gently open and close her hand hourly to prevent stiffness. Caution her to keep her hand and wrist dry. For example, advise her to secure a plastic bag over the dressing when she bathes or showers.

If the doctor directs her to change the dressing and clean the incisional area, show her how. First, though, suggest that she ask for help from a friend or family member. Then describe how to remove the old dressing with nonsterile gloves and then change to sterile gloves before cleansing the incision. Show her and her helper how to use a sterile gauze pad and sterile water to wipe gently from the top to the bottom of the incision. Finally, demonstrate how to apply a new adhesive bandage or a dressing provided by the doctor.

Alert the patient to the signs of infection—redness, warmth, swelling, or pus at the incisional site—and instruct her to call the doctor immediately if these occur. Remind her to make an appointment to have the sutures removed in 10 to 14 days.

Other care measures

Because an underlying systemic condition (such as obesity, pregnancy, diabetes, leukemia, renal disease, or Raynaud's syndrome) can exacerbate carpal tunnel syndrome, review the patient's history carefully to assess her learning needs. For example, encourage overweight patients to begin a nutritionally balanced, medically supervised, weight-loss program. Urge diabetics to monitor blood glucose levels regularly, to exercise, and to follow their dietary regimens. Remember to inform pregnant patients that in many instances carpal tunnel syndrome resolves on its own after delivery.

Further readings

Bear-Lehman, J., et al. "Primary Carpal Tunnel Syndrome: How Are We Managing It?" *Canadian Journal of Occupational Therapy* 55(5):243-48, December 1988.

deCarteret, J.C. "Carpal Tunnel Syndrome As an Occupational Illness," *Washington Nurse* 17(2):22, March 1987.

Falkenburg, S.A. "Choosing Hand Splints to Aid Carpal Tunnel Syndrome Recovery," *Occupational Health Safety* 56(5):60, 63-64, May 1987.

Fodor, J., et al. "Carpal Tunnel Syndrome: The Role of Radiography," *Radiology Technology* 58(6):497-502, July-August 1987.

Gordon, C., et al. "Electrodiagnostic Characteristics of Acute Carpal Tunnel Syndrome," *Archives of Physical Medicine and Rehabilitation* 68(9):545-48, September 1987.

Gordon, C., et al. "Wrist Ratio Correlation with Carpal Tunnel Syndrome in Industry," *American Journal of Physical Medicine and Rehabilitation* 67(6):270-72, December 1988.

Jupiter, J.B., and Krushell, R.J. "Evaluating Hand Injuries," *Emergency Medicine* 19(19):58-62, 64-65, 69+, November 15, 1987.

Schenck, R.R. "Carpal Tunnel Syndrome: 'Industrial Epidemic'," *American Association of Occupational Health Nurses Journal* 37(6):226-31, 242-44, June 1989.

Wild, E., et al. "Analysis of Wrist Injuries in Workers Engaged in Repetitive Tasks," *American Association of Occupational Health Nurses Journal* 35(8):356-66, August 1987.

Relieving symptoms of carpal tunnel syndrome

Dear Patient:

If you're having symptoms of carpal tunnel syndrome, you know how disabling they can be. You know, too, that strain on your wrist nerve triggers your discomfort. To get relief and prevent permanent damage, you need to *stop* or *cut back* on the activity producing the strain.

Of course, that's easier said than done. If the activities that produce strain are related to your job or hobbies, stopping or decreasing them takes careful planning. Use the following suggestions to help.

Make changes at work

Modify your work habits and work area. If you work on an assembly line, do piece work, or have a repetitive job, ask your supervisor to help you change or eliminate activities that strain your wrist. For example:
• Make sure any tools you use fit your hand correctly so you don't need to twist your wrist too much when turning, gripping, or squeezing objects.
• If you must lift and move objects, use both hands rather than the hand with carpal tunnel syndrome.
• Install a padded armrest at your work station to relieve the stress on your hands, wrists, and shoulders.
• Arrange to rotate your duties, or find a different technique for doing your job that puts less stress on your wrist.
• If you work at a typewriter, computer, or another type of terminal, try lowering the height of your work table to de-

crease the angle of wrist flexion.
• Raise your chair or sit on a pillow if you can't adjust your work table. Just be sure to support your feet to promote good posture and good circulation in your lower legs.

Wear a restraining device

Wear a splint or a specially designed glove whenever you perform repetitive activities — or all the time, if your doctor advises. These devices are available by prescription from medical supply stores.

Slow down

Slow down when performing repetitive activities with your hands. For example, if knitting causes symptoms, you can knit at a slower pace. But if you do piece work or if you work on an assembly line and a machine paces your work, discuss the problem with your supervisor or union representative.

Do hand exercises

Your doctor, nurse, or physical therapist can teach you special exercises to strengthen all your hand and wrist muscles. If all your muscles are strong, you'll put less strain on one particular muscle or group of muscles.

Reduce swelling

If fluid retention aggravates your symptoms, ask your doctor about taking diuretics to relieve some of the swelling in the carpal tunnel. Or drink plenty of fluids. Coffee and tea are natural diuretics. Elevating your hand may also help relieve swelling temporarily.

PATIENT-TEACHING AID

Selecting a splint or a glove

Dear Patient:

Restraining your hand and wrist can promote healing and reduce the nerve and tissue swelling caused by carpal tunnel syndrome. Two types of restraining devices are available — splints and protective gloves.

Although these devices may feel awkward at first, they can let you perform most tasks when properly fitted. At the same time, they'll help to limit your hand and wrist activity. A proper fit may require one or two medical visits.

Depending on which device your doctor orders, use these guidelines to help make your selection.

About splints
When selecting a splint, look for certain features. An effective splint should:
• immobilize your wrist and support your palm, but it shouldn't pinch your fingers or prevent you from bending them comfortably.
• be lightweight and allow you to work comfortably and efficiently.

• position your thumb away from your fingers, allowing some thumb-to-index finger motion but limiting thumb-to-little finger motion.
• have an absorbent lining and be made of a material (for example, a porous or elasticized material) that allows the skin to "breathe."
• have padding over the muscular areas inside your hand to absorb vibrations.

About protective gloves
When selecting a protective glove, keep these features in mind. An effective glove should:
• absorb perspiration with a washable lining and be made of a material that "breathes."
• contain internal seams that don't bulge, chafe, bind, constrict blood circulation, or reduce your dexterity.
• be easy to put on and remove.
• adjust easily for comfortable and proper fit.
• feel comfortable to wear on the job and be sturdy enough to withstand the rigors of work.

SPLINT

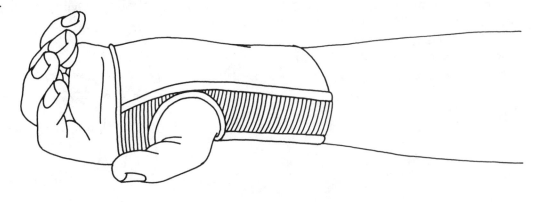

Exercises for patients with carpal tunnel syndrome

Dear Patient:

If you're limiting your hand motions to relieve carpal tunnel syndrome, you'll need to exercise your wrist, hand, fingers, and thumb daily to maintain muscle tone. Your doctor, nurse, or physical therapist will show you how to support, control, and move your hand correctly. Do your exercises with the affected hand and, if needed, with the other hand.

Wrist and hand exercises

1 Extend your arm—palm down, fingers straight. Keep your palm flat. Slowly raise your fingers as far as they'll comfortably go. Avoid flexing your wrist. Then slowly lower your fingers as far downward as they'll comfortably go.

2 Keeping your arm in the extended position, wave or rock your hand from side to side. Then gently twist your hand from side to side. Next, move it in small circles in one direction and then the opposite direction.

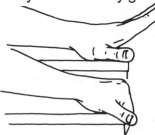

Fingers and thumb exercises

1 With a rubberband around your fingers for mild resistance, spread your fingers as far apart as possible. Then bring them back together. Now make a fist.

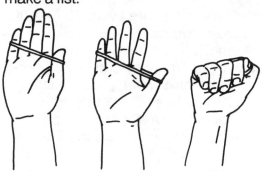

2 Hold up your hand and touch your little finger and thumb together. Repeat this movement, touching your other three fingers to your thumb.

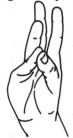

3 Finally, bend all your fingers up and down, as though waving goodbye.

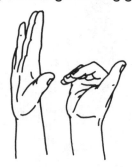

Tendinitis and bursitis

When teaching about tendinitis and bursitis, you'll be dealing with patients whose primary concerns are relief from discomfort and restoration of mobility. After all, the pain caused by these common disorders can disrupt sleep, daily activities, and job performance.

Begin by helping the patient understand the source of his pain and the rationale for therapy. Discuss the effect of prescribed medications, and show him how to apply heat or cold to relieve symptoms. If appropriate, teach him or his caregiver how to use a sling or other immobilizing device to rest his sore joint.

Once the patient's pain is under control, your next teaching hurdle is persuading him to comply with exercises that promote joint mobility and prevent muscle atrophy. You'll also need to review life-style changes to avoid recurrence of his disorder.

Discuss the disorder

Depending on which inflammatory disorder your patient has, explain that tendinitis affects the tendons, the fibrous bands that connect muscle to bone, whereas bursitis affects the bursae, the fluid-filled synovial sacs that cushion and lubricate body joints. The bursae, located throughout the body, ease movement by reducing friction and pressure between muscles or between muscle and bone (see *Anatomy of a joint: A look at tendons and bursae*, page 446).

Tendinitis, a painful inflammation or tear in a tendon, may result from trauma (such as strain during sports activity), postural malalignment, abnormal body development, hypermobility, or as a complication of another disease. It most commonly affects the shoulder, hip, heel (Achilles tendinitis), or hamstring. And it can afflict anyone who performs an activity that overloads a tendon or repeatedly stresses a joint, although it's more common in older people. The disorder causes localized pain around the affected area and restricted joint movement. Initially, swelling results from fluid accumulation. Then as the disorder progresses, calcium deposits in and around the tendon cause further swelling and immobility.

Bursitis refers to inflammation that results in swelling of one or more bursae, causing sudden or gradual pain and limiting joint motion. It can result from any activity that chronically irritates the bursae—from recurring trauma that puts stress or pressure on a joint to an inflammatory disease, such as gout or rheumatoid arthritis. Common stressors include repetitive kneeling, such as

---

Nancy Rae Mitchell, RN, MSN, assistant professor of nursing at California State University, Bakersfield, wrote this chapter.

CHECKLIST

Teaching topics in tendinitis and bursitis

☐ Explanation of the disorder and its symptoms
☐ Risk of complications, such as adhesive capsulitis
☐ Exercises to maintain joint range of motion
☐ Corticosteroids and other drugs to relieve pain and inflammation
☐ Heat or cold treatments
☐ Correct use of slings or other immobilizers
☐ Life-style changes to prevent recurrent inflammation
☐ Sources of information and support

Anatomy of a joint: A look at tendons and bursae

When discussing tendinitis or bursitis with your patient, explain how tendons and bursae facilitate movement. Review this illustration of the shoulder to describe how the tendons, like stiff rubber bands, hold and move muscles and bones together. Then point out how the bursae, located at friction points around joints and between tendons, cartilage, or bone, keep these body parts cushioned and lubricated so they move freely.

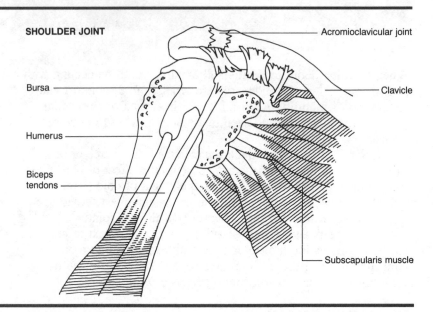

SHOULDER JOINT

Acromioclavicular joint

Bursa

Clavicle

Humerus

Biceps tendons

Subscapularis muscle

from carpet laying ("housemaid's knee"), jogging in worn-out shoes on hard asphalt surfaces (ankle or foot bursitis), and prolonged sitting, with crossed legs, on hard surfaces (hip bursitis). Septic bursitis may result from a wound infection or from bacterial invasion of the skin over the bursa.

Complications

Untreated, tendinitis can produce severe pain as calcium erodes into adjacent bursae, causing acute calcific bursitis with swelling, warmth, and redness involving the surrounding skin. Likewise, untreated bursitis can cause extreme pain and restricted joint movement. Be sure to warn the patient that failure to comply with therapy, especially prescribed exercises, may lead to joint immobility. In particular, warn the patient with shoulder tendinitis or bursitis that he may develop "frozen shoulder" (adhesive capsulitis). This may require surgery to free, or "unlock," the joint.

Describe the diagnostic workup

Inform the patient that a thorough medical history and physical examination are the basis for diagnosis. However, blood and other diagnostic tests, such as arthrocentesis, ultrasonography, or arthrography, may be ordered to rule out other causes (see *Explaining arthrography*).

Blood tests

If appropriate, prepare the patient for such tests as a complete blood count, HLA-B27 typing, rheumatoid factor, and C-reactive protein. If the patient has bursitis, explain that the doctor will assess serum uric acid levels to rule out gout.

Arthrocentesis

If the doctor suspects a joint infection, prepare the patient for arthrocentesis to detect microorganisms and other causes of infection or inflammation. Tell him that during arthrocentesis, he'll be asked to assume a position and then to remain still. After cleaning the skin over the joint, the doctor will insert a needle, withdraw some fluid, and apply a small bandage to the puncture site. The test takes about 10 minutes. After it, tell the patient to rest the affected area and to use cold packs to reduce pain, swelling, and stiffness. Instruct him to report any increased pain, tenderness, swelling, warmth, redness, or fever, which may signal infection.

Ultrasonography

Explain to the patient that this noninvasive test uses high-frequency sound waves to help diagnose bursitis. Inform him that the doctor or technician will apply a cool gel (a sound-wave conductant) to the painful area. Then the technician will move a transducer over the area, and images of the tissues will appear on a screen. Assure him that the procedure is painless and brief.

Teach about treatments

Explain that treatment aims to relieve symptoms and maintain joint mobility while the inflamed tendon or bursa heals. Help the patient identify ways to modify his life-style to avoid activities that may aggravate his disorder. Encourage him to follow a program of prescribed exercise to maintain range of motion in his joint. Make sure he knows how to apply ice or heat for symptomatic relief, and review instructions for taking medications.

Activity

If the patient's tendinitis or bursitis stems from recurring joint trauma or overuse, discuss how he can modify or eliminate pain-producing activities. For example, if the patient develops Achilles tendinitis, you may need to recommend that he wear well-cushioned shoes, lose excess weight, and pursue recreational activities that don't require weight-bearing, such as swimming. Caution him to stop using an affected joint as soon as it begins to hurt. Explain that pain signals excessive stress on a joint.

Show the patient how to do therapeutic exercises, if prescribed. If he has shoulder pain, give him a copy of the teaching aid *Exercises to ease your aching shoulder,* pages 450 and 451. To minimize pain during exercise, encourage him to apply heat to the affected joint beforehand. Or if ordered, suggest that he take a mild analgesic, such as acetaminophen (Tylenol), about an hour before exercise. If he experiences pain after exercise, suggest that he apply a cold pack, wrapped in a towel, to his sore joint.

Medication

Point out that although drug therapy can't cure tendinitis or bursitis, it can minimize discomfort. Then, as appropriate, discuss corticosteroids and nonsteroidal anti-inflammatory drugs (NSAIDs), including aspirin.

If the doctor plans to inject a corticosteroid into the joint

Explaining arthrography

If the patient's shoulder or knee fails to respond to conservative treatment, arthrography may be performed. Explain to the patient that this radiographic test involves injecting air or a radiopaque contrast medium into the affected joint to help identify abnormalities. Tell him that the test takes about an hour and is usually performed by a radiologist.

Describe how the doctor cleans and numbs the test area. Then explain that he'll insert a needle into the joint, first to aspirate fluid for analysis and then to inject air (for contrast) or a contrast medium. If he uses contrast medium, he'll manipulate the joint to ensure even distribution of the substance. Then he'll take a series of X-rays.

Afterward, the doctor may advise compression—wrapping the joint with an elastic bandage—for several days. If he does, show the patient how to wrap the bandage, and advise him to rest the joint for about 12 hours, as ordered. Tell him that he may use ice for swelling and an analgesic to relieve pain. Inform him that he may notice crackling or clicking noises for 1 or 2 days. If the noises persist, instruct him to notify the doctor.

Teaching about joint injections

Is your patient with tendinitis or bursitis having a joint injection? Here are some teaching points to cover as you explain the procedure.

Benefits
Inform the patient that the doctor delivers medication through a needle directly into the joint cavity to treat tendinitis or into the bursal sac to treat bursitis. Explain that the medication relieves pain by reducing inflammation and swelling. This will help maintain mobility, preserve function, and prevent contractures and muscle atrophy from disuse.

The procedure
Tell the patient that the procedure is relatively quick and simple but may be painful. Inform him that he'll be positioned comfortably. Then the doctor will clean and drape the injection site. Stress that the patient stay still as the doctor gives him a local anesthetic and injects the medication.

When the doctor withdraws the needle, he'll apply pressure on the injection site. He may massage the joint to enhance absorption or ask the patient to gently flex the joint.

Aftercare
Tell the patient to rest the affected joint for 24 hours and, as possible, to sit rather than stand if he had the injection in his leg. At home, advise him to apply cold — not heat — to relieve residual soreness. Explain that pain should diminish, if not immediately, within 2 days.

cavity to treat tendinitis or into the bursal sac to treat bursitis, explain that this procedure can provide long-term relief of pain and inflammation. As you prepare the patient, mention that the injected medication will be confined to his joint or bursa. Rarely, the drug may leak into the patient's circulation, causing systemic disturbances. Instruct him to report blurred vision, mood changes, frequent urination, increased thirst, rash or hives, or persistent pain at the injection site. For more information, see *Teaching about joint injections.*

If the patient's taking aspirin or another NSAID, such as naproxen (Naprosyn) or piroxicam (Feldene), explain that the prescribed drug reduces pain and inflammation. Tell him to report signs and symptoms of GI upset, such as nausea, vomiting, anorexia, or diarrhea. Urge him to call the doctor immediately if he has black, tarry stools or if his vomit contains blood or resembles coffee grounds—key signs of GI bleeding. Also tell him to report unintentional weight gain. Warn him to avoid taking aspirin along with other NSAIDs because this increases the risk of adverse reactions. To minimize gastric irritation, advise him to avoid alcoholic beverages and to take the drug with food or antacids.

Procedures
Several procedures, ranging from cold and heat applications to immobilization, may offer relief while the inflamed area heals.

Treatments with cold
If the doctor orders cold treatment to relieve swelling and pain, show the patient how to use a commercial cold pack. Or explain that he can fill a plastic bag with ice, squeeze the air out, and wrap the ice pack in a towel or pillowcase before applying (to prevent frostbite). If the affected joint is hard to cover with an ice pack, suggest freezing a wet towel just until it's malleable. Tell him to put the frozen towel inside a pillowcase or a dry towel before molding it around the sore area. Caution him always to remove ice after 20 minutes to prevent skin damage. Then instruct him to reapply ice as often as his doctor recommends.

Treatments with heat
If the doctor orders heat treatment to improve blood flow, promote muscle relaxation, and lessen discomfort, discuss how to use dry heat, such as a heating pad, or moist heat, such as a warm, wet towel. If the patient uses a heating pad or a hot-water bottle, tell him to check his skin under the device frequently to prevent burns. To keep a moist towel warm, suggest using it under a hot-water bottle or waterproof heating pad. (The water bottle or heating pad shouldn't be as hot as when used for dry heat.) Discuss the value of soaking sore joints in a basin or tub of warm water. Then instruct him to limit all forms of heat therapy to 20 minutes. Tell him to repeat heat application as directed by his doctor.

Immobilization
Teach the patient how to wear a splint, brace, or other joint immobilizer, if appropriate. If the doctor orders a sling, give the patient a copy of the teaching aid *How to apply a sling,* page 452.

Show him how to judge when the sling or other supportive device is too tight by checking for swelling or a prickling sensation in his fingers or toes. Teach him how to prevent skin irritation and to inspect his skin for redness under the device every 8 hours, or as often as the doctor recommends.

Surgery

Tell the patient with tendinitis that surgery usually isn't necessary, unless the tendon ruptures completely. However, if more conservative treatments fail to relieve symptoms, he may need surgery to repair the tendon or to remove calcium deposits.

If the patient has chronic bursitis or a frozen shoulder, explain that surgery to remove the inflamed bursal sac may be necessary. Tell him that his affected part may be immobilized after surgery until the wound heals. Later, the doctor may prescribe an exercise routine to prevent immobility.

Other care measures

Tell the patient to elevate a swollen heel, knee, or elbow. Explain that elevation helps to reduce swelling and pain. For elbow bursitis, suggest wrapping the joint snugly in a compression bandage for 24 to 48 hours to prevent excessive fluid accumulation, which causes pressure and pain.

Urge the patient to comply with follow-up appointments until the inflammation completely resolves. Teach him how to prevent recurrence by modifying activities that lead to joint stress and overuse. Review how to practice proper body mechanics, relieve pressure on weight-bearing joints, and avoid repeated bending and stooping and excessive lifting and stretching.

Sources of information and support

American Association of Orthopaedic Medicine
926 East McDowell Road, #202 Phoenix, Ariz. 85006
(602) 254-5315

American Osteopathic Academy of Sports Medicine
7201 Harvest Hill, Madison, Wis. 53717
(608) 831-4400

Further readings

Birrer, R.B., et al. "Syndromes of Chronic Use and Overuse," *Patient Care* 23(12):215-17, 221-22, 225, July 15, 1989.
Heller, M.B. "Local Injection Therapy: Techniques That Work in Tendinitis/ Bursitis Syndrome," *Consultant* 27(12):107-09, 113-14, 116-17, December 1987.
Jensen, K., and DiFabio, R.P. "Evaluation of Eccentric Exercise in Treatment of Patellar Tendinitis," *Physical Therapy* 69(3):211-16, March 1989.
Puffer, J.C., and Zachazewski, J.E. "Management of Overuse Injuries," *American Family Physician* 38(3):225-32, September 1988.
Riddle, D.L., and Freeman, D.B. "Management of a Patient with a Diagnosis of Bilateral Plantar Fasciitis and Achilles Tendinitis," *Physical Therapy* 68(12):1913-16, December 1988.
Simon, R.R. "Joint Pain Without Trauma," *Emergency Medicine* 19(13):22-26, 28-29, 32, July 15, 1987.

Exercises to ease your aching shoulder

Dear Patient:

These exercises can help you keep your shoulder relaxed, so it doesn't stiffen. Try to do your exercises once a day or as often as your doctor or physical therapist directs.

Arm circling

Stand sideways next to a table or the back of a chair. Hold on with your unaffected arm for support. Now, bend forward at the waist. Let your sore arm hang down like a pendulum.

Make slow circles with your sore arm. Gradually increase the size of the circles until you can swing your arm in large clockwise circles in front of you. Then reverse the direction and make counterclockwise circles.

As your shoulder inflammation subsides, the doctor may ask you to increase the number of times you do this exercise. Ask him or the physical therapist if you should use weights while you do this exercise.

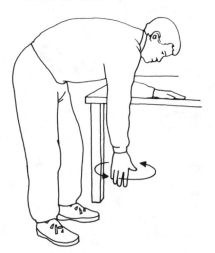

Finger climbing

Stand facing a wall, an arm's length away. Place the hand of your sore arm on the wall and slowly walk your index and middle fingers up the wall as high as you can without discomfort. Hold this position for a few seconds, then walk your fingers down again. Repeat as often as your doctor instructs.

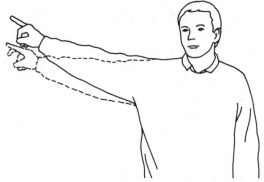

Next, stand sideways with your sore shoulder facing the wall about an arm's length away. Repeat the exercise. As your fingers climb higher, sidestep closer to the wall to allow your shoulder the maximum range of motion. Each day, try to reach a higher point.

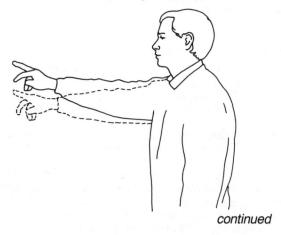

continued

Exercises to ease your aching shoulder — *continued*

Elbow raising

Place the hand of your sore arm on the opposite shoulder. Using your unaffected hand, gently push the elbow of your sore arm straight up as far as you can without discomfort. Then lower your elbow to the starting position. Each day, try to hold your elbow up a little longer, until you can hold the position for a few minutes.

upward. When you've raised your sore arm as high as you can without discomfort, hold the position for a few seconds. Then let the arm drop slowly.

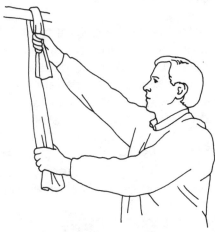

Arm extensions with a broomstick

Grasp a broomstick (or cane or yardstick) with both hands at hip level and raise it up over your head. Then, lower it behind your head to the back of your neck. Hold the position for as long as you comfortably can, then reverse the procedure. Each day, try to hold the broom behind your head a little longer, until you can hold the position for several minutes.

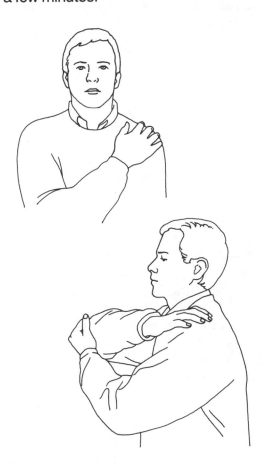

Arm lifting with a pulley

Drape a bath towel over a secure shower rod, or attach a pulley and rope in an open doorway. Grab an end of the towel or rope with each hand. Using your unaffected arm, gently pull on the towel or rope, lifting your sore arm

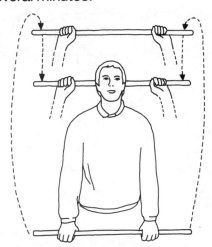

PATIENT-TEACHING AID

How to apply a sling

Dear Caregiver:

The doctor wants the patient to wear a sling temporarily to support and rest his sore shoulder. Ask the doctor when and how often the patient can remove the sling. Follow these directions to help him put on the sling.

1 A sling looks like a triangular scarf. Place the triangle's center point at the elbow of the patient's affected arm. The longest side of the triangle should be parallel to his body.

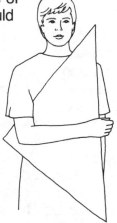

2 Drape the upper point over the unaffected shoulder. Help the patient bend the elbow of his affected arm at a 90-degree angle, with his thumb pointing up. Place the lower point of the triangle over the affected shoulder, enclosing the forearm in the sling.

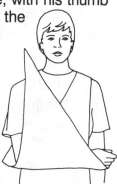

3 Now, knot the two ends of the sling loosely around his neck. Always position the knot to the side—never in the back of his neck. To keep the knot securely in place and to prevent skin irritation, place the sling outside his collar or insert a gauze pad under the knot.

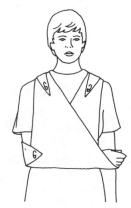

4 If the knot is uncomfortable, pin each point to the opposite side. Make sure that the edge of the sling extends to the first joint of the little finger. This holds the wrist in line with the arm to prevent wrist damage. Now, use a safety pin to fasten the overflap at the elbow to the sling fabric. This will keep the sling from falling off.

Sprains and strains

Because a sprain or a strain may seem like a minor injury to many patients, you'll need to stress the importance of rehabilitation in regaining normal strength in the injured limb. You'll also need to convince active patients to immobilize or protect the injured body part while it heals. Athletes, in particular, may pose special problems if they're eager to resume training or competition.

Regardless of the patient's attitude about his injury, you'll need to define a sprain and a strain and point out possible complications if the patient doesn't protect and rehabilitate the injured limb. Describe necessary diagnostic tests and treatments, including activity limitations, analgesic and anti-inflammatory medication, and immobilization devices. If necessary, explain surgery to repair a torn ligament.

Discuss the disorder

Tell the patient that a *sprain* refers to stretching or tearing the capsule or ligament surrounding a joint, causing acute pain and swelling. An ankle sprain, for instance, may occur when the patient twists his ankle during a fall or while stepping on an uneven surface. In a knee sprain, the patient sustains a sudden forceful blow that causes him to twist his knee while it's bearing weight and his foot is in a stable position. This can occur during a sport, such as football or skiing, or in a motor vehicle accident. Warn the patient that once he injures his knee, he's vulnerable to reinjury. To reinforce your teaching, give him a copy of the patient-teaching aid *Taking care of your knees,* pages 458 and 459.

Inform the patient that a *strain* is a partial, microscopic tear in a muscle or tendon or both. An *acute* strain results from a sudden forced movement that overstretches a muscle or tendon. At the moment of an acute strain, the patient may feel no pain; instead, it may develop later with continued activity. As a result of the tear, the tissue bleeds into the surrounding tissues, causing swelling. A *chronic* strain stems from the cumulative effect of repeated muscle overuse. Such strains commonly result from injury during sports, such as tennis, golf, or basketball. The patient can also suffer a strain when he uses poor body mechanics in lifting or carrying. (For more information, see *Sprains and strains: An inside view,* page 454, and *Classifying sprains and strains,* page 455.)

Mary Faut Rodts, RN, MS, ONC, who wrote this chapter, is an assistant professor at Rush College of Nursing, Rush University, Chicago.

CHECKLIST

Teaching topics in sprains and strains

☐ Explanation of the injury: sprain or strain
☐ Complications, including impaired circulation, nerve damage, and loss of function in the affected area
☐ Preparation for diagnostic tests, such as X-rays
☐ Anti-inflammatory and analgesic drugs to relieve swelling and pain
☐ Treatments, such as rest, ice, compression, and elevation
☐ Physical therapy for rehabilitation
☐ Immobilization devices, such as elastic bandages, casts, and crutches
☐ Surgery for severe sprains
☐ Sources of information and support

Sprains and strains: An inside view

Except for possible swelling and discoloration, your patient can't actually see a strain or a sprain. But he can surely feel them because a *sprain* is the stretching or tearing of a ligament—the fibrous tissue that binds joints together. A *strain,* whether acute or chronic, is a partial muscle tear. A strain may also affect tendons—the fibrous tissue that connects muscle to bone. Here's what they look like "inside."

KNEE SPRAIN

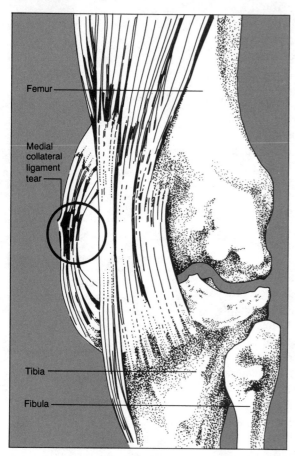

Femur

Medial collateral ligament tear

Tibia

Fibula

CALF STRAIN

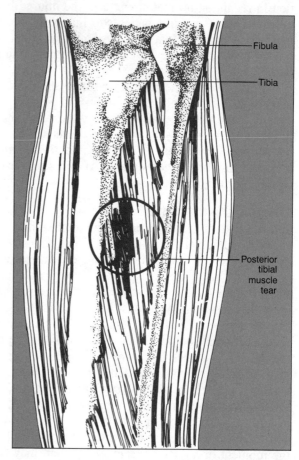

Fibula

Tibia

Posterior tibial muscle tear

Complications

Emphasize to the patient the importance of following the doctor's instructions carefully to minimize swelling, a common problem with sprains and strains. Explain that lack of compliance can lead to severe swelling, which can impair circulation and cause nerve damage and loss of function in the affected area.

Tell the patient that even a mild or moderate sprain (Grade I or II) can cause joint instability and loss of function if he doesn't undergo adequate rehabilitation. Warn that permanent instability can result if a severe sprain, such as a complete anterior cruciate tear, isn't surgically repaired.

Describe the diagnostic workup

Tell the patient that the doctor will perform a thorough physical examination of the injured area to evaluate joint stability. He may also order an X-ray, computed tomography (CT) scan, or magnetic resonance imaging (MRI) to evaluate the injury's severity and location.

Inform the patient that X-rays may reveal bone separation, fractures, or joint instability. Explain that while X-ray tests cause no pain, stress X-rays (taken with the injured part in the most stressful position that pain permits) cause discomfort. They may be needed, however, to evaluate ligament laxity. If the doctor orders a CT scan or MRI, assure the patient that these tests are painless. Be sure he understands the test's purpose and what happens before, during, and after each test.

Teach about treatments

Emphasize the patient's contribution to recovery when you discuss activity restrictions and, later, rehabilitation goals. Discuss the medications his doctor will prescribe for pain and inflammation. Describe procedures used to treat these injuries, including application of ice and heat, elevation of the affected area, and use of an elastic bandage. Tell him about immobilization devices and crutches. If appropriate, prepare him for surgery for a severe sprain.

Activity

Instruct the patient to rest the injured limb for the first 24 hours after injury. After that, he may resume some activities, using a sling, wrap, cast, or crutches. Discourage activities that risk further injury until healing and rehabilitation are complete.

Prepare the patient for rehabilitation to help him regain normal function. How soon he'll begin depends on the injury. For example, the patient with a strain can start exercising sooner than a patient with a sprain that requires healing of the torn ligament. Explain prescribed exercises, which usually begin with simple range-of-motion exercises followed by isometric exercises in the injured limb. Then, as healing progresses, he'll include regular conditioning and strengthening exercises. Stress the importance of exercising the uninjured extremities while the injured limb heals to prevent loss of muscle tone and vascular problems. Tell the patient that he can return to athletic activities once healing and rehabilitation are complete.

Medication

Inform the patient that his doctor may prescribe analgesics to relieve pain and nonsteroidal anti-inflammatory drugs (NSAIDs) to decrease inflammation. Review dosages and adverse reactions for these drugs. Instruct him to take NSAIDs with meals to prevent GI distress. Ask about factors that may heighten his risk for GI distress, such as previous sensitivity to salicylates or a history of

Classifying sprains and strains

Tell your patient that sprains and strains are classified by the extent of tissue damage.

Sprains
In a sprain, injuries are classified as:
Grade I (mild) — minor or partial ligament tear with normal joint stability and function
Grade II (moderate) — partial ligament tear with mild joint laxity and some function loss
Grade III (severe) — complete ligament tear or complete separation of ligament from bone, causing total joint laxity and function loss.

Strains
In a strain, degrees of injury include:
Grade I (mild) — microscopic muscle or tendon tear or both with no loss of strength
Grade II (moderate) — incomplete muscle or tendon tear or both with bleeding into muscle tissue and some loss of strength
Grade III (severe) — complete muscle or tendon tear or both (rupture), usually resulting from separation of muscle from muscle, muscle from tendon, or tendon from bone.

Managing ankle sprains

Describe the treatment for the patient's ankle injury. Inform him that treatment depends on the extent of injury.

Grade I (mild)
Tell the patient to apply ice, to elevate his ankle for 24 to 48 hours, and to use a compression dressing (elastic bandage). Give him crutches to assist with weight-bearing. Explain that he may resume normal activity when the pain goes away.

Grade II (moderate)
Tell the patient to apply ice and to elevate his ankle for 24 to 48 hours after injury. Then the doctor will prescribe crutches and a padded posterior splint or an aircast for 4 weeks. Advise the patient to perform ice massage soon after the sprain, followed by range-of-motion exercises, twice daily.

Tell him that he can stop using the crutches when the pain diminishes. When he regains his full range of motion and his pain disappears, the doctor will remove the aircast.

Grade III (severe)
Tell the patient to apply ice and to elevate his ankle for 24 to 48 hours. The doctor will apply a short-leg walking cast for 3 weeks, and the patient may resume partial weight-bearing with crutches, as necessary, until the pain decreases.

When the cast is removed, encourage the patient to follow a rehabilitation program, consisting of ice massage and range-of-motion exercises for 3 more weeks. Tell him that during this time an aircast will protect his ankle.

ulcers. Warn him to immediately discontinue the medication and notify the doctor if nausea, vomiting, abdominal pain, or dark stools occur.

Procedures
Teach the patient the mnemonic *RICE (Rest, Ice, Compression, and Elevation)* to help him remember what to do during the first few days after a sprain or a strain. Then instruct him about any immobilization device the doctor has prescribed.

RICE. Inform the patient that rest and ice reduce pain and swelling. Tell him to place ice in a plastic bag, to wrap the bag in a towel, and to place the bag over the most tender area of the injury. Instruct him to use it for 48 hours, applying it at 30-minute intervals, and moving it every 5 minutes to avoid frostbite. Afterward, he may use a heating pad for up to 30 minutes periodically to make him more comfortable.

Advise the patient to reduce swelling by elevating the injured extremity above heart level for the first 24 hours after an injury. Next, explain that wrapping the injured part in an elastic bandage to compress the tissues will also help reduce swelling. Give the patient a copy of the teaching aid *How to apply an elastic bandage,* page 460.

Immobilization. Inform the patient that usually the doctor will order an immobilization device to relieve pain and promote healing. Such a device supports or immobilizes the injured body part. The type of device used hinges on the severity of his injury and his degree of disability.

If the patient has a Grade II sprain, the doctor may order an aircast—an inflatable device with an adjustable, rigid, lightweight shell (see *Managing ankle sprains*). Tell him that the aircast easily conforms to the extremity's shape and size. Another advantage: it's removable to allow for hygiene and early range-of-motion exercises.

If the patient has a Grade III sprain, tell him that the doctor may recommend a plaster or fiberglass cast to provide more rigid support. Explain that he'll wear it for 3 to 4 weeks. After the cast is applied, tell the patient to carefully monitor his neurovascular status by checking pulses, warmth, color, mobility, and sensory function around the sprain site. Also warn him to note any increased swelling. These signs suggest an overly tight cast.

Explain that a plaster or fiberglass cast will feel warm as it dries. Depending on its thickness, a plaster cast may take up to 24 hours to dry completely; a fiberglass cast dries in minutes. Tell him not to put weight on the cast until it's completely dry. Weight-bearing reshapes the cast and may produce pressure points. Tell him that the cast should remain uncovered as it dries—exposure to air speeds drying. If his uncovered leg or hand feels cold, tell him to warm the area with a sock or mitten, and to check his neurovascular status frequently. Give the patient copies of the teaching aids *How to care for your cast,* pages 423 to 425, and *Troubleshooting your casted limb,* pages 426 and 427.

Tell the patient that his doctor may recommend crutches for a lower extremity injury to allow for minimal or no weight-bearing until his discomfort diminishes.

Surgery

Explain that surgery may be necessary for a sprain that causes joint instability. Tell the patient that the surgeon will explore the torn capsule or ligament and repair it with sutures. The patient will need to wear a cast or brace for about 6 weeks after surgery. After a successful repair, if ordered, the patient may begin early range-of-motion exercises.

Other care measures

Encourage the patient to express his concerns about his condition. If necessary, advise him to consult a community health nurse to assess his home environment and to provide follow-up care.

Sources of information and support

American Academy of Orthopaedic Surgeons
222 S. Prospect Avenue, Park Ridge, Ill. 60068
(708) 823-7186

American College of Sports Medicine
401 West Michigan Street, Indianapolis, Ind. 46202-3233
(317) 637-9200

American Physical Therapy Association
1111 North Fairfax Street, Alexandria, Va. 22314
(703) 684-2782

National Association of Orthopaedic Nurses
Box 56, North Woodbury Road, Pitman, N.J. 08071
(609) 582-0111

Further readings

Cote, D.J., et al. "Comparison of Three Treatment Procedures for Minimizing Ankle Sprain Swelling," *Physical Therapy* 68(7):1072-76, July 1988.
Mulvey, T. "Anatomy and Pathology of the Shoulder Complex," *Orthopedic Nursing* 7(3):23-28, May-June 1988.
Sonzogni, J.J., Jr. "A Trio of Summer Sports Injuries," *Emergency Medicine* 20(13):52-53, 55-56, July 15, 1988.
Webster, B. "Treating Sports Injuries," *Occupational Health* (London) 40(5):542-44, May 1988.
Wood, P. "A Repetitive Problem...Repetition Strain Injury," *Nursing Times* 84(7):41-43, February 17-23, 1988.

Taking care of your knees

Dear Patient:

Now that you've hurt your knee, you're more likely to hurt it again. Here are some tips for preventing a new injury and for recognizing and caring for a knee injury if you should hurt yourself again.

Preventing knee injuries

Build up your leg muscles. Remember, the stronger your leg muscles — especially your quadriceps (front thigh muscles) and your hamstrings (back thigh muscles) — the less vulnerable your knee. Try isometric exercise,

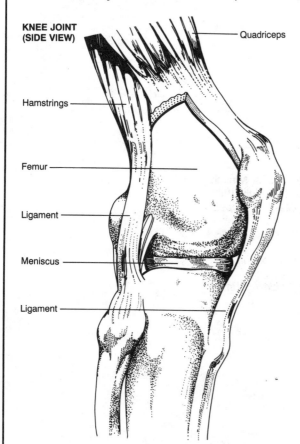

KNEE JOINT (SIDE VIEW)

Quadriceps

Hamstrings

Femur

Ligament

Meniscus

Ligament

weight training (using Nautilus or similar equipment), or sports such as swimming or biking. Consult your doctor about which exercise or equipment is best for you.

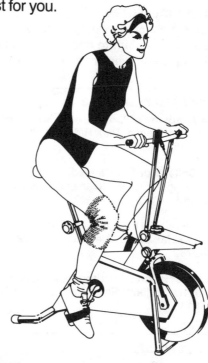

Maintain a normal weight for your height and frame. Being overweight increases your risk of reinjuring your knee.

Don't engage in sports activities until your strength returns and you can fully bend and stretch your knee without pain or swelling. If you begin too soon, you're likely to reinjure your knee.

Until your knee fully heals, wrap it with tape or an elastic bandage when you exercise or play sports. Although this won't add strength, it may remind you to be cautious.

continued

Taking care of your knees — *continued*

Wear smooth-soled athletic shoes if you play sports on artificial turf. Don't wear cleats. They boost your injury risk by anchoring your foot to the playing surface with each step. Then your leg has less "give" when your knee comes in contact with a person, an object, or the ground.

If you take up a new sport, choose one that fits your skills and experience. Work into it slowly. Warm up carefully with conditioning exercises, and don't try to do too much, too soon. Remember, tired muscles are weak muscles. Without muscle support, your reinjury risk increases.

Recognizing a knee injury

You know your knee is injured and you should see a doctor when you:
• have pain and swelling
• feel something moving abnormally inside your knee
• wobble or sense that your knee's unstable
• hear (or someone else hears) a "pop" around your knee
• sense numbness or tingling in your toes or feet. *Important:* Call your doctor without delay if this happens, even if you're not in pain.

Caring for a knee injury

If you do reinjure your knee, remember "RICE": *r*est, *i*ce, *c*ompression, *e*levation. Follow these steps to reduce pain and swelling.
• Rest your knee by getting off your feet and staying off them for at least 24 hours.
• Apply an ice pack to your knee for about 20 minutes every half hour for a day or more.

• Use a compression device, such as an elastic bandage, to support injured tissues and reduce swelling. Take care not to restrict your circulation by wrapping the bandage too tightly.

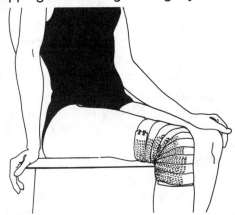

• Elevate your knee — ideally above heart level. This also helps control swelling.

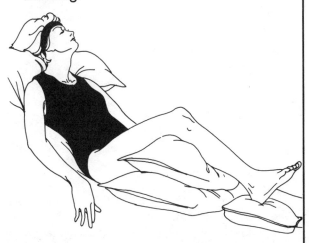

• Call your doctor. Depending on your injury's severity, he may suggest removing fluid from your knee (for severe swelling and inflammation). Or he may recommend rest and isometric exercises, starting 1 to 2 days after the injury, and more active exercise, starting once pain and swelling decrease.

How to apply an elastic bandage

Dear Patient:

An elastic bandage compresses the tissues around a sprain or a strain to help prevent swelling and provide support. The directions below explain how to wrap an elastic bandage around an ankle. You can modify them for wrapping your knee, wrist, elbow, or hand.

1 With one hand, hold the loose end of the elastic bandage on the top of your foot between your instep and toes. With the other hand, wrap the bandage twice around your foot, gradually moving toward your ankle. Make sure to overlap the bandage in spiral fashion.

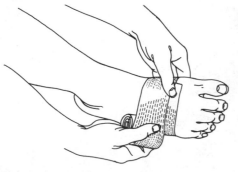

2 After wrapping your foot twice, move your hand to support your heel. Use your other hand to wrap the bandage in figure-eight fashion, leaving your heel uncovered.

To do this, angle the bandage up, cross it over the foot, and pass it behind the ankle. Next, angle the bandage down, cross it over the top of your foot, and pass it under your foot to complete the figure-eight turn (see top of next column). Do this step twice.

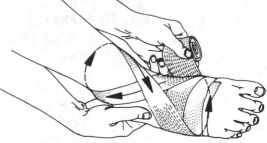

3 Now, circle the bandage around your calf, moving toward your knee. Overlap the elastic as you wrap. Stop just below the knee. Don't wrap downward.

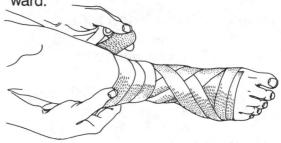

4 Secure the end of the bandage with a metal clip or adhesive tape.

Comfort and safety tips

Aim for a snug, not a tight, fit. Never wrap the bandage so tightly that it restricts or cuts off your circulation. If you're stretching the bandage material, chances are you're wrapping it too tightly.

Promote circulation by removing and rewrapping your bandage at least twice daily.

Remove the bandage immediately if you have any numbness or tingling. When these symptoms disappear, you can reapply the bandage. If numbness or tingling doesn't stop, call your doctor.

Eye, Ear, Nose, and Throat Conditions

Contents

Cataracts

Because surgery alone can correct cataracts, your teaching will focus on the procedure and aftercare. And because most patients are admitted and discharged the same day, you'll have to accomplish a great deal in a short time. That's why preparing and implementing a concise and efficient teaching plan becomes crucial. (See *Teaching the cataract patient,* page 464.)

Although cataracts occur so commonly that your patient probably knows someone who's had them, he may not understand what a cataract is. So you'll need to define the disorder for him, describe diagnostic tests, and explain surgery. Then you'll outline postoperative care measures to safeguard his newly improved vision.

Discuss the disorder

Dispel the common misconception that a cataract is a growth or a film on the eye. Explain that a cataract is a clouding of the normally transparent eye lens. Then describe how the eye's lens, like a camera's, focuses images. But instead of focusing images on film, the eye's cornea and lens focus images on the retina. When a clouded lens blocks light, the resultant image appears fuzzy (see *How a cataract blurs vision,* page 465).

Inform your patient that cataracts take many years to develop and are usually associated with aging. They may occur in both eyes, progressing at different rates. Usually, clouding starts in a small part of the lens. That's why vision remains virtually unaffected at first. Because cataracts are characterized by painless and progressive vision loss, most people wait to seek medical help until their vision becomes so poor that performing ordinary activities becomes difficult.

Complications

Advise the patient that a cataract eventually impairs vision drastically, causing blindness. Surgery to remove the cataract restores vision. An untreated cataract can also lead to glaucoma if the lens swells or, rarely, to an inflamed iris.

Describe the diagnostic workup

Teach the patient about tests that will be performed before surgery, including routine visual acuity tests, slit-lamp examination and tonometry, indirect ophthalmoscopy, keratometry, and ocular

Heather Boyd-Monk, RN, SRN, BSN, and **Joanne Patzek DaCunha, RN, BS,** contributed to this chapter. Ms. Boyd-Monk is the assistant director of nursing for education programs, Wills Eye Hospital, and a clinical instructor in the department of nursing, Thomas Jefferson University Hospital, Philadelphia. Ms. DaCunha is a clinical editor at Springhouse Corporation, Springhouse, Pa.

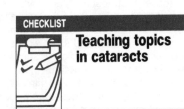

CHECKLIST

Teaching topics in cataracts

☐ Explanation of cataracts
☐ Preparation for diagnostic tests, such as a visual acuity test, slit-lamp examination, tonometry, indirect ophthalmoscopy, keratometry and ultrasonography
☐ Surgical lens removal
☐ Lens replacement options: intraocular lens, contact lens, and cataract eyeglasses
☐ Aftercare instructions, including eye shield application, eye drop administration, and activity restrictions
☐ Sources of information and support

Teaching the cataract patient

A standard teaching plan can help you organize the brief time you'll have to teach a cataract patient. Then, once you finish assessing your patient's learning needs, you'll modify the plan accordingly.

Assess first
Suppose you're caring for Vera Coyle, a 73-year-old, retired lab technician. While you're taking her history, she remarks, "I think I need new glasses. My old ones are so scratched and foggy, I can hardly read the newspaper or do my needlework. I had my daughter bring me here. I'm afraid to drive."

As Mrs. Coyle talks, you notice several bruises on her arms and legs. When you ask about them, she chatters, "I'm always bumping into things—like the door to the linen closet. The other day I tripped going up the stairs and hurt my knee."

When the doctor examines Mrs. Coyle, he diagnoses a cataract in her right eye and recommends surgery to remove the clouded lens and to implant a synthetic lens called an intraocular lens implant. He tells her that only occasionally are cataract glasses or contact lenses used to correct vision, although she'll still need corrective lenses for reading and close work. Surprised by the diagnosis, Mrs. Coyle asks for a few days to decide about the surgery.

Later, as you talk with her and her daughter, you discover that despite Mrs. Coyle's scientific background, she mistakenly thinks that a cataract grows over the eye. She doesn't understand what cataract surgery involves, and she's worried about using the contact lens that the doctor said she could get 6 to 8 weeks after the operation.

She says, "I came here thinking I needed new glasses. Now I find I need an operation. I'm not certain, at my age, that I can do this. I guess I need to know more about this implant thing."

What are Mrs. Coyle's learning needs?
To decide what to teach Mrs. Coyle, compare what she already knows—about cataracts, the surgery to remove them, and aftercare—with the content of a standard teaching plan. Then include or modify teaching points as needed. A standard teaching plan for a cataract patient covers:
• anatomy of the eye and how the lens works
• definition of a cataract, including causes, pathophysiology, and symptoms
• diagnostic tests, such as slit-lamp examination, keratometry, and ocular ultrasonography
• surgery and lens replacement options
• postoperative care measures and precautions.

After talking with Mrs. Coyle, you know you won't have to cover signs and symptoms; they're what brought her to the doctor. And she's just undergone the diagnostic procedures. You know she's adaptable and alert because she's not unreasonably upset about the sudden diagnosis. She's already mentioned that she needs information to help her decide about the surgery. You conclude that you'll focus a teaching plan for Mrs. Coyle on a clear definition of cataracts, an explanation of how they interfere with sight, a brief review of the surgical procedure with full explanation of lens replacement, and precise postoperative care instructions.

Set learning outcomes
Now that you've identified Mrs. Coyle's learning needs, list the outcomes on which you agree. Use the standard teaching plan as a guide. For example, Mrs. Coyle will be able to:

```
-define a cataract in simple terms
-describe how the eye lens functions
-explain how an intraocular lens implant re-
stores distance vision
-show how to apply an eye shield and use eye
drops
-list postoperative precautions.
```

Select teaching tools and techniques
To teach Mrs. Coyle, you choose a short explanation of a cataract, a brief discussion of eye lens function, and a demonstration of eye-drop and eye-shield application, and postoperative precautions—for example, how to keep soap and water out of her eyes to prevent infection or accidental damage. You may use large-print pamphlets, such visual aids as an eye model and a camera, bold posters or flip charts, an eye shield, and an empty eye-drop bottle. You'll reinforce your teaching with printed patient-teaching aids that Mrs. Coyle can review at home.

Because Mrs. Coyle is talkative, you'll need to time the teaching session carefully.

Evaluate your teaching
Appropriate evaluation methods include direct observation and discussion, sometimes using questions and answers, such as about lens replacement and coping with altered vision postoperatively. You might also use simulation of typical problems Mrs. Coyle may encounter after surgery. For example, you could act out how to overcome depth perception loss, covering one of your eyes with a shield.

Can Mrs. Coyle apply an eye shield and eye drops? Does she understand postoperative precautions? Return demonstration can help you evaluate these learning goals.

How a cataract blurs vision

Help your patient understand how a cataract blurs his vision by showing him how the normal and the clouded lens focus light.

Normal eye
Light shining on the cornea passes through the pupil and the clear lens and is focused upside down on the retina. The retina converts light into electrical impulses, and the

optic nerve collects and sends these impulses to the brain, which interprets the image the right way up.

Eye with cataract
Light shining through the cornea is blocked by a cloudy lens. As a result, a blurred image is cast onto the retina, and a hazy image is sent to the brain.

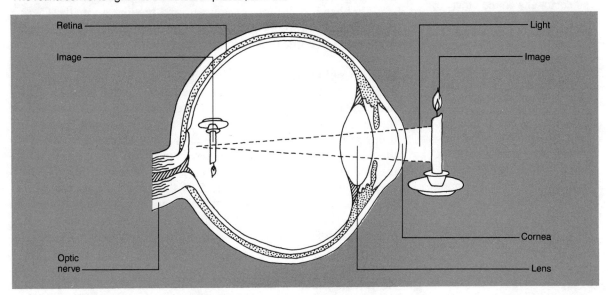

ultrasonography. These tests confirm the diagnosis and determine whether surgery is feasible. When the patient is having an intraocular lens implanted during surgery, the doctor will also measure the length of the eyeball and the curvature of the cornea. Some tests will be repeated after surgery to check the patient's vision.

Visual acuity test
Tell the patient that this brief test checks his distance and near vision and confirms the amount of vision lost. To test distance vision, the patient reads the Snellen eye chart from a distance of 20′ (6 meters), starting with the smallest line that he can see clearly.

To test near vision, he reads a card with print in graded sizes (Jaeger card) from a distance of about 14″ (36 cm). Explain that he'll read first with one eye, next with the other eye, then with both eyes—both with and without corrective lenses.

Slit-lamp examination
Explain that this test allows the doctor to examine the front of the eye and also helps diagnose a cataract. It takes 5 to 10 minutes and it's painless. Any patient who's had an eye examination is fa-

Learning about the slit-lamp examination

Tell the patient that the slit lamp allows the doctor to evaluate abnormalities in the front of the eye. During the examination the patient sits at the slit lamp with his chin on a support and his forehead resting against a bar. The doctor sits on the other side of the slit lamp and examines the patient's eyes through a microscope-like device.

Explain that the doctor will shine minute beams of light into the patient's eye. (To diagnose a cataract, the doctor shines the beam of light to see where it is blocked by the cloudy lens.) Instruct the patient to remain as motionless as possible and to move his eyes as directed.

miliar with the slit lamp, although the doctor probably didn't identify the apparatus by name. For more information, see *Learning about the slit-lamp examination*.

Tonometry

Inform the patient that tonometry is part of the routine slit-lamp examination. The tonometer, attached to the slit lamp, measures intraocular pressure. The test takes only a few minutes. Using special eyedrops, the doctor first numbs the patient's eyes. Then he presses the tonometer gently against the surface of each eyeball and gauges intraocular pressure. Instruct the patient to look straight ahead, hold both eyes open, and breathe normally. Caution him not to rub his eyes for at least 20 minutes after the test. This prevents corneal abrasions.

Indirect ophthalmoscopy

Explain that this test determines whether the retina is intact to make cataract surgery feasible. (Surgery improves vision only if the retina is functioning.) First the doctor or nurse instills eye drops to dilate the pupils, which takes 20 to 45 minutes. When the pupils are dilated, the brief test begins. Tell the patient that the doctor will ask him to focus on a spot on the ceiling. The doctor then holds a lens over each of the patient's eyes and views the retina through an indirect ophthalmoscope, which he wears on his head. If he can't see the retina because a cataract obscures it, he may perform ocular ultrasonography.

Keratometry

Advise the patient that in this brief, painless procedure, the doctor measures the corneal curvature. This permits him to calculate the power of the intraocular lens implant. Tell the patient that to ensure an accurate measurement, the doctor will perform keratometry before any ultrasound tests, which may briefly change the cornea's shape.

Ocular ultrasonography

Tell the patient that the doctor may use two kinds of ocular ultrasonography to evaluate eye structures: A-scan and B-scan. Either scan takes about 15 minutes. During the scan, a small transducer directs high-frequency sound waves at eye structures. When the sound waves strike the structures, they rebound to the transducer and are displayed as images on an oscilloscope's screen. A-scan images appear as waveform spikes; B-scan images form a dot pattern.

A-scan ultrasonography. Explain that the doctor uses this test to assess the eyeball's length and to determine the power of the intraocular lens. First he numbs the eye with drops, then places the clear plastic transducer tip directly on the eyeball.

B-scan ultrasonography. Inform the patient that the doctor uses this test to evaluate the retina when a cataract obscures it and indirect ophthalmoscopy can't be done. First the doctor coats the eyelid with a water-soluble conductant jelly. Then he places the transducer on the eyelid and instructs the patient to move his eyes or change his gaze. The movement helps identify structures within the eye.

Teach about treatments

Inform the patient that surgery is the only way to treat a cataract and restore sight. Explain that most cataracts are removed during same-day surgery (although patients with concurrent disorders may stay overnight for observation). Describe the procedure and the patient's options for lens replacement (see *Describing lens replacement options,* page 468). Mention that most patients (95%) will have an intraocular lens implant.

Then teach the patient how to care for his eye when he goes home. Remind him to arrange for someone to accompany him to and from the hospital because after surgery he'll need help with transportation home.

Preoperative teaching

Describe how the surgeon removes the lens and implants an intraocular lens. Tell the patient that before surgery, you'll give him eye drops to dilate his pupil and to reduce the risk of infection.

As appropriate, discuss anesthesia. If the patient's having a local anesthetic, explain that he'll be awake during surgery. Inform him that the surgeon will give him about three injections of a numbing solution above and below his eye. His eye will be open throughout the surgery, but the anesthetic blocks the optic nerve, so he won't *see* the operation. He'll be aware of the operating room's bright lights. Tell him that his other eye will be patched closed to prevent movement.

Then, standing at the head of the operating table, the surgeon will instruct the patient to lie still and be silent—talking can cause eye movement. Tell the patient that during a brief procedure the surgeon will remove the cloudy lens. Then his eye will be irrigated with a solution to prevent infection.

When the procedure's over, the surgeon will patch the patient's eye. Periodically, the nurse will instill eye drops to prevent infection. Explain that he'll be allowed out of bed immediately after surgery. And if he's an outpatient, he'll be discharged in a few hours when the anesthetic wears off.

Postoperative teaching

Inform the patient that for 6 to 24 hours after surgery, he'll have a patch and a shield on his eye until he sees the doctor the next day. Then for 4 to 6 weeks, he will wear the shield at bedtime and glasses during the daytime to protect his eye. (Make sure to tell him that the doctor will prescribe reading glasses so that he can see things up close.)

Next, instruct the patient to sleep on his unaffected side, and teach him how to apply the shield. (See *How to remove and apply an eye shield,* page 470.) Then review eye-drop administration.

Describing lens replacement options

When explaining cataract surgery, be sure your patient understands that removing the clouded lens won't restore his vision on its own. He'll need a device to replace the missing lens. Most frequently, the doctor uses an intraocular lens implant to correct vision. Occasionally, a contact lens or cataract glasses may be options, although doctors seldom prescribe cataract glasses.

Explain that without a lens implant, vision will be blurred after surgery. Add that the patient must wait between 4 and 8 weeks after surgery until the doctor can prescribe contact lenses or reading glasses or both. As appropriate, review these options with your patient.

Intraocular lens implant
Inform the patient that with this lens he'll probably have clear distance vision immediately, but he'll need reading glasses for near vision. Note that the lens implant, which corrects visual acuity to 20/20 in some patients, provides normal depth perception and peripheral vision with no distortion.

Contact lens
Tell the patient planning to wear a contact lens that it provides normal depth perception and peripheral vision. Caution him that not everyone can wear a lens comfortably. Moreover, learning to insert and remove the lens requires patience, perseverance, and a steady hand. Then explain how to clean and care for the lens, mentioning that even an extended-wear lens, which he can wear continually for up to 7 days, must be checked, cleaned, and reinserted by the doctor at regular intervals. Tell him to expect minimal distortion.

Cataract glasses
Outline the drawbacks of cataract eyeglasses, especially if the patient's other eye is normal. For example, they decrease peripheral vision and affect depth perception because the thick lenses magnify images 20 to 35 times. Warn the patient to take extra care crossing streets and navigating stairways. Also mention that some patients have headaches, dizziness, and nausea until they get used to the glasses.

IMPLANTED INTRAOCULAR LENS

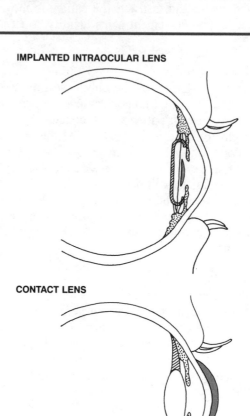

CONTACT LENS

CATARACT GLASSES

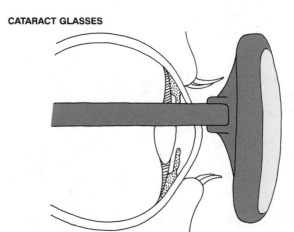

Explain that the doctor may order antibiotic eye drops to prevent infection and corticosteroid eye drops to prevent inflammation. Caution the patient to report acute eye pain to his doctor at once.

Finally, review postoperative activity precautions to prevent increasing intraocular pressure and accidental damage. For example, remind the patient *not* to:
- sleep on the affected side
- lift heavy objects for several weeks
- get soap or unsterile water in his eyes (suggest he tilt his head back to wash and rinse his hair)
- strain during defecation.

Tell him that he'll return to the doctor's office for another slit-lamp examination and tonometry test to evaluate the results of the surgery.

Sources of information and support

American Society of Cataract and Refractive Surgery
3702 Pender Drive, Suite 250, Fairfax, Va. 22030
(703) 591-2220

Better Vision Institute
2020 K Street, NW, Suite 800, Washington, D.C. 20006
(202) 223-2776

Eye Care
1319 F Street, NW, Washington, D.C. 20004
(202) 628-3816

Further readings

Andrews, C.L. "Nursing Care of the Cataract Patient in an Ambulatory Surgery Center," *Ophthalmic Nursing Forum* 3(3):1-8, March 1987.
Borders, C.R. "Cataract Surgery: Who's a Candidate?" *Patient Care* 20(13):46-50, 55, 58-59, 62, 68, 71, August 15, 1986.
Frank, A., and Werfel, N. "ECCE with Phacoemulsification and Flexible IOL Implantation," *Today's OR Nurse* 10(6):30-35, 38-40, June 1988.
Rigler, S. "Personalizing 'Routine' Cataract and IOL Surgery...Intraocular Lens," *Today's OR Nurse* 9(11):20-21, 44-46, November 1987.
West, K. "ABCs of Cataract Surgery Preparation...Assessment, Briefing, and Counseling." *Journal of Ophthalmic Nursing Technology* 6(4):156-58, July-August 1987.
Zavon, B., and Slater, N. "A Surgical Counseling Plan for Patients Undergoing Cataract Surgery," *Journal of Ophthalmic Nursing Technology* 7(2):68-71, March-April 1988.

How to remove and apply an eye shield

Dear Patient:

Your doctor wants you to remove the eye shield (and the patch) that he placed on your eye after surgery. For the next 4 to 6 weeks, he wants you to protect your eye with the eye shield at night. This will prevent rubbing or bumping your eye during sleep.

Removing the shield and patch

1 Wash your hands thoroughly with soap and water.

2 Use a downward motion to peel the tape off your forehead. Gently remove the shield and patch from your eye and continue to peel the tape downward to your cheek. Now, remove the tape from the shield and discard the patch.

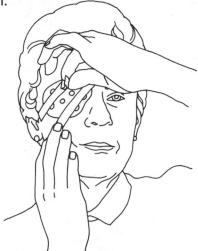

3 If the doctor has ordered eye drops, insert them now.

Applying the shield

Before using the eye shield at bedtime, wash your hands. Place the shield over the affected eye. Then secure it with two parallel strips of hypoallergenic tape, taping from the middle of your forehead to your cheekbone. Make sure that you leave a space between the strips of tape so that you can see through the shield.

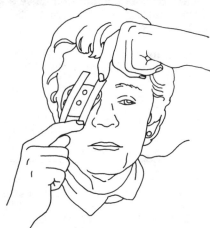

When you get up in the morning, carefully remove the shield. Keep it in a convenient place ready to apply again the next night or anytime you lie down.

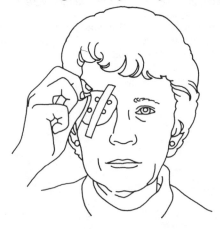

Retinal tear and detachment

Because a retinal tear or detachment demands immediate treatment, your teaching must be brief and reassuring but firm. If the patient only has symptoms such as visual floaters or light flashes, he'll probably be stunned by the need for urgent treatment and the high risk of partial or total vision loss. After treatment, your teaching can address restrictions to ensure healing without complications.

Discuss the disorder

Begin by explaining that the retina, which lines two-thirds of the inner eyeball, is the part of the eye that perceives light. A hole or tear in the retina allows a jellylike substance called vitreous humor to leak between the retina's sensory and pigment layers. This separates—or *detaches*—the retina from its blood supply. Without adequate circulation, the retina can't function properly and vision loss results.

Discuss the cause, if known, of the patient's retinal detachment. Such detachment usually results from degenerative changes of aging, which cause a spontaneous retinal hole. Contributing factors include myopia, cataract surgery, and trauma. Retinal detachment also may result from fluid accumulation in the subretinal space because of inflammation, tumors, or systemic diseases. Or, it may stem from traction placed on the retina by vitreous bands or membranes associated with proliferative diabetic retinopathy, posterior uveitis, or a foreign body lodged in the eye.

Review the patient's symptoms. Initially, he may complain of floating spots in his vision and recurrent flashes of light. As detachment progresses, he'll notice gradual, painless vision loss. He may describe the experience as looking through a veil or a cobweb.

Complications

Point out that retinal detachment rarely heals spontaneously. Tell the patient that he'll lose his vision without surgical reattachment of the retina.

Describe the diagnostic workup

Prepare the patient for direct and indirect ophthalmoscopy to detect retinal detachment, and slit-lamp examination to "sketch" the detachment if one is found.

Joanne Patzek DaCunha, RN, BSN, and **Patricia L. Radzewicz, RN, BSN,** contributed to this chapter. Ms. DaCunha is a clinical editor with Springhouse Corporation, Springhouse, Pa. Ms. Radzewicz was head nurse, EENT unit, at the University of Illinois, Chicago.

CHECKLIST

Teaching topics in retinal tear and detachment

☐ Explanation of retinal tear and detachment, including causes and symptoms
☐ Risk of vision loss without treatment
☐ Preparation for direct or indirect ophthalmoscopy, slit-lamp examination, or other eye tests
☐ Cryotherapy, photocoagulation, or diathermy to repair retinal tear or detachment
☐ Scleral buckling or laser surgery to repair retinal detachment
☐ Activity restrictions after treatment
☐ Eyedrops and their administration
☐ Coping with depth-perception loss
☐ Source of information and support

Direct and indirect ophthalmoscopy

Explain that direct and indirect ophthalmoscopy are used to search the retina for holes and tears. Both tests permit the doctor to see inside the eye and both take about 5 minutes. Advise the patient that first the doctor may instill eyedrops to dilate the pupils. (This gives him a clearer view.) Reassure the patient that although the eyedrops may sting, he should feel no discomfort during the test.

Explain that for *direct* ophthalmoscopy, the doctor peers into the eye through a hand-held ophthalmoscope. Tell the patient that he'll sit upright and stare straight ahead while a bright light shines into his eye.

For *indirect* ophthalmoscopy, tell the patient that he'll lie back and look at the ceiling. Then the doctor, wearing a head-lamp, will shine light into the patient's eye while he studies its interior through a hand-held magnifying lens.

Slit-lamp examination

If the doctor performs a slit-lamp examination, explain that this test allows him to measure a retinal detachment and view other abnormalities inside the eye. Tell the patient that during the test, he will sit on one side of the slit lamp, with his chin on a support and his forehead resting against a bar. The doctor will sit on the other side, looking into the patient's eyes through a microscope-like device. During the examination, the doctor may shine a thin beam of bright light into the patient's eyes. Instruct him to remain as motionless as possible and to move his eyes as the doctor directs.

Teach about treatments

Explain that treatment aims to repair the retinal hole or tear, then to reattach the retina surgically. Results depend on the detachment's extent and location. If the surgeon repairs a detachment in the peripheral retina (associated with nearsightedness), the patient usually regains normal vision. If the detachment involves the macular area, central visual acuity may be poor after surgery. To promote recovery, teach the patient how to instill eyedrops after he's discharged and tell him why he must avoid vigorous physical activity.

Procedures

If appropriate, tell the patient that he may need cryotherapy, photocoagulation, or diathermy to seal the retinal hole or tear. Inform him that he'll probably go home a few hours after the procedure. Suggest acetaminophen (Tylenol) for any discomfort. Then make sure he knows how to give himself eyedrops.

Instruct the patient to avoid vigorous physical activity, bending over, straining, and lifting heavy objects, as they increase intraocular pressure. If elevated, intraocular pressure impairs the

Scleral buckling: Two-step treatment for retinal detachment

Inform the patient that treating retinal detachment is a two-step process. First, the surgeon repairs the retinal hole or tear; then he reattaches the retina.

Repairing the retinal hole or tear
Using cryotherapy, photocoagulation, or diathermy, the surgeon creates a sterile inflammatory reaction that seals the retinal hole or tear and achieves retinal readherence.

Reattaching the retina
The surgeon then performs scleral buckling. Tell the patient that this procedure applies external pressure to the separated retinal layers to reunite the retina with its blood supply.

First the surgeon severs the superior rectus muscle. This allows him to place a silicone plate (or sponge) called an explant over the site of readherence. He keeps the explant in place with a circling band. The pressure exerted on the explant indents or "buckles" the eyeball, gently pushing the choroid and retina closer together.

This reunites the retina with its blood supply and prevents vitreous humor from seeping between the detached retinal layers. Seepage can lead to further detachment and possible blindness.

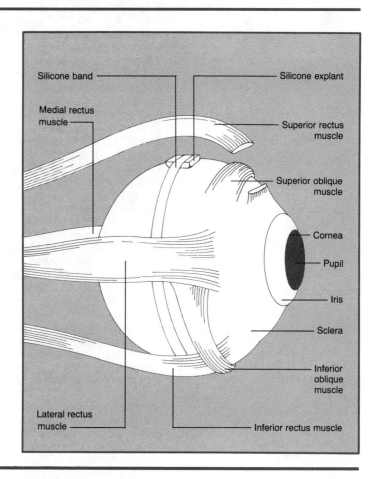

optic nerve's blood supply, which can damage his vision if not corrected.

Surgery
Teach the patient that scleral buckling can reattach the retina. (See *Scleral buckling: Two-step treatment for retinal detachment*.) Before surgery, tell the patient that the doctor may order bed rest and patches on both eyes to minimize eye movement. He also may recommend special positioning for the patient's head to prevent the detachment from spreading to the macula. Explain these measures to the patient.

Postoperatively, inform the patient that he'll be on bed rest with bathroom privileges for several days, then he'll gradually progress to ambulation. Explain that he must comply with positioning instructions after surgery to ensure that his retina remains attached. Advise him to avoid activities that raise intraocular pressure, such as hard coughing or sneezing and bending or straining

Teaching about laser surgery for retinal disorders

Your patient may wonder if laser surgery is for real. Assure him that this proven space-age technique can indeed repair retinal tears and detachments — quickly — with minimal pain and complications.

Explain laser surgery
Discuss how laser treatment generates focused, or monochromatic, light waves. Then it amplifies their power by deflecting them off mirrors to obtain a finely focused, high-energy beam.

To mend retinal holes, tears, and detachments, eye surgeons use heat-generating thermal lasers to achieve photocoagulation or photovaporization. For example, the argon laser produces a short-wavelength, blue-green beam that's highly effective on blood and pigment, making it ideal for repairing the vascular retina or for containing an existing localized detachment with laser burn scars. This limits its size and prevents further damage.

Identify benefits and risks
Inform the patient that laser surgery avoids the common complications of more invasive surgery, such as hemorrhage and infection. Add that it causes less pain and discomfort. Then mention its risks — increased intraocular pressure, iritis, bleeding, pitting of the eye's lens, and, rarely, cataract formation.

Describe the procedure
Inform the patient that he'll have anesthetic eyedrops instilled before treatment. Then he'll wear a special contact lens to keep his eye open throughout the procedure. Tell him that the lens also absorbs some of the thermal energy generated by the laser.

Explain that during the treatment he'll sit at a slit lamp, facing the doctor. Stress the importance of sitting still throughout the procedure. Agree on a signal that the patient will use if he must move, for example, to sneeze.

Next, describe the periodic flashing lights that he'll see as the surgeon uses the laser beam. Assure the patient that the actual procedure lasts only minutes, if that. And after a brief time in the recovery room, he can go home.

Cover aftercare
Tell the patient that typically after treatment, his eye may look bloodshot, and his eyelid may turn black and blue. Explain that he may experience blurred vision and decreased night vision. Also mention that he may see spots before his eyes. Possibly, the bright laser light may trigger a transient headache. Then before he goes home, have him show you how he instills his prescribed eyedrops to protect against infection. And advise him to:
• keep his doctor's appointment for his 24-hour checkup (and other regularly scheduled appointments)
• notify the doctor at once if he has bleeding or his vision is significantly decreased
• avoid activities that increase intraocular pressure, especially using epinephrine-containing nose drops or sprays. He shouldn't strain during defecation, which increases venous pressure in his head, neck, and eyes. If necessary, suggest that he use a stool softener to avoid constipation. Instruct him to keep his head up, to move slowly, and to avoid bending over or moving suddenly.
• sleep with extra pillows under his head to reduce intraocular pressure
• engage in light exercise, such as walking, to promote circulation
• wear sunglasses if the sun bothers his eyes.

during defecation. Emphasize that he mustn't squint or rub or squeeze his eyes. Explain that this can rupture the suture line or cause a new retinal detachment.

If appropriate, tell the patient about laser surgery, an alternative treatment to repair retinal tears and detachment. (See *Teaching about laser surgery for retinal disorders*.)

Other care measures

If the patient has an eye patch, caution him to move about carefully because his depth perception will be impaired. Then give him a copy of the teaching aid *Adjusting to a depth-perception loss*, page 476.

After discharge, the patient will instill his own eye preparations to prevent infection, so show him the proper technique. Mention that the doctor may suggest taking acetaminophen at home to relieve discomfort.

Suggest that the patient avoid crowds to minimize jostling and refrain from reading and writing, which demand rapid eye movement. Advise him to wear dark glasses to reduce photophobia. Instruct him to promptly report any severe or increasing pain; this may indicate increased intraocular pressure or uveitis. Warn him to report any sudden vision changes immediately, and remind him to return for checkups, as ordered.

Provide emotional support; the patient may be distraught about his possible loss of vision. Allow him to air his concerns, and respond to his questions.

Source of information and support

National Eye Institute, National Institutes of Health
9000 Rockville Pike, Building 31, Room 6A32, Bethesda, Md. 20892
(301) 496-5248

Further readings

Boyd-Monk, H., and Steinmetz, C.G. *Nursing Care of the Eye.* East Norwalk, Conn.: Appleton and Lange, 1987.
Clanton, C., and Means, M.E. "Retinal Reattachment: Quality and Appropriateness of Care," *Journal of Ophthalmic Nursing and Technology* 7(4):130-33, July-August 1988.
Gardner, T.W., and Shoch, D.E. *Handbook of Ophthalmology: A Practical Guide.* East Norwalk, Conn.: Appleton and Lange, 1987.
Newell, F.W. *Ophthalmology Principles and Concepts,* 6th ed. St. Louis: C.V. Mosby Co., 1986.
Stein, H.A., and Slatt, B. *The Ophthalmic Assistant: Fundamentals and Clinical Practice.* St. Louis: C.V. Mosby Co., 1988.
Vaughan, D., and Asbury, T. *General Ophthalmology,* 11th ed. East Norwalk, Conn.: Appleton and Lange, 1986.

Adjusting to a depth-perception loss

Dear Patient:

If you're wearing an eye patch after retinal surgery, you may notice some loss of depth perception. To prevent accidents, be especially careful when you walk around or when you climb stairs. Think before you move. Don't assume an object is where it's supposed to be—make sure it's there. These safety tips will guide you.

Sitting down
Slowly approach the chair or other seat. Then turn around and walk backward until the backs of your knees touch the seat. With one hand, grasp the chair's armrest or a nearby table for support. Then sit down.

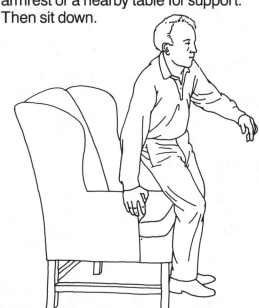

Pouring liquids
Place an empty glass or cup on the counter. Grasp the beverage container with one hand. With your free hand, lo-

cate your glass or cup. Now place the mouth of the beverage container on the edge of your glass, and pour slowly. Watch closely how much you pour. For coffee, juice, or other beverages, fill your cup or glass only one-half to two-thirds full. This will prevent overflows or spills as you lift the glass to your mouth.

Climbing stairs
First grasp the stairs' handrail. Next, use the toe of your foot to locate the riser of the first stair. Lift your foot and place it on the stair. Repeat this procedure as you climb. Use the same method to step up onto a curb.

Descending stairs
Before descending, grasp the handrail. Then use your heel to locate the edge of the top stair. Next, slowly lower your foot and place it on the stair. Repeat this procedure as you descend. The same procedure will help you step off a curb safely.

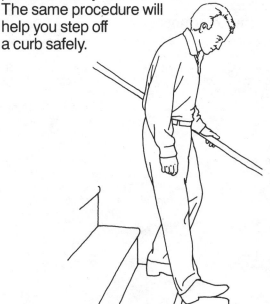

Conjunctivitis

The most common eye disorder in the Western Hemisphere, conjunctivitis strikes all age groups, from newborns to elderly persons. As a result, you'll have many opportunities for patient teaching. What should you emphasize? To help you decide, you'll need to understand the various forms and causes of conjunctivitis. For instance, when conjunctivitis results from bacterial or viral infection, you'll stress proper hand washing and other measures to prevent contagion. You'll include directions for applying prescribed eyedrops and ointment and discuss possible adverse drug effects. If appropriate, you'll cover self-care measures, such as the use of cold compresses to relieve irritated eyes.

Although usually self-limiting, some forms of conjunctivitis may become chronic—causing permanent vision loss in severe cases. Bear in mind that thorough teaching can help the patient minimize potential complications and prevent recurrences.

Discuss the disorder

Inform the patient that conjunctivitis is a catchall term for various disorders that cause conjunctival inflammation. Explain that the conjunctiva is a mucous membrane that lines the inner eyelids and covers the white of the eyeball or sclera. (See *Reviewing conjunctival anatomy*, page 478.) Mention that the popular term "pinkeye" denotes a key sign of conjunctivitis—hyperemia or eye redness. (See *Hyperemia in conjunctivitis*, page 479.)

Tell the patient that conjunctivitis commonly results from bacterial or viral infections. Other causes include an allergic reaction or a chemical or mechanical irritation of the eyes. If the patient's condition has been diagnosed, discuss his form of the disorder in more detail.

Bacterial conjunctivitis

Inform the patient that bacterial conjunctivitis typically develops suddenly, causing eye redness, burning, tearing, and a sticky, mucopurulent eye discharge. He may complain that his eyelids feel stuck together when he wakes up, or he may have the sensation of a foreign body in his eye. The most common causative microorganisms are *Staphylococcus, Pneumococcus, Haemophilus,* and *Moraxella.*

Assure the patient that the infection lasts only about 2 weeks and won't affect his vision. If he complains of blurring when you're checking his vision, advise him to blink several times. This should remove mucus and clear his sight. Warn him that bacterial

CHECKLIST

Teaching topics in conjunctivitis

☐ An explanation of the major types of conjunctivitis, including causes and symptoms
☐ Preparation for diagnostic tests, such as slit-lamp examination
☐ Correct application of eyedrops and ointments
☐ Instructions to prevent the spread of infectious conjunctivitis, such as proper hand washing and other hygienic measures
☐ Self-care measures to soothe eye irritation, such as cold compresses and artificial tears
☐ Source of information and support

Heather Boyd-Monk, SRN, RN, BSN, assistant director of nursing for education programs at Wills Eye Hospital, Philadelphia, wrote this chapter.

Reviewing conjunctival anatomy

Inform the patient that the conjunctiva lining the upper and lower eyelids is called the *palpebral* conjunctiva. The conjunctiva covering the sclera (white of the eyeball) is the *bulbar* conjunctiva.

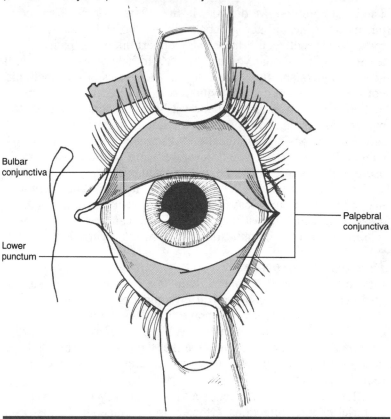

conjunctivitis can easily and rapidly spread to his other eye or to family members.

Caution the patient that bacterial conjunctivitis can become chronic unless treated properly. Chronic conjunctivitis, in turn, may cause dry eyes, scarring, and in severe cases, loss of vision.

Viral conjunctivitis
Tell the patient that viral infections produce copious tearing and swollen preauricular lymph nodes (located just in front of the ears). Explain that common causative agents include several adenovirus types and herpes simplex virus.

Pharyngoconjunctival fever. This form is the most common adenoviral infection in children. Tell the child's parents or caregiver that signs and symptoms—conjunctivitis, pharyngitis (sore throat), and fever—usually develop 2 to 10 days after exposure to the virus (adenovirus type 3). Associated signs and symptoms include runny nose and eyes, GI disturbances, swollen preauricular lymph nodes, or even meningeal symptoms, such as headache, neck ache, fever, or seizures.

Add that this form usually affects only one eye and lasts about 3 weeks. Warn the parents that the disorder is most prevalent during the summer and that swimming pools are a likely source of infection.

Epidemic keratoconjunctivitis (EKC). In this highly contagious form of conjunctivitis, signs and symptoms include eye redness, profuse tearing, blurred vision, and pain from corneal involvement. Warn the patient that the condition tends to occur in large outbreaks because immunity to the virus (adenovirus type 8) is very low. Tell him that the infection typically lasts from 2 to 8 weeks, or longer.

Herpes simplex conjunctivitis. Increasingly common, this viral disease causes eye redness, a foreign body sensation, and pain from corneal involvement. Inform the patient that the infection usually affects only one eye. Mention that herpes simplex isn't highly contagious.

Allergic conjunctivitis
Explain that allergic conjunctivitis results from eye exposure to an allergen, such as airborne pollen or mold. This disorder may also be associated with wearing contact lenses.

Hay fever conjunctivitis. If the patient suffers from hay fever, he may have itchy, burning eyes.

Vernal conjunctivitis. This form of allergic conjunctivitis occurs during spring and summer months in temperate climates. The typical patient is a preadolescent male whose main symptoms are itchy eyes, a stringy, mucoid eye discharge, and pain associated with corneal involvement. Vernal conjunctivitis usually affects both eyes, and inflammation may last 1 to 2 weeks. Explain to the patient or his parents that symptoms are likely to recur annually until he reaches maturity. In some cases, the disorder becomes chronic.

Giant papillary conjunctivitis (GPC). Increasingly common among wearers of hard or soft contact lenses, this allergic condition may develop after weeks or years of normal lens wear. Although its exact cause is unclear, GPC may occur when contact lenses or lens solutions irritate the eyes, causing a hypersensitivity reaction.

Primary signs and symptoms include gradual lens intolerance, blurred vision, increased mucus discharge from the eyes, slight swelling of the upper eyelid, a foreign body sensation, and itchy eyes. Advise the patient that the doctor will examine his eyes and may recommend that he temporarily discontinue wearing his lenses. Eventually he may need to replace his lenses and switch to a preservative-free lens solution.

Chemical conjunctivitis
This form of conjunctivitis may occur in newborns treated with Credé's method to prevent infant blindness. In Credé's method, the newborn's eyes are treated shortly after birth with an anti-infective ophthalmic ointment, such as erythromycin. Tell the parents that this prevents conjunctivitis from infectious microorganisms (such as gonococci and chlamydiae), which may

Hyperemia in conjunctivitis

Your patient may ask why his eye is so red. Tell him that eye redness (hyperemia) is a key sign of conjunctivitis. Hyperemia is caused by local relaxation of the arterioles. Assure him that the condition is not painful and will clear up when his conjunctivitis resolves.

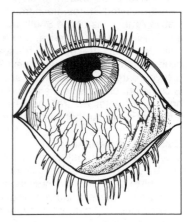

Teaching about trachoma

You can assure your patients that conjunctivitis rarely leads to vision loss. Trachoma, however, is a major exception. This chronic form of keratoconjunctivitis is usually confined to the eye, but can also localize in the urethra.

Although the infection itself is self-limiting, it causes permanent corneal and conjunctival damage. Severe trachoma may lead to blindness, especially if a secondary bacterial infection develops.

In the United States, trachoma is prevalent among Native Americans of the Southwest; it's also prevalent in Africa, Latin America, and Asia, particularly in children. In fact, trachoma is the leading cause of blindness in the world's underdeveloped areas.

If you care for patients in an area where trachoma is common, emphasize the importance of early diagnosis and treatment. Treatment before scarring ensures recovery but not immunity from reinfection.

Causes and transmission
Inform the patient that trachoma results from infection by *Chlamydia trachomatis,* an organism once thought to be a virus but now thought to be related to bacteria. These chlamydial organisms, described as nonmotile, obligate intracellular parasites, are transmitted from eye to eye by flies and gnats in endemic areas.

Trachoma is spread by close contact between family members or among schoolchildren. Other predisposing factors include poverty and poor hygiene from lack of water.

How the disorder progresses
Trachoma begins with a mild infection resembling bacterial conjunctivitis. Clinical features include visible conjunctival follicles, red and edematous eyelids, pain, photophobia, tearing, and exudation.

After about 1 month, conjunctival follicles enlarge into inflamed papillae that later become yellow or gray. At this stage, small blood vessels invade the cornea under the upper eyelid.

Eventually, severe scarring and contraction of the eyelids cause entropion; the eyelids turn inward and the lashes rub against the cornea, producing corneal scarring and visual distortion. Severe conjunctival scarring may obstruct the lacrimal ducts and cause dry eyes.

Treatment
Primary treatment of trachoma consists of 3 to 4 weeks of topical or systemic antibiotic therapy with tetracycline, erythromycin, and sulfacetamide. (Tetracycline is contraindicated in pregnant patients because it may adversely affect the fetus, and in children under age 7, in whom it may discolor teeth permanently.) Severe entropion requires surgical correction.

Prevention
Emphasize the importance of hand washing and making the best use of available water supplies to maintain good personal hygiene. To prevent trachoma, warn patients not to allow flies or gnats to settle around the eyes.

Because no definitive preventive measure exists (vaccines offer temporary and partial protection, at best), stress strict compliance with the prescribed drug therapy.

If ordered, teach the patient or family members how to instill eye drops correctly.

---

have been acquired from the mother during passage through the birth canal. A 1% silver nitrate solution, once commonly prescribed, is rarely used today because it doesn't prevent chlamydial infections. If the newborn's eyes become red or swollen after the procedure, tell the parents that these symptoms usually resolve spontaneously.

If appropriate, discuss a chronic form of keratoconjunctivitis called trachoma. A chlamydial infection, this disease occurs mostly in underdeveloped areas of the world. For more information, see *Teaching about trachoma.*

Describe the diagnostic workup
Inform the patient that a thorough medical history and eye examination are essential for diagnosing conjunctivitis. Prepare him for a slit-lamp examination, explaining that this procedure allows the doctor to visualize abnormalities in the front of the eye.

Describe what happens during the examination. The patient

will sit on one side of the slit lamp with his chin on a support and his forehead resting against a bar. The doctor will sit on the other side of the slit lamp and look into the patient's eye through a microscope. Then the doctor will shine a thin beam of bright light into the patient's eye. Instruct the patient to remain as motionless as possible and to move his eyes as the doctor directs.

Explain that the slit-lamp examination can help diagnose several forms of conjunctivitis. In vernal conjunctivitis, the test may reveal a shield-shaped defect in the upper third of the cornea, resulting from epithelial thinning. The doctor also examines the conjunctiva with the slit lamp. For example, a cobblestone appearance under the upper eyelid indicates vernal conjunctivitis or GPC (see *Conjunctival papillae*).

If the doctor suspects a virulent bacterial infection, he may order a culture and sensitivity test to identify the microorganism. Tell the patient that the doctor will use a cotton-tipped applicator to remove a sample of eye discharge, or that he'll take a scraping of the conjunctiva inside the patient's lower eyelid. Assure him that these procedures aren't painful.

Teach about treatments
Discuss the prescribed medication for the patient's form of conjunctivitis. Remember to cover any special instructions.

Medication
If the patient has a bacterial infection, tell him that the doctor will prescribe antibiotic or sulfonamide eyedrops or ointment. Ophthalmic anti-infectives include sulfacetamide, sulfisoxazole, neomycin, chloramphenicol, or chlortetracycline. For refractory conjunctivitis, the doctor may prescribe tobramycin or gentamicin. For gonococcal infections, he may order systemic penicillin or a cephalosporin.

Teach the patient how to give himself eyedrops or ointment. Provide a copy of *How to use eye ointment,* page 484. Urge him to call the doctor if he experiences signs of sensitivity, such as itching eyelids or constant burning. Tell him always to wash his hands before and after application. Instruct him not to touch the tip of the tube or dropper to his eye or the surrounding tissue.

For herpes simplex viral infections, inform the patient that the doctor may prescribe an antiviral ointment, such as trifluridine, vidarabine, or idoxuridine. If the patient is using idoxuridine, instruct him to apply the medicine exactly as prescribed and for no longer than his doctor orders. Tell him not to use an old solution, which may cause eye burning and be ineffective. Instruct him to call the doctor if his eyes burn or his eyelids itch or swell.

If the patient is using vidarabine, caution him not to exceed the recommended dosage. Explain that this ointment, like idoxuridine, may cause temporary blurred vision. Warn him not to drive a car or operate machinery as long as cloudy vision persists. If trifluridine is prescribed, tell the patient to notify the doctor if his condition doesn't improve in 7 days or if his eyes become irritated.

Conjunctival papillae

Tell the patient that bumps (or papillae) that appear in the conjunctiva of the upper eyelid are a telltale sign of vernal conjunctivitis or giant papillary conjunctivitis. The cobblestone appearance represents swollen lymph tissue within the conjunctival membrane.

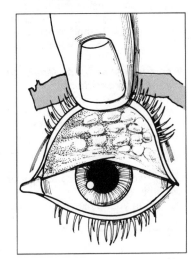

INQUIRY

Questions patients ask about conjunctivitis

Why do I get pinkeye so often?
Pinkeye results from a viral or a bacterial infection. Without realizing it, you may be contaminating your eyes with infected fingers, towels, washcloths, contact lenses, or eye makeup. To prevent recurrent infections, you mustn't touch or rub either the infected or the uninfected eye with your fingers. And don't share washcloths and towels with family members. Also make a habit of washing your hands frequently.

If someone else in my family gets pinkeye, can they use my medicine?
No, they shouldn't share your medicine. The doctor prescribed your medicine especially for your condition. Just because another family member has similar symptoms doesn't mean he has the same type of pinkeye—or should use the same medicine as you.

Can I use the same eyedrops or ointment if I get pinkeye again?
No. When your pinkeye has improved, throw your medicine away. Leftover medicine may lose its effectiveness with time. Moreover, it can become contaminated with harmful germs. Besides, your new symptoms may stem from another type of conjunctivitis and require different medicine. See a doctor about your new symptoms—don't try to diagnose and treat yourself.

Ever since I began wearing soft contact lenses I've had a series of pinkeye infections. Do you think my lenses are causing these infections?
Your lenses probably aren't, but your cleaning methods or solution may be. Make sure to precisely follow the manufacturer's directions for the lens cleaning solution.

Also check the product's expiration date to be certain that your solution isn't too old. If it's too old, it may be ineffective or contaminated.

And *never* moisten your lenses with anything but a sterile solution. For instance, don't moisten them with saliva before putting them in your eyes.

Although adenoviral forms of conjunctivitis (such as pharyngoconjunctival fever or EKC) resist treatment, tell the patient that his doctor may prescribe antibiotic eyedrops to prevent a secondary bacterial infection.

Teach the patient with allergic conjunctivitis about medications to prevent or relieve his symptoms. To reduce inflammation, the doctor may prescribe corticosteroid eyedrops. Instruct him to use the drops exactly as directed. Long-term use may cause cataracts or increased intraocular pressure.

To alleviate allergic symptoms, the doctor may prescribe ophthalmic cromolyn sodium 4%. Instruct the patient to take this drug exactly as prescribed; regular use is required for prophylaxis. The doctor also may prescribe topical decongestants to relieve eye redness and swelling and systemic antihistamines to control general allergic symptoms.

Other care measures
Educate the patient about self-care measures to make him more comfortable and to prevent the transmission of infection.

Enhancing comfort. If the patient has viral or allergic conjunctivitis, tell him that cold compresses may help relieve eye irritation. Also suggest artificial tears, available in drugstores without a doctor's prescription. Tell him that artificial tears are especially soothing if kept refrigerated.

If the patient's medication makes his eyes sensitive to bright light, suggest that he wear sunglasses. Advise the patient with allergic conjunctivitis that an air conditioner or air purifier may improve his well-being.

Preventing contagion. If the patient has a contagious form of conjunctivitis, emphasize and demonstrate proper hand washing to prevent spreading infection. Give him a copy of the patient-teaching aid *Tips for proper hand washing,* page 114. Advise him to avoid touching both the infected and the uninfected eye. If he forgets, stress the importance of washing his hands before and after touching his eyes.

Teach the patient and his family not to share washcloths, towels, pillows, eating utensils, eye medications, or makeup. (See *Questions patients ask about conjunctivitis.*) Recommend using paper towels instead of washcloths or cloth towels for washing and drying his hands and face. If he must use cloth towels and washcloths, advise him to set some aside for his exclusive use and not to share them with another family member. Tell him to wash his cloth towels, washcloths, and linens separately from the family's laundry—using hot water and detergent. Suggest that he use facial tissues instead of handkerchiefs.

Wearing contact lenses may also transmit infection. Instruct the patient to avoid wearing them until his eye is completely healed to avoid spreading infection to the other eye. Once the infection clears up, he should thoroughly clean his contact lenses and lens case before using them again.

Tell the female patient that she may become allergic to her eye makeup. Suggest changing to a hypoallergenic brand or temporarily avoiding eye cosmetics to see if the symptoms resolve. Eye makeup also can become a breeding ground for infectious microorganisms, so warn the patient not to share her cosmetics.

Follow-up care. Stress the importance of follow-up medical appointments. Also instruct the patient to call the doctor if his symptoms persist more than 2 weeks or if he experiences worsening eye redness or pain, blurred vision, light sensitivity, or repeated blinking.

Source of information and support

National Eye Institute, National Institutes of Health
9000 Rockville Pike, Building 31, Room A34, Bethesda, Md. 20892
(301) 496-2234

Further readings

Arentsen, J.J. "The Dry Eye," *Journal of Ophthalmic Nursing Technology* 6(4):134-37, July-August 1987.
Chess, J. "Diagnosis and Treatment of Red Eye," *Physician Assistant* 12 (9):110-11, 115-17, 119, September 1988.
Goldstein, J. "Pharmacology of Ophthalmic Drugs: Anti-inflammatory and Anti-infective Agents, Part 2," *Journal of Ophthalmic Nursing Technology* 6(5):193-97, September-October 1987.
Lawlor, M.C. "Common Ocular Injuries and Disorders: Red Eye," *Journal of Emergency Nursing* 15(1):36-43, January-February 1989.
Taylor, P.B., and Nozik, R.A. "Conjunctivitis: Causes and Management," *Hospital Medicine* 23(12):58, 61-63, 67-68, December 1987.

PATIENT-TEACHING AID

How to use eye ointment

Dear Patient:

Your doctor has prescribed this eye ointment for you:

Name of medicine: _____.
Use this ointment _____times
a day in your _____eye.

Here's how to apply the ointment:

1 Wash your hands thoroughly. Then hold the ointment in your hand for several minutes to warm it before use.

2 Moisten a rayon ball or tissue with water and clean any secretions from around your eye. Wipe outward in one motion, starting at the side near the nose. Remember to avoid touching the uninfected eye.

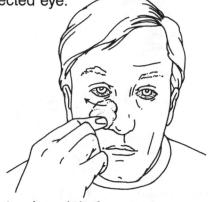

3 Now, stand or sit before a mirror or lie on your back, whichever's most comfortable.

4 Gently pull down your lower eyelid. Tilt your head back slightly and look at the ceiling.

5 Squeeze a small amount of ointment (about ¼ inch to ½ inch) inside the conjunctival sac between your lower eyelid and the white of your eyeball. Steady your hand by resting two fingers against your cheek or nose. It's best to hold the tube close to its tip so you don't accidentally poke your eye with the applicator tip.

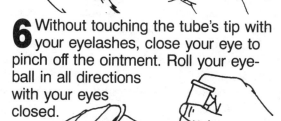

6 Without touching the tube's tip with your eyelashes, close your eye to pinch off the ointment. Roll your eyeball in all directions with your eyes closed.

7 Recap the medication. If you're using more than one ointment, wait about 10 minutes before you use the next one. Don't worry if you have blurred vision temporarily after you use the ointment; this is normal.

Otitis externa

Most commonly affecting swimmers during the summer, otitis externa can actually strike anyone throughout the year. However, if your patient has this infection of the external auditory canal during hot weather or is a competitive swimmer, your most difficult teaching task may involve persuading him to stay out of the water until the infection resolves. You may also need to discourage him from using cotton-tipped swabs or sharp objects to clean the ear canal. What's more, your teaching must cover instillation of eardrops and preventive measures because otitis externa can persist and recur.

Discuss the disorder

Using a picture or a model of the ear, point out where otitis externa occurs as you discuss causes, predisposing factors, and common symptoms (for more information, see *Swimmer's ear: Where it hurts,* page 486). Tell the patient that the disorder can be acute or chronic.

Explain that otitis externa usually results from an excessively moist ear canal or from trauma. Common predisposing factors include swimming in contaminated water, excessive wearing of earplugs or earphones, chronic discharge from a ruptured eardrum, use of sharp objects or cotton-tipped swabs to clean the ear canal, or exposure to irritants, such as hair sprays or dyes, which may cause the patient to scratch his ear. Both moisture and trauma create ideal growing conditions for bacteria or fungi.

Inform the patient that chronic otitis externa may be associated with skin conditions, such as seborrhea or psoriasis, which recur and cause inflammation.

Tell the patient that symptoms of otitis externa include mild to severe ear itching or pain (or both) aggravated by jaw motion or pressure on the pinna or on the tragus. What's more, he may have a swollen, inflamed ear canal, ear discharge, and partial hearing loss.

Complications

Warn the patient that without effective treatment otitis externa can lead to complete closure of the ear canal, causing significant hearing loss. If the infection affects the middle ear, he may experience otitis media (see "Otitis media," pages 491 to 496, for more information). In severe otitis externa, cellulitis may develop, requiring oral or parenteral antibiotic therapy.

Pamela J. Currie, RN, MSN, CRNP, who wrote this chapter, is a nurse practitioner at the University of Pennsylvania Student Health Service, Philadelphia.

CHECKLIST

Teaching topics in otitis externa

☐ Causes, predisposing factors, and signs and symptoms for acute and chronic otitis externa
☐ Complications—namely, hearing loss and cellulitis
☐ The diagnostic workup, including otoscopy, culture for bacteria, and audiometry, if necessary
☐ Activity restrictions, such as no swimming during active infection
☐ Medications—antibiotics and corticosteroids, antifungals, and analgesics
☐ Proper eardrop instillation
☐ Applying heat for pain relief and measures to prevent infection recurrence—especially in children

Swimmer's ear: Where it hurts

Show your patient the areas affected by otitis externa (swimmer's ear). Explain that he may have a sore, swollen ear canal — which can result in impaired hearing — a painful tragus, and discharge.

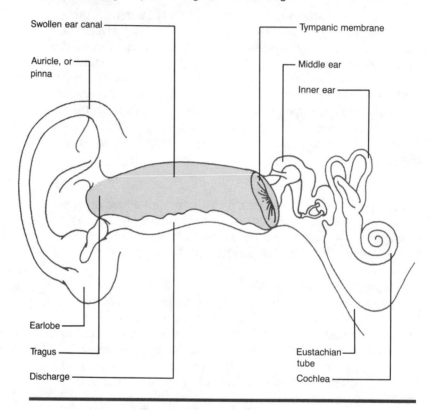

Swollen ear canal

Auricle, or pinna

Earlobe

Tragus

Discharge

Tympanic membrane

Middle ear

Inner ear

Eustachian tube

Cochlea

Describe the diagnostic workup
To rule out ceruminosis, which can cause symptoms similar to otitis externa, the doctor will check for excessive earwax as he examines the patient's ears. If discharge is present, the doctor may obtain a culture specimen. If he suspects a hearing loss, he may also order audiometric tests.

Otoscopy
Explain that the doctor will view the ear canal and the tympanic membrane (eardrum) with an otoscope, looking for signs of infection. Reassure the patient that the examination should cause little discomfort (depending on the severity of his disorder) and should take less than 5 minutes. Forewarn him that his ear will be gently pulled upward and backward to straighten the ear canal and to ease otoscope insertion. Once the doctor positions the otoscope, he'll examine the inside of the patient's ear. To encourage a child's cooperation and allay his fears, let him hold the otoscope while you explain its use.

Culture for bacteria
Inform the patient that the doctor may culture a specimen of ear discharge to identify the causative microorganism and guide selection of antimicrobial therapy. Mention that he'll feel the nurse or doctor lightly scrape his ear with a blunt instrument. After that, the specimen cells will be applied to a culture medium and analyzed in the laboratory.

Audiometric tests
Tell the patient that audiometric tests detect hearing loss and measure its severity. Mention that testing takes about 20 minutes. Explain that each ear will be tested separately. First, the examiner will check the patient's ears with an otoscope. Then he'll press on the ears to detect whether the ear canal will close under pressure from earphones. If necessary during the test, the ear canal can be held open with a stiff-walled plastic tube.

Describe the earphones through which the examiner will transmit sounds of varying intensity. Inform the patient that the examiner will send the tone first to the ear that hears better. This will familiarize the patient with the tone. Instruct him to signal (or press a response button) whenever he hears the tone, emphasizing that he should respond even if the tone sounds faint. If the patient has been exposed to loud noises within the last 16 hours—loud enough to cause tinnitus or make face-to-face communication difficult—the test may be postponed.

Teach about treatments
Treatment involves avoiding the conditions that cause the disorder, using medications to fight infection, and taking measures to relieve discomfort.

Activity
Advise the patient to avoid swimming until otitis externa resolves.

Medication
Inform the patient that the doctor may prescribe antibiotic-corticosteroid eardrops (such as Cortisporin) or antifungal eardrops (such as Otic Domeboro). Typically, the patient will need to instill the eardrops several times a day. Instruct him how to use eardrops; if the patient is a child, give the parents directions as well as a copy of the teaching aid *Giving eardrops to a child,* page 489. Tell the patient to contact the doctor if he has signs and symptoms of local sensitivity to the eardrops—for example, local swelling, increased itching, or hives.

If appropriate, explain that the doctor may insert an earwick to help transport the medication throughout the patient's ear canal. Mention that the earwick may first be moistened with Burow's solution to dry the ear. Then the earwick may be removed, or it may remain in the ear, and the patient may be directed to moisten it periodically with medication. Tell him to ask the doctor how often to remoisten it. Typically, the earwick remains in place for 24 to 48 hours.

Tell the patient that acetaminophen may help relieve pain. If cellulitis develops, treatment may include systemic antibiotics.

Other care measures

Tell the patient that warm compresses or a heating pad applied to the affected ear may relieve pain. To prevent burns, however, clearly instruct him to use the heating pad only on the low setting and to leave it in place for no more than 15 minutes. Caution him not to fall asleep with the heating pad on.

Instruct the patient not to get shower or bath water in his ears. Recommend that he use water-repellent earplugs during bathing for at least 1 week during active infection.

Discuss measures to prevent reinfection, such as:
• using water-repellent earplugs while swimming
• swimming with the head above water
• wearing petrolatum-coated lamb's wool earplugs while showering or bathing
• instilling 1 or 2 drops of a drying solution (equal amounts of household vinegar, household alcohol, and sterile water) in the ear after swimming or showering to help evaporate excess moisture.

Finally, offer the parents of a child with recurrent otitis externa a copy of *How to prevent swimmer's ear,* page 490.

Further readings

Dudley, J.P. "Ear, Nose, Throat, and Sinus Infections," *Topics in Emergency Medicine* 10(4):43-51, January 1989.

Fekety, R., et al. "Prophylaxis for Children and Travelers," *Patient Care* 23(9):104-08, May 15, 1989.

Kroll, S.S., and Gerow, F.J. "Sulfamylon Allergy Simulating Chondritis," *Plastic and Reconstructive Surgery* 80(2):298-99, August 1987.

Meyers, B.R., et al. "Malignant External Otitis. Comparison of Monotherapy vs. Combination Therapy," *Archives of Otolaryngology Head and Neck Surgery* 113(9):974-78, September 1987.

Moser, R. "Ear Infections in Children: Controversies in Care," *Physician Assistant* 13(1):23-24, 26, 28-32+, January 1989.

Schwartz, R.H. "A Practical Approach to Chronic Otitis," *Patient Care* 21(12):91-94, 97-98, 101-03+, July 15, 1987.

Slack, R.W. "A Study of Three Preparations in the Treatment of Otitis Externa," *Journal of Laryngology and Otology* 101(6):533-35, June 1987.

Giving eardrops to a child

Dear Parent or Caregiver:

To treat your child's ear infection, the doctor has prescribed eardrops. Use them exactly as directed on the label.

Getting ready

1 First wash your hands thoroughly. Then examine the medicine. Does it look discolored or contain sediment? If it does, notify the doctor and have the prescription refilled. If it looks normal, you can proceed.

2 Warm the medicine (for your child's comfort) by holding the bottle in your hands for about 2 minutes.

3 Then shake the bottle (if directed), open it, and fill the dropper by squeezing the bulb. Place the open bottle and dropper within easy reach.

Giving eardrops

1 Have your child lie on his side to expose the ear you're treating. Now gently pull the top of his ear up and back. This will straighten his ear canal.

2 Position the filled dropper above — but not touching — the opening of your child's ear canal. Gently squeeze the dropper's bulb once to release 1 drop.

Watch the drop slide into the ear canal. Or have your child tell you when he feels the drop enter his ear.

Then, gently squeeze the dropper's bulb to release the number of drops prescribed.

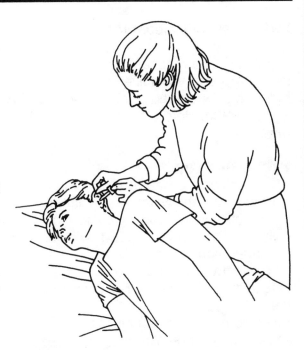

3 Continue holding your child's ear as the eardrops disappear down the ear canal. Now, massage the area in front of his ear. Ask him to tell you when he no longer feels the drops moving in his ear. Then release his ear.

4 Tell your child to remain on his side and to avoid touching his ear for about 10 minutes. If your child's active, place an eardrop-moistened cotton plug in his ear to help keep the medicine in his ear canal. Don't use dry cotton because it may absorb the medicine.

If both ears require medicine, repeat the procedure in your child's other ear. Finally, return the dropper to the medicine bottle (or recap the dropper bottle).

Store the bottle away from light and extreme heat.

How to prevent swimmer's ear

Dear Parent or Caregiver:

If your child has repeated bouts of swimmer's ear, you'd like to prevent it before it gets started or stop it before it gets worse. Here are some hints that may help.

Prevention tips

• Cut back on the time you allow your child to stay in the water — especially if the infection keeps coming back. Typically, you should let your child swim for no longer than 1 hour.

• Allow between 1 and 2 hours for his ears to dry before letting him go back in the water.

• If he complains of water in the ear, show him how to shake or tap his head

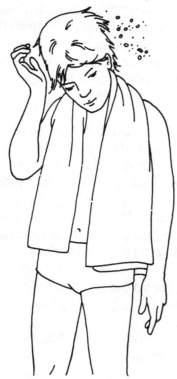

to release water trapped in his ear canal. Then show him how to blot the excess water with the corner of a towel.

• Let your child take short baths or showers every day, but insist he dry his ears afterward using a small dab of cotton rather than a cotton-tipped swab. (Swabs are too big for a child's ears. They can injure the ear canal and make an infection worse.)

• Try using a drying solution made of equal parts water, vinegar, and rubbing alcohol. Put a few drops in your child's ear after he showers, after he swims, and when he goes to bed. Let the solution stay in the ear for at least 5 minutes each time.

Gently wiggle his ear to help the drops seep deeper into the ear canal. This will help to evaporate moisture remaining in your child's ear canal.

Nipping swimmer's ear in the bud

Despite these measures, if your child's ear starts itching or causes him pain, follow these simple steps to keep it from getting worse:

• Call your child's doctor, who may prescribe medicine or may advise you to put a homemade drying solution in your child's ear.

• Keep your child out of the water for at least 1 week — longer if pain, itching, and swelling don't clear up within that time.

• Dry your child's ears immediately after he showers or bathes and shampoos his hair. Then give eardrops as directed by the doctor.

Otitis media

Although otitis media can strike at any age, it most commonly affects infants and children. In fact, acute otitis media represents one of the most common pediatric diagnoses. As a result, you'll largely direct your teaching to parents and, if appropriate, to their children. Expect that parents may be worried and frustrated because otitis media tends to recur. Respond by clearly explaining common symptoms of recurrence. Stress that they can help avoid recurrence of otitis media by seeking prompt treatment for their child and ensuring that he completes the entire course of antibiotic therapy.

You'll also need to help parents understand the disorder by explaining the causes of otitis media, such as bacterial infection and eustachian tube obstruction. Then you'll cover test preparation, surgery, if needed, and other care measures.

Discuss the disorder

Inform the patient (or his parents) that otitis media refers to inflammation of the middle ear. It's associated with fluid accumulation. (See *Where fluid collects in otitis media*, page 492.) Explain that *acute otitis media* usually results from bacterial infection, which produces a buildup of purulent fluid. Bacteria ascend from the nasopharynx through the eustachian tube to the normally sterile middle ear. Because children normally have a shorter and more horizontal eustachian tube than adults, they're predisposed to middle ear infections. Mention that swimming, diving, and flying (especially if the patient has an upper respiratory tract infection) increase the risk of ascending bacterial infection.

Confirm the classic signs and symptoms of acute otitis media: earache, fever, irritability, and hearing loss. In children, especially, a common sign is ear tugging. Other complaints include dizziness, nausea, and possibly tinnitus. If the eardrum ruptures, drainage may occur. If appropriate, tell the patient that *chronic otitis media* is characterized by painless, purulent discharge and moderate to severe hearing loss.

Explain that *serous otitis media* refers to the accumulation of nonpurulent fluid in the middle ear. This usually results from eustachian tube obstruction, which may be secondary to a viral upper respiratory tract infection or an allergy. It may also follow barotrauma. This pressure injury stems from the inability to equalize pressures between the environment and the middle ear. For example, barotrauma may occur in an airline passenger during

Pamela J. Currie, RN, MSN, CRNP, who wrote this chapter, is a nurse practitioner affiliated with the University of Pennsylvania Student Health Service, Philadelphia.

CHECKLIST

Teaching topics in otitis media

☐ An explanation of acute otitis media and of serous otitis media, along with signs and symptoms
☐ Complications, including ruptured eardrum, mastoiditis, and permanent hearing loss
☐ Preparation for tests, such as otoscopy, tympanometry, and audiometry
☐ Activity restrictions on swimming and on plane travel
☐ Medication, chiefly antibiotics
☐ Myringotomy and tympanostomy tube placement, if necessary
☐ Other care measures, including application of local heat

Where fluid collects in otitis media

Show the patient or his parents where fluid collects in the middle ear. Then tell why this happens.

Explain that the eustachian tube normally equalizes pressure in the middle ear. However, obstruction of the eustachian tube or abnormal reflux can cause a vacuum in the middle ear space, hindering drainage of secretions and allowing them to collect. If the secretions remain sterile, the fluid may be thin and watery (in serous otitis media). Or if infectious organisms enter the middle ear space, the fluid may contain pus (in acute otitis media).

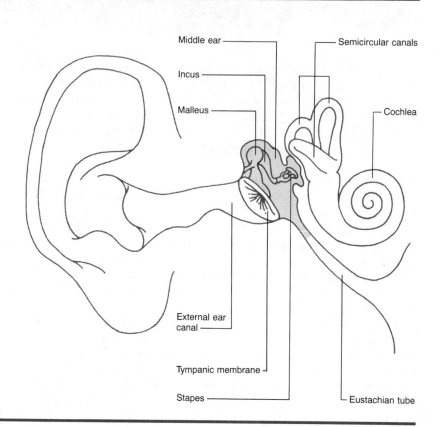

Middle ear

Incus

Malleus

Semicircular canals

Cochlea

External ear canal

Tympanic membrane

Stapes

Eustachian tube

rapid descent if he has an upper respiratory tract infection.

Common symptoms include a mild earache, a feeling of fullness or popping in the ear, and diminished hearing.

Complications

Warn the patient or his parents that untreated or inadequately treated otitis media can result in a torn or ruptured eardrum. If fluid discharge is present, otitis externa can occur. Other possible complications include mastoiditis, meningitis, cholesteatomas, and permanent hearing loss.

Describe the diagnostic workup

Tell the patient that the doctor may perform an otoscopic examination and may schedule tympanometry and other audiometric tests to evaluate the middle ear.

Otoscopy

Show the patient an otoscope, and inform him that the doctor will use this instrument to inspect the eardrum and the middle ear for signs of otitis media. Add that the doctor may use an insufflation tube to check the eardrum's mobility. Reassure the patient that this painless procedure takes fewer than 5 minutes.

Explain that the doctor will gently pull the ear upward and backward (to straighten the ear canal), insert the otoscope, and look inside the ear. If the patient is a child, let him hold the otoscope while you explain how the doctor will use it.

Tympanometry

Inform the patient that tympanometry will be ordered to assess his hearing loss and evaluate the middle ear's condition. This test measures the flow of sound energy into the ear and the ear canal's response to changes in air pressure. It helps evaluate how well the tympanic membrane functions in conducting sound to the inner ear. Explain that a middle ear infection can affect tympanic membrane function.

Tell the patient that the test takes 2 or 3 minutes. First, using an otoscope, the examiner will inspect the patient's ear canal for impacted cerumen (earwax) or other obstructions. Then he'll measure the ear canal's size and shape and select the right-sized test instrument (called a probe cuff). Next, the patient will feel the examiner gently position a probe in the ear canal by pulling upward and backward on the auricle. Mention that silicone putty may be used to secure the probe in a snug, leakproof seal and to ensure accurate test results. Tell him that he may feel transient dizziness but no other discomfort. Reassure him that the probe won't harm his ear.

When the test begins, the examiner will measure the middle ear's reflexes to air pressure changes and to sound variations. Then he'll record the results (called a tympanogram) transmitted by the probe. Instruct the patient not to move, speak, or swallow during the test. Caution him not to be startled when he hears the loud tone that's part of the reflex-eliciting measurement.

Audiometry

Tell the patient that audiometry can detect hearing loss and measure its degree. Explain that testing takes about 20 minutes and that the examiner tests each ear separately, starting with the ear that hears better. Before the test, he'll use an otoscope to inspect the patient's ears for impacted cerumen. Then he'll press on the ears to detect whether the canals will close from the pressure of the earphones worn during the test. (If the canals do close, the examiner may insert a stiff-walled plastic tube into the ear to prevent closure during the test.)

Describe the earphones through which the patient will hear sounds of varying intensity during the test. Then tell him that the examiner will transmit a tone to the better-hearing ear to familiarize the patient with the sounds. Instruct the patient to signal (or press a response button) each time he hears this tone. Emphasize that he should respond even when the tone sounds faint. Advise him that the test will be postponed if he's been exposed to loud noises within the last 16 hours (loud enough to cause tinnitus or make face-to-face communication difficult).

Teach about treatments

Although the doctor may advise rest for otitis media, you'll focus your teaching on the mainstay of treatment: medication. For some patients, you may need to discuss ear surgery, and all patients will need to learn self-care measures.

Activity

Advise the patient to rest until his fever and pain subside. Also instruct him to avoid swimming, diving, and, if possible, flying—especially if he's had an upper respiratory tract infection.

Medication

Inform the patient that treatment for *acute otitis media* consists mainly of antibiotics, such as amoxicillin, ampicillin, and erythromycin (often combined with sulfamethoxazole). Other prescribed antibiotics include cefaclor, amoxicillin and clavulanate potassium, and cefixime. (For more information, see *Teaching about antibiotics for acute otitis media.*)

Instruct the patient to take the medication exactly as directed for as long as prescribed, usually about 7 to 10 days. If appropriate, explain that lower doses of antibiotics may be prescribed prophylactically for recurrent acute otitis media, especially in children.

Inform the patient that decongestants may reduce swelling and eustachian tube obstruction, and acetaminophen may relieve pain and control fever. Warn parents not to give children aspirin because of its suspected association with Reye's syndrome.

Tell the patient with *serous otitis media* that treatment may include decongestants and antihistamines, especially if allergies trigger the disorder or if he must travel by plane. For pain relief, an analgesic, such as benzocaine (Auralgan) or similar eardrops, may be used, but only if the eardrum is intact. Teach the patient how to instill eardrops. Or if the patient is a child, give the parents directions as well as a copy of the teaching aid *Giving eardrops to a child,* page 489.

Surgery

Explain that the most common and effective surgery for recurrent otitis media is myringotomy. (Occasionally, adenoidectomy may be performed in recurrent otitis media, but some experts dispute its effectiveness.) Myringotomy incises the tympanic membrane, releasing fluid from the middle ear and relieving pain and pressure against the tympanic membrane. The procedure may also prevent a ruptured eardrum.

Tell the patient that he'll receive a general anesthetic before myringotomy. (An infant or young child, however, may not receive an anesthetic, so advise the parents that the pain will be brief.) Afterward, he may have a dressing to absorb drainage. Show him how to change the dressing and, of course, caution him to wash his hands before and after each change to prevent infection. Inform him that the incision usually heals in 2 or 3 weeks. Instruct the patient (or his parents) to notify the doctor if his ear

Teaching about antibiotics for acute otitis media

DRUGS	ADVERSE REACTIONS	TEACHING POINTS
amoxicillin (Amoxil) **amoxicillin and clavulanate potassium** (Augmentin)	• Watch for abdominal cramps, severe diarrhea, signs of hypersensitivity (for example, hives, itching, rash, and wheezing), and excessive, unusual thirst or weight loss. • Other reactions include flatulence, headache, mild diarrhea, nausea, sore mouth or tongue, and vomiting.	• Instruct the patient to complete the prescribed course of therapy. Remind him to take every dose. • If the drug causes GI upset, advise him to take it with meals. • If he's taking the drug in suspension form, remind him to check the label for storage instructions.
ampicillin (Omnipen, Polycillin)	• Watch for abdominal cramps, severe diarrhea, signs of hypersensitivity (for example, hives, itching, rash, and wheezing), and excessive, unusual thirst or weight loss. • Other reactions include flatulence, headache, mild diarrhea, nausea, sore mouth or tongue, and vomiting.	• Instruct the patient to complete the prescribed course of therapy. Remind him to take every dose. • Tell him to take the drug on an empty stomach 1 hour before or 2 hours after a meal. • Advise the female patient taking this drug to avoid using oral contraceptives. Suggest using another birth control method. • If the patient's taking the drug in suspension form, remind him to check the label for storage instructions.
cefaclor (Ceclor) **cefixime** (Suprax)	• Watch for abdominal pain and distention; diarrhea (severe, watery, perhaps bloody); fever; hives, itching, or rash; nausea or vomiting; unusual fatigue, thirst, weakness, or weight loss; and wheezing. • Other reactions include mild diarrhea, mild GI upset, and sore mouth or tongue.	• Instruct the patient to complete the prescribed course of therapy. Remind him to take every dose. • Suggest taking the drug with food or milk to decrease GI upset. • Tell him to store the reconstituted suspension form in the refrigerator and to shake the drug well before taking a dose. Inform him that the suspension form is stable for 14 days if refrigerated. • If the drug triggers diarrhea, tell the patient to contact the doctor before taking any antidiarrheal medicine.
erythromycin (E-Mycin, Erythrocin, Ilosone, Pediamycin)	• Watch for dark- or amber-colored urine, fever, pale stools, severe abdominal pain, unusual fatigue or weakness, and yellow-hued eyes or skin (more common with Ilosone). • Other reactions include abdominal cramps, diarrhea, nausea, sore mouth or tongue, and vomiting.	• Instruct the patient to complete the prescribed course of therapy. Remind him to take every dose. • Advise him to take the drug 1 hour before or 2 hours after meals. If the doctor prescribes enteric-coated, estolate, or ethylsuccinate drug forms, the patient can take the drug without regard to meals.
co-trimoxazole (trimethoprim-sulfamethoxazole) (Bactrim, Septra) **sulfamethoxazole** (Gantanol)	• Watch for aching joints or muscles, fatigue, fever, hypersensitivity signs (skin blisters, peeling, rashes, and redness), pallor, unusual bleeding or bruising, weakness, and yellow-hued eyes or skin. • Other reactions include anorexia, diarrhea, dizziness, headache, nausea, photosensitivity, and vomiting.	• Instruct the patient (or the patient's caregiver) to complete the entire prescribed course of therapy. Remind him to take every dose. • Advise him to take the drug on an empty stomach 1 hour before or 2 hours after meals. • Tell him to drink a full glass of water with each dose and extra water daily to prevent formation of urine crystals. • Caution him to avoid direct sunlight and ultraviolet light to prevent a photosensitivity reaction. • If appropriate, advise him to notify his surgeon that he's taking this drug before he receives a general anesthetic. • Explain that "DS" on the drug label may mean "double strength."

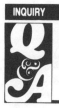

Questions parents ask about otitis media

The doctor says my child has a temporary hearing loss. When will his hearing return?
Your child's hearing should return to normal once his infection or eustachian tube blockage is relieved. Make sure he takes his medication as the doctor directs. If he's having surgery, remember to follow the doctor's directions afterwards. If his condition remains hard to treat, hearing improvement may take longer.

How many times must my child get an ear infection before the doctor will recommend tubes?
The doctor usually advises placement of the tympanostomy tubes you're talking about after a child's been treated with antibiotics for 1 to 3 months without improved hearing. Or he may recommend their use after a child has had numerous and frequent ear infections even without a hearing loss.

Now that my child has tubes in his ears, how will I know if he has an infection?
If the tubes function normally, you'll see drainage from the outer ear canal. However, if the tubes are clogged, your child may respond as usual to infection. That is, he may tug at his ear, feel feverish, and act restless and irritable.

drains for more than 1 week or if the drainage color changes.

If the doctor inserts a pressure-equalizing tube (called a tympanostomy tube) through the tympanic membrane after myringotomy, explain that the tube stays in place for 6 to 12 months unless the doctor removes it sooner. Usually, however, the tube falls out (toward the outer ear) on its own. Advise the patient to notify the doctor when the tympanostomy tube falls out. He should also notify the doctor if he has any ear pain, fever, or pus-filled ear discharge. These effects may signal a blocked tube or a reinfection. (For more information, see *Questions parents ask about otitis media*.)

After a myringotomy and tympanostomy tube insertion, tell the patient that many doctors permit swimming without protecting the ears. And unless he swims in contaminated water, he's unlikely to be reinfected, but he should consult his doctor to be sure. Warn him not to get soapy bath or shampoo water in his ear canal. Suggest that he use petrolatum-coated, cotton earplugs during showers or baths.

Other care measures
Show the patient how to soothe the affected ear by applying heat locally. Caution parents to apply heat cautiously to a child's ear to avoid burns. Also teach parents to hold their infant in an upright position during bottle feeding to help maintain eustachian tube patency.

Instruct the patient to seek prompt treatment for upper respiratory tract infections. Also teach him to practice self-inflation of the eustachian tube to relieve pressure during airplane travel. Tell him to pinch his nose shut, then take a deep breath, close his mouth, and try to blow his nose while keeping it shut. Or advise him to swallow or yawn during a flight.

Further readings
Carlin, S.A., et al. "Early Recurrences of Otitis Media: Reinfection or Relapse?" *Journal of Pediatrics* 110(1):20-25, January 1987 (published erratum appears in *Journal of Pediatrics* 110(4):668, April 1987).

Dyson, A.T., et al. "Speech Characteristics of Children After Otitis Media," *Journal of Pediatric Health Care* 1(5):261-65, September-October 1987.

Fireman, P. "Newer Concepts in Otitis Media," *Hospital Practice* 22(11):85-91, November 30, 1987.

Jones, S.L., et al. "A Nursing Intervention to Increase Compliance in Otitis Media Patients," *Applied Nursing Research* 2(2):68-73, May 1989.

Schwartz, R.H. "The Reevaluation Visit for Acute Otitis Media," *Journal of Family Practice* 24(2):145-48, February 1987.

Von, T., et al. "The Effects of Chronic Otitis Media on Motor Performance in 5- and 6-Year-Old Children," *American Journal of Occupational Therapy* 42(7):421-26, July 1988.

Epistaxis

A common occurrence both in children and adults, epistaxis (nosebleed) usually can be treated at home, although many patients seek treatment at the doctor's office or emergency department. Because blood loss (even a small amount) can be frightening, you may center your initial teaching on decreasing patient anxiety and discussing ways to control the bleeding. This becomes especially important when you consider that an anxious patient may hyperventilate and aspirate blood from his nose.

Later, you'll teach the patient to recognize when he needs medical attention for epistaxis. You'll explain that after locating the source of bleeding, treatment consists of controlling the bleeding by various means, such as cauterization, nasal packing, and arterial embolization or ligation.

Discuss the disorder

Inform the patient that epistaxis refers to any bleeding from the nasal cavity. The bleeding may be acute or recurrent and anterior or posterior. The frequency of bleeding, the site, and the cause determine the disorder's seriousness.

Tell the patient that the nasal cavity's rich arterial blood supply makes it susceptible to epistaxis. Explain that the internal and external carotid arteries supply blood to the posterior part of the nasal cavity. In the anterior nasal cavity, branches of these two arteries anastomose, creating a highly vascular area known as Kiesselbach's (or Little's) area. This is the site of most episodes of epistaxis, referred to as *anterior epistaxis*. Although less common, *posterior epistaxis* is considered more serious because it may involve the larger arteries.

Teach the patient that the causes of epistaxis may be *external* or *internal*. External causes include nose picking, nose blowing, and traumatic injury from a blow to the nose or from a foreign body inserted in the nose. External causes also include environmental factors (such as forced-air heating, which dries the nasal mucosa and leads to cracking and bleeding) and inhaled irritants, which cause nasal blood vessels to dilate and to become more fragile.

Internal causes of epistaxis include infection, neoplasm, or a vascular disorder (such as hypertension). Anticoagulation therapy, chronic aspirin use, sclerotic vessel disease (such as arteriosclerosis), Hodgkin's disease, vitamin K deficiency, rheumatic fever, and blood dyscrasias (for example, hemophilia, purpura, leukemia, and some anemias) may predispose the patient to epistaxis. Additionally, hematopoietic, idiopathic, and hereditary disorders,

CHECKLIST

Teaching topics in epistaxis

☐ External and internal causes of epistaxis
☐ The difference between anterior and posterior epistaxis
☐ Complications of severe epistaxis
☐ Blood studies and other diagnostic tests, such as sinus X-ray, computed tomography scan, and carotid angiography
☐ Activity restrictions
☐ Medications to control bleeding
☐ Manual compression to stop epistaxis in children
☐ Other treatments to control bleeding, such as cauterization, balloon compression, nasal packing, arterial embolization, and arterial ligation
☐ Home care measures, including ice packs, medicated gauze, and humidifiers
☐ Source of information and support

Debra Harris Lillback, RN, BSN, MSN, who wrote this chapter, is the coordinator of quality assessment at Crozer-Chester Medical Center in Upland, Pa.

such as telangiectasia (Osler-Weber-Rendu disease), may cause epistaxis. So can acute or chronic infections, such as sinusitis, which produce congestion and eventual capillary bleeding. Rarely, ectopic endometrial nasal tissue from endometriosis may cause nasal bleeding during menstruation (for more information, see *Questions patients ask about nosebleeds*).

Complications
Stress that failure to control epistaxis may result in significant blood loss and subsequent low blood pressure, impaired respiratory status, and even shock (especially from massive blood loss with posterior epistaxis). Profuse posterior epistaxis may be complicated by aspiration, and cumulative complications may even lead to life-threatening respiratory or cardiac arrest.

Describe the diagnostic workup
Prepare the patient for diagnostic procedures to locate the bleeding and identify its cause. The doctor will compile a health history and perform a physical examination. He'll also inspect the patient's nasal cavity and evaluate his blood pressure (to detect possible hypertension). Discuss other tests that he may order, such as routine blood tests, sinus X-rays, computed tomography (CT) scan, and carotid angiography.

Blood studies
If the doctor orders blood tests, such as a complete blood count, platelet count, prothrombin time, and activated partial thromboplastin time, explain that these studies will help estimate blood loss and rule out a hematopoietic or coagulation disorder as the cause of bleeding. Prepare the patient for venipuncture.

If the patient's treatment program includes nasal packing for posterior epistaxis, tell the patient that arterial blood gases may be measured to monitor air exchange and oxygen levels in his blood. Tell him who will perform the arterial puncture and when. Instruct him to breathe normally during the test. Forewarn him that he may feel a brief cramping or a throbbing sensation at the puncture site (radial, femoral, or brachial artery).

Sinus X-rays
Inform the patient that a sinus X-ray may reveal whether a sinus neoplasm or an infection causes his nose to bleed. X-ray images will be taken from several angles. Reassure him that the procedure takes only a few minutes and should cause no discomfort. Instruct him to remove any dentures, jewelry, or metal objects that may obscure the images and distort the test findings.

CT scan
Explain that a CT scan can detect tumors or vascular abnormalities that may cause epistaxis. Inform the patient that the test is painless and takes between 30 and 60 minutes. If the doctor will be using a contrast medium, instruct the patient not to eat or drink anything for 4 hours before the test.

Then preview what happens during the test. Tell the patient

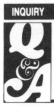

Questions patients ask about nosebleeds

Why do I always seem to get nosebleeds in the spring?
An allergy may trigger springtime nosebleeds. This is especially true if a winter of forced-air heating leaves your nasal cavity dry and irritated and prone to bleeding.

To prevent nosebleeds, try to avoid known irritants. Also consider adding moisture to the air you breathe with a room or whole-house humidifier. Another home remedy may help too. Just dab a small amount of petroleum jelly inside your nose to help keep it moist. If you think you have an allergy, talk with your doctor before you begin taking any medications to control it.

My sister thinks I must have high blood pressure because I get nosebleeds. Is she right?
Not necessarily. Experts disagree on whether high blood pressure causes nosebleeds or is the symptom of other causes that lead to them. In patients who have high blood pressure, blood vessel degeneration from arteriosclerosis is the primary cause of nosebleeds. Hypertensive patients usually have more serious nosebleeds because of increased pressure on the blood vessels. As a result, they often require medical treatment to stop the bleeding. Consult your doctor to identify the exact cause of your nosebleeds. Then comply with his recommendations to keep the nosebleeds from recurring.

Sometimes I vomit when I have a nosebleed. Why does this happen?
Swallowing blood from a nosebleed can upset your stomach and cause vomiting. Prevent this by sitting up rather than lying down during a nosebleed and by holding your head slightly forward. Also spit out—rather than swallow—any blood that comes into your mouth. Finally, avoid drinking fluids if you have any blood in your mouth, throat, or stomach. Doing so may cause vomiting.

---

that he'll be positioned on a movable X-ray table with a strap placed across his head to restrict any movement. The table will then slide into the scanner's circular opening. If a contrast medium is ordered, the patient will receive it intravenously. The infusion takes about 5 minutes. Instruct him to immediately report any discomfort—for example, a feeling of warmth or itching. Assure him that the technician can see and hear him from an adjacent room. Describe the noises that he'll hear as the scanner revolves around him.

Carotid angiography
Explain that this radiologic test outlines the external and internal carotid arteries to help define the bleeding source. Estimate the time the test will take (30 minutes to 4 hours), depending on the blood vessels examined. Inform the patient that an area on his skin will be shaved and cleaned. Then he'll receive a local anesthetic, and a catheter will be introduced into a blood vessel.

During the test, a dyelike contrast medium will be injected through the catheter into the arteries. Then several X-rays will be taken to follow the dye's passage through the blood vessels. Warn the patient that he may feel flushed or nauseated or notice an unusual taste in his mouth when he receives the contrast medium. Reassure him that these sensations should subside quickly. Inform him that he may be asked to assume various positions; otherwise, direct him to stay still to avoid blurring the images.

Describe what happens after the test, beginning with the catheter's removal. Tell the patient that he'll have pressure applied to the insertion site for about 15 to 30 minutes. Afterward, a bulky dressing will be applied. To provide additional pressure, a sandbag will be rested against the dressing.

Teach about treatments

Explain treatments to stop the nosebleed and prevent recurrent bleeding. Specific measures include manual compression to stop the bleeding, medication to constrict nasal blood vessels, and avoidance of activities that may traumatize the nose. As appropriate, describe additional procedures, such as chemical or electrocautery, balloon compression, nasal packing, arterial embolization, or surgical ligation.

Activity

Urge the patient to avoid activities that may injure his nose—contact sports, for example. If he can't avoid such activities, encourage him to wear protective equipment, such as a helmet, a face protector, or an inhalation mask.

Instruct him to limit his activity both during and after a nosebleed and to sit down rather than lie down during a nosebleed. Caution him not to blow his nose forcefully.

Medication

Teach the patient about drugs to help control bleeding. For example, the doctor may use a cotton ball or cotton-tipped applicator to apply a vasoconstrictor (such as epinephrine) to the bleeding site to constrict the blood vessels and reduce the bleeding.

Procedures

Discuss various procedures that control bleeding, including manual compression, cauterization by chemical or electrocautery, balloon compression, and nasal packing. If these measures fail and bleeding persists or if the patient bleeds profusely, explain that arterial embolization may be necessary.

Manual compression. Show the patient how to perform manual compression at the first sign of bleeding. Direct him to sit up, lean forward, and grasp the entire lower half of his nose between his thumb and fingers. Tell him to firmly compress both sides of his nose against the nasal septum for about 10 minutes. This will allow the blood to clot. If the bleeding restarts after he releases the pressure, explain that a large clot may be keeping the broken blood vessel from retracting. In this case, instruct him to blow his nose vigorously to dislodge the clot and then to repeat the compression procedure for another 10 minutes or longer.

Uncontrollable epistaxis may result from ineffective compression or from severe anterior or posterior epistaxis (or both). Urge the patient to continue compressing his nose and to seek medical attention without delay if bleeding persists. If the patient is a young child, give his parents a copy of the teaching aid *Teaching a child how to stop a nosebleed,* page 504.

Cauterization. Inform the patient that the doctor may use either *chemical cautery* or *electrocautery* to stop epistaxis. Before cauterization, he may apply an anesthetic (such as xylocaine) to initiate vasoconstriction and pain relief. Next, he may apply an absorbable material to the area to decrease bleeding. Explain that chemical cauterizing agents include silver nitrate, trichloroacetic acid, or chromic acid, which the doctor will apply to the bleeding site with a wooden or wire applicator. In electrocautery, the doctor will use a wire applicator to apply a thermal or high-frequency current to the bleeding site. Reassure the patient that both methods cause minimal discomfort and take only a few minutes to perform. Instruct him not to disturb the cauterized site because the area easily can bleed again.

Balloon compression. An alternative to cauterization or nasal packing, balloon compression may be used to stop epistaxis (see *Understanding balloon compression for epistaxis,* page 502). Inform the patient that he'll be hospitalized for the procedure and that he'll stay in bed for 24 to 48 hours after the balloon is inserted. During this time, the nurse will offer him cool liquids to drink and ice chips to suck. She'll apply an ice pack to his neck to reduce the blood flow to his head, and as ordered, give him a sedative to help him to rest. Warn the patient that his nose may continue to ooze. Tell him to report any breathing difficulty.

Inform the patient that he may require rest for another 24 hours after the balloon's removed and before being discharged. Instruct him not to blow his nose until the doctor gives permission. Even then, instruct him to blow his nose gently.

Nasal packing. If direct pressure and cauterization fail to stop the bleeding, the doctor may insert nasal packing. Tell the patient that first he may receive a sedative or a tranquilizer. Then he'll sit down and lean slightly forward. The doctor will anesthetize the patient's nasal passages with a vasoconstrictive agent (which may also help to control bleeding). As soon as the anesthetic takes effect, the doctor will suction blood clots and debris from the patient's nose and locate the bleeding site. If the patient has anterior epistaxis, explain that the doctor will use forceps to layer petrolatum or iodoform gauze strips horizontally inside the nasal cavity. He'll leave one end of the gauze at the tip of the nostril to allow easy removal of the packing.

If the patient has posterior epistaxis, the doctor will insert a lubricated catheter into the patient's nose and advance it into the nasopharynx. Instruct the patient to pant to minimize gagging. When the catheter reaches the nasopharynx, the doctor will pull it out through the mouth and secure it to sutures tied around a roll of gauze. Then the doctor will withdraw the catheter through the nose. This action pulls the packing into proper position behind the soft palate and against the posterior septum. Inform the patient that the doctor will inspect the patient's mouth to make sure that the packing clears the uvula. Then he'll detach the catheter from the packing and secure the packing with tape and dental rolls.

Tell the patient that he must be hospitalized for this procedure and that he'll remain in bed for 2 to 4 days after the packing is inserted. Advise him that he may be sedated to help him rest. Instruct him to ring for help if he has any breathing difficulty.

Advise the patient that before his discharge he may need to rest for another day after the packing's removed. Caution him not

Understanding balloon compression for epistaxis

When a patient has epistaxis severe enough to require medical attention, chances are he's going to be upset and afraid—especially if the doctor chooses a nasal balloon catheter to stop the bleeding. Help relieve the patient's anxiety by discussing how the device works, how it's inserted, and how it's removed.

Describe the device
Tell the patient that the doctor may select a single- or double-cuffed nasal balloon catheter to control posterior epistaxis. Both devices rely on pressure to compress bleeding blood vessels.

Once inflated, the single-cuffed device compresses the blood vessels while a soft, collapsible outer bulb prevents the device from sliding out of place. When the doctor inflates the double-cuffed catheter, the posterior cuff secures the catheter in the nasopharynx, and the anterior cuff compresses the bleeding blood vessels. Reassure the patient that this device has a central airway so that he can breathe more naturally.

Explain insertion
Inform the patient that first the doctor will lubricate the catheter with an antibiotic ointment and then will slide the catheter into the patient's nostril. Next, through a valve in the catheter, the doctor will inflate the balloon cuff with a sterile saline solution. Then he may secure the catheter's outer tip to the patient's nose with tape.

Tell the patient that the nurse will check the catheter's placement. Mention that a small amount of discharge normally appears around the catheter.

Discuss removal
When the bleeding's controlled, the doctor will use a syringe to withdraw the saline solution from the balloon. Then he'll gently withdraw the catheter.

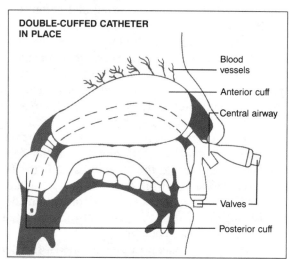

SINGLE-CUFFED CATHETER IN PLACE — Blood vessels, Cuff, Valve, Bulb

DOUBLE-CUFFED CATHETER IN PLACE — Blood vessels, Anterior cuff, Central airway, Valves, Posterior cuff

to blow his nose for the next 2 or 3 days because this may provoke new bleeding. Inform him that he can expect slight oozing of bloodstained fluid from his nose for the next few days. Direct him to report any frank bleeding.

Arterial embolization. If the doctor can't locate the specific arterial bleeding site quickly, he may perform arterial embolization. First, prepare the patient to undergo carotid angiography to find the bleeding blood vessel. Explain that he'll receive a local anesthetic, and a catheter will be introduced into a blood vessel. Then a contrast medium will be injected through the catheter into the arteries. X-rays will be taken to follow the dye's passage to the bleeding blood vessel. Next, the doctor will inject a clot-forming material into the artery via the catheter. The clot thus formed will stop the bleeding.

After the procedure, pressure will be applied to the catheter insertion site for 15 to 30 minutes. Then a dressing will be applied, and a sandbag will be pressed against the dressing.

Surgery
Advise the patient that he may need surgery to ligate the blood vessel responsible for severe bleeding or for bleeding that conservative treatment fails to stop. If the patient's having external carotid arterial ligation, inform him that the doctor will make an incision in the patient's neck. If the anterior ethmoidal artery is involved, the surgeon will make an incision along the outside edge of the patient's eye.

Inform the patient that he'll receive a sedative before the procedure and a local anesthetic for the surgery itself. Tell him that afterward he'll remain in the hospital for 24 to 48 hours for observation.

Other care measures
Demonstrate home care measures to control epistaxis. Show the patient how to apply ice packs to the back of the neck during a bleeding episode. Explain that cold helps to constrict the vessels supplying blood to the nose and, in turn, slows or stops the bleeding. Also show him how to press gauze impregnated with an antibiotic drug, such as bacitracin (Bacitin), over the bleeding site. Explain that this moistens nasal mucosa and helps prevent recurrent bleeding. To keep his nasal mucosa from drying out further, advise him to use a cool-mist humidifier to add moisture to the air in his home.

Finally, if the patient has had severe bleeding, explain that he may need intravenous therapy (to reestablish adequate hydration and restore fluid balances) or even a blood transfusion.

Source of information and support
National Institute of Allergy and Infectious Diseases
9000 Rockville Pike
Building 31, Room 7A-03, Bethesda, Md. 20205
(301) 496-5717

Further readings

Chait, R.H., and White, J.D. "Emergency Management of Epistaxis," *Emergency Medical Services* 16(9):55-57, 85, October 1987.

Guarisco, J.L., and Graham III, H.D. "Epistaxis in Children: Causes, Diagnosis, and Treatment," *Ear, Nose, and Throat Journal* 68(7):522, 528-30, 532+, July 1989.

Harvey, M. "Controlling Nasal Haemorrhage: The Brighton Epistaxis Balloon," *Nursing Times* 83(13):48-49, April 1-7, 1987.

"Hemotympanum with an Intact Skull," *Emergency Medicine* 21(5):63, March 15, 1989.

Hicks, J.N., and Vitek, G. "Transarterial Embolization to Control Posterior Epistaxis," *Laryngoscope* 99(10, part 1):1027-29, October 1989.

Lockhart, J.S., and Griffin, C. "Action STAT! Epistaxis," *Nursing86* 16(11):33, November 1986.

Teaching a child how to stop a nosebleed

Dear Parent:

Even a minor bump on your child's nose can start a nosebleed. To keep your child from panicking, teach him how to stop the bleeding. Here are some steps to follow.

Apply pressure
When your child's nose bleeds, show him how to pinch the lower half of his nose tightly shut between his thumb and fingers. Tell him to breathe through his mouth while he holds his nose like this for about 10 minutes.

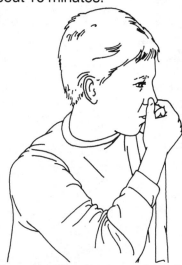

If his hand or fingers tire, advise him to switch hands by placing the thumb and fingers of his rested hand above the fingers of his tired hand. Tell him to start pinching with the rested hand as he lets go with his tired hand. Then he can slide his fingers down his nose until they're pinching the lower half of his nose as before.

Practice pinching each other's noses.

This way you'll both learn how much pressure to apply. And you'll know how your fingers feel when they're in the right position.

Watch to be sure your child compresses the entire lower half of his nose — not just the tip.

Sit still, be calm — and other tips
Teach your child to sit down — quietly and calmly — whenever his nose starts to bleed. Show him how to tilt his head slightly forward so that he doesn't swallow or choke on his blood.

Warn him not to tilt his head backward, not to lie down, and not to stuff a tissue in his nose.

Direct him to spit out any blood that gets in his mouth or throat. Tell him to spit into a container if possible. This will allow you or another supervising adult to estimate the blood loss.

Reassure your child that he can resume playing when the bleeding stops. Ask him to play *quietly,* not vigorously, to keep the bleeding from starting again.

Remind him not to pick or blow his nose after a nosebleed because the bleeding may recur.

Get help
Instruct your child to get help from an adult if a nosebleed doesn't stop after 10 minutes or if bleeding starts again. Direct him to stay calm and to walk (not run) to find help if he has to. Tell him to hold his head straight or bent slightly downward and to keep applying pressure on his nose until he finds help.

Allergic rhinitis

Plagued by fitful sneezing and a stuffy, itchy nose, the patient with allergic rhinitis usually feels miserable but doesn't know why. You'll need to teach him what causes this disorder and how it differs from the common cold, for which it's often mistaken.

Prepare the patient for tests to confirm the diagnosis and to identify the allergens responsible for this disorder. Then teach him how to control his symptoms with medications and careful avoidance of environmental allergens. If appropriate, explain immunotherapy that can desensitize him to specific allergens. Reassure him that with proper treatment he can minimize or even eliminate his signs and symptoms.

Discuss the disorder

Inform the patient that allergic rhinitis is an allergic response to airborne allergens. It's characterized by inflamed nasal mucous membranes. Describe how the nose normally functions and how allergic rhinitis disrupts this complex mechanism (see *Understanding how the nose functions,* page 506).

Explain that in allergic rhinitis the immune system produces antibodies against seemingly harmless substances (called antigens or allergens), such as dust, pollen, or mold. Then, subsequent antigen-antibody interaction triggers the allergic response, causing the mast cells in the nose and surrounding tissues to release histamine and other potent chemicals.

Ask the patient to review his symptoms. He'll probably report nasal stuffiness, a runny nose, postnasal drip, sneezing, reddened and teary eyes, sinus pain, and an itchy nose and palate. Note that symptoms primarily affect the nose and eyes but may also involve the sinuses and ears.

Discuss the two major forms of allergic rhinitis. In *seasonal allergic rhinitis,* better known as hay fever, symptoms are more common during certain seasons of the year. In *perennial allergic rhinitis,* symptoms occur year-round. The perennial form may cause chronic nasal obstruction (commonly extending to the eustachian tube), particularly in children. To help the patient identify his specific allergens, discuss the annual appearance of major pollens and molds (for more information, see *Seasonal suspects: Identifying allergens year-round,* page 507).

Allergic rhinitis usually first appears during childhood or adolescence but affects all ages. If your patient's a child or a teen-

Sandra Ludwig Nettina, RN, MSN, CRNP, who wrote this chapter, is a nurse practitioner in Ellicott City, Md.

CHECKLIST

Teaching topics in allergic rhinitis

☐ Explanation of allergic rhinitis, its cause, and signs and symptoms
☐ The types of allergic rhinitis, including seasonal and perennial
☐ Seasonal patterns for major allergens
☐ Detecting allergic rhinitis in children
☐ Diagnostic tests, such as skin testing and nasal cytology
☐ Medication to control signs and symptoms
☐ Immunotherapy
☐ Reducing environmental exposure to allergens
☐ Sources of information and support

Understanding how the nose functions

Does your patient know that his nose isn't just a sense organ? Tell him that the nose filters, warms, and moistens inspired air. Then explain how allergic rhinitis disrupts this organ's functioning.

Inside the nasal cavity
Begin by explaining that the inside of the nose is called the *nasal cavity.* Tell the patient that this cavity lies above the hard palate (or roof of the mouth) and below the cranial cavity. Air enters the nose through the two *anterior nares*, passes into a widened area called the *vestibule,* and travels through a slitlike nasal passage to the nasopharynx.

Nasal mucosa
Inform the patient that a mucus-secreting membrane called the *nasal mucosa* lines the nasal cavity. From this mucosa, minute hairlike *cilia* wave in constant motion, trapping inspired foreign particles (dust, bacteria, and viruses) and sweeping them backward to the throat to be swallowed.

Tell the patient that bony turbinates (superior, middle, and inferior) separate the inner nose into passageways. Covered with nasal mucosa, these structures project into the nasal cavity, providing additional surface area to help clean, humidify, and warm inspired air.

Allergic response
As your patient can surely attest, the nose is a highly sensitive organ. Inform him that the nasal mucous membranes react to various environmental factors, which may include allergens, such as pollen and mold, or irritants, such as cigarette smoke or formaldehyde. When they encounter substances that interfere with proper functioning, the turbinates swell and mucus production increases in an effort to carry away offending irritants. The result: sneezing, nasal stuffiness, itching, a runny nose, and other symptoms.

LATERAL CROSS-SECTION: NASAL CAVITY

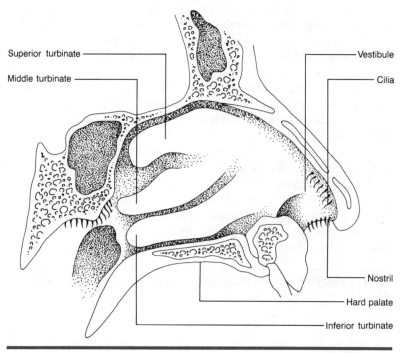

ager, help him and his parents to distinguish between allergic rhinitis and an upper respiratory tract infection. Give them a copy of the teaching aid *Detecting hay fever in your child,* page 512.

Reassure the patient that allergic rhinitis doesn't lead to asthma, eczema, or other allergic conditions or complications. Also point out that allergy symptoms tend to diminish as the patient ages.

Describe the diagnostic workup

Explain that the doctor can usually diagnose allergic rhinitis from an examination of the nose with a nasal speculum. Emphasize the importance of the health history in determining the possible cause of the patient's symptoms. Assist the patient to keep a record of his symptoms by giving him a copy of the patient-teaching aid *Keeping an allergy diary,* page 513.

Prepare the patient for skin tests to determine his sensitivity to specific allergens and for nasal specimen cytology to check for allergy-related inflammation, as ordered.

Nasal examination

Inform the patient that the doctor may first spray a decongestant into the patient's nose. Then, using a nasal speculum, the doctor will inspect the nasal tissues. Describe how nasal examination helps differentiate an allergy from an upper respiratory tract infection, such as a cold. In allergic rhinitis, the nasal mucosa usually appears swollen, pale, and gray. In the common cold, it is typically swollen and red.

Skin tests

Tell the patient that the doctor may perform skin tests to help pinpoint the allergens responsible for his symptoms. Explain that these tests involve exposing the skin to an extract of the suspected allergen. The doctor then checks for skin reactions that indicate hypersensitivity or allergy. Warn the patient that if he has a reaction, his skin may itch—but caution him not to scratch the area.

If the patient's scheduled for patch testing, explain that a sample series of common allergens will be applied (with patches taped to the skin) to his upper back or forearm. Instruct him to discontinue antihistamine medications for at least 48 hours before the test, longer if he's taking astemizole (Hismanal). Tell him that he must return several days after patch application so the doctor can examine his skin for reactions. Inform him that a positive patch test proves that he has a contact sensitivity but doesn't necessarily prove that the test substance causes his allergic rhinitis.

If the patient's having intradermal testing, explain that the doctor will use a very small needle to inject allergen extracts beneath the patient's outer skin layer. After about 15 to 20 minutes, the doctor will examine the area. Redness or swelling (called a wheal or hive) at the site constitutes a positive reaction.

Nasal specimen cytology

Teach the patient that this test involves collecting a sample of nasal discharge or mucosa for laboratory analysis. To collect a speci-

---

Seasonal suspects: Identifying allergens year-round

Encourage your patient to watch for a seasonal pattern in his allergic rhinitis signs and symptoms. Use the information below to help him identify the offending allergens.

Seasonal patterns for tree and grass pollens vary throughout the country and somewhat from year to year. If the patient's allergic to multiple allergens, he may have difficulty deducing what causes his signs and symptoms. For a definitive diagnosis, refer him to an allergist.

Spring allergens
If the patient's signs and symptoms worsen a month or so before new leaves unfold, he may be allergic to tree pollens. Elm, maple, oak, sycamore, ash, pecan, mountain cedar, and walnut trees are potential culprits.

Summer allergens
If the patient suffers more from June to August, he may be hypersensitive to grass pollen. Bermuda grass ranks as a common offender, with sheep sorrel, English plantain, and other pollen-producing grasses and plants running close behind.

Fall allergens
Ragweed pollen, the most notorious fall allergen, causes signs and symptoms from August to October, depending on the region. Point out that sagebrush, Russian thistle, and other pollen-shedding plants also may trigger fall allergies.

Year-round allergens
If the patient sniffs and sneezes year-round, he may be allergic to dust mites, animal dander, cigarette smoke, or other allergens that persist in his environment. Mold spores also may provoke perennial allergy, but this occurs more commonly in summer and fall.

men of nasal discharge, instruct the patient to blow his nose into waxed paper. To obtain a sample of nasal mucosa, explain that the doctor will gently scrape the inferior turbinate inside the patient's nose with a curette. Reassure him that nasal scraping will cause no pain or bleeding and that the curette will be advanced only slightly into his nose. Describe how the specimen will be stained and examined under a microscope. The presence of eosinophils indicates allergic rhinitis; the presence of polymorphonuclear leukocytes indicates infection.

Teach about treatments
Explain that allergy signs and symptoms can be controlled with medications and life-style changes to avoid airborne allergens. Long-term management also may include immunotherapy.

Medication
Discuss various medications to relieve signs and symptoms, including antihistamines, corticosteroids, decongestants, and cromolyn sodium. Tell the patient that medications may be oral or nasal, prescription or nonprescription, and taken intermittently or continuously. For more information, see *Teaching about drugs for allergic rhinitis.*

Stress that nonprescription medications can be as potent and effective as prescription drugs in their ability to relieve signs and symptoms or trigger adverse effects.

To relieve nasal irritation and crusting, advise the patient to use a saline-based nasal spray or drops. Suggest that he buy a commercially prepared product or make his own solution by mixing ¼ teaspoon salt in 1 cup of warm water. Tell him to use a syringe to irrigate his nose and to lean over the sink to drain the discharge. Or advise him to instill a fine spray into each nostril with a spray bottle. Caution him to discard any unused homemade saline solution because it may harbor microorganisms.

Procedures
If conservative treatments aren't effective, the patient may be a candidate for immunotherapy ("allergy shots"). Explain that this treatment involves desensitizing the immune system to specific allergens. Inform the patient that he'll be injected with a purified extract of the allergen in increasingly stronger doses. Gradually, his immune system will become more tolerant of the allergen until it no longer triggers an allergic reaction when he's exposed to it in his environment. Injections may continue weekly for 1 to 3 years, depending on the patient's response.

Urge the patient to keep scheduled appointments for immunotherapy. Emphasize that he'll need to stay in the doctor's office for 20 to 30 minutes after each injection to be monitored for anaphylaxis. Make sure he understands that immunotherapy is not a cure and that his signs and symptoms may recur.

Other care measures
When the patient can identify specific allergens, he can avoid them—or many of them. Encourage him to concentrate on keep-

Teaching about drugs for allergic rhinitis

DRUG	ADVERSE REACTIONS	TEACHING POINTS
Antihistamines		
astemizole (Hismanal) **azatadine** (Optimine) **brompheniramine** (Chlorphed, Dimetane) **chlorpheniramine** (Chlor-trimeton, Teldrin) **clemastine** (Tavist) **cyproheptadine** (Periactin) **dexchlorpheniramine** (Dexclor, Polaramine) **diphenhydramine** (Benadryl, Benylin) **terfenadine** (Seldane) **tripelennamine** (PBZ)	• Watch for dizziness, fainting, fever, gastric distress, hallucinations, severe drowsiness, severe dry mouth or throat, sore throat, unusual bleeding or bruising, and unusual fatigue or weakness. • Other reactions include anorexia; blurred vision; insomnia; irritability; mild drowsiness; mild dry mouth, nose, or throat; nasal stuffiness, thickened bronchial secretions; and tremor.	• Advise the patient to use any of the following measures to relieve a dry mouth: warm water rinses, artificial saliva, ice chips, or sugarless gum or candy. • Caution him to avoid overusing mouthwash, which may add to mouth dryness (alcohol content) and destroy normal flora, setting the stage for dental caries. • Remind him to take astemizole on an empty stomach, at least 2 hours after a meal, and to avoid eating for at least 1 hour after taking dose. • Warn him to avoid activities that require alertness, such as driving a car or operating machinery, until he knows how the drug affects the central nervous system (CNS). • Advise him that GI distress may be reduced by taking the drug with food or milk. • Caution him to consult his doctor before using alcoholic beverages, tranquilizers, sedatives, pain relievers, sleeping medications, or other CNS depressants because these agents may increase sedation. • Warn him to stop taking antihistamines 3 or 4 days before diagnostic skin (allergy) tests to ensure the validity of his test response. • Instruct him to notify his doctor before discontinuing the drug for any reason. • Tell him that terfenadine and astemizole cause less drowsiness than other antihistamines. • Because long-term use can cause blood abnormalities, urge him to comply with scheduled blood tests.
Corticosteroids (inhaled)		
beclomethasone dipropionate (Beconase, Vancenase) **dexamethasone** (Decadron Turbinaire) **flunisolide** (Nasalide)	• Watch for bleeding from or ulceration of nasal passages, chest tightness, confusion, depression, dizziness, dyspnea, fainting, fatigue, fever, gastric distress, insomnia, itching, mouth and throat lesions, weakness, and wheezing. • Other reactions include altered taste perception, appetite increases, burning nose, dry mouth and throat, hoarseness, and local fungal infections.	• Instruct the patient to use the drug only as directed. Inform him that the full therapeutic effect may be delayed and requires regular use of the inhaler as directed by the doctor. • Encourage the patient with blocked nasal passages to use an oral decongestant 30 minutes before (or a nasal decongestant 5 minutes before) intranasal corticosteroid administration to ensure adequate penetration. Advise him to clear nasal passages of secretions before using the inhalable form of the drug. • Ask him to read the manufacturer's instructions and demonstrate how to use the inhaler. Assist him until he shows he can use the inhaler properly. • Tell him that oral fungal infections can be prevented by following inhalations with a glass of water. • Advise him to clean the inhaler according to the manufacturer's instructions. • Tell him to inform his doctor if he notices a decreased response to the drug; an adjustment in dosage or discontinuation of the drug may be necessary. Warn him not to exceed the recommended dosage on his own. • Instruct him to observe for adverse effects, and if fever or local irritation develops, to discontinue the drug and notify the doctor.

continued

Teaching about drugs for allergic rhinitis — *continued*

DRUG	ADVERSE REACTIONS	TEACHING POINTS
Decongestants (nasal)		
naphazoline (Privine) **oxymetazoline** (Afrin, Dristan) **phenylephrine hydrochloride** (Allerest, Neo-Synephrine, Sinex)	• Watch for behavioral disturbances, blurred vision, increased blood pressure, painful or difficult urination, palpitations, seizures, and weakness. • Other reactions include dizziness, drowsiness, dry nose and throat, facial twitching, headache, increased nasal discharge, insomnia, nasal stinging, ocular irritation and tearing, pallor, photophobia, rebound nasal congestion or irritation (with excessive or long-term use), sneezing, sweating, and tremor.	• Instruct the patient to rinse the tip of the spray bottle or nose dropper with hot water and dry it with a clean tissue. Or advise him to wipe the tip of the nasal jelly container with clean, damp tissues. • Direct him to blow his nose gently to clear nasal passages well before using medication. • If the patient's using nose drops, teach him how to instill them correctly. Tell him to tilt his head back while sitting or standing up, or to lie on a bed with his head tilted back over the bedside. Urge him to stay in position for a few minutes after instillation to permit the drug to permeate his nose. • If he's using a nasal spray, show him how to instill it. Tell him to hold his head upright, squeeze the spray bottle quickly and firmly to introduce 1 or 2 sprays into each nostril, wait 3 to 5 minutes, blow his nose, and repeat the dose. • If he's using nasal jelly, direct him to place it in each nostril and sniff it well back into his nose. • Tell him that increased fluid intake helps to liquefy his nasal secretions. • Warn him to consult his doctor or pharmacist before using other nonprescription drugs because many contain sympathomimetics, which can cause hazardous reactions. • Emphasize that only one person should use a particular nose dropper or nasal spray device. • Advise him not to exceed the recommended dosage and to use the drug only when needed because rebound congestion may result from overuse. • Tell him that his nasal mucosa may sting, burn, or dry out. • Warn him that excessive use may cause irregular heartbeats and hypotensive symptoms, such as dizziness and weakness. • Caution the patient with hypertension to use this drug only as directed by his doctor.
Decongestants (oral)		
phenylpropanolamine (Propagest, Rhindecon) **pseudoephedrine hydrochloride** (Nucofed, PediaCare, Sudafed)	• Watch for breathing difficulty, hallucinations, increased blood pressure, palpitations or other irregular heartbeats, and seizures. • Other reactions include anorexia, anxiety, dizziness, drowsiness, dry mouth, excitability, fear, headache, insomnia, light-headedness, nausea, restlessness, tremor, vomiting, and weakness.	• If the patient has difficulty swallowing capsules, suggest that he open the drug capsules and mix the contents with applesauce, jelly, honey, or syrup. The long-acting mixture must be swallowed without chewing or crushing. • Advise him to take his last daily dose 2 or 3 hours before bedtime to avoid possible insomnia. • Tell the patient that a dry mouth can be relieved by using ice chips, sugarless gum, or sugarless hard candy. • Instruct him to take a missed dose if he remembers within 1 hour. After 1 hour, advise him to skip the dose and resume his regular dosage. Warn him not to double-dose. • Tell him to store this drug away from heat and light and safely out of the reach of children. • Advise consulting his doctor or pharmacist before using other nonprescription drugs. Many contain sympathomimetics, which can cause hazardous reactions. • Warn him that drug effectiveness may diminish with long-term use. • If the patient has hypertension, caution him to use this drug only as directed by the doctor.

continued

Teaching about drugs for allergic rhinitis — *continued*

DRUG	ADVERSE REACTIONS	TEACHING POINTS
Miscellaneous		
cromolyn sodium (Nasalcrom)	• Watch for anaphylaxis (angioedema, chest tightness, hives, increased wheezing), nausea, nosebleeds, painful urination, severe headache, and vomiting. • Other reactions include a bad taste in the mouth, cough, dizziness, joint pain and swelling, mild headache, nasal burning, nasal congestion, and sneezing.	• Instruct the patient to administer the drug at regular intervals to ensure effectiveness. • Direct him to clear his nasal passages by blowing his nose before administering the drug. • Mention that therapeutic effects may not occur for 2 to 4 weeks after initiating therapy. • If the patient is taking prescribed adrenocorticoids, tell him to continue taking them during cromolyn therapy unless otherwise instructed by the doctor. • If the patient also uses a prescribed nasal decongestant, advise him to take a dose about 5 minutes before he takes cromolyn (unless otherwise indicated). This helps to distribute cromolyn sodium in the airway.

ing his bedroom allergen-free if that's where he spends the most time. Give him a copy of the patient-teaching aid *Allergy-proofing your surroundings,* page 514.

Caution the patient not to smoke tobacco, which can further irritate the respiratory system. Also advise him to avoid alcoholic beverages, which cause nasal congestion and impede breathing. Recommend that he get plenty of rest and avoid stress. Point out that anxiety or anger may intensify an allergy attack. As a last resort, suggest drastic life-style changes, such as relocation to a pollen-free area.

Sources of information and support

Allergy Association
P.O. Box 7273, Menlo Park, Calif. 94026
(415) 322-1663

Asthma and Allergy Foundation of America
1717 Massachusetts Avenue, Suite 305, Washington, D.C. 20036
(202) 265-0265

National Institute of Allergy and Infectious Disease
9000 Rockville Pike, Building 31, Room 7A-03, Bethesda, Md. 20205
(301) 496-5717

Further readings

Bunch, D. "Air Pollution and Respiratory Health," *AARC Times* 13(12):26-28, 30, December 1989.
Culver, S., and Parks, B.R., Jr. "Antihistamines in Allergic Rhinitis," *Pediatric Nursing* 15(6):615-16, November-December 1989.
Jacobs, R., et al. "Rhinitis: Not Just Hay Fever," *Patient Care* 23(6):168-70, 173-76, 181-84, March 30, 1989.
Lieberman, P. "Rhinitis: Allergic and Nonallergic," *Hospital Practice* 23(6):117-20, 123-29, 132+, June 15, 1988.
Mazow, J.B. "Allergic Rhinitis: Formulating the Best Treatment Plan," *Consultant* 29(4):143-44, 149-50, 155, April 29, 1989.
Rashotte, J. "The Seasonal Invader...Respiratory Syncytial Virus," *Canadian Nurse* 85(10):28-32, November 1989.

Detecting hay fever in your child

Dear Parent:

When your child sneezes and has a runny nose, you may think he's catching a cold. But keep in mind that hay fever—also called allergic rhinitis—can cause similar symptoms. Take this home quiz to help you distinguish between a cold and hay fever.

Noticing suspicious symptoms

Does your child repeatedly use his fingers or the heel of his hand to wipe his nose upward? (This action, called the *allergic salute,* relieves itching and opens the nasal passages.)

Yes ☐   No ☐

Can you see a horizontal crease near the tip of your child's nose from repeated rubbing?

Yes ☐   No ☐

Does your child keep wrinkling his nose like a rabbit to relieve itching?

Yes ☐   No ☐

Does your child have dark semicircles or half-moon-shaped shadows (also called *allergic shiners*) under his eyes? (This sign results from swelling and congested blood vessels.)

Yes ☐   No ☐

Do you notice any consistent pattern to your child's symptoms? Are his symptoms worse at certain times of the year or after he plays in a dusty attic or a moldy cellar, in a pile of leaves, or with a dog or cat?

Yes ☐   No ☐

Is your child's nose runny? Does the skin under his nose look crusted, red, or cracked?

Yes ☐   No ☐

Does your child breathe noisily? Or does he persistently breathe through his mouth? Are his lips dry?

Yes ☐   No ☐

Does your child frequently make a clucking sound or thrust his tongue forward to relieve itchiness in the roof of his mouth?

Yes ☐   No ☐

Does your child say that he feels like throwing up—or does he vomit often? (These symptoms may result from swallowing nasal secretions.)

Yes ☐   No ☐

Does your child sound hoarse? Does he frequently clear his throat or cough?

Yes ☐   No ☐

What the answers mean

If you answered "yes" to some or all of these questions, suspect hay fever. Discuss these symptoms with your child's doctor. Only he can confirm the diagnosis. If your child does have hay fever, follow your doctor's instructions for treating it.

Keeping an allergy diary

Dear Patient:

To help you track down the cause of your allergy, keep a record of your symptoms for at least 1 week. Each time your allergy acts up, make a note of where you were and what you were doing at the time. Also note any actions you took to relieve your symptoms and how well these measures worked. Take your diary with you the next time you see the doctor.

Date and time						
Where were you when symptoms occurred?						
What were you doing at the time?						
What were your symptoms?						
How bad were they? 1: mild 2: moderate 3: severe 4: disabling						
How long did your symptoms last?						
What did you do to relieve your symptoms?						
Did you feel better?						

Allergy-proofing your surroundings

Dear Patient:

Here's an inexpensive, safe, and effective treatment for an allergy: Simply avoid the substances that cause your symptoms. Maybe you can't remove all of them from your environment, but you can limit your exposure to them and minimize your symptoms. Here's what to do.

In your bedroom

• Remove dust catchers, such as knick-knacks, stuffed animals, wall hangings, and books.
• If you're allergic to animal dander, keep furry pets—dogs, cats, gerbils, and hamsters—out of the bedroom.
• Use blankets made of synthetic materials rather than wool.
• Replace feather pillows and comforters with those filled with Dacron, nylon, or other polyester fibers.
• Encase your mattress and boxspring in airtight vinyl covers.
• Remove plants or an aquarium from the room because these may increase mold spores in the air.

Throughout your house

• Dust at least two or three times weekly. Use a damp mop or cloth instead of a broom, which can raise dust.
• Use an electronic air cleaner to remove mold, house dust, and pollens from the air. Be sure to wash or replace the filter periodically.
• In warm weather, close the windows and use an air conditioner.

• Clean air-conditioner and heat outlet filters regularly.

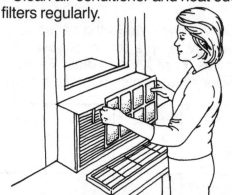

• Remove heavy rugs and draperies that catch and hold dust. Replace them with washable curtains and cotton throw rugs.
• Keep humidity low to reduce mold spores. Use a dehumidifier. Clean bathrooms frequently.
• Cover upholstered furniture with vinyl sheeting or slipcovers that can be washed frequently.
• Ban smoking and the use of aerosol or scented products in your home.

Outdoors

• Don't landscape your home with pollen-bearing trees, such as elm, maple, birch, poplar, ash, oak, walnut, sycamore, or cypress.
• Rake fallen leaves so that mold won't grow on them.
• Wear a dust mask when you cut the grass.
• Plan vacations and outings to avoid major allergen seasons. Remember that when allergy season is in full swing, pollen counts are usually lower in urban areas.

Pharyngitis

A sore throat—the hallmark of pharyngitis—is one of the most common medical complaints, especially in children. Because most cases are relatively mild, you'll focus your teaching on comfort measures to ease the symptoms, how to prevent transmission of the infection, and when the patient may return to work or school.

Teach the patient about the cause of his pharyngitis, its mode of transmission, and possible complications. Explain the purpose of diagnostic tests, if indicated, and the use of medications and self-care measures. Reassure him that his pharyngitis should resolve quickly and without complications if he complies with treatment. (For more information, see *Teaching the patient with streptococcal pharyngitis,* page 516.)

Discuss the disorder
Inform the patient that pharyngitis is a medical term for a sore throat, or inflammation of the pharynx. Explain that viruses, bacteria or, in chronic cases, irritants (such as cigarette smoke) can cause the inflammation.

Viral pharyngitis
Tell the patient that the most common cause of a sore throat is a virus, such as rhinovirus, coronavirus, and adenovirus. All of these viral agents are associated with the common cold. Other causative viruses include influenza viruses, herpesvirus (which commonly causes generalized oral lesions), and the Epstein-Barr virus (which occurs with mononucleosis).

Explain that establishing the identity of causative viruses usually isn't necessary because there are no specific treatments. Teach the patient that the symptoms of viral pharyngitis include upper respiratory congestion, runny nose, scratchy throat, a cough associated with postnasal drip, and itchy, watery eyes. He may also have swollen posterior cervical lymph nodes on the sides of his neck, slightly behind the midline of the neck. Though generally not severe, his symptoms may last up to 10 days. Mention that viral pharyngitis is usually milder than the bacterial form.

Bacterial pharyngitis
Tell the patient that about 10% of all sore throats are "strep throats." They're caused by group A beta-hemolytic streptococci (most commonly *Streptococcus pyogenes*). This type of pharyngitis is most common in children, especially during epidemics.

Sandra Ludwig Nettina, RN,C, MSN, CRNP, who wrote this chapter, is an independent nurse consultant in Ellicott City, Md.

CHECKLIST

Teaching topics in pharyngitis

☐ Definition of pharyngitis and overview of the types, primarily viral or bacterial
☐ How infectious pharyngitis is spread
☐ Importance of diagnosis and treatment of group A streptococcal pharyngitis to prevent complications
☐ Warning signs and symptoms of complications
☐ Preparation for throat culture and venipuncture, if indicated
☐ Instructions for increased fluid intake
☐ Use of medications, such as antibiotics, antipyretics, and analgesics
☐ Self-care measures, such as gargling and humidification, and measures to prevent infection transmission

Teaching the patient with streptococcal pharyngitis

Use a standard teaching plan to help you organize the brief time you'll have to teach the patient how to relieve the discomfort of pharyngitis and prevent transmitting his infection. After you've assessed the patient, you'll modify the plan to meet his individual needs. Here are some guidelines.

Assess the patient's complaint
Suppose you're caring for Peter Fritz, a 39-year-old laborer who has diabetes mellitus. He has come to the community health clinic complaining of a severe sore throat, headache, and muscle aches. When you ask him about his symptoms, he says, "I'm just worn out, and I've had chills and a fever for the past 2 days." His wife, who has accompanied him to the clinic, mentions that she has just recovered from a cold that lasted for 3 weeks.

You note that Mr. Fritz's temperature is 102° F. (38.9° C.). Examining him, you find that his anterior cervical lymph nodes are enlarged. As you gently palpate them, he exclaims, "Hey, that's sore!" When you inspect his throat, you note a purulent exudate.

Determine Mr. Fritz's learning needs
Compare what Mr. Fritz already knows about pharyngitis with the contents of a standard teaching plan, including:
• types and causes of pharyngitis
• signs and symptoms of pharyngitis
• diagnostic tests, such as a throat culture
• treatments, including activity and diet modifications, medications, gargling, and humidification.

After you examine and talk with Mr. Fritz, you decide to focus your teaching specifically on streptococcal pharyngitis. You plan to teach him about the cause of this form of pharyngitis and how a throat culture is obtained. Because his condition is contagious, he'll need to learn how the infection is transmitted and what he can do to prevent spreading it to others. Once the doctor has prescribed drug therapy, you'll reinforce how and when to take medications

and possible adverse reactions. You'll also discuss self-care measures to improve his condition, such as gargling and modifying his usual activities and daily diet.

Set learning outcomes
Enlist Mr. Fritz's cooperation in developing appropriate learning outcomes. Specifically, he'll be able to:

-state the cause of streptococcal pharyngitis
-explain how the infection is spread
-discuss when it's safe to resume contact with others
-prepare a salt solution to use as a gargle
-list foods (in addition to fluids) he can consume to increase his fluid intake
-demonstrate proper hand-washing techniques.

Select teaching tools and techniques
Use *brief explanations* to teach Mr. Fritz what causes streptococcal pharyngitis, how the infection spreads, when he can resume contact with others, and possible adverse drug reactions to watch for. Then use *demonstration* to teach him the proper way to wash his hands. Also show him how to prepare a salt solution and gargle.

Enhance your teaching with *pamphlets* and *equipment,* such as household measuring devices. Reinforce your teaching with printed *patient-teaching aids* that Mr. Fritz can review at home.

Evaluate your teaching
After your teaching, does Mr. Fritz know the cause of streptococcal pharyngitis? Can he discuss how the microorganisms are spread and how to prevent transmission? To evaluate your teaching, use *question-and-answer discussion.* For instance, ask him what role fomites play in the infection chain. *Return demonstration* will help you assess his grasp of skills—for example, mixing and using a salt-solution gargle.

Describe the signs and symptoms of streptococcal pharyngitis. Besides a sore throat, the patient may have a fever; a yellow, white, or gray exudate (purulent and patchy) inside the throat; and enlarged, tender anterior cervical lymph nodes on the sides of his neck. They're in front of the midline under the angle of the jaw. He may also suffer from a headache, muscle aches, and chills. Warn him that he may have difficulty swallowing and that the symptoms usually last about 5 days. Emphasize that this type of pharyngitis requires prompt treatment with antibiotics to prevent complications.

Point out that other forms of bacterial pharyngitis, although less common, also respond to antibiotic treatment. Other causative bacteria include streptococci from groups C and G (which may mimic group A infections but are not associated with the complication of rheumatic fever); mixed anaerobic bacteria (which cause gingivitis as well as pharyngitis); *Neisseria gonorrheae* (which is transmitted through oral sexual activity with an infected partner); *Mycoplasma pneumoniae* (which may be associated with pneumonia or bullous myringitis); and *Corynebacterium diphtheriae* (which causes diphtheria and produces a membranous exudate on the pharynx and a toxic systemic infection). Mention that non-group A streptococcal and mycoplasma pharyngitis are fairly common; however, these infections often resolve without diagnosis or treatment.

Other forms of pharyngitis
If the patient's symptoms seem severe but he doesn't have a bacterial infection, urge him to be examined for mononucleosis. Teach him to watch for and report these signs and symptoms: throat pain and swelling, an exudate on the inside of his throat, profound fatigue, swollen lymph nodes, and fever. He may also have an enlarged spleen or liver.

Mention that, in rare instances, an overgrowth of *Candida albicans* (thrush) may cause pharyngitis, especially in a patient whose normal oral flora has been altered by antibiotic therapy, immunosuppressive therapy, or a debilitating illness. Inform the patient that thrush is a fungal infection that responds well to antifungal medications.

How pharyngitis spreads
Explain that coughing, sneezing, or breathing near another person causes microorganisms to be dispersed in tiny airborne droplets. Transmission occurs when these droplets come into contact with another person's mucous membranes or with fomites (surfaces such as the patient's fingers, a used tissue, toys, or books) on which the microorganisms can live until picked up by another host.

Because pharyngitis has an incubation period of several days to several weeks, the infection is contagious even before symptoms occur. Advise the patient that after symptoms emerge he can resume contact with others in 24 to 48 hours. Explain that once his immune system is fully activated or he has begun antibiotic therapy, he is much less contagious.

Complications
Tell the patient that complications rarely result from viral pharyngitis. However, advise him that untreated bacterial pharyngitis—especially group A streptococcal pharyngitis—can cause sinusitis, otitis media, mastoiditis, cervical adenitis, and peritonsillar abscess. If you suspect bacterial pharyngitis, alert him to the signs and symptoms of these complications so that he'll know when to seek additional medical attention (see *When to call the doctor*). Warn him that these complications require prolonged antibiotic therapy and perhaps even hospitalization.

When to call the doctor

Pharyngitis commonly resolves without medical intervention. However, teach the patient to seek medical attention if he has a history of rheumatic fever, a known exposure to group A streptococcal infection, or if his signs and symptoms don't resolve within 10 days. Also tell him to watch for and report the following:
- blood in the urine
- earache
- inability to swallow
- joint pain
- oral temperature above 101° F. (38.3° C.)
- persistent hoarseness
- profound fatigue
- rash
- very swollen, tender lymph nodes.

Rheumatic fever: Still a risk?

Inform the patient that the chance of developing rheumatic fever as an aftermath of strep throat is small: The incidence is about 0.5 to 1 case per 100,000 persons. However, the risk still does exist.

Several outbreaks of rheumatic fever during 1985 and 1986 (in western Pennsylvania, Salt Lake City, and Columbus, Ohio) reminded health care workers that this complication can still occur—especially in children.

The link with strep throat
Explain that rheumatic fever occurs when the immune system reacts to a group A streptococcal infection by producing antibodies that cause inflammation in the joints and heart muscle. This may take place a few days to 6 weeks after the acute infection.

Avoiding the risk
Stress that the best insurance against rheumatic fever is correct diagnosis and treatment of group A beta-hemolytic streptococcal pharyngitis. Emphasize that compliance with antibiotic therapy—even if it isn't started for a week after onset of symptoms—will prevent rheumatic fever.

Inform the patient that more serious complications, such as rheumatic fever and glomerulonephritis, may result from an abnormal immune response to group A streptococcal pharyngitis. Glomerulonephritis is a form of renal failure that occurs 1 to 3 weeks after a streptococcal infection. With diuretics and supportive therapy, this complication usually resolves without renal damage. Rheumatic fever is a rare complication that causes arthritis and inflammation of the heart muscle several days to 6 weeks following group A streptococcal infection. (See *Rheumatic fever: Still a risk?*)

Describe the diagnostic workup
Dispel the misconception that all sore throats are strep throats that require testing with a throat culture and treatment with penicillin. If the patient has no fever, exudate, or swollen lymph nodes on the front of his neck—and if he has coldlike symptoms—then he probably has viral pharyngitis, and no testing is necessary.

However, the person with coldlike symptoms will need a throat culture if group A streptococcal pharyngitis is a possibility—for example, if the patient is under age 25 (especially a child) and has a sore throat; if he's over age 25 and has been exposed to the infection; or if he has a history of rheumatic fever or diabetes mellitus.

If the patient requires a *throat culture,* explain that this test identifies the specific bacteria causing his sore throat. Inform him that the specimen will be cultured in the laboratory and the results will be available in 24 to 48 hours. If *rapid streptococcal antigen testing* is available, tell him that the results will be available within 10 minutes. Although less sensitive than the culture method, the rapid streptococcal tests are highly specific for group A streptococcus.

Explain that the throat culture may be obtained by the doctor or the nurse, who will use a cotton-tipped swab to obtain the specimen from the back of the pharyngeal wall and the tonsils. Warn the patient that the procedure may make him gag briefly.

If the patient has symptoms of mononucleosis, prepare him for a venipuncture to obtain a blood sample for a *complete blood count* (CBC) and a *monospot screening test*. Explain that the results from the CBC are usually available the next day, but those from the monospot screening may take several days.

Teach about treatments

Explain that treatment includes rest, medications to control fever and pain, antibiotic therapy (for a bacterial infection), and self-care measures, such as gargling and humidification.

Activity

Advise the patient to restrict his activity based on his own tolerance. If he has a fever or feels fatigued, instruct him not to exert himself. Additional rest will make him feel better and may help his immune system to fight the infection. If he has mononucleosis, caution him to avoid contact sports. Explain that this illness may cause an enlarged spleen, making it more susceptible to injury.

Diet

Tell the patient to follow a liquid or soft diet while his throat is sore and swallowing is difficult. Instruct him to drink at least eight glasses of fluid a day to prevent dehydration associated with his fever. Point out that soft foods, such as ice cream, gelatin, pudding, and yogurt, are easier to swallow than liquids and count as fluids because they become liquid at room temperature.

Medication

Explain that the use of medications depends on the form of pharyngitis. (See *Questions patients ask about a sore throat*, page 520.) For bacterial pharyngitis, antibiotics are prescribed; for viral pharyngitis, palliative medications are used until the infection resolves. In group A streptococcal pharyngitis, the doctor may prescribe an oral form of penicillin, such as penicillin VK, ampicillin, or amoxicillin, which the patient will take for 10 days. Instruct him to take the drug on an empty stomach and to take all of the medication prescribed, even after he starts to feel better. Or instead of oral penicillin, the doctor may administer one I.M. injection of penicillin G benzathine, a long-acting form of the drug.

If the patient is allergic to penicillin, he may be treated with erythromycin. Instruct him to take the medication with meals to prevent abdominal cramping, nausea, and diarrhea.

Regardless of the antibiotic prescribed, instruct the patient to stop taking the drug and to call his doctor if he develops a rash, facial swelling, or difficulty breathing—signs of a possible allergic reaction. Warn the female patient that antibiotics may reduce the

Questions patients ask about a sore throat

What's the difference between a sore throat and a strep throat?
A sore throat is a general term for a symptom you experience; a strep throat is a specific type of sore throat. Don't mix up the two terms—they're not interchangeable. Strep throat is caused by infection with streptococcal bacteria; it requires antibiotic treatment. Other types of sore throat vary in their causes and treatments.

I've been told I'm a strep carrier. What does this mean?
Some people harbor streptococcal bacteria in their throats—even though they lack symptoms or have completed antibiotic treatment. You may remain a carrier for several months or longer following an acute strep infection. While you're a carrier, the harmful bacteria are greatly reduced in strength and number, so prolonged antibiotic treatment isn't necessary. Be assured that your risk of spreading the infection to others is small.

At the end of my workday, my throat hurts. Why?
Irritants in your workplace may be to blame. Perhaps you're breathing chemical fumes that directly irritate your throat or cause postnasal drip, which in turn causes a sore throat. Ask other workers if they have similar symptoms; if the irritant is strong, others will be affected, too. Alternatively, you may be allergic to some substance in your workplace. Consult a doctor who will help you identify the offending substance and recommend treatment, if necessary.

---

effectiveness of oral contraceptives. Point out that she may need to use a backup method of birth control throughout the menstrual cycle in which she is taking the antibiotic.

If the patient is taking nystatin for candidal pharyngitis, instruct him to make sure his mouth is free of food debris before taking the drug. However, caution him against using mouthwashes because they may further alter his oral flora. Teach him to hold the liquid suspension in his mouth for a few minutes before swallowing to maximize drug contact with his mucosal surfaces. Also tell him not to drink anything for 30 minutes afterward to prevent washing away the medication. If the patient is an infant, instruct the parents to swab nystatin onto the infant's oral mucosal surfaces. Mention that adverse effects from nystatin are rare.

Advise the patient with streptococcal pharyngitis to take aspirin or acetaminophen (Tylenol) to reduce his fever and control minor pain. Instruct parents to give their children acetaminophen because aspirin has been associated with Reye's syndrome when given to children with the flu or chicken pox. Advise all patients to avoid overdosage and to keep the medication out of children's reach because acetaminophen toxicity results in severe liver damage.

Recommend taking aspirin or acetaminophen every 4 to 6 hours to reduce a fever over 101° F. (38.3° C.) or 30 minutes to 1 hour before eating or drinking to decrease the pain of swallowing. If the patient takes a stronger analgesic, such as ibuprofen or another nonsteroidal anti-inflammatory agent, warn him to take the drug with food to avoid gastric distress. If codeine sulfate is prescribed for a dry, nonproductive cough, warn him not to drive or operate machinery if the drug makes him drowsy.

To help the patient swallow, suggest that he gargle with a 20% xylocaine viscous solution. Warn him not to exceed the recommended dosage. Caution him to wait for 15 minutes after gargling before eating or drinking. Explain that the drug may anesthetize his tongue, increasing his risk of hurting himself while chewing, and decrease his protective airway reflexes, increasing his risk of choking.

If the patient uses nonprescription throat lozenges and anesthetic sprays to control pain, warn him to use the medications only as directed.

Other care measures
Point out that treatment of pharyngitis largely depends on self-care measures, such as gargling. Tell the patient that gargling will rinse exudate away from his pharynx and may remove the bacteria or virus causing the infection as well. Instruct him to gargle three to four times daily with salt water (1 teaspoon of salt in a glass of lukewarm water). If the patient is a child, give the parents a copy of the patient-teaching aid *Teaching your child to gargle,* page 522.

Teach the patient proper hand-washing techniques and respiratory hygienic measures, such as covering his nose and mouth when coughing or sneezing, to prevent spreading his infection. Give him a copy of the patient-teaching aid *Tips for proper hand-washing,* page 114.

Instruct the patient to humidify his environment with a vaporizer or humidifier, especially if he's using indoor heat, which dries the air. Explain that adequate humidity is less irritating to inflamed mucous membranes. Tell him to clean the humidifier and refill it according to the manufacturer's instructions. Other measures he may use to increase humidity are to open the windows (taking care not to cause a draft); place open containers of water near heat sources; and take a shower or stand in a steamy bathroom.

If the patient who has frequent bouts of pharyngitis inquires about having his tonsils removed, explain why this procedure is no longer routinely performed. (See *Will a tonsillectomy prevent pharyngitis?*)

Will a tonsillectomy prevent pharyngitis?

If your patient has frequent bouts of pharyngitis, he may ask if having his tonsils removed will prevent recurrence. The answer, simply, is no.

Advise patients and parents that a tonsillectomy—the surgical removal of the palatine tonsils—was commonly performed on children 25 years ago, but it is not routinely done today. Explain that pharyngitis may still occur even if his tonsils are removed. Also, the tonsils, which are made of lymph tissue, actually help to protect the body from systemic infections.

Mention that occasionally a tonsillectomy is indicated because the tonsils are chronically enlarged and interfere with breathing or swallowing. However, the procedure is not advised for children under age 3.

Further readings
Bisno, A.L., et al. "The Rise and Fall (and Rise?) of Rheumatic Fever," *JAMA* 259(5):728-29, February 5, 1988.
Centor, R.M., et al. "Sore Throat: Streptococcal or Not?" *Patient Care* 21(18):28-34, 37+, November 15, 1987.
Guroy, M.E., and Murray, H.W. "Management of Pharyngitis," *Physician Assistant* 12(12):30, 35-37, 41-42, December 1988.
Massell, B.F., et al. "Penicillin and the Marked Decrease in Morbidity and Mortality from Rheumatic Fever in the United States," *New England Journal of Medicine* 318(5):280-86, February 4, 1988.
Matson, C. "Streptococcal Pharyngitis," *Consultant* 28(12):23-28, December 1988.

PATIENT-TEACHING AID

Teaching your child to gargle

Dear Parent:

Gargling may soothe your child's sore throat by rinsing away debris and germs from the back of her throat. Teach your child to gargle three or four times a day until her sore throat resolves. Just follow these steps.

1 Mix 1 ounce of mouthwash with 5 ounces of lukewarm tap water in a cup or glass. Or mix 1 teaspoon of salt in 6 ounces of lukewarm water.

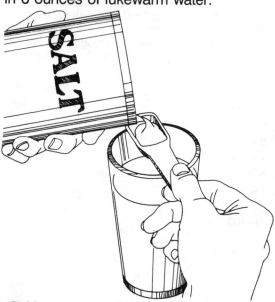

2 Have your child sit or stand in front of the sink. If this isn't practical, hold a basin or bowl in front of her.

3 Tell your child to take a large sip of solution as if she were drinking—but not to swallow it. She should take and hold about 1 ounce of solution in her mouth at a time.

4 Instruct your child to tilt her head backward and to open her mouth and breathe out through her mouth.

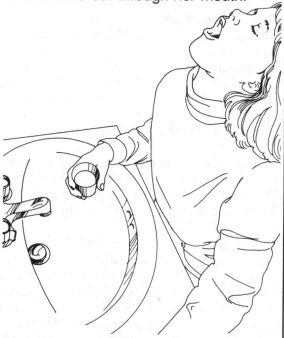

This will create the gargling action. Warn her that the solution will bubble up from the back of her throat. To avoid choking, caution her to breathe out gently and not to breathe in. Encourage her to keep the solution in her mouth for at least 15 seconds.

5 After about 15 seconds, tell your child to lean forward and spit the solution into the basin or sink. It may be mixed with tinges of saliva, blood, or pus.

6 Repeat these steps until you've used all the solution.

Laryngitis

Because hoarseness—the cardinal sign of laryngitis—usually resolves with minimal treatment, you'll focus your teaching on self-care measures, such as voice rest. Also explain the varied causes of laryngitis, and help the patient to identify and avoid activities or irritants that trigger his signs and symptoms.

However, because persistent hoarseness may be a sign of a more serious condition, such as laryngeal cancer, you'll need to teach the patient when to seek a more thorough examination. At that time, you'll explain diagnostic tests to evaluate the larynx.

Discuss the disorder
Inform the patient that laryngitis refers to acute or chronic inflammation of the larynx or voice box. The larynx, comprised of muscle and cartilage, is located between the epiglottis and trachea.

Describe how laryngitis causes hoarseness. Explain that the larynx contains two vocal cords. These folds of tissue line the inner walls of the larynx and stretch in various ways to make the different speech sounds. In laryngitis, infection or irritation results in swollen, inflamed vocal cords. When the patient speaks, air passes over the swollen cords, distorting his voice and making him sound hoarse.

Acute laryngitis
Teach the patient that acute laryngitis lasts from a few days to a week. It usually results from bacterial or viral infection, voice strain, irritation from cigarette smoke or fumes or, rarely, traumatic injury from or aspiration of caustic chemicals.

Inform the patient that acute laryngitis usually begins with hoarseness, ranging from mild to complete voice loss. Associated signs and symptoms depend on the cause. For example, if he has signs and symptoms of an upper respiratory tract infection—sore throat, nasal congestion, runny nose, mild cough, and watery eyes—along with hoarseness, tell him that a viral infection is the probable cause. However, if his hoarseness is accompanied by a fever, persistent cough, and difficult breathing, he may have a bacterial infection.

Point out that excessive use of the voice also can cause acute laryngitis. Voice strain may be associated with the patient's work (teaching, coaching, or singing, for example) or with recreational activities, such as cheering at a sporting event. Suspect voice strain if his only signs and symptoms are hoarseness and throat pain, with no signs of infection.

Sandra Ludwig Nettina, RN,C, MSN, CRNP, who wrote this chapter, is an independent nurse consultant in Ellicott City, Md.

CHECKLIST

Teaching topics in laryngitis

☐ Definition of laryngitis and how it causes hoarseness
☐ Two forms of laryngitis, acute and chronic, and causes
☐ Warning signs for airway obstruction
☐ Preparation for indirect laryngoscopy or endoscopic examination, if ordered
☐ Voice restriction to rest vocal cords
☐ Medications for symptomatic relief
☐ Other care measures: humidification and communication aids

Understanding the endoscopic examination

Teach the patient that this procedure involves passing a snakelike fiberscope through his nose and down into his larynx. Explain that the instrument has a light on one end and an eyepiece on the other and that, once the instrument is inserted, the doctor can see the patient's vocal cords. Tell the patient that he'll be asked to talk or cough so that the doctor can visualize and examine the action of the cords.

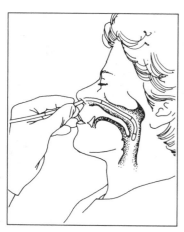

Chronic laryngitis
If the patient's signs and symptoms persist for more than 2 weeks, help him to identify possible causes, such as smoking, repeated voice strain, frequent exposure to inhaled irritants, or chronic upper respiratory tract infections (sinusitis, bronchitis, or allergic rhinitis, for example). Mention that continuing hoarseness also may be a sign of laryngeal cancer or, rarely, hypothyroidism.

Complications
Although uncommon, severe swelling of the vocal cords from allergic reaction, infection, or trauma can cause airway obstruction unless treated promptly. Instruct the patient to seek immediate medical attention if he has difficulty breathing, his breathing becomes noisy, or he feels his throat is closing. Warn him that severe laryngitis may require hospitalization and, perhaps, a tracheotomy if his airway is obstructed.

Describe the diagnostic workup
Explain that the diagnosis hinges on the patient's history and signs and symptoms. Stress that information about his occupation, habits, and recreational activities is essential to determine the cause of his laryngitis. Diagnostic tests are usually not necessary; however, if he has signs and symptoms of pharyngitis or an upper respiratory tract infection, the doctor may order a throat culture.

Inform the patient that his doctor may perform indirect laryngoscopy or endoscopic examination if his hoarseness lasts more than 10 to 14 days, has no obvious cause, or doesn't respond to treatment.

Indirect laryngoscopy
This procedure allows the doctor to look at the patient's larynx to help determine the cause of his signs and symptoms and to rule out a serious lesion, such as cancer. Assure him that the procedure is painless and that a local anesthetic will prevent him from gagging. Mention that indirect laryngoscopy is usually done in the doctor's office. Give him a copy of the patient-teaching aid *Learning about indirect laryngoscopy,* page 526.

Endoscopic examination
Mention that the doctor may use a flexible fiberscope (a fiberoptic endoscope) to visualize the larynx. (See *Understanding the endoscopic examination.*) Explain that sedation usually isn't necessary, but a small amount of anesthetic may be sprayed into the patient's nose. Tell him that he'll sit up straight with his head supported by a head rest during the procedure. He'll be asked to breathe through his nose while a thin, flexible tube is inserted into his nostril.

Teach about treatments
Explain that laryngitis usually resolves with minimal treatment. Inform the patient that treatment focuses on avoiding irritants and resting the voice so that his larynx has a chance to heal. Other self-care measures include using a humidifier and sucking on throat lozenges. (See *Questions patients ask about treating laryngi-*

tis.) If he has a bacterial infection, tell him that he'll need antibiotic therapy.

Activity
Advise the patient that he need not limit his physical activity unless he feels excessively fatigued. Resting his voice is the key to treatment. Instruct him to talk as little as possible—and not to sing or yell—for several days, or until the hoarseness resolves. If his occupation or recreational pursuits require him to use his voice, tell him to limit these activities for 2 to 5 days.

Diet
Although the patient need not follow a special diet, instruct him to drink at least eight glasses of nonalcoholic, noncaffeinated fluid a day. Explain that this will ensure adequate hydration.

Medication
Teach the patient about medications to provide symptomatic relief. These include nonprescription analgesics and throat lozenges for a sore throat. If the doctor prescribes an antibiotic to treat a bacterial infection, remind the patient to complete the full course of therapy, even after he feels better. Warn the patient to avoid taking antihistamines and decongestants, which dry mucous membranes and therefore may worsen his laryngitis.

Other care measures
Recommend that the patient use a vaporizer or humidifier at night to relieve irritation and inflammation of laryngeal mucous membranes. Advise him to read and follow the manufacturer's operating and cleaning directions carefully. Remind him to clean and empty the unit daily. In a humidifier, germs can breed and thrive in any remaining water. In a vaporizer, mineral deposits from hard water may build up and block steam flow. Caution him to place the unit on a flat surface several feet away from where he'll be, to keep the power cord safely away from objects such as radiators and heaters, and to unplug the unit when it's not in use. Tell him to use humidification whenever he runs his heater or air conditioner because these systems dry the air.

If the patient is hospitalized for severe, acute laryngitis, encourage him to communicate by writing on a communication board or pad of paper, or by shaking his head "yes" or "no."

Stress that if the patient's hoarseness doesn't resolve in a week, he should seek a more thorough examination to rule out a serious condition, such as laryngeal cancer.

Further readings
Blitzer, A. "Dysphonia: Is It from Voice Abuse—or Something More Serious?" *Consultant* 28(3):141-43, 147, March 1988.

Chasin, W.D., et al. "What a Problem Voice Tells You," *Patient Care* 21(3):60-62, 67-69, 73-74+, February 15, 1987.

Nelson, G.B. "Assessment and Intervention for Communication Problems in Home Health Care," *Journal of Home Health Care Practice* 1(1):61-76, November 1988.

INQUIRY

Questions patients ask about treating laryngitis

Will gargling help me get my voice back?
No. The larynx is below the epiglottis, which separates the throat from the windpipe. Therefore, gargling solution never reaches the larynx. But gargling may soothe your throat if it's sore.

Will cough medicine help my condition?
Only if you're coughing or clearing your throat frequently because of an allergy or a cold. If frequent coughing and throat clearing are irritating the inflamed larynx, then a cough suppressant may help.

If I quit smoking, will this help my throat?
Definitely. Laryngitis is an inflammation of the larynx, and cigarette smoke irritates the inflamed larynx. The key to treatment is avoiding irritants that contribute to inflammation.

Learning about indirect laryngoscopy

Dear Patient:

To evaluate your hoarseness, the doctor must examine your larynx. He can't do this by looking directly down your throat. Instead, he'll use a lighted mirror to examine your larynx indirectly.

Laryngoscopy takes about 1 minute. It doesn't hurt and it's quite safe.

Before the test
You may wish to avoid eating and drinking for several hours before the test. This will help to ensure that you won't vomit when the doctor passes a mirror down your throat. If you wear dentures, remove them just before the examination.

During the test
You'll be asked to sit upright and lean forward with your chin thrust out. This position helps make the larynx visible. Remember to remain in this position throughout the test.

If you have a sensitive gag reflex, the doctor will spray a local anesthetic on the back of your throat to numb the area and prevent gagging. You may notice an unpleasant taste, or you may have a sensation of swelling in the back of your throat and difficulty in swallowing.

Next, someone will position a light source behind you and to one side. This light will reflect off a mirror strapped to the doctor's forehead.

The doctor will ask you to open your mouth wide and stick out your tongue as far as possible. He'll grasp your tongue

with a piece of gauze, or he'll use a tongue blade to gently pull it forward.

Then the doctor will insert a warm mirror with a long handle into the back of your throat. Be sure to keep your mouth open and to breathe through your nose. Then he may ask you to speak or make certain sounds so that he can evaluate the movement of your larynx.

Throughout the test, try to relax and concentrate on your breathing. Be assured that the examination won't hinder your breathing.

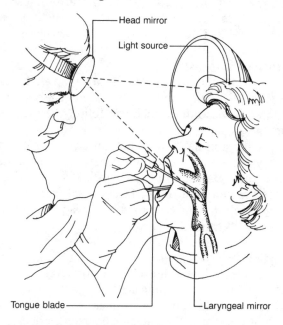

Labels: Head mirror, Light source, Tongue blade, Laryngeal mirror

After the test
If you've had a local anesthetic, you won't be allowed to eat or drink until the anesthetic wears off and your gag reflex returns, usually in about 2 hours. Then you may resume your normal diet, beginning with sips of water.

11

Skin Conditions

Contents

Pressure sores

Painful, slow healing, and easily infected, pressure sores are fully preventable. Unfortunately, a bedridden patient may be too ill to learn about preventive measures. As a result, much of your teaching will be directed at the caregiver.

Early in the patient's illness, explain to the patient and caregiver how pressure sores (also called decubitus ulcers or bedsores) develop and how infection can set in. Underscore the importance of preventive measures, such as turning and repositioning, range-of-motion (ROM) exercises, and proper nutrition and skin care. Keep in mind that complying with these measures will be difficult. Until the patient or caregiver actually sees a sore develop, he may not heed your instructions.

If a pressure sore does develop, you'll need to teach your patient and his caregiver to perform a daily inspection of body sites where sores commonly develop. Reinforce your early preventive teaching so that he doesn't develop more. Then describe the four stages of pressure sores, how to examine sores, and what to do to encourage healing. Treatment measures, in fact, may be easier to teach than preventive ones. Why? Reversing visible pathology may seem more urgent than preventing pressure sores.

Discuss the disorder

Explain how a pressure sore develops. As the sore's name suggests, *pressure* is the primary cause. Prolonged sitting or lying in one position exerts pressure on the skin, especially over bony prominences. This pressure reduces local blood flow, depriving skin cells of life-sustaining oxygen and nutrients. Skin damage results if pressure persists for more than 2 hours.

Point to and name bony prominences where circulation could be easily compromised (see *Pressure points: Common sites for sores,* page 530). Warn your patient that pressure from wrinkles in sheets and clothing, ill-fitting braces and casts, or even crumbs in bed could exacerbate his problems.

If your patient has trouble understanding the effects of pressure, ask him if he's ever had a "pins-and-needles" feeling from sitting with his foot tucked under him. Explain that this feeling resulted from temporary disruption of blood flow, and that the same principle applies to pressure sores. However, if your patient is acutely ill or has had a cerebrovascular accident or other disorder that diminishes sensation or prohibits movement, he may not feel pressure. For this patient, teaching preventive measures to his caregiver is especially important.

CHECKLIST

Teaching topics in pressure sores

☐ Major causes of pressure sores: pressure, shearing force, and moisture
☐ Risk factors
☐ Infection as a complication
☐ Sites, signs, and stages of pressure sore development
☐ Importance of repositioning and range-of-motion exercises for prevention and healing
☐ Pressure relief devices
☐ Role of diet in preventing and healing pressure sores
☐ Cleansers, treatments, and dressings
☐ Debridement or skin graft surgery, if indicated
☐ Skin care

Patricia L. Hartzell, RN, BS, NHA, who wrote this chapter, is director of nursing, Kendal at Longwood, Kennett Square, Pa.

Pressure points: Common sites for sores

Sores may develop at pressure points, which are shown in these illustrations. To help prevent them, emphasize the importance of frequent repositioning and carefully checking the skin for any changes.

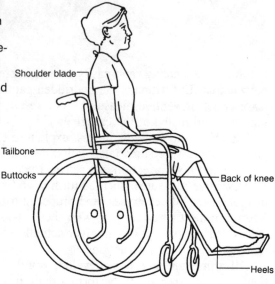

Shoulder blade

Tailbone

Buttocks

Back of knee

Heels

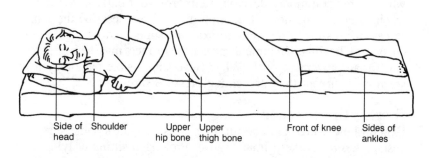

Side of head — Shoulder — Upper hip bone — Upper thigh bone — Front of knee — Sides of ankles

Shearing force, the force applied when tissue layers move over one another, can also cause pressure sores. This force stretches the skin, compressing local circulation. It can result, for instance, from raising the head of the bed, as gravity tends to pull the patient downward. Friction adds to the problem if the patient slides himself up in bed rather than lifts his hips.

Moisture is another cause of pressure sores. Whether from perspiration or incontinence, moisture softens skin layers and provides an environment for bacterial growth, leading to skin breakdown.

Explain that in addition to these three causes, certain conditions increase the patient's chances for developing pressure sores (see *Who's at risk for pressure sores?*).

Complications
Once the patient develops pressure sores, warn him that they require aggressive treatment to stop them from worsening. If treatment is delayed or inadequate, local infection can result, possibly leading to bacteremia and septicemia.

Who's at risk for pressure sores?

Besides pressure, shearing force, and moisture, several conditions can predispose patients to pressure sores and delay healing. These include poor nutrition, diabetes mellitus, paralysis, cardiovascular disorders, and even the aging process itself. Additional risk factors include obesity, insufficient weight, edema, anemia, poor hygiene, and exposure to chemicals.

Describe the diagnostic workup

Tell the patient and his caregiver that diagnosis is based on observation. Point out that early identification may halt progression of sores. Give them a handy checklist as a reminder to observe vulnerable areas regularly and to practice other preventive measures (see *Pressure sore record sheet,* pages 536 and 537). If the patient is alone, he could use a hand mirror to check hard-to-see areas. If he finds writing difficult, he could tape-record his observations.

Inform the patient that a developing pressure sore appears as a pink, red, or even dusky skin discoloration that doesn't disappear even after pressure is relieved. Other signs include warmth in the area, paleness with possible swelling, cyanosis, and blistering. A deep ulcer may first appear with only slight discoloration or a small opening surrounded by tissue that feels hard.

If a pressure sore progresses, one or more breaks in the skin of varying depth and size will occur, with or without drainage. Instruct the caregiver to measure the sore's width and length, using a disposable ruler. To measure depth, instruct him to gently insert a sterile, cotton-tipped applicator into the sore at its deepest point, then remove the applicator, and use the ruler to measure the depth reached. Tell him to record the sore's location; its depth, width, and length; and its stage (see *Four stages of pressure sores*). If the pressure sore is open or draining, he should record

Four stages of pressure sores

Teach your patient the four stages of pressure sores. Advise him to inspect his body daily and to contact the doctor immediately if he spots a new sore, or enlargement or signs of infection in an existing sore.

Stage 1
In this stage, skin stays red for 5 minutes after removal of pressure and may develop an abrasion of the epidermis. (A black person's skin may look purple.) The skin also feels warm and firm. The sore is usually reversible if you remove pressure.

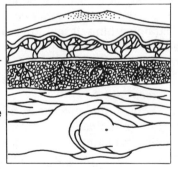

Stage 2
Breaks appear in the skin, and discoloration may occur. Penetrating to the subcutaneous fat layer, the sore is painful and may be visibly swollen. If pressure is removed, the sore may heal in 1 to 2 weeks.

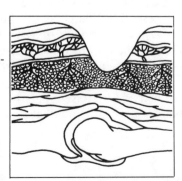

Stage 3
A hole develops that oozes foul-smelling yellow or green fluid. Extending into the muscle, the sore may develop a black, leathery crust or eschar at its edges and eventually at the center. The sore isn't painful. Healing may take months.

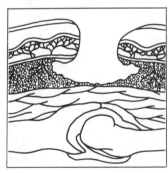

Stage 4
The sore destroys tissue from the skin to the bone and becomes necrotic. Findings include foul drainage and deep tunnels that extend from the sore. Months or even a year may elapse before the sore heals.

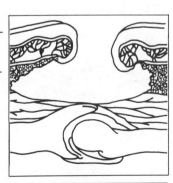

Turning schedule

As ordered, advise the caregiver to turn and reposition the patient every 2 hours—on his side and then on his back, on his stomach, and onto his other side.

Tell the caregiver to adjust the schedule for comfortable positioning to coincide with the patient's activities, such as positioning him on his back when he eats.

Suggest using two clocks, as shown here, to help remember which position to use.

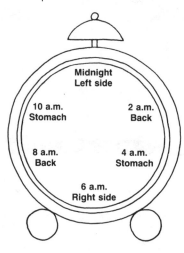

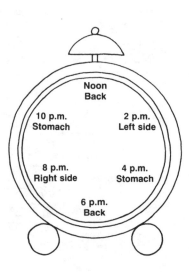

the drainage amount and color and the sore's status (infected, healing, or unchanged) at every dressing change. Stress the importance of recording these observations throughout treatment.

Teach about treatment

First and foremost is prevention. Teach your patient and his caregiver that movement and exercise improve circulation and prevent sores. Emphasize how a healthful diet keeps skin healthy and better able to resist breakdown. Also teach about protective skin care. If a pressure sore does develop, instruct the patient in proper cleansing, treatment, and dressing procedures.

Activity

Teach the patient and his caregiver turning and repositioning techniques and active or passive ROM exercises to help prevent pressure sores and relieve pain from existing sores.

Turning and repositioning. Teach the patient and his caregiver techniques for turning and repositioning in bed, so that every 2 hours the patient is in a different position (see *Turning schedule*). If appropriate, encourage the patient to turn himself; making the effort will help maintain his strength. Tell the caregiver to make sure the patient is comfortable (not in a jackknife position) after turning. Provide a copy of the patient-teaching aid *How to reposition a person in bed,* page 538.

Advise the caregiver to place pillows or rolled-up towels next to areas on the patient where pressure sores are most likely to develop. Suggest propping a footboard (padded with a towel, if necessary) at a 90-degree (right angle) or at least a 60-degree angle so the patient can rest his feet against it when lying on his back.

Tell the caregiver to turn the bedridden patient toward him to prevent a fall from the bed. Suggest using a turning sheet, placing it under the patient's body at its heaviest points—between the shoulders and the hips (see *Pressure relief devices*). Caution the caregiver to avoid straining himself and to get help, if necessary.

Explain to the wheelchair-bound patient where vulnerable pressure points are, and teach him how to shift and reposition his weight, and how to do wheelchair push-ups (see *Changing your position in a wheelchair,* page 539).

ROM exercises. Explain the importance of performing ROM exercises regularly. Inform the patient and his caregiver that movement keeps blood circulating, which helps keep skin healthy. Exercises are especially important and are done passively if the patient can't move areas of his body because of paralysis, numbness, or unconsciousness. Give the patient or his caregiver a copy of the teaching aid *Performing passive range-of-motion exercises,* pages 540 and 541. Ask them to record exercise sessions, noting anything unusual—if the patient is able to assist in bending a joint, for example, or if any exercise causes pain. Encourage the patient to get out of bed and exercise regularly if possible. Stress that any activity helps reduce the time that pressure is exerted on any one area.

Pressure relief devices

Special pads, mattresses, and beds can help relieve pressure for the patient who is confined to one position for long periods.

Gel flotation pads
These pads disperse pressure over a wide surface area.

Water mattress or pads
A wave effect continuously provides even distribution of body weight.

Alternating-pressure mattress
Alternating deflation and inflation of mattress tubes change areas of pressure.

Convoluted foam mattress or pads
Elevated foam areas cushion skin, minimizing pressure. Depressed areas relieve pressure.

Spanco mattress
This mattress, made of polyester fibers with silicon tubes, decreases pressure without restricting position.

Sheepskin pad
This type of pad prevents pressure and absorbs moisture. It must be in direct contact with the skin.

Foam rubber
Cut to just the right size and shape, foam rubber cushions individual areas.

Clinitron bed
This bed contains beads that move under an airflow to support the patient, thus eliminating shearing force and friction.

Stryker or Foster frame or CircOlectric bed
These devices relieve pressure by turning the patient.

Lift sheet or mechanical lifting device
Lift sheets and other devices prevent shearing by lifting the patient rather than dragging him across the bed.

Padding
Pillows, towels, and soft blankets can reduce pressure in body hollows.

Foot cradle
This device lifts the bedclothes to relieve pressure over the feet.

Diet

Tell your patient that a balanced diet, especially one that promotes healthy skin, is critical in preventing and treating pressure sores. Warn him that once a pressure sore forms, it won't heal if he isn't getting adequate nutrition. Encourage him to eat foods rich in protein and certain minerals and vitamins.

Explain that iron helps transport vital nutrients to skin cells. It's most plentiful in meats, dark green vegetables, and enriched breads and cereals. Mention that zinc helps heal pressure sores and promotes healthy skin. Good sources of zinc are meats, oysters, and whole-grain breads and cereals.

Inform the patient that vitamin C aids wound healing, promotes iron absorption, and helps the skin form collagen for healthy connective tissue. Food sources for vitamin C include citrus fruits, strawberries, cantaloupe, sweet peppers, tomatoes, cabbage, potatoes, and broccoli. Also important are the B vitamins, which aid in skin cell growth and help the body metabolize protein. The best food sources for the B vitamins are meats, poultry, fish, whole-grain breads and cereals, dairy foods, and green, leafy vegetables, such as spinach.

Also explain the importance of adequate fluid intake and maintaining desirable weight.

Treating pressure sores

Teach the patient and his caregiver about stage-related treatments for pressure sores. Stage 1 treatments prevent skin breakdown and improve circulation. Stage 2 treatments, used with stage 1 treatments, prevent further skin damage. Those at stages 3 and 4 treat and prevent infection and remove necrotic tissue.

STAGE 1 TREATMENTS

Lubricants (Lubriderm)
Lubricants increase tissue pliability and stimulate local circulation. Instruct the caregiver to massage the lotion gently over the affected area. Vigorous massage can further damage skin.

Clear plastic dressings (Op-Site)
This dressing adheres to the skin, protecting against friction. Permeable to moisture vapor, it allows oxygen to enter but keeps germs and water out. If the caregiver has trouble securing the dressing in a moist area, advise him to dry the area first with a hair dryer.

Gelatin-type wafers (DuoDerm, Johnson & Johnson ulcer dressing)
These wafers promote healing and protect the skin.

Vasodilator sprays (Proderm)
These sprays act as a lubricant and increase local blood supply.

Whirlpool baths
Besides cleansing the skin, whirlpool baths stimulate circulation. Warn the patient not to use a whirlpool bath too frequently because it may dry his skin.

STAGE 2 TREATMENTS

Normal saline solution or water
Normal saline solution or water cleanses the sore and prevents infection. Tell the caregiver to cleanse the sore gently to avoid further skin damage.

Hydrogen peroxide
A 25% solution cleanses the sore, removes debris, and prevents infection. The caregiver should follow cleansing with a saline rinse.

STAGES 3 AND 4 TREATMENTS

Hydrogen peroxide
A 50% solution cleanses the sore, acts as an antibacterial agent, and lifts debris to the surface. The caregiver should follow cleansing with a normal saline rinse.

Povidone-iodine solution (Betadine)
A 50% solution cleanses the sore and fights infection. Warn the caregiver not to use this treatment if the patient is allergic to iodine.

Granular absorbent dressing (DuoDerm granules or Debrisan beads)
This treatment draws drainage from the sore. Instruct the caregiver to apply the powder form directly to the sore. Warn against using this treatment on a healing sore because it may damage new tissue.

Gel-like absorbent (Bard absorptive dressing)
This dressing liquefies on contact with drainage, which helps draw exudate from the sore.

Enzymatic ointment (Elase, Travase)
This ointment breaks down dead tissue to aid drainage.

Healing gel or ointment (Carrington Wound Gel, Special Care Gel)
This treatment encourages new cell formation.

Sodium chloride–impregnated dressing (Mesalt)
This treatment and dressing cleanses deep or infected sores by wicking drainage, debris, and bacteria from the sore, while maintaining a moist environment, which promotes healing. Tell the caregiver to anchor this dressing with hypoallergenic tape or Mefix, an adhesive fabric that conforms to body contours.

Gauze dressings
Gauze adheres to dead tissue, allowing its removal along with the old dressing. Tell the caregiver to avoid Telfa-like dressings because they won't adhere to dead tissue.

Wet-to-dry dressings
Teach the caregiver how to make a wet-to-dry dressing. Tell him to soak gauze in a normal saline solution or an antiseptic solution. As the dressing dries, it adheres to the sore. When it's removed, debris comes with it.

Skin treatments

Once a pressure sore has developed, explain specific treatments (see *Treating pressure sores*). Inform the patient that the treatment depends on the sore's stage. Besides the treatments listed in the chart, mention that a heat lamp may be used to dry moist areas and increase local circulation. Tell the caregiver to use only a 25-watt light bulb (as the doctor directs) at a distance of 18″ (46 cm) to 24″ (61 cm) from the affected skin area for no longer than 20 minutes. Warn the caregiver that increasing the duration, reducing the distance, or increasing the wattage may result in burns. Stress that the caregiver stay with the patient during treatment. Also provide copies of the patient-teaching aids *Applying a dressing*, pages 542 and 543, and *Applying a special wound-cleaning agent*, page 544.

Be sure the patient and his caregiver can recognize and record signs of healing because the doctor may want to change the treatment. Such signs include a reduction in the sore's size and drainage and the appearance of healthy-looking granulation tissue (looks grayish red, bleeds easily, and is easily injured).

Provide instruction on caring for delicate skin. Explain that cleansing with a gentle soap removes irritants and bacteria. Tell the caregiver to pat rather than rub skin dry and to give special attention to drying skin folds. Advise gently massaging in lotion or oil on damp skin to retain moisture. Suggest rubbing in powder at bony prominences and at skin folds to absorb moisture and reduce friction. (Rubbing in the powder avoids caking and irritation.)

If the doctor recommends debridement (mechanical, chemical, or surgical removal of necrotic tissue) or skin graft surgery, explain the procedure and why it's being performed.

Other care measures

If the patient has trouble with incontinence, urge his caregiver to toilet him frequently. Warn that prolonged contact with urine or feces can cause chemical irritation and maceration. Advise using a single layer of padding for urine and fecal incontinence. Excessive padding increases perspiration, leading to maceration. It also increases the likelihood of wrinkling, which can cause skin irritation from added pressure.

Further readings

Barnes, S.H. "Patient/Family Education for the Patient with a Pressure Necrosis," *Nursing Clinics of North America* 22(2):463-74, June 1987.

Dimant, J., and Francis, M.E. "Pressure Sore Prevention and Management," *Journal of Gerontological Nursing* 14(8):37-38, August 1988.

Exton-Smith, N. "The Patient's Not for Turning," *Nursing Times* 83(42):42-44, October 21-27, 1987.

Gould, D. "Patients and Pressure Sores," *Nursing Times* 83(47):48-51, November 25-December 1, 1987.

Sebern, M. "Home-Team Strategies for Treating Pressure Sores," *Nursing87* 17(4):50-53, April 1987.

Waterlow, J. "Prevention Is Cheaper Than Cure," *Nursing Times* 84(25):69-70, June 22-28, 1988.

Pressure sore record sheet

Dear Patient:

Use this chart to remind you to check your skin daily for pressure sores. They may develop at spots where bones are prominent and close to the skin, such as at your elbow, shoulder, hip, knee, or ankle.

Every day mark the block for each body site with N (normal), R (red), or M (moist). If a sore is developing, contact your doctor.

Also use this chart to keep track of the treatments and prevention techniques you're using, including skin care, exercise, and diet.

Date													
SKIN INSPECTION													
Back of head													
Left side of head													
Right side of head													
Rim of left ear													
Rim of right ear													
Left shoulder													
Right shoulder													
Left elbow													
Right elbow													
Left side of middle back													
Right side of middle back													
Left hip													
Right hip													
Front of left knee													
Front of right knee													
Inner left knee													
Inner right knee													

continued

PATIENT-TEACHING AID

Pressure sore record sheet — *continued*

Date																

SKIN INSPECTION — *continued*

Outer left knee																
Outer right knee																
Inner left ankle																
Inner right ankle																
Outer left ankle																
Outer right ankle																
Left heel																
Right heel																
Tailbone area																

SKIN CARE

Pressure relief device used? (Yes/No)																
Skin massage with lotion? (Yes/No)																
Treatment as ordered? (Yes/No)																

EXERCISE

Number of times out of bed?																
Number of times turned while in bed?																
Range-of-motion exercises performed? (Yes/No)																

DIET (percentage of food served that was actually eaten)

100%																
75%																
50%																
Less than 50%																

PATIENT-TEACHING AID

How to reposition a person in bed

Dear Caregiver:

You'll use three positions when turning and repositioning a person in bed: back, side, and stomach. Follow these instructions.

Back positioning
Place a flat, firm pillow under the person's head so that his neck is straight and in line with his spine. Then lift his heels slightly by placing a thin blanket under his calves. Slightly bend his elbows, and rest his hands on his hips. Straighten his legs, and place his feet (toes pointing up) on a padded board resting against the foot of the bed at a 60-degree or 90-degree angle.

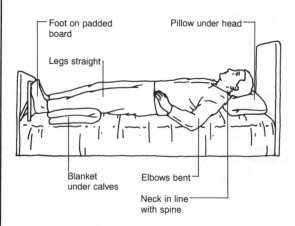

Foot on padded board
Legs straight
Pillow under head
Blanket under calves
Elbows bent
Neck in line with spine

Side positioning
After you've turned the person onto his side, place his head in line with his spine. Support his head and neck with a firm, flat pillow. Next, support his back with a pillow, and have him wrap his arms around another pillow. Then move his upper leg forward until his knee is bent, to raise it above his lower leg. Place a pillow under this leg to keep it at hip level. Slightly bend the lower knee and place a folded towel (or blanket or piece of foam rubber) under it to keep his ankle off the bed.

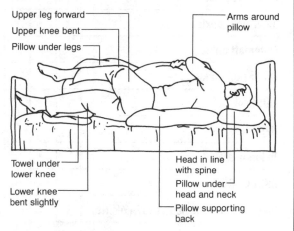

Upper leg forward
Upper knee bent
Pillow under legs
Arms around pillow
Towel under lower knee
Lower knee bent slightly
Head in line with spine
Pillow under head and neck
Pillow supporting back

Stomach positioning
After turning the person onto his stomach, turn his head to one side and place a pillow or folded towel under his cheek. Then move his arms up so that his bent elbows are in line with his shoulders. Next, place folded towels beneath his chest and stomach. Finally, straighten his legs. Support his ankles and raise his toes off the bed by using a rolled towel or small rolled blanket.

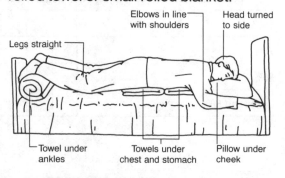

Elbows in line with shoulders
Head turned to side
Legs straight
Towel under ankles
Towels under chest and stomach
Pillow under cheek

Changing your position in a wheelchair

Dear Patient:

Sitting for a long time in a wheelchair can cause pressure sores. You can see from the illustration where pressure sores are most likely to develop. However, by shifting your weight and doing push-ups, you can relieve pressure on those spots and prevent pressure sores.

PRESSURE POINTS

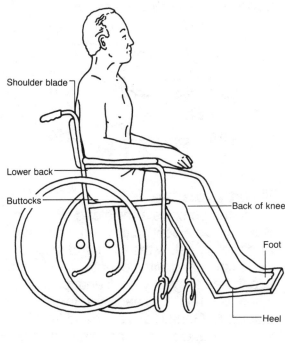

Shifting your weight

A wheelchair is much more confining than a bed, so you have fewer options for changing your position. But you should try (or ask your caregiver) to shift your weight from buttock to buttock at least once every hour. When you shift the weight to one buttock, hold the position for 1 minute and then shift to the other side and hold for a minute.

Doing push-ups

If you can move your arms, try these wheelchair push-ups. Grip the arms of the chair and push down hard with your hands and arms to try to raise your upper body off the seat. If you can, use this same technique for shifting your weight.

PUSHING DOWN AND RAISING YOUR UPPER BODY

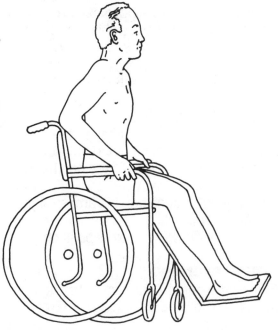

Performing passive range-of-motion exercises

Dear Caregiver:

Passive range-of-motion exercises are important if the person in your care can't exercise part of his body. Even though these exercises are called "passive," have the person help as much as possible because any movement can improve his muscle tone and strength. Your doctor, nurse, or therapist will need to show you how to support, control, and move each joint properly as you perform the exercise.

Repeat the exercises for the prescribed number of times.

Neck exercise
Lay the patient on his back, with his head flat (no pillow). With one hand, support the back of his head; with your other hand, support his chin. Extend his neck by moving his head backward, so he's looking at the ceiling. Next, bring his head forward until his chin comes as close to his chest as possible without causing discomfort. Now, turn his head to the left and to the right.

Shoulder exercise
With the patient sitting or lying down, extend his arm straight out to the side, with his palm facing up. Place one hand under the elbow; use your other hand to grip his wrist. Then keep his arm straight and bring it up until it reaches his ear. Return the arm to its original position.

Elbow exercise
Extend the person's arm straight out to the side, with his palm facing up. Grasp

his wrist to keep his hand from drooping. Now, bend the arm at the elbow and bring his hand up toward the shoulder and then back to its original position. Repeat with the other arm.

Forearm exercise
Place the person's arms along his sides. Grasp the wrist and hand of one arm. Keeping the person's elbow on the bed, raise his hand and gently twist it so his palm is up. Then twist it so the palm is down. Repeat with the other arm.

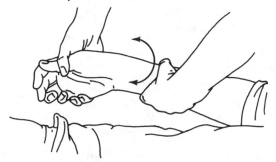

Wrist exercise
Place the person's arms along his sides. Keeping his elbow on the bed, hold one arm slightly below the wrist and raise it. Grasp the hand with your other hand, lift it, and bend it gently back and forth. Then rock the hand back and forth sideways. Gently twist the hand from side to side. Do the same thing with the other hand.

Finger exercise
Place the person's arms along his sides. With one of your hands grasp one of his, keeping his wrist straight. With your other hand, gently straighten out his

continued

PATIENT-TEACHING AID

Performing passive range-of-motion exercises — *continued*

fingers. Now, working from his little finger to his thumb, spread each pair of adjoining fingers apart and then bring them back together. Then pinch the thumb together with each of his fingers, one finger at a time. Repeat with the other hand.

Hip and knee exercise
Straighten the person's legs flat on the bed. Place one hand under his ankle and the other under his knee. Then bend his knee toward his chest.

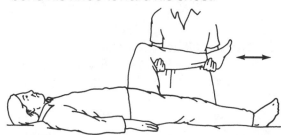

Bring his leg down and straighten it and then gently move it out to the side away from his other leg. Gently move it back to the center and then over and across the other leg. Then, back to the center. Repeat with his other leg.

Ankle exercise
Straighten the person's legs on the bed. Place one hand under his heel and the other against the ball of his foot. Push the ball of his foot gently toward his head as you pull his heel down.

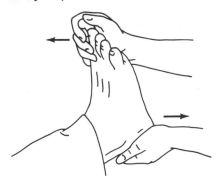

Next, pull his toes down toward the bed while you push his heel up.

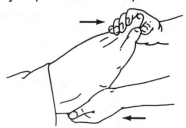

Finally, straighten the foot and move it gently from side to side. Repeat with the other foot.

Foot exercise
Begin by straightening the person's legs flat on the bed. Place one hand under one of his heels and the other under the ball of his foot. Gently twist his sole inward toward the other foot, back to the center, and then outward. Repeat this exercise with the other foot.

Toe exercises
Straighten the person's legs flat on the bed. Support his heel or ankle with one hand and use the other hand to curl his toes toward his sole. Straighten his toes and then bend them gently back toward the top of his foot and straighten them again.

   Next, working from the little toe to the big toe, spread each pair of adjoining toes apart. Then bring them back together.

   Repeat these exercises with the toes of the other foot.

Applying a dressing

Dear Caregiver:

Follow this step-by-step guide to cleaning, treating, and dressing a person's pressure sore.

Assemble the equipment

Gather the equipment: dressings (gauze pads or transparent adhesive dressings are most common), scissors, hypoallergenic tape, cleaning solution (such as peroxide or Betadine solution), antibacterial ointment if ordered, two bowls in which to pour the cleansers, sterile gloves, plastic disposable bags, and baby oil.

Have the new dressing ready before you take off the old one. Cut strips of hypoallergenic tape in advance, too. Pour boiling water in the bowls to sterilize them, and discard the water. Then pour sterile water in one bowl and the cleaning solution in the other.

Position the person so you can reach the sore easily.

Remove the old dressing

Wash your hands thoroughly. Carefully remove the tape from the person's skin. If this is painful, moisten the tape with baby oil before you remove it. If the skin under the tape is inflamed, don't apply the new tape there. Remove the old dressing, but don't touch any part of it that touched the sore. Check the amount and color of any drainage on it. Fold its edges together, place it in a disposable bag, and close the bag.

Check the sore

Inspect for swelling, redness, drainage, or pus—signs of probable infection. Is the sore healing?

Whether the sore appears to be infected, healing, or unchanged since the last dressing change, write down what you see; do this every time you change the dressing. *Do not touch the sore.*

Put on sterile gloves

Now remove all hand jewelry and wash your hands thoroughly before handling the sterile gloves.

Start with the glove for the hand you use most often. Grasp it by its cuff with your thumb and forefinger, and lift it from its wrapper. Be careful to touch only the inside of the glove (to keep the outside surface sterile). Now slip it on.

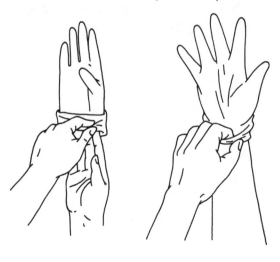

continued

Applying a dressing — *continued*

Now pick up the second glove by slipping your gloved fingers under its cuff.

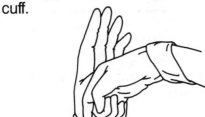

Pull on the second glove.

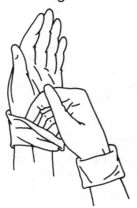

Clean the sore

Saturate a gauze pad with Betadine or peroxide. Now lightly scrub both the sore and the area around it.

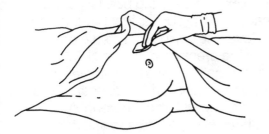

Saturate a second gauze pad in the sterile water. Wring it out over the sore, as shown in the illustration at the top of the next column.

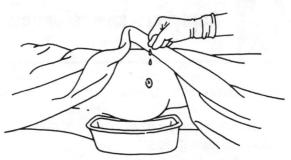

Use another gauze pad to gently blot dry the sore and the skin around it. Dispose of all pads in a disposable bag.

Put on the new dressing

If you're applying a *gauze dressing,* be careful not to touch any area of it that will touch the sore. If the doctor has ordered it, squeeze an antibacterial ointment onto the dressing before applying it. Tape the dressing securely in place.

If you're applying a *transparent adhesive dressing,* take the packet it comes in and remove part of the protective paper; then use your thumb to press that part of the dressing onto the skin near the sore. Peel the remaining paper off the dressing and smooth it over the sore and surrounding skin.

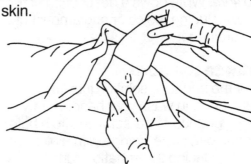

Press down all four sides of the dressing to prevent leakage.

After you've finished applying the dressing, take off your gloves, throw them away in a disposable bag, seal the bag, and wash your hands thoroughly.

Applying a special wound-cleaning agent

Dear Caregiver:

Follow these steps to apply a special wound-cleaning agent.

Assemble the equipment

You'll need several 4-inch by 4-inch sterile gauze pads, a 5-inch by 9-inch sterile dressing, hypoallergenic tape, bed-saver pads, an irrigation syringe, irrigating solution (usually sterile water) and a container to pour it into, a container to catch irrigation runoff, a wound-cleaning agent (beads or paste) prepared as directed, sterile disposable gloves, and a disposable bag.

Check the sore

Remove the old dressing and check it for drainage or pus. Then fold its sides together with the soiled side in and put it in the disposable bag. Carefully inspect the sore for signs of infection: redness, swelling, drainage, or pus. *Don't touch the sore.* Write down a description of the sore, including the color and amount of any drainage.

Irrigate the sore

Pour the irrigating solution into its container and wash your hands. Draw about 1 ounce of the solution into a bulb syringe or a large syringe with a plunger.

After placing the irrigation-runoff container against the skin below the base of the sore, hold the syringe with its tip about 2 inches from the sore, and squirt all the solution into the sore. Be sure to remove *all* the old paste and debris from the sore; if necessary,

irrigate the sore again. Don't touch the sore with the syringe tip, or it will be contaminated and unusable for future dressing changes.

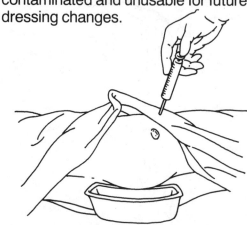

Put on the sterile gloves. Then wrap a sterile gauze pad around your finger and gently pat dry the area around the sore. But leave the sore moist to stimulate the action of the beads or paste. Then throw the pad in the disposable bag.

Put on the cleaning agent

If you're using wound-cleaning paste, apply it with a sterile gauze pad into the sore—at least ¼-inch deep. If you're using wound-cleaning beads, pour the beads into the sore at least ¼-inch deep.

Cover the sore with a sterile dressing. Tape the dressing down on all four sides. Finally, take off the sterile gloves, throw them away in the disposable bag, and wash your hands thoroughly.

Check every 8 hours to see if the wound-cleaning agent has changed color. If it has, remove the beads or paste by irrigating again. If it hasn't, change the beads or paste every 12 hours.

Herpes zoster

Commonly known as shingles, herpes zoster will test your teaching skills. Because this disorder can cause extreme pain, you may need to spend extra time teaching about analgesic measures and reassuring the patient that herpetic pain usually goes away. Initially, you'll discuss the cause of herpes zoster and its course. You'll also inform the patient about drug therapy. Because the disorder may be associated with inadequate immune defenses, you'll need to emphasize the importance of recognizing and avoiding infection.

If you care for elderly patients or those with serious immunosuppressive illnesses, you're likely to have many opportunities for teaching about herpes zoster. That's because the disorder has become increasingly common with the increased numbers of elderly and immunocompromised patients—cancer survivors, transplant recipients, and those with acquired immunodeficiency syndrome (AIDS).

Discuss the disorder

Tell the patient that herpes zoster results from the varicella zoster virus—the same virus that gave him chicken pox as a child. Explain that during the course of chicken pox the virus invades the peripheral nerves and remains dormant in the nervous system. As long as the immune system functions properly, the virus stays suppressed. However, the virus may be reactivated if the immune system deteriorates from age, disease, drug therapy, radiation, or trauma.

Confirm the patient's signs and symptoms. Initially, he'll experience mild fever, fatigue, and pain, tingling, or burning along the course of the affected nerve pathways. A rash may appear at the same time or follow in 4 or 5 days. The fever subsides when the rash appears as red patches. Within 1 or 2 days, the rash develops into blisters, which may remain small or coalesce into large eruptions. Characteristically, the rash is confined to one or two neighboring thoracic or lumbar dermatomes, and the virus spreads in a bandlike manner along the dermatome. Occasionally, herpes zoster travels along the fifth cranial nerve (the trigeminal nerve), producing lesions on the face and head (see *Herpes zoster sites,* page 546).

Inform the patient that blisters may continue to appear for several days and may last from 1 to 2 weeks. As the attack progresses, the blisters fill with pus. Eventually they crust and form scabs, and usually heal completely within a month of the initial

CHECKLIST

Teaching topics in herpes zoster

☐ What causes herpes zoster
☐ Signs and symptoms and course of herpes zoster infection
☐ Complications, such as postherpetic neuralgia
☐ Tests, such as the Tzanck test, to confirm diagnosis
☐ Drug therapy with acyclovir, analgesics, antihistamines, and other drugs
☐ Other care measures, including infection prevention

Beth A. Bravante, RN,C, MSN, who wrote this chapter, is a certified registered nurse practitioner at Temple University Hospital in Philadelphia.

Herpes zoster sites

The herpes zoster virus infects the nerves that innervate the skin, the eyes, and the ears. Each nerve (tagged for its corresponding vertebral source) emanates from the spine, banding and branching about the body to innervate a skin area called a dermatome.

Show your patient how the herpes zoster rash erupts along the course of the affected nerve fibers, covering the skin in one or several of the derma-

tomes shown below.

Explain that the thoracic (T) and lumbar (L) dermatomes are most commonly affected, but other dermatomes, such as those covering the cervical (C) and the sacral (S) areas can be affected too. In fact, the herpes zoster rash can occur anywhere on the face or body.

Keep in mind that dermatome levels are variable and overlap.

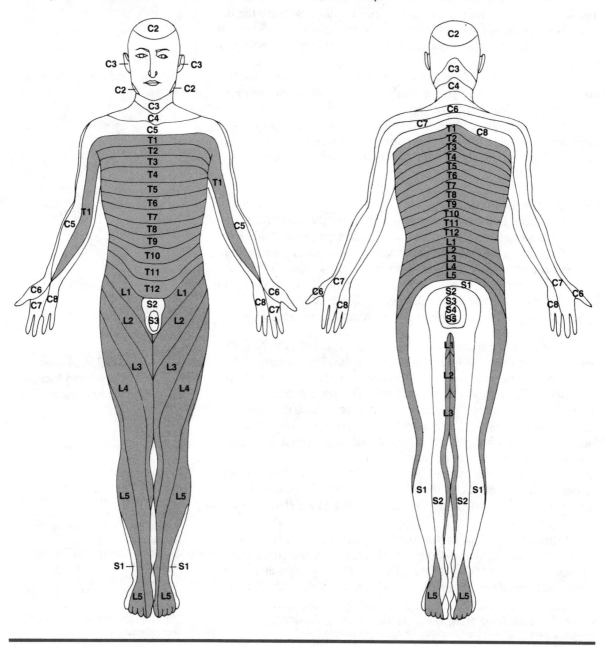

eruption. Explain that if the lesions are deep or become infected, scarring may occur.

Pruritus, pain, and tingling may occur along the nerve pathway 1 to 4 days before eruption of the lesions and continue. Reassure the patient that these signs and symptoms usually resolve in a few weeks.

Tell the patient that herpes zoster can affect the eye (herpes zoster ophthalmicus), producing conjunctivitis, scleritis, keratitis, or iridocyclitis. If the disease involves the eighth cranial nerve and the ear (Ramsay Hunt syndrome), the patient will experience ear pain (often severe) and blisters on the external ear and on the eardrum. Symptoms may also include hearing loss, tinnitus, vertigo, loss of taste, and facial paralysis. Hearing loss and tinnitus may be prolonged but are usually reversible; facial paralysis and loss of taste may be permanent.

Complications

Inform the patient that despite excellent medical care, long-lasting or serious complications of a herpes zoster attack sometimes occur. The most common complication is persistent pain in the area of the skin lesions or the affected dermatome, known as postherpetic neuralgia. About 3% of all patients and up to 50% of patients over age 70 may continue to experience aching, burning, or itching sensations more than a month after the initial rash clears up.

In some patients, pain may persist for about 15 years. If pain fails to respond to conventional drug therapy, the patient may experience sleep and appetite disturbances, excessive fatigue, and depression.

In severely immunocompromised patients, the zoster rash may spread over the entire body, much like chicken pox. This form of the disease, called disseminated herpes zoster, is usually accompanied by fever and malaise, and may ultimately infect the central nervous system and lungs. AIDS patients are particularly vulnerable to disseminated disease.

Describe the diagnostic workup

Tell the patient that the doctor can diagnose herpes zoster from a thorough health history and a physical examination. He can confirm the diagnosis once the rash develops. Before the rash appears, however, accompanying pain may mimic that of other disorders, such as appendicitis, peptic ulcer, pleurisy, and herniated disk.

Explain that the doctor may use the cutaneous *Pap smear* or the *Tzanck test* to confirm the diagnosis. Each test involves scraping exudate from an open vesicle, smearing the material on a slide, and staining the smear for microscopic examination. Multinucleated giant cells and intranuclear inclusion bodies confirm a herpes infection. However, the tests don't distinguish herpes zoster from herpes simplex, so the doctor may order other tests—a *culture,* for example.

Teach about treatments

Inform the patient that treatment consists primarily of drug therapy to relieve pain and promote healing of the skin lesions. In addition, stress measures to prevent infection, especially in immunocompromised patients.

Medication

Teach the patient about medications used to treat herpes zoster, including acyclovir, aspirin and other analgesics, silver sulfadiazine, tricyclic antidepressants, and capsaicin.

Acyclovir. Inform the patient that acyclovir (Zovirax) is the drug of choice. The drug inhibits the herpes zoster virus. And although it can't cure the disease, it can relieve pain and promote healing. Therapy should be initiated as early as possible after the onset of signs and symptoms of the virus. For safety and effectiveness, advise the patient to take acyclovir exactly as the doctor directs. Use the patient-teaching aid *Learning about acyclovir,* page 566, to give the patient more information.

Aspirin and other analgesics. Tell the patient that aspirin or, in severe or unresponsive cases, narcotic analgesics may control the pain associated with herpes zoster. In postherpetic neuralgia, narcotic analgesics should be avoided because of the danger of addiction with long-term use. (The patient with a proven allergy to tartrazine dye should avoid aspirin.) Alert the patient who is receiving high-dose aspirin therapy to signs of GI bleeding, such as vomit or stools that obviously contain blood and vomit or stools that look like coffee grounds. Advise him to report these signs to the doctor immediately. Also describe other reportable signs—petechiae, easy bruising, or bleeding gums, for example. To prevent accidental poisoning, instruct him to keep aspirin (and all other medications) in child-resistant containers out of the reach of children.

Silver sulfadiazine. Tell the patient that silver sulfadiazine (Silvadene), an anti-infective cream commonly used in treating burns, appears to relieve pain and dry herpes zoster blisters. Reassure him that this cream won't stain his skin. Show him how to wash his hands before applying the cream. Or suggest that he apply the cream with a disposable finger cot or glove. Also caution him to discard any cream that has become discolored. If he notices increased itching or a new rash or burning sensation, advise him to consult the doctor.

Tricyclic antidepressants. Inform the patient that a tricyclic antidepressant, such as amitriptyline (Elavil, Endep), may be prescribed to relieve pain, especially that of postherpetic neuralgia. Explain that this medicine also alleviates the insomnia and depression that may accompany severe pain.

Caution the patient, however, that adverse reactions to the medication may involve several organ systems. For example, cardiovascular system effects include dysrhythmias, ECG changes, hypertension, orthostatic hypotension, palpitations, tachycardia—even myocardial infarction or stroke.

Many patients also experience central nervous system effects, such as drowsiness, confusion, dizziness, extrapyramidal symptoms (tics and tremors, for example), headache, nervousness or anxiety, peripheral neuropathy, seizures, vivid dreams, and weakness. Dry mouth remains a common complaint along with excessive perspiration.

Eyesight and hearing may be affected, producing blurred vision, increased intraocular pressure, mydriasis, or tinnitus. The patient may also lose his appetite, feel nauseated or even vomit, become constipated, have difficulty urinating, or develop jaundice. Mention that rarely patients experience excessive sensitivity to light, or they experience other hypersensitivity reactions, including rashes or drug fever.

Discuss ways of minimizing these adverse effects. For example, advise the patient to lie down for 30 minutes after taking the first dose and to get up slowly to prevent orthostatic hypotension. Suggest that he take the medication with milk or food to minimize GI upset. Sugarless gum, hard candy, or ice chips may relieve dry mouth. Recommend he take a full dose at bedtime if daytime sleepiness becomes a problem. Advise him to avoid tasks that require mental alertness, such as driving an automobile or truck. Warn him to avoid alcohol, other medications, and excessive exposure to sunlight (and suggest he wear a sunscreen if he works out-of-doors). Caution him to follow dosage instructions exactly and to avoid increasing or decreasing the dose without consulting the doctor. Emphasize that he mustn't stop taking the drug suddenly because he may experience unpleasant effects, such as headache, malaise, and nausea.

Capsaicin. Tell the patient that capsaicin (Axsain, Zostrix) relieves peripheral neuropathy and postherpetic neuralgia. Explain that topical application 3 to 4 times daily should provide pain relief in 2 to 4 weeks. Advise him to rub enough cream into his skin to cover the painful area but not enough to form a caked residue. Point out that he may experience a temporary burning sensation and reddening of the skin during the first several days of use. Remind him that applying capsaicin fewer than 3 times daily may not provide effective pain relief and may prolong the burning sensation.

Other care measures

Advise the patient to apply cool compresses for additional relief from pain and itching. Repeatedly reassure him that herpetic pain will eventually subside. To promote healing and avoid infection, warn him not to scratch the lesions. Instruct him to notify the doctor if pain continues more than 2 months after the rash disappears—or if he has sleep disturbances, loses his appetite, or tires easily after the rash clears up.

Explain that because the patient's immune system is impaired or suppressed he is more vulnerable to infections. Teach him ways to recognize and prevent infection. Review the classic signs and symptoms of infection:

- fever
- warmth, redness, swelling, tenderness, or pain in any body area
- persistent or productive cough
- drainage from any opening or wound.

Then discuss what the patient can do to prevent infection. Recommend that he get an adequate amount of sleep, exercise regularly, and eat a well-balanced diet. Advise him to stay away from anyone with a known infection (a cold, for example). Recommend that he avoid crowds, especially during flu outbreaks. Demonstrate how he should examine his body and mouth daily for signs of infection. Also show him proper hand-washing techniques. Then recommend that he wash his hands before eating and after using the toilet, blowing his nose, stroking a pet, or handling money.

Explain that infants, young children, and adults with illnesses that suppress the immune system (such as AIDS) can contract chicken pox from someone with herpes zoster. So caution the patient to avoid contact with these individuals whenever possible.

Finally, if appropriate, inform the patient of the association between disseminated herpes zoster and human immunodeficiency virus (HIV) infection, also known as AIDS-related complex or ARC. Urge him to obtain proper HIV testing.

Further readings

Andiman, R.M., and Leicht, S.S. "Herpes Zoster on the Increase," *Patient Care* 22(8):71-73, 77, 83-87, April 30, 1988.

Hammond, E. "Herpes Zoster Infections in Children with Hodgkin's Disease," *Journal of the Association of Pediatric Oncology Nurses* 4(1-2):23-29, 1987.

Lefort, S.M. "Herpes Zoster and Postherpetic Neuralgia: The Need for Early Intervention in the Elderly," *Nurse Practitioner* 14(3):30, 35-36, 38, March 1989.

McGowan, J.E., Jr. "Infection Control: New Problem Organisms for Infection Control," *Infection Control and Hospital Epidemiology* 10(6):267-69, June 1989.

McKinney, W.P., et al. "Susceptibility of Hospital-based Health Care Personnel to Varicella Zoster Virus Infections," *American Journal of Infection Control* 17(1):26-30, February 1989.

"Questions and Answers About Shingles," *Patient Care* 22(8):133-34, April 30, 1988.

Photosensitivity reactions

Many people associate a suntan with youth and good health. In fact, the opposite is true: Long-term exposure to ultraviolet radiation causes premature aging of the skin and skin cancer. Because sunburn represents the most common photosensitivity reaction, your foremost teaching goal is to convince patients to protect themselves from overexposure to sunlight.

Luckily, because the media focus so much attention on the adverse effects of sun exposure, persuading people to protect themselves from the sun is easier today than it was years ago. For some people, though, old habits die hard; so your teaching needs to reinforce positive behaviors and clear up misconceptions. Emphasize these points: the signs and symptoms of photosensitivity reactions, complications of sun overexposure, sunscreen use, and skin inspection for changes from sun overexposure.

Discuss the disorder

Inform the patient that photosensitivity is an adverse reaction to natural or artificial light or to light and certain chemicals (including some medications). Then as appropriate, discuss the following risk factors associated with photosensitivity:
- *occupation.* People who work outdoors, such as farmers and construction workers, possess a higher risk than office workers.
- *life-style.* People who spend their leisure time outdoors, such as skiers or beachgoers, have a higher risk than those with indoor interests, such as stamp collectors and moviegoers.
- *age.* Infants and elderly people possess a higher risk because they have the most delicate skin structures.
- *environmental factors, such as altitude and latitude.* The higher the altitude and the closer to the equator, the greater the risk of damage from direct ultraviolet rays.
- *ozone layer density.* Ozone blocks dangerous ultraviolet-C rays from reaching the earth. However, in certain areas, holes in the ozone layer allow these rays to reach the earth, which can lead to severe photosensitivity reactions and skin damage.

Next, identify the kinds of photosensitivity reactions: sunburn, phototoxic reactions, and photoallergic reactions. Inform the patient that *sunburn* results from unprotected exposure to the sun's ultraviolet rays. (See *How ultraviolet rays damage the skin*, page 552.) The most common photosensitivity reaction, sunburn produces skin redness, swelling, itching, blistering, and peeling.

Explain that a *phototoxic reaction* results from exposure to sunlight teamed with certain medications, such as antihistamines

Joanne Muir, RN,C, BSN, and **Cheryl H. Yarboro, RN, BSPA,** wrote this chapter. Both are rheumatology advanced clinical nurses at the National Institutes of Health, Bethesda, Md.

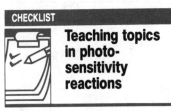

CHECKLIST

Teaching topics in photo-sensitivity reactions

☐ Types of photosensitivity reactions and their causes, signs, and symptoms
☐ Risk factors for photosensitivity reactions
☐ Complications of sun overexposure, including premature skin aging and skin cancer
☐ Diagnosis by physical examination and, if necessary, punch biopsy
☐ Promoting adequate hydration
☐ How sunscreens work and how to apply them
☐ Importance of wearing protective clothing when outdoors during periods of intense sunlight
☐ How to care for sunburned skin
☐ How to check for signs of skin cancer
☐ Avoiding other sources of harmful light, including sunlamps and tanning salons
☐ Sources of information and support

How ultraviolet rays damage the skin

A suntan may look good, but it truly isn't good for anyone. Teach your patient that the sun's ultraviolet-B (UVB) rays penetrate superficial skin, causing the outermost layer to burn, blister, dry, and peel. Emphasize that these rays also change and darken the protective melanin in epidermal cells. In response to the damage, blood volume in the area increases, resulting in red, swollen, sore skin that's painful on touch.

Meanwhile, ultraviolet-A (UVA) rays penetrate deeper into connective tissue, damaging the proteins that keep the skin flexible and youthful looking. These rays may also inhibit the enzymes necessary to repair the cells damaged by UVB rays, contributing to skin cancer.

Eventually, ultraviolet rays cause further skin changes, including a loss of elasticity and a diminished vascular network. The result: thick, wrinkled skin at best, and skin cancer at worst. To help the patient understand the potential harm from ultraviolet rays, use this illustration to show him the changes that occur with sunburned and sun-damaged skin.

NORMAL SKIN

Normal vascular network

SUNBURNED SKIN

Dry and peeling outer skin layer

Darkening and other changes of epidermal melanin

Swollen and reddened papillary dermis

Increased blood volume in vascular network

SUN-AGED SKIN

Thickened and wrinkled outer skin layer

Degeneration of elastic tissue and decreased vascular network

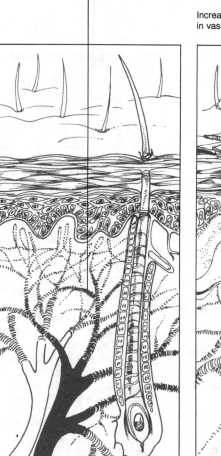
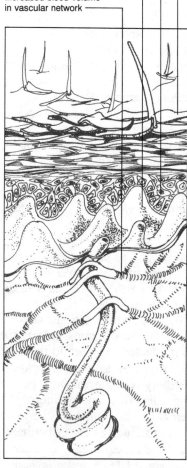
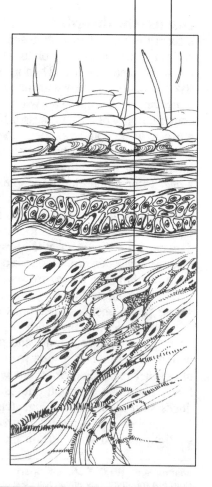

and antimicrobials. (See *Photosensitivity triggers,* pages 554 and 555.) Other offending chemicals include dyes, coal tar, and oil of bergamot (used in perfumes, soaps, and lotions). Dose-related, a phototoxic reaction causes a burning sensation followed by redness, swelling, peeling, and hyperpigmentation. An example is berlock dermatitis (caused by oil of bergamot), which produces an acute reaction with red blisters that later become hyperpigmented.

Certain foods that touch the skin while the patient's in the sun can cause a phototoxic reaction. These foods include carrots, celery, parsnips, and limes.

Tell the patient that a third type of photosensitivity reaction, called a *photoallergic reaction,* is an acquired immune response. It can arise after even slight exposure to light. For example, polymorphous light eruption produces redness, papules, blisters, urticaria, and eczema on exposed areas starting 2 hours to 5 days after light exposure and persisting for up to 2 weeks. Another form, called solar urticaria, begins just minutes after exposure and lasts about an hour, causing burning, itching, redness, and wheals.

Complications

Emphasize that the long-term complications from repeated photosensitivity reactions, mainly sunburn, include premature aging of the skin (wrinkling and a dry, leathery appearance) and skin cancer.

Discuss the risk of skin cancer in more detail. Tell the patient that basal cell carcinoma, the most common form, occurs most often on exposed areas, such as the face, head, and neck. With prompt detection and treatment, this cancer is highly curable. Mention, though, that repeated surgery can cause deformity on conspicuous skin areas. Malignant melanomas may also develop from sun exposure. And although improving, the prognosis for malignant melanoma remains relatively poor.

Inform the patient that other diseases, such as systemic lupus erythematosus, can be aggravated by sunlight. Also mention the potential for infection, which may be introduced through scratching sunburned skin.

Describe the diagnostic workup

Inform the patient that a physical examination confirms photosensitivity reactions. The doctor inspects the skin for rashes, darkened skin areas, freckles, and moles in exposed areas and compares it with the skin in sun-protected areas. If a skin area looks suspicious, he may perform a punch biopsy, obtaining a tissue sample for histologic analysis. Tell the patient that the 15-minute test can be done in the doctor's office, and results are usually available in a day.

Skin biopsy

Inform the patient that a punch biopsy helps diagnose skin damage caused by the sun. First the doctor cleans the biopsy site and administers a local anesthetic to numb it. He pulls the skin surrounding the lesion taut, firmly presses the punch into the lesion, then rotates it to obtain a tissue specimen. He lifts out the tissue

Photosensitivity triggers

Caution the patient that sun exposure combined with certain chemical agents may cause a photosensitivity reaction. These agents include medications, cosmetics, perfumes, deodorant soaps, shampoos, and even some sunscreen preparations.

Review the following list of the most common sensitizing agents. That way, you'll be in a position to advise the patient who's using any of these to check with his doctor if he intends to spend time in the sun or if redness, itching, or a rash develops after sun exposure. Caution him, however, not to stop taking a prescribed drug on his own. Also advise him to read ingredient labels carefully before buying or using cosmetics, soaps, or lotions.

Antihistamines

cyproheptadine (Periactin)
diphenhydramine (Allerdryl 50, Benadryl)

promethazine (Phenergan, Prometh-50)
trimeprazine tartrate (Temaril)

Antimicrobials

demeclocycline (Declomycin)
doxycycline hyclate (Doryx, Vibramycin)
griseofulvin (Fulvicin-U/F, Grisactin)
methacycline (Rondomycin)
minocycline (Minocin)
nalidixic acid (NegGram)
oxytetracycline (Terramycin)
oxytetracycline with sulfamethizole and phenazopyridine
   (Urobiotic-250)
sulfacytine (Renoquid)

sulfadoxine and pyrimethamine (Fansidar)
sulfamethizole (Proklar-M, Thiosulfil)
sulfamethoxazole (Gantanol)
sulfamethoxazole and trimethoprim (Bactrim, Cotrim)
sulfasalazine (Azulfidine)
sulfathiazole with sulfacetamide and sulfabenzamide
   (Sultrin, Triple Sulfa, Trysul)
sulfisoxazole (Gantrisin)
tetracycline (Achromycin V)

Antineoplastic drugs

dacarbazine (DTIC-Dome)
fluorouracil (Adrucil, Efudex, Fluoroplex)
methotrexate sodium (Folex, Mexate)

procarbazine (Matulane)
vinblastine (Velban)

Cardiovascular drugs

acetazolamide (Diamox)
bendroflumethiazide (Naturetin)
benzthiazide (Exna)
captopril (Capoten)
chlorothiazide (Diuril)
furosemide (Lasix)
hydralazine (Apresoline)
hydrochlorothiazide (Esidrix, HydroDIURIL)
hydroflumethiazide (Diucardin, Saluron)
methyclothiazide (Aquatensen, Enduron)

metolazone (Diulo, Zaroxolyn)
polythiazide (Renese)
procainamide (Pronestyl)
quinethazone (Hydromox)
quinidine gluconate (Quinalan)
quinidine sulfate (Cin-Quin)
spironolactone and hydrochlorothiazide (Aldactazide)
triamterene and hydrochlorothiazide (Dyazide, Maxzide)
trichlormethiazide (Metahydrin, Naqua)

Nonsteroidal anti-inflammatory drugs

ketoprofen (Orudis)
naproxen (Anaprox, Naprosyn)

piroxicam (Feldene)
sulindac (Clinoril)

Oral hypoglycemics

acetohexamide (Dymelor)
chlorpropamide (Diabinese, Glucamide)
glipizide (Glucotrol)

glyburide (DiaBeta, Micronase)
tolazamide (Tolinase)
tolbutamide (Orinase)

continued

Photosensitivity triggers—*continued*

Psychoactive drugs

amitriptyline (Elavil, Endep)
amoxapine (Asendin)
chlorpromazine (Thorazine)
chlorprothixene (Taractan)
desipramine (Norpramin, Pertofrane)
doxepin (Adapin, Sinequan)
fluphenazine (Permitil, Prolixin)
haloperidol (Haldol)
imipramine (Janimine, Tofranil)
isocarboxazid (Marplan)

maprotiline (Ludiomil)
nortriptyline (Aventyl, Pamelor)
perphenazine (Trilafon)
perphenazine and amitriptyline (Etrafon, Triavil)
prochlorperazine (Compazine)
protriptyline (Vivactil)
thioridazine (Mellaril)
thiothixene (Navane)
trifluoperazine (Stelazine)
trimipramine maleate (Surmontil)

Topical agents

6-acetoxy-2,4,-dimethyl-*m*-dioxane (preservative)
benzophenones
cinnamates
hexachlorophene (pHisoHex)
6-methylcoumarin (in perfumes, shaving lotions, sunscreens)

musk ambrette (in perfume)
oils of bergamot, cedar, citron, lavender, lime, sandalwood
oxybenzone
para-aminobenzoic acid (PABA)
PABA esters

Other drugs

amiodarone (Cordarone)
carbamazepine (Tegretol)
gold salts (Myochrysine, Solganal)

isotretinoin (Accutane)
oral contraceptives

plug with forceps or a needle. Then he sends the specimen to the pathology laboratory for analysis. Last, he applies an adhesive bandage or one or two sutures, depending on the punch size.

Explain that in hard-to-diagnose conditions, the doctor may perform a photo patch test of the skin on the patient's back. This determines if he's allergic to light.

Teach about treatments

Inform the patient that treatment focuses on prevention. Suggest that he first identify his skin type (see *Categorizing photosensitivity,* page 556). Then he needs to avoid overexposure to the sun—for example, by applying sunscreens, wearing protective clothing, and reducing exposure time during peak sunshine hours. Periodically, he should check his skin carefully for cancer signs. Other measures include increasing fluids and avoiding certain medications, other chemicals, and substances while he's in the sun. When a photosensitivity reaction does develop, treatment includes ointments and other soothing measures for a sunburn (see the patient-teaching aid *How to treat a sunburn,* page 559).

Fluids

Advise the patient to drink plenty of fluids while he's outdoors in the sun and whenever he gets a sunburn to replenish fluid lost through perspiration and dehydration.

Categorizing photosensitivity

The American Academy of Dermatology categorizes photosensitivity by skin types that range from I to VI. A patient with fair, sensitive skin has skin type I; a patient with dark, insensitive skin has skin type VI. Use the following chart to help your patient estimate his photosensitivity. Then offer this rule of thumb for choosing sunscreens with numbered sun protection factors: The fairer the patient's skin, the higher the sun protection factor needed.

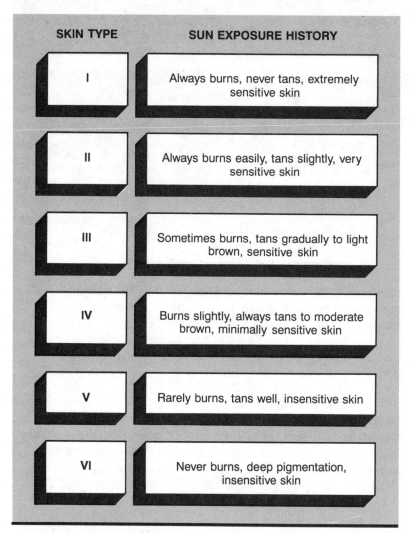

SKIN TYPE	SUN EXPOSURE HISTORY
I	Always burns, never tans, extremely sensitive skin
II	Always burns easily, tans slightly, very sensitive skin
III	Sometimes burns, tans gradually to light brown, sensitive skin
IV	Burns slightly, always tans to moderate brown, minimally sensitive skin
V	Rarely burns, tans well, insensitive skin
VI	Never burns, deep pigmentation, insensitive skin

Medication
Tell the patient to protect his skin from sun damage by applying generous amounts of sunscreen. Explain that sunscreens are graded by their sun protection factors (SPFs), which can range from 2 to 50. These numbers refer to how long the sunscreen protects the skin from burning. For example, by applying a sunscreen with an SPF of 2, a person who usually burns after 30 minutes can presumably stay in the sun twice as long without burning.

Inform the patient that the American Academy of Dermatology and the Skin Cancer Foundation recommend using a sunscreen with an SPF of 15 or higher *for all skin types*. Advise him to apply it generously to dry skin in exposed areas 15 to 30 minutes before going outside. This allows the sunscreen time to penetrate and bind to the skin. Tell him to reapply the sunscreen at least every 2 hours while he's outdoors—more often if he's perspiring or swimming, even if he uses a water-resistant lotion.

Remind him to use the sunscreen on his ears, nose, and especially his lips—skin cancer that occurs on the lips tends to spread more easily than skin cancer in other areas. Tell him that products with a SPF factor of 15 are now available in stick form for the lips. Or he can use an opaque sunblock, such as zinc oxide, on highly sensitive areas.

Advise the patient to select a sunscreen that contains para-aminobenzoic acid (PABA) or a PABA substitute (benzophenones, cinnamates, and salicylates) because this ingredient offers the most protection against skin damage and cancer.

But because PABA protects only against ultraviolet-B (UVB) rays, suggest that he buy a broad-spectrum sunscreen that also protects against ultraviolet-A (UVA) rays. These sunscreens contain benzophenones, oxybenzone, methoxybenzone, sulfisobenzone, and butyl methoxydibenzoylmethane (Parsol 1789). Of course, if a particular sunscreen has an unpleasant odor, attracts insects, stains clothing, or causes a rash or other allergic reaction, suggest that the patient try a different brand, checking the ingredients first.

Also tell the patient that sunscreen use can't be started too early. If appropriate, advise him to teach his children and teenagers about sun protection and to begin applying sunscreens to infants by age 6 months. Half of lifetime ultraviolet radiation exposure occurs by age 18. In fact, just one severe childhood or adolescent sunburn doubles the risk of skin cancer.

Other care measures
Give the patient easy-to-follow guidelines to ensure protection from ultraviolet radiation. Reassure the patient who must work outdoors or who simply enjoys being outside that he needn't restrict his activities as long as he protects himself from the sun. He should limit sun exposure between 10 a.m. and 3 p.m., when ultraviolet rays are the most intense. Caution him that even on overcast days, 80% of the sun's radiation passes through the clouds. Even sitting in the shade or under an umbrella may not completely protect him because sand, water, concrete, and snow reflect the light. Besides, UVA rays remain strong all day and prove as damaging in winter as in summer.

Suggest that for maximum protection, the patient should wear protective clothing while outside—long-sleeved shirts and long pants made of tightly woven, dark-colored fabrics (blue denim is best), a wide-brimmed hat or visor, and good-quality sunglasses (see *Why wear sunglasses?*). Most important, remind him to apply sunscreen before going outside.

Why wear sunglasses?

As you discuss ways the patient can protect his skin from the sun's harmful effects, advise him to protect his eyes too. Here's why. Current studies suggest that ultraviolet radiation penetrates the eye's clear lens and contributes to premature cataracts, especially in people with light-colored eyes.

Advise the patient to choose sunglasses that filter out ultraviolet rays.

Stress the importance of checking his skin for changes in freckles and moles that can signal cancer. Tell the patient to report any changes in mole color, size, or shape, the appearance of irregular borders, any persistent waxy lumps or rough, red patches, or any sores that don't heal. (See the patient-teaching aid *How to examine your skin,* page 560.)

Inform the patient that sunlight isn't the only kind of light that can damage his skin. Sunlamps and tanning lights also emit harmful ultraviolet rays. Tanning salons use lamps that emit predominantly UVA rays without UVB rays, leading some salons to advertise that this light produces a suntan safely. Caution your patient that no suntan is safe. Warn him that all ultraviolet rays can trigger photosensitivity reactions and skin damage. Point out exposure to UVA radiation over time can suppress the immune system, injure the eyes, and augment damage from UVB rays.

Rarely, some people are also sensitive to fluorescent lights. If your patient has this sensitivity, tell him that he can buy plastic tubes that slide over the bulbs. These tubes permit light to shine through, but they filter out the ultraviolet wavelengths responsible for triggering this sensitivity.

Sources of information and support

American Academy of Dermatology
1567 Maple Avenue, Evanston, Ill. 60201
(312) 869-3954

American Cancer Society
1599 Clifton Rd., NE, Atlanta, Ga. 30329
(404) 320-3333

Cancer Information Service, National Cancer Institute
Fox Chase Cancer Center, 7701 Burholme Ave., Philadelphia, Pa. 19111
(800) 4-CANCER

Skin Cancer Foundation
245 Fifth Ave., New York, N.Y. 10016
(212) 725-5176

Further readings

Coody, D. "There Is No Such Thing As a Good Tan," *Journal of Pediatric Health Care* 1(3):125-32, May-June 1987.

Epstein, J.H., and Silverman, R.A. "Blocking Ultraviolet Damage to the Skin," *Patient Care* 21(12):26-29, 32-33, 36, July 15, 1987.

Lawler, P.E. "Be Sunsible: Steps Toward Safety in the Sun," *Oncology Nursing Forum* 16(3):424-27, May-June 1989.

"Photosensitivity from Thiazide Diuretics," *Nurses Drug Alert* 12(4):29, April 1988.

"Sunscreen Agents," *Australia Nurses Journal* 18(7):29-30, February 1989.

Thompson, R.C. "Out of the Bronzed Age," *FDA Consumer* 21(5):20-23, June 1987.

How to treat a sunburn

Dear Patient:

A bad case of sunburn doesn't have to get worse. Use these tips to soothe your skin and to promote healing.

Use ointments
Apply a first-aid ointment containing a local anesthetic, or use a sunburn spray or cream.

Caution: Read labels carefully. Avoid using any preparation that contains agents that your skin is sensitive to.

Apply compresses
Apply cool compresses of Burow's Solution, Domeboro Powder (both are available in drugstores), witch hazel, or baking soda. Dissolve powder forms in tepid water according to directions on the label. Use the compresses for 15 minutes several times a day. Make sure the compresses stay damp enough to feel soothing, but not so wet that they drip.

Bathe or shower
Take cool baths or showers to reduce pain and possibly reduce blistering. Consider adding baking soda to the bath water. This may relieve stinging or itching from sunburn. After bathing, keep your skin well moisturized.

Take pain medication
Take aspirin to relieve swelling, redness, and pain. If you can't take aspirin, try an aspirin substitute — for example, acetaminophen (Tylenol) — to relieve some discomfort. Acetaminophen won't reduce swelling and redness.

Prevent other problems
Drink plenty of fluids to replace those lost through perspiration. This helps prevent dehydration.

Stay out of the sun until your skin heals completely. Sunburned skin is more susceptible to a second serious burn.

If you're not feeling better in 2 or 3 days, see your doctor. He may prescribe a medicine to help.

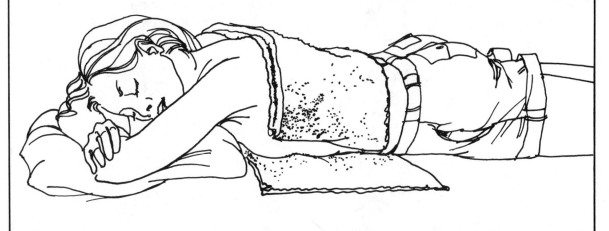

How to examine your skin

Dear Patient:

It's a good idea to examine your skin every month. That's because persistent sun exposure or photosensitivity reactions can lead to skin cancer. See your doctor if you notice suspicious-looking changes in the size, texture, or color of a mole or if you have a sore that doesn't heal. Detected early, most skin cancers are curable.

Check your skin right after a bath or shower. Stand before a full-length mirror in a well-lighted room. Keep a small mirror handy for seeing behind you and for examining hard-to-see spots. Note any freckles, moles, blemishes, and birthmarks, remembering where they are and what they look like. Then proceed:

1 Standing unclothed in front of the mirror, check the front of your body. Turn to each side and look over your shoulder to see behind you. Use your hand mirror also. Then lift your arms and examine the sides of your body.

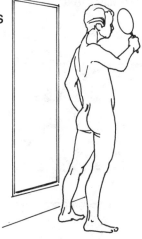

2 Inspect your arms and hands. Check the backs of your hands, your palms, your fingers, and both sides of your forearms and upper arms.

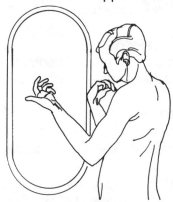

3 Examine your legs, checking the fronts, backs, and sides. Look between your buttocks and around the genital area.

4 Next, move close to the mirror to look carefully at your neck, face, lips, eyes, ears, nose, and scalp. Part your hair with a comb to see better.

5 Now, sit down. Bend your knees to bring your feet close to you. Examine your soles, insteps, ankles, and between your toes.

Herpes simplex

The discomfort and social stigma associated with the herpes simplex virus (HSV) present a formidable teaching challenge. Besides educating the patient about his disease, you'll be called on to help him cope with the emotional distress that having herpes may generate.

Your teaching will help the patient understand how he contracted the disease, learn to use medication and take other measures to relieve symptoms, recognize factors that trigger recurrent disease, and avoid transmitting HSV.

Discuss the disorder

Inform the patient that millions of people suffer from herpes. Experts estimate that about 20 million have genital herpes; even more sustain cold sores. Explain that HSV—also called *Herpesvirus hominis*—is highly contagious. The type-1 strain (HSV-1) usually produces lesions on the skin or the mucous membranes of the lips and mouth (gingivostomatitis). The type-2 strain (HSV-2) produces lesions on the genitals and other nearby areas. HSV-1 is commonly spread by oral contact with an infected person or through respiratory secretions, whereas HSV-2 is transmitted by sexual contact. Emphasize that both HSV-1 and HSV-2 remain contagious whether the carrier has active lesions or no signs and symptoms at all.

Herpes simplex virus type 1

If your patient has an HSV-1 infection, explain that initial symptoms usually include a sore throat (pharyngitis) or oral lesions or both. The virus may also involve the eye's conjunctiva and cornea (keratoconjunctivitis). Other signs and symptoms may include fever, chills, muscle aches, and swollen neck lymph nodes—especially if the patient has infected, draining tonsils. The lesions—commonly called cold sores or fever blisters—ulcerate, turning yellow and scabrous. These sores crust in about 2 days and begin healing without scarring in about 10 days.

Explain that an HSV-1 infection may recur, with tingling, burning, or itching sensations usually preceding the characteristic eruptions by 1 or 2 days.

Herpes simplex virus type 2

If your patient has genital herpes caused by HSV-2, explain that the initial infection usually occurs from 2 to 20 days after expo-

Beth A. Bravante, RN,C, MSN, who wrote this chapter, is a certified registered nurse practitioner at Temple University Hospital in Philadelphia.

CHECKLIST

Teaching topics in herpes simplex

☐ Recognizing signs and symptoms of herpes simplex virus (HSV) infections—HSV-1 and HSV-2
☐ How HSV infection spreads
☐ Recurrence and trigger factors
☐ Complications, such as ocular herpes, increased cancer risks, and spontaneous abortion
☐ Drug therapy, such as acyclovir and vidarabine
☐ Comfort measures, such as bed rest and sitz baths
☐ Preventing HSV transmission
☐ Source of information and support

Genital herpes cycle

Inform the patient that after the initial genital herpes infection, a latency period follows. During this time, the virus enters the nerves surrounding the lesions and remains there permanently. Intermittent viral shedding may take place in the latency period.

Explain that repeated herpetic outbreaks may develop at any time, again followed by a latent stage when healing's complete. The frequency of these outbreaks varies—recurring as often as three to eight times yearly. Although the cycle continues indefinitely, some people remain symptom-free for years.

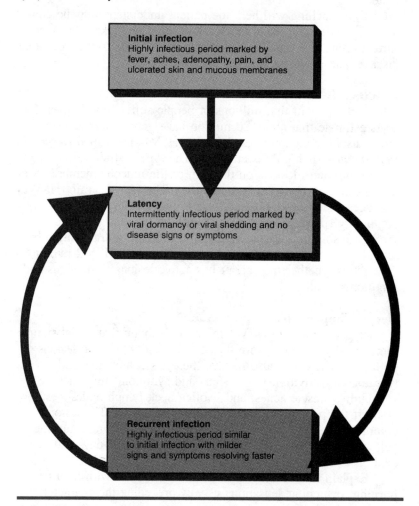

Initial infection
Highly infectious period marked by fever, aches, adenopathy, pain, and ulcerated skin and mucous membranes

Latency
Intermittently infectious period marked by viral dormancy or viral shedding and no disease signs or symptoms

Recurrent infection
Highly infectious period similar to initial infection with milder signs and symptoms resolving faster

sure. Add that tingling or burning sensations may precede the clusters of small, fluid- or pus-filled blisters that develop on the vulva, vagina, penis, buttocks, thighs, or legs. Many patients also experience itching, genital irritation, vaginal or urethral discharge, swollen inguinal lymph nodes, and tender upper inner thighs. The painful lesions ulcerate, crust, and finally heal without scarring in 3 to 6 weeks.

Explain that recurring episodes of genital herpes usually

cause less pain than the initial infection and last between 7 and 10 days (see *Genital herpes cycle*). Discuss trigger factors, such as physical or emotional stress, sunlight, menstrual cycle changes, and sexual intercourse.

Complications

Inform the patient that inadequate measures to contain herpes simplex may lead to its spread and complications. For example, accidental self-inoculation by HSV-1 or HSV-2 can cause infection of the fingers, called herpetic whitlow. Spread to the eyes, herpes simplex can cause keratitis and visual impairment.

If your patient is a woman with genital herpes, tell her that urine retention is a common complication, resulting from difficult and painful urination. Explain that genital herpes is associated with an increased risk of cervical cancer, spontaneous abortion, and neonatal infection in infants whose mothers transmitted herpes during vaginal birth. Rare complications include viral encephalitis, congenital infections, and erythema multiforme.

Describe the diagnostic workup

Tell the patient that HSV is usually diagnosed from the patient's health history and physical examination. Inform him that a *Tzanck test* may confirm the diagnosis. Explain that the doctor will scrape some material from the base of an open blister, smear it on a slide, and stain it for microscopic examination. The test will confirm the presence of an HSV infection, but it can't distinguish among HSV-1, HSV-2, and herpes zoster (or shingles). The doctor may also examine a *blood sample* for the presence of antibody to HSV, or he may order a *viral culture* of material scraped from an open blister. Inform the patient that the culture will confirm an HSV infection and differentiate between HSV-1 and HSV-2.

Teach about treatments

Although HSV infections are incurable, drug therapy and other treatments, such as bed rest, can reduce pain, prevent the spread of lesions, and possibly decrease recurrences. Besides explaining treatments and comfort measures, familiarize the patient with measures to prevent transmitting the disease.

Activity and diet

If the patient has a severe case of herpes simplex, with many painful lesions, recommend bed rest for 1 or 2 days. If urination causes pain, the patient may avoid consuming fluids. Explain that urinating less frequently can place him at risk for a urinary tract infection. Encourage him to drink 10 to 12 glasses of water or other fluids daily.

Medication

Outline how to take medications prescribed for HSV infections, including antiviral agents, analgesics, and, possibly, lysine. Teach the patient that medications can't cure herpes, but they can relieve some symptoms.

Relieving cold sores

Although there's no cure for a cold sore, suggest these measures to relieve accompanying discomfort:
• Apply cool compresses.
• Take aspirin or other pain medication as directed.
• Avoid irritating food and beverages, such as grapefruit juice, which has a high acid content.
• Use an over-the-counter cold sore remedy recommended by the doctor, such as Campho-Phenique or Blistex.
• Call the doctor if the cold sore doesn't heal in 10 days or if symptoms recur frequently.

Antiviral agents. *Acyclovir* (Zovirax) is the drug of choice for treating genital herpes. And though this drug won't speed healing or prevent recurrences, it may decrease the outbreak's severity and the duration of viral shedding. Review administration and adverse effects with the patient, and provide a copy of the patient-teaching aid *Learning about acyclovir,* page 566.

If the patient's taking topical *vidarabine* (Vira-A Ophthalmic) for ocular herpes, explain that this eye ointment may relieve symptoms of recurrent keratitis. Tell him the drug may increase tearing or make him feel like something's in his eyes. If he experiences burning, increased sensitivity to light, itching, pain, redness, or new eye problems after using vidarabine, urge him to contact the doctor.

Instruct the patient to follow application directions exactly and not to exceed the recommended dosage. Caution him to wash his hands before using the drug, not to touch the tube to his eye or surrounding areas, and to store the ointment according to label directions. Remind him to discard the ointment after treatment's complete. Suggest he wear sunglasses if light bothers his eyes during treatment. Offer him the patient-teaching aid *How to use eye ointment,* page 484.

Analgesics. Explain that the doctor may recommend aspirin or acetaminophen (Tylenol) to relieve pain and reduce fever. Review typical adverse effects, such as GI upset, associated with these drugs. Warn parents to avoid giving aspirin to a child with cold sores to reduce the risk of Reye's syndrome.

Tell the patient that the doctor may prescribe a topical anesthetic, such as *lidocaine* (Stanacaine, Xylocaine Jelly), for painful skin lesions or a lidocaine mouthwash for mouth and throat ulcers (for more information, see *Relieving cold sores*). This drug, which gives temporary relief, may make eating and drinking less painful, promoting adequate hydration.

Lysine. Advise the patient that the amino acid lysine may offer effective prophylaxis against recurrent herpes outbreaks. Explain that taking lysine in response to prodromal symptoms, such as burning, itching, or tingling, may limit or prevent lesions. Encourage the patient with recurrent infections to drink milk and to eat such lysine-rich foods as chicken, fish, pork, and legumes.

Other care measures
Suggest washing herpetic lesions several times daily with mild, unscented soap and warm water. Caution the patient to pat the lesions dry and to avoid scratching them.

To obtain additional pain relief for genital lesions, suggest the patient apply compresses soaked in a drying substance—Burow's solution, for example. For women, suggest pouring warm water over the vulva or urinating in a portable sitz bath. Explain that keeping the lesions clean and dry will help prevent spreading. Advise the patient to wear cotton underpants to help absorb excess moisture.

Point out other ways to avoid transmitting infection. For instance, encourage the patient to wash his bed linens, clothes, and eating utensils separately from those of other family members. Demonstrate proper hand-washing techniques, and caution him not to let others use his personal items, such as his towel, washcloth, soap, toothbrush, toothpaste, or drinking cup.

Discuss how genital herpes affects sexual relationships (see *Sex and genital herpes*), and offer guidelines on preventing its spread during intercourse. Because genital herpes increases the risk of cervical cancer, recommend that women with herpes have a Pap smear every 6 to 12 months.

Keep in mind that HSV infections may exact a high emotional toll. Feelings of loneliness, anger, and self-pity are common among patients with genital herpes. Invite the patient to share his concerns with you, the doctor, or a support group. Your open, nonjudgmental instruction can help him channel his distress constructively as he adjusts to living with his disease. And providing a sympathetic, supportive forum for his fears and problems can go a long way toward making him feel less like a victim and an outcast.

Source of information and support
American Social Health Association
(Herpes Resource Center)
P.O. Box 13827, Research Triangle Park, N.C. 27709
(919) 361-2742

Further readings
Bhasker, S., et al. "A Practical, High-Yield Mouth Exam," *Patient Care* 24(2):53-57, 60, 62, January 30, 1990.
Bleich, L. "Nongenital Herpes Simplex Virus: Obstetrical Significance," *Journal of Nurse-Midwifery* 32(6):339-48, November-December 1987.
Breslin, E. "Genital Herpes Simplex," *Nursing Clinics of North America* 23(4):907-15, December 1988.
Brock, B.V., et al. "Frequency of Asymptomatic Shedding of Herpes Simplex Virus in Women with Genital Herpes," *Journal of the American Medical Association* 26(3):418-20, January 19, 1990.
Chenitz, W.C., and Swanson, J.M. "Counseling Clients with Genital Herpes," *Journal of Psychosocial and Nursing Mental Health Services* 27(9):11-17, 32-33, September 1989.
"Cold Sores and Canker Sores," *Harvard Medical School Health Letter* 14(10):6-7, August 1989.
Feder, H.M., Jr., et al. "Common Questions About Herpes Simplex," *Hospital Practice* 24(1A):50, 52, 55-56, January 30, 1989.
"Herpes Simplex Infections," *Occupational Health* (London) 41(4):102-03, April 1989.

Sex and genital herpes

Genital herpes can cause long-term sexual problems. The person who has herpes may fear that he's a source of danger to his partner. He may retreat from revealing his condition to his partner. Or he may hesitate to initiate a relationship.

To compound the problem, the patient's herpes-free partner always runs the risk of acquiring the disease through sexual intercourse.

Offer your patient acceptance and support as he deals with his dilemma: how to have a meaningful sex life without transmitting a lifelong disease. Suggest a few guidelines:
• Avoid having sexual intercourse from the disease's prodromal stage until 10 days after the lesions heal. Though herpes can be transmitted at any time, chances are that transmission occurs less frequently during symptom-free periods.
• Understand that the use of condoms doesn't guarantee protection against herpes, but it does increase safety.
• Approach relationships with honesty, but avoid shocking revelations like, "I have something terrible to tell you." Rather, broach the subject of herpes with discretion at a convenient time. Use neutral words and terms. For instance, think of herpes as "intermittently self-limiting" rather than "incurable."

Learning about acyclovir

Dear Patient:

Taken as directed, acyclovir (also called Zovirax) inhibits viral activity. That means that this drug will help you heal — by relieving discomfort and shortening the length of your infection. But it won't kill your virus. When you stop taking acyclovir, your symptoms may flare up, and you may have occasional outbreaks in the future.

Follow instructions exactly

For safety and effectiveness, take acyclovir exactly as your doctor directs. If you're using acyclovir *ointment,* wear a disposable glove or finger cot to apply it.

If you're taking *tablets or capsules,* take them with food to avoid stomach upset, try not to miss any doses, and don't take them longer or more often than directed.

If you forget a dose, take it as soon as possible. If it's nearly time for your next dose, though, skip the dose and go back to your usual schedule. *Never* take a double dose.

Remember to take acyclovir until the prescription's finished, even if your symptoms begin to disappear.

Report side effects

Call the doctor immediately if you're taking acyclovir *capsules or tablets* and you notice a rash or experience changes in your menstrual periods.

With this form of the drug, you should also watch for headaches, joint pain, acne, and trouble with sleeping. You may even lose your appetite, feel nauseated, or vomit.

If acyclovir makes you feel dizzy, don't drive. And don't do other tasks that require alertness until you feel better.

Call the doctor if you take acyclovir by *injection* and you have these symptoms: a rash, hallucinations (seeing, hearing, or feeling things that aren't there), trembling, confusion, or blood in your urine.

If you're using *ointment,* you may notice signs of infection or irritation, including burning, itching, blistering, or peeling.

Soon after treatment starts, your gums may bleed or swell and feel tender. Brushing and flossing your teeth and massaging your gums regularly may help. Also, see your dentist routinely to have your teeth cleaned. Check with your doctor or your dentist if you have other dental problems or if you have questions about proper care.

Special instructions

• Store acyclovir away from heat, dampness, and direct light. These can cause the medicine to break down. So don't keep acyclovir in the bathroom or near the kitchen sink or stove.
• Throw away unused or old medicine.
• Keep acyclovir, including discarded medicine, away from children.
• Acyclovir won't keep you from passing herpes to others. (If you have genital herpes, avoid sex until you're symptom-free.)
• Call your doctor if your symptoms get worse or don't improve in a few days.

Psoriasis

Although psoriasis isn't contagious or life-threatening, its unsightly skin lesions can cause discomfort and embarrassment. You'll be challenged to teach the patient to cope with this incurable and frustrating skin condition.

Initially, your teaching may focus on describing the remissions and recurrences that characterize psoriasis. Then you'll point out factors that cause flare-ups. You'll also review treatment options, such as skin care, medications, ultraviolet (UV) light therapy, support groups, and psoriasis treatment centers. (For more information, see *Teaching the newly diagnosed psoriasis patient,* page 568.)

Discuss the disorder

Inform the patient that psoriasis is a chronic skin disease, which is characterized by abnormally accelerated growth and multiplication of epidermal cells. Whereas normal skin cells reproduce every 28 days, skin cells affected by psoriasis may reproduce as frequently as every 4 days. Consequently, dead skin cells accumulate rapidly, emerging as dry, silvery scales atop patchy erythematous lesions. Called plaques, these characteristic lesions usually affect the elbows, knees, and scalp, but they can appear anywhere. Removal of the scales typically reveals tiny punctate bleeding spots known as Auspitz's sign.

Explain that psoriatic plaques affect the scalp in about 50% of patients. The disease usually spares the face, but the plaques may appear behind the ears. In a few patients, psoriasis may affect the nails, producing pitting, discoloration, and hyperkeratosis and separation of the nail from the nail bed.

Discuss the acute phase, which involves general skin reddening. About half of all patients report accompanying itching, which may be intense—especially at night. As the rash progresses, the cracked, encrusted plaques may cause pain. Furthermore, the rash may mimic that of other diseases, such as seborrhea, allergic skin reactions, and secondary syphilis. This can lead to social isolation and misunderstanding.

Tell the patient that the disease typically alternates between recurrences and remissions. During remission, symptoms disappear. The patient may express frustration and hopelessness during recurrences. Unfortunately, these responses may intensify his symptoms and decrease the effectiveness of treatment.

Joanne Lavin, RN, EdD, and **Joan E. Mason, RN, EdM,** wrote this chapter. Ms. Lavin is an assistant professor at Kingsborough Community College in Brooklyn, N.Y. Ms. Mason is a clinical editor and consultant for Springhouse Corp., Springhouse, Pa.

CHECKLIST

Teaching topics in psoriasis

☐ Explanation of psoriasis and its course, including alternating remissions and recurrences
☐ Types of psoriasis
☐ Factors that trigger flare-ups, such as stress, sunburn, and skin injury
☐ Drug treatment, including tar preparations, topical corticosteroids, anthralin, methotrexate, and etretinate
☐ Ultraviolet light therapy
☐ Skin care, including cleansing, dressings, and measures to relieve itching
☐ Managing psoriasis of the scalp and nails
☐ Preventing flare-ups
☐ Coping with the psychosocial effects of psoriasis
☐ Sources of information and support

Teaching the newly diagnosed psoriasis patient

At first, the patient who learns he has psoriasis may feel uncomfortable and self-conscious. Later, he may also feel annoyed and frustrated by time-consuming daily skin treatment. What approach can you take to teach him to cope with and care for psoriasis? To find out, refer to a standard teaching plan. This will help you identify his specific learning needs. Then modify the plan accordingly.

Assess first
Your patient, John Jones, is a 26-year-old boat sales-man and an avid water-skier. About 2 months ago, he noticed red, itchy patches, covered with silvery scales, developing on his elbows, knees, and scalp. The doctor diagnosed psoriasis and prescribed daily bathing with a tar gel followed by application of a hy-drocortisone cream to the affected areas.

John has returned to the doctor today because the itchy psoriasis plaques have spread to his legs, chest, and back. He confesses that his compliance with the prescribed treatment has been spotty. "I don't have time to sit in a bathtub all day," he com-plains.

As you and John talk further, you learn that he's missed work all week because he's embarrassed about his appearance. "With my skin looking like this, I'd probably be asked to leave the sales floor."

The doctor confirms that John's psoriasis is worse. He asks you to teach John about the disease and to review the treatment regimen thoroughly in hopes of promoting compliance.

Define learning needs next
To decide what to teach John, compare what he al-ready knows about psoriasis with the content of a standard teaching plan, which includes:
• the course of the disease
• types of psoriasis
• what triggers flare-ups
• drug treatment, such as tar preparations and topi-cal corticosteroids, and procedures, such as ultravi-olet (UV) light therapy
• skin care (cleansing and controlling itching)
• prevention of flare-ups
• coping skills to deal with the psychological effects of psoriasis.

From talking with John, you realize that he knows little about the recurring nature of psoriasis, and he's angry and resentful about his treatment plan. Clearly, he needs to learn more about all of the topics in the standard teaching plan. Your first goal is to help John understand the disease process and why he needs

to comply with treatment measures. You'll highlight this by reviewing the skin care routine in detail.

In addition, you recognize that he needs an outlet to express his feelings about the impact psoriasis has had on his life-style. You'll need to emphasize ways to maintain a normal personal and professional life.

Agree on learning outcomes
Guided by the standard teaching plan, you and John review learning outcomes. Together, you agree that he'll be able to:

```
-describe the course of psoriasis
-recite the steps in his treatment regimen
-demonstrate skin care techniques, such as
cleansing methods, applying medications, and
wearing occlusive dressings
-list ways to prevent flare-ups
-state why he needs regular follow-up care
-name steps he'll take to maintain his social
life and job standing.
```

Choose teaching tools and techniques
Start with a short *discussion* of psoriasis and its characteristics, including factors that trigger the dis-ease, medications, UV light therapy, and skin care regimens. Be sure to allow plenty of time for *ques-tions and answers*. Encourage John to express his feelings about how psoriasis affects his life-style.

Use *demonstration* to teach about skin care proce-dures, such as cleansing and applying medication. Again, urge John to ask questions and discuss his feelings.

Vary your teaching with *visual aids*—booklets, dia-grams, videotapes, and printed instructions for skin treatment. These tools will reinforce your teaching and help John retain what he's learned.

Evaluate your teaching effectiveness
How effective was your teaching? Use *questions and answers* to assess whether John understands pso-riasis and how well he follows treatment. Can he name the key features of psoriasis? Also find out if he's coping more effectively with the effects of pso-riasis. Has he missed much work? Also ask how he protects his skin when (and if) he water-skis.

Use *return demonstration* to ensure that John can perform skin care routines, such as applying medica-tions and occlusive dressings. Based on your find-ings, estimate his progress and if necessary, redirect your teaching.

Outline the types of psoriasis (see *Identifying the types of psoriasis,* page 570). As appropriate, distinguish further among mild, moderate, and severe disease forms (see *Psoriasis: Mild to severe*). Most patients have mild-to-moderate psoriasis, which doesn't affect their general health.

Explain that the cause of psoriasis is unknown although researchers do think that a biochemical malfunction triggers abnormal cell division. Mention too that psoriasis tends to run in families, suggesting a genetic predisposition to the disease. Alcohol, endocrine imbalances, infection, pregnancy, skin injuries, emotional stress, and environmental factors, such as cold weather and sunburn, may trigger recurrences. Point out that the disease affects men and women equally and typically begins between ages 5 and 40, although it may occur at any age.

Complications
Stress that compliance with the prescribed treatment regimen reduces the patient's risk for infection. Point out that infection increases his discomfort and retards healing. Also emphasize that compliance with treatment may speed remission, thereby avoiding the social isolation and depression that may accompany and complicate psoriasis.

Describe the diagnostic workup
Explain that a health history and physical examination usually are all that's needed to diagnose psoriasis. For some patients, though, a skin biopsy may be ordered to confirm the diagnosis or to rule out another disorder. For the same reason, the patient may have routine chest X-rays, blood tests, and urinalyses. If the doctor suspects an infection, advise the patient that a microscopic examination and Gram stain of the skin scales may identify the causative organism.

Teach about treatments
Describe the treatment regimen for psoriasis, including activity and dietary recommendations, medications, and procedures such as UV light therapy and UV light combined with various medications. Explain that these measures help control abnormal skin cell proliferation, heal plaques, and prevent new lesions. Reinforce the patient's coping skills to boost his self-esteem. And discuss ways to reduce flare-ups—for example, by practicing stress-reduction techniques (for more information, see *Stress and psoriasis—a vicious cycle,* page 571).

Activity
Tell the patient that he probably doesn't need to limit his activities. If fatigue or severe pain accompanies flare-ups, advise him to rest. Also recommend regular rest periods for the patient with psoriatic arthritis.

Diet
Caution the patient to avoid certain foods and beverages that may aggravate psoriasis (meat, seafood, and alcohol, for example).

Psoriasis: Mild to severe

Discuss with the patient the varying degrees of psoriasis.

Mild
The patient with mild psoriasis usually exhibits plaques that are scattered over a small skin area and rarely require long-term medical attention. For example, a patient with quarter-sized plaques on his elbows or knees has mild psoriasis.

Moderate
A patient with moderate psoriasis has more and larger plaques—up to several centimeters in diameter. Psoriasis involving most of the scalp would be called moderate. The patient typically expresses as much concern about his appearance as about discomfort resulting from symptoms.

Severe
In severe psoriasis, plaques can cover at least half of the body. Examples include erythrodermic or pustular forms of the disease, palmoplantar psoriasis, and psoriatic arthritis.

Identifying the types of psoriasis

Psoriasis occurs in various forms—ranging from one or two localized plaques to widespread lesions and crippling arthritis.

Erythrodermic psoriasis
Inform the patient that erythrodermic psoriasis is marked by extensive flushing all over the body, which may or may not result in scaling. The rash may begin rapidly to signal new psoriasis, it may develop gradually in chronic psoriasis, or it may occur as an adverse reaction to a drug.

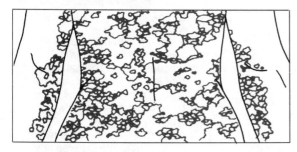

Guttate psoriasis
Explain that this type of psoriasis typically affects children and young adults. Erupting in drop-sized plaques over the trunk, arms, legs, and sometimes the scalp, this rash of plaques generalizes in several days. It's commonly associated with upper respiratory tract streptococcal infections.

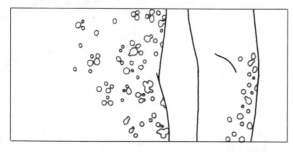

Inverse psoriasis
Tell the patient that smooth, dry, bright red plaques characterize inverse psoriasis. Located in skin folds (the armpits and groin, for example), the plaques fissure easily.

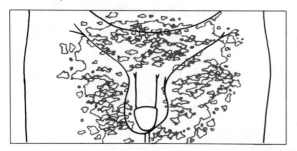

Psoriasis vulgaris
Teach the patient that psoriasis vulgaris is the most common type. It begins with red, dotlike lesions that gradually enlarge and produce dry, silvery scales. The plaques usually appear symmetrically on the knees, elbows, extremities, genitals, scalp, and nails.

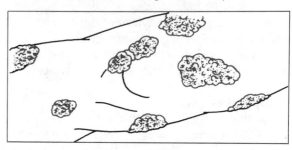

Pustular psoriasis
Describe pustular psoriasis as an eruption of local or extensive small, raised, pus-filled plaques. Precursors include emotional stress, sweat, infections, or adverse drug reactions.

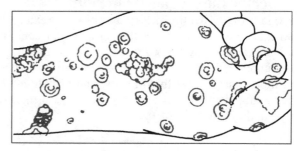

Psoriatic arthritis
Inform the patient that psoriatic arthritis develops in about 10% of psoriasis patients. Commonly affecting the terminal joints of the fingers and toes, the disease also attacks the lower back, wrists, knees, or ankles, causing pain, swelling, and sometimes crippling. Blood tests detect no rheumatoid factor—the key to distinguishing psoriatic arthritis from rheumatoid arthritis.

Family history, nail malformation, and distal interphalangeal joint involvement also characterize this disorder.

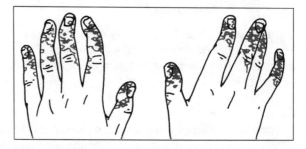

Suggest that he keep a record of his diet and eliminate any foods that prove to trigger flare-ups.

Medication

Teach the patient to use psoriasis medications properly. For example, if he's using special shampoos for scalp psoriasis, advise him that he may need to change or alternate products if he develops tolerance to the medicine. As appropriate, discuss such medications as coal tar preparations, topical corticosteroids, anthralin, methotrexate, and etretinate.

Coal tar preparations. Explain that coal tar products (AquaTar, Estar Gel, Fototar, psoriGel, T/Derm, and others) retard skin cell growth and relieve inflammation, itching, and scaling. Marketed as creams, ointments, gels, bath solutions or emulsions, oils, and shampoos, most can be purchased without a prescription.

Instruct the patient to use a coal tar preparation daily at bedtime. Advise him to apply the medicine in the direction of hair growth to prevent folliculitis. Caution him, though, not to apply the medicine to his face, armpits, groin, or other skin folds. The preparation may cause redness and burning in these sensitive areas. Forewarn him that coal tar will stain sheets, towels, and nightclothes. Suggest that he allow the medicine to air-dry before dressing. Make sure to review measures for avoiding too much sun because coal tar preparations increase photosensitivity.

Topical corticosteroids. Inform the patient that topical corticosteroids are the treatment of choice for mild-to-moderate psoriasis of the trunk, arms, and legs. Explain that these drugs decrease epidermal cell growth and reduce inflammation. They may also relieve symptoms by inducing vasoconstriction. Instruct the patient to contact the doctor as soon as possible if he notices signs of infection, such as painful, pus-containing blisters, or signs of irritation, including blistering, burning, itching, or peeling, after using these topical agents. Mention that treatment commonly combines topical corticosteroids with emollients, tar preparations, and UV light therapy. For many patients, this regimen minimizes adverse reactions and treatment expense.

Explain that topical corticosteroids don't cure psoriatic plaques. They do, however, convert the plaques into thin, flat, less noticeable, and less annoying patches. Caution the patient that relief with these drugs may be temporary and that rapid relapse typically occurs when therapy stops. Discontinuing potent topical corticosteroids occasionally transforms stable, chronic, plaque-type psoriasis into generalized pustular psoriasis. For this reason, topical corticosteroids alone aren't usually prescribed for long-term treatment. Because systemic corticosteroids can cause similar adverse reactions, they're rarely used to treat psoriasis.

If the patient has mild psoriasis involving the extremities, tell him that 0.025% triamcinolone acetonide ointment (Aristocort, Kenalog, or Trymex) may provide relief. Facial, groin, or axillary plaques may respond to 1% desonide cream (DesOwen, Tridesilon) or alclometasone dipropionate (Aclovate). More potent topical preparations, such as 0.1% betamethasone valerate (Betatrex, Val-

Stress and psoriasis – a vicious cycle

Stress exacerbates psoriasis – and the discomfort and disfigurement of psoriasis cause stress. Help the patient break this vicious cycle by explaining how stress and psoriasis interact (either singly or simultaneously) on three levels.

Physical level
The effects of psoriasis on the body – scaling, itching, bleeding plaques – cause discomfort, which can lead to anxiety and fatigue. Worry over the progress of the disease may create additional stress, which may lead to appetite loss and sleep disturbances. Furthermore, inadequate nutrition and rest intensify physical stress.

Emotional level
Psoriasis can lead to an altered self-image. Anger, frustration, and hopelessness may cause the patient to withdraw from personal and professional relationships. In turn, this isolation adds to the patient's emotional burden and low self-esteem and creates more stress.

Social level
Without a support system, the patient may be devastated by negative experiences in daily life. For example, if psoriasis affects his scalp, he may complain that the barber refuses to cut his hair. The patient may conclude that he's all alone in his struggle with psoriasis.

isone) or 0.1% triamcinolone acetonide (Aristocort, Kenalog, Triaderm), may be prescribed for moderate psoriasis.

Demonstrate the downward stroke used for applying a topical corticosteroid. Make sure to instruct the patient to wash his hands thoroughly before and after using the medicine. Caution him to avoid touching his eyes because repeated eye exposure to these drugs has been associated with cataract formation.

Advise the patient to contact the doctor immediately if infection or irritation develops during topical corticosteroid use. Tell him to watch for such signs and symptoms as pain, redness, pus-filled blisters, itching, and peeling. Caution him to use these medications only for the time prescribed because prolonged use can cause atrophy, skin discoloration, striae, telangiectasis, and possible drug tolerance (or resistance to therapy).

Anthralin. Inform the patient that anthralin (Anthra-Derm, Drithocreme, or Lasan) may help heal large plaques that don't respond to coal tar or topical corticosteroid preparations. This topical psoriatic agent inhibits skin cell proliferation without being absorbed systemically.

Explain that the patient's tolerance of the drug and the severity of his psoriasis determine the drug strength he'll use. Mention that he'll use a less concentrated anthralin preparation as his skin heals. Once the plaques shrink, anthralin therapy can stop, and routine skin care can resume. Give the patient a copy of the teaching aid *Learning about anthralin,* page 577. Review the instructions with him and answer any questions.

Methotrexate. A drug that inhibits cell replication, methotrexate (Folex, Mexate) may relieve severe, unresponsive psoriasis. Tell the patient to report chills, diarrhea, fever, mouth or lip sores, reddened skin, stomach pain, and unusual bleeding or bruising to the doctor immediately. Also instruct him to contact the doctor if other adverse effects develop while he's taking this drug.

Because alcohol increases the risk of hepatotoxicity, warn the patient to avoid drinking alcoholic beverages while taking methotrexate. Advise him to check with the doctor before taking any medication and to avoid over-the-counter analgesics, such as aspirin and ibuprofen (Advil, Nuprin). Explain that these drugs may raise plasma concentrations of methotrexate to toxic levels. Also advise the patient to consult the doctor before having any immunizations during or after methotrexate treatment. Caution him also to avoid people with contagious diseases, if possible, because the drug can lower his white blood cell count.

Because methotrexate may cause photosensitivity reactions, instruct the patient to take precautions to avoid excessive exposure to sunlight. For example, suggest that he wear a wide-brimmed hat and sunglasses. Finally, because methotrexate lowers platelet counts—and thereby increases bleeding risks—instruct the patient to consult the doctor before undergoing surgery or dental work. Also advise him to use a soft toothbrush and to exercise care when using a toothpick or dental floss.

Etretinate. Inform the patient that this potent retinoic acid derivative may be prescribed for severe psoriasis that's resistant to other drugs or treatments. Especially effective for treating pustular and erythrodermic psoriasis, etretinate (Tegison) may also relieve extensive plaque-type psoriasis—although recurrences within 2 months after therapy ends are common.

Emphasize that this potent teratogen may remain in the body for up to 3 years after treatment ends. That's why the drug shouldn't be used by women who are pregnant, who intend to become pregnant, or who use unreliable contraception. Drug studies indicate that etretinate doesn't affect a man's sperm, although it does have a negative effect on spermatogenesis in laboratory animals.

Instruct the patient to report these reactions immediately: dark-colored urine, flulike symptoms, vision changes (especially blurred or double vision), and yellowing of the eyes or skin. Other drug-related effects include abdominal pain, bone or joint pain, chapped lips, dry nose and mouth, eye irritation, fatigue, hair thinning, muscle aches, photosensitivity, and unusual bleeding.

Inform the patient that his psoriasis may appear to worsen during the first month of treatment, possibly with skin redness or itching, but this usually subsides with continued use. Reassure him that this is common, and 2 to 3 months may pass before he notices an improvement. Advise him to contact the doctor if skin irritation or other psoriatic symptoms grow severe.

To relieve dry mouth, suggest using sugarless hard candy, chewing gum, or ice chips. If dry mouth persists after 2 weeks, advise the patient to consult the doctor or dentist because this condition increases the risk of periodontal disease.

Procedures

In controlled amounts, UV light—either from artificial sources or from natural sunlight—suppresses skin cell replication and controls psoriatic symptoms. Caution the patient, however, that too much UV light can exacerbate his disease, probably because normal skin cells reproduce more quickly to repair the damage. Of the three UV light wavelengths—UVA (short wave), UVB (middle wave), and UVC (long wave)—UVB is most commonly used to treat psoriasis. If appropriate, discuss procedures that combine UV light with drug therapies, such as coal tar preparations or psoralen, to increase treatment effectiveness.

UVB light therapy. UVB therapy is considered the most effective and least risky treatment for moderate-to-severe psoriasis. Explain that inpatient or outpatient UVB light therapy may be used daily during a flare-up. Once the flare-up resolves, the treatments may taper off. If the patient's skin turns severely red or burns, however, treatment may stop temporarily for 1 to 2 days.

Tell the patient that the light may be natural from the sun or contained in a body-sized, tubelike UV light treatment chamber. Smaller light devices may be used to treat hands, feet, or other sites of localized plaques. For more information, see *What happens during UV light treatments,* page 574.

What happens during UV light treatments

If your patient's having ultraviolet (UV) light therapy, tell him that this procedure may help to relieve and control psoriasis.

Prepare the patient to undergo brief daily treatments. The entire treatment course may last 1 to 3 weeks (depending on results). Explain that he'll stand inside a body-sized UV light chamber (similar to the one shown), or he'll use a small light chamber for hands or feet or other body parts. For the body-sized chamber, he'll remove any clothing that covers the plaques. In this way he'll expose affected skin to the banks of fluorescent lights surrounding him.

Explain that a special coating on these lights guarantees that the appropriate UV wavelength reaches his skin. Reassure him that exposure will be electronically timed to ensure safety. The first session usually lasts between 15 and 30 seconds.

Because a mild sunburn produces the best response, exposure time will gradually increase until the light turns the patient's skin pink. If he has dark skin, making minimal color changes hard to observe, ask him to recall whether he felt a mild sunburn after his last treatment. Emphasize that he'll wear dark, polarized goggles to protect his eyes from damage during treatments.

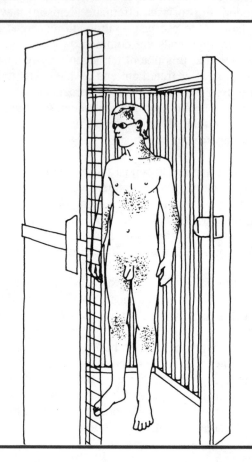

Explain that soaking in warm water for 30 minutes before therapy will help to remove scales and enhance light penetration. After the treatment course, point out that maintenance UVB light therapy (in the treatment center, the doctor's office, or at home) may prolong remission.

Goeckerman therapy. Inform the patient that this procedure combines topical coal tar treatment with UVA or UVB light therapy to increase the effectiveness of each. Used mostly during flare-ups, Goeckerman therapy also may be effective for extended periods to treat chronic, resistant plaques.

Review instructions for applying an ⅛-inch-thick layer of 1% or 5% crude coal tar ointment to the plaques. Instruct the patient to leave the ointment on his skin for 12 to 14 hours. Then before he bathes, advise him to remove the ointment with clean towels or sheets saturated in olive or mineral oil. Next, he'll receive a UV light treatment equivalent to between 20 and 30 minutes of sunlight. Inform him that his skin will turn slightly red or pink 12 hours later. Symptoms should begin subsiding within 5 days. Caution him that this treatment procedure may produce a burn much like sunburn. Also point out that long-term, continued treatment increases his risk of skin cancer.

Modified Goeckerman therapy. Tell the patient that using UVB light therapy after applying topical drugs, such as coal tar preparations (such as Estar Gel), corticosteroids, or kerolytic agents, rather than crude coal tar ointment constitutes modified Goeckerman therapy. Although this treatment may relieve psoriasis faster than does standard Goeckerman therapy, remission may be briefer.

Ingram therapy. Explain that this procedure uses anthralin rather than a tar preparation. Instruct the patient to apply anthralin to his plaques and to leave it on as directed (usually between 8 and 12 hours). Next, he should remove the anthralin with mineral oil. Then, after bathing, he'll receive a UVB light treatment. With Ingram therapy, the normal skin surrounding the plaques is protected by a layer of zinc oxide or petrolatum. Tell the patient that his symptoms should improve within 4 weeks.

Photochemotherapy. Inform the patient that photochemotherapy (PUVA) combines UVA light treatment with psoralen—either orally or topically. Explain that psoralen, a photosensitizing agent, increases sensitivity to UVA light. Point out that UVA light alone doesn't relieve psoriasis. Combined with psoralen, however, UVA light treatments block skin cell replication. Psoriasis vulgaris, which responds poorly to topical corticosteroids, anthralin, or coal tar treatments, may respond to PUVA therapy. Tell the patient that he may need about 30 treatments before symptoms clear totally.

Instruct the patient either to take psoralen tablets or to apply topical psoralen 2 to 3 hours before his UVA light treatment. Tell him that his initial exposure may last only a few minutes. Explain that the exposure time will lengthen incrementally, based on how much melanin his skin contains, his usual response to sunlight, and his sunburn history. Point out that because skin redness may peak from 48 to 72 hours after the treatment, he'll receive PUVA treatments every other day or twice weekly.

Mention that he'll wear special glasses, or goggles, to protect his eyes during the light treatment. Instruct him also to keep his eyes closed during the treatment. Because psoralen remains active for at least 24 hours, remind him to protect his skin and eyes from sunlight and artificial UVA light sources for at least a day after the PUVA session. Recommend wearing long-sleeved clothing (to avoid sunburn) and sunglasses (to prevent corneal and retinal damage) that filter out UV light (both indoors and outdoors).

List the possible adverse effects of PUVA treatment, including short-term nausea, itching, and skin redness. Advise the patient to take the psoralen with milk or food to minimize nausea. Other risks are the same as those associated with overexposure to sunlight, including cataracts, freckling, premature skin aging, and an increased risk of skin cancer.

Other care measures
Instruct the patient to avoid scratching the plaques. Suggest that he divert his attention from his discomfort by reading, playing a game, watching television, talking on the phone, or listening to music. To avoid scratching, recommend that he wear gloves or a

576 Psoriasis

Managing nail and scalp psoriasis

If psoriasis affects your patient's nails and scalp, support his perseverance with treatment for these frustrating conditions.

Nail care
Inform the patient that nail psoriasis will improve as skin plaques diminish. Tell him that the doctor may treat nail psoriasis with a 1% solution of fluorouracil (Efudex, Fluoroplex), which is applied to the nails twice a day for 3 to 6 months. Explain that improvement will be slow because the nail impedes topical drug penetration.

Advise the patient to remove debris under the nails, if possible. The doctor may then recommend wrapping them with a corticosteroid-impregnated tape. This may also offer some relief.

Scalp care
To relieve mild scaling, instruct the patient to lather with a tar shampoo (such as Polytar or Sebutone) and then apply a steroid lotion (such as Synalar or Diprosone).

To relieve heavy scaling, tell the patient to apply mineral oil or P & S Liquid (an oil-based salicylic acid) overnight under an occlusive dressing (such as a plastic shower cap) to loosen thick scales. Advise him to follow the overnight oil treatment with a tar-based shampoo and gentle combing to release heavy scales. Severe scalp psoriasis may respond to a steroidal lotion or solution and an occlusive dressing after the shampoo.

Inform the patient that the doctor may initiate an overnight treatment of anthralin (Lasan) ointment followed by a morning shampoo to reduce thick, chronic scales. He'll continue the treatment until scales diminish.

special plastic suit. Applying ice cubes or mentholated shaving cream may also provide relief. Recommend using a room humidifier in the winter. This may prevent skin dryness, which increases itching.

Emphasize prevention. Discuss measures to prevent flare-ups. For example, advise the patient to avoid activities that could injure his skin, and emphasize meticulous compliance with his daily skin care regimen. Also give him a copy of the patient-teaching aid *Daily skin care for psoriasis,* page 578. If appropriate, review *Managing nail and scalp psoriasis.*

Promote coping and self-esteem. The patient may need your help in dealing with social and professional problems. For example, he may lose interest in sex because he feels embarrassed about his appearance. If he thinks his appearance inhibits his drive or responses, suggest that he try undressing after turning out the lights, or having sex in a dimly lit or dark room. Or offer this possibility: Tell him to apply a scented emollient (such as Alpha Keri lotion or bath oil) to soften and smooth his skin before intimacy.

If he's concerned that his appearance negatively affects his career, advise him to cover up plaques with long-sleeved or turtleneck shirts. Encourage him to voice his feelings about how psoriasis affects his work and social activities. If he expresses interest, refer him to appropriate agencies and support groups. Also, encourage him to stick to his treatment regimen and to attend follow-up appointments.

Sources of information and support

National Psoriasis Foundation
6443 West Beaverton Highway, Suite 210, Portland, Ore. 97221
(503) 297-1545

Psoriasis Research Association
107 Vista del Grande, San Carlos, Calif. 94070
(415) 593-1394

Psoriasis Research Institute
P.O. Box V, Stanford, Calif. 94305
(415) 326-1848

Further readings

Abel, E.A., et al. "Insights Into Psoriasis Management," *Patient Care* 23(19):102-05, 108, 111-13, November 30, 1989.
Coleman, D.A., et al. "A Worse-Case Guide for Any Case of Psoriasis," *RN* 51(3):39-43, March 1988.
Dunn, M.L., et al. "Treatment Options for Psoriasis," *American Journal of Nursing* 88(8):1082-87, 1090-91, August 1988.
Hall, J.C. "Improving Control of a Recalcitrant Condition," *Consultant* 27(12):67-68, 71, December 1987.
Lombardo, B., et al. "Group Support for Derm Patients," *American Journal of Nursing* 88(8):1088-91, August 1988.

Learning about anthralin

Dear Patient:

The doctor has prescribed anthralin (also called Anthra-Derm, Drithocreme, or Dritho-Scalp) to relieve your psoriasis symptoms. This drug works by blocking the abnormal growth of skin cells. Review these tips for using anthralin effectively.

Follow instructions exactly

Use anthralin exactly as the doctor directs. If you miss a dose, apply it as soon as possible. However, if it's almost time for your next dose, skip the missed dose and go back to your regular schedule. Never apply a double dose or an extra dose.

If the doctor has prescribed short-contact treatment, apply a thin layer of anthralin to the affected skin or scalp. Gently rub in the medicine. Allow it to remain on your skin for 20 to 30 minutes. Then remove it by bathing or shampooing (if you're treating your scalp).

If the doctor has prescribed overnight treatment, gently apply a thin layer of anthralin cream or ointment to the affected skin areas. Remove *anthralin cream* the next morning by bathing or shampooing. Remove *anthralin ointment* with warm mineral oil. Then bathe or shampoo. If you apply the drug to your scalp, dry and part your hair and then rub the anthralin cream into your hair. Follow the instructions given to remove the cream.

Report side effects

Call the doctor if your skin becomes red or irritated or if you notice a rash after applying this medicine.

Prevent staining

Anthralin will stain your skin, hair, clothing, bed linens, bathtub, and shower. Skin or hair stains will wear off in 2 to 3 weeks after you stop using anthralin. To protect your hands, wear plastic gloves when you apply anthralin.

To protect your bed linens and nightclothes, ask the doctor about wearing a plastic shower cap or protective dressings at bedtime.

To protect your bathtub and shower, wash anthralin from the porcelain or tile with hot water and a household cleanser immediately after use.

Special instructions

- Keep this medicine away from your eyes and other mucous membranes, such as your mouth and the inside of your nose.
- Don't use anthralin on your face or sex organs or in skin folds and creases, such as the groin or underarms.
- Avoid applying anthralin to blistered, raw, or oozing skin.
- Spread on petroleum jelly to protect the normal skin surrounding the treated areas.

Daily skin care for psoriasis

Dear Patient:

To prevent infection and promote healing, you'll need to observe a daily skin care routine. Follow the doctor's instructions, and review the tips below.

Soaking in the tub

A daily tub soak will help to remove scales and relieve itching. Add an oatmeal preparation (such as Aveeno) or a tar gel (such as AquaTar, Estar Gel, or psoriGel) to your bathwater to soothe your skin.

Once you've added a small amount of the bath product to your water, relax and soak for about 20 minutes. Soaking adds moisture to your skin and promotes absorption of tar gels.

While you soak, use a soft brush to gently loosen psoriasis scales.

After bathing, pat tender skin dry with a soft towel. Remember to pat gently to avoid injury and prevent irritation.

Shampooing

If psoriasis affects your scalp, the doctor may recommend a daily shampoo with a tar-based medicine. If so, work the shampoo into your scalp and leave it on for at least 10 minutes before you rinse your hair. After shampooing, remove the scales with a fine-toothed comb.

Tip: If you have severe scaling, apply mineral oil or a prescribed medicine overnight to help loosen the scales so that you can remove them during your morning shampoo.

Applying medicine

Once you're dried off, apply your prescribed medicine. If you notice any unusual redness or burning, stop using the medicine and notify the doctor.

Memorize the directions on your medicine label — especially if you need to reapply your medicine 2 or 3 times a day.

If you're applying a *topical corticosteroid,* you can increase its absorption by using an occlusive dressing. Depending on the site and size of the treated area, you may cover up with plastic gloves, plastic wrap, or a vinyl exercise suit.

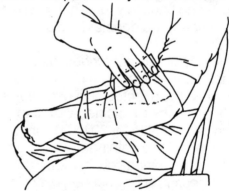

Apply your medicine at bedtime. Then cover the area with the plastic dressing and secure the dressing with tape. You'll remove the dressing the next morning.

If you're using a *tar-based product, never* wear a plastic dressing. This could cause a severe burn.

If the doctor recommends a combination of tar and a topical corticosteroid (for increased effectiveness), apply one on top of the other. Again, *avoid using a plastic dressing.*

Dermatitis

With dermatitis, patients are usually so uncomfortable that they seek medical attention right away, only to learn that relief from this skin inflammation may become a life-long struggle. Your goals, then, are to teach them how to recognize dermatitis and relieve pruritus, and thus promote healing. To accomplish these goals, you'll help them identify aggravating factors by exploring their occupations, life-styles, hobbies, and stressors. Most important, you'll teach a meticulous skin care regimen that includes medications, baths, and dressings. You'll also discuss the pathophysiology of dermatitis, how to identify the disorder, and the role of activity and diet.

Discuss the disorder

Because dermatitis has many names, your patient may be confused about exactly what he has. Tell him that the popular term for dermatitis is "eczema." Then, as appropriate, explain that the most common types are *atopic dermatitis,* caused by an inherited immunologic response, and *contact dermatitis,* caused by an acquired immunologic response. Atopic dermatitis may last through a lifetime of exacerbations and remissions; contact dermatitis is usually incidental. In both disorders, pruritic skin causes the patient to scratch, which produces a rash and lesions. The rash and lesions, in turn, cause pruritus and perpetuate the cycle.

Inform the patient that *atopic dermatitis* may be related to immunoglobulin gamma E (IgE) and cell-mediated hypersensitivity combined with decreased sebum production and increased transepidermal water loss. Typically beginning between ages 2 and 6 months, atopic dermatitis affects 9 of every 1,000 persons. In infants, erythematous, papulovesicular (red, blisterlike), exudative lesions appear on the face, arms, and legs (see *Lesion patterns in pediatric atopic dermatitis,* page 580). Explain that remission sometimes occurs spontaneously around ages 2 or 3, but that dermatitis may recur when the patient encounters aggravating factors (see *What triggers atopic dermatitis?* page 581). Older patients usually have a history of asthma, allergic rhinitis, or familial allergies.

Explain the acute form of atopic dermatitis: a red, bumpy, swollen rash that itches intensely. Scratching the rash produces oozing, crusted lesions. Explain its chronic form, which is characterized by barklike skin with thickened lesions and hypopigmented (white) and hyperpigmented (brown) areas. Besides having sensitive skin, patients with atopic dermatitis experience increased

Marcia Jo Hill, RN, MSN, who wrote this chapter, is manager of dermatologic therapeutics at Methodist Hospital, Houston.

CHECKLIST

Teaching topics in dermatitis

☐ Explanation of the type of dermatitis: atopic or contact, including causes and signs and symptoms
☐ Preventing complications—permanent skin damage and skin infections—by compliance with treatment
☐ Diagnosis by appearance and by patch testing to identify allergens
☐ Activity restrictions and diet's role in treatment
☐ Medications, including antihistamines, topical corticosteroids, and emollients
☐ How to take a therapeutic bath and how to care for the skin
☐ How to apply a total body wrap
☐ How to apply wet-to-dry dressings
☐ Importance of identifying and avoiding known allergens and aggravating factors
☐ Sources of information and support

Lesion patterns in pediatric atopic dermatitis

Depending on the child's age, the rash and lesions in atopic dermatitis form a characteristic pattern. Use this chart to prepare the parents for the lesions' approximate progression over 4 years.

AGE 2 to 9 MONTHS

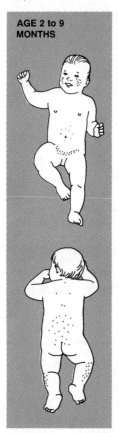
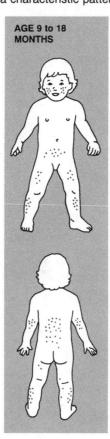

AGE 9 to 18 MONTHS

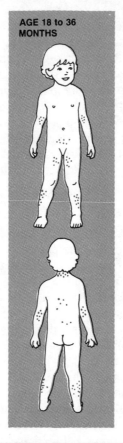

AGE 18 to 36 MONTHS

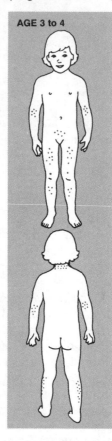

AGE 3 to 4

OLDER THAN AGE 4

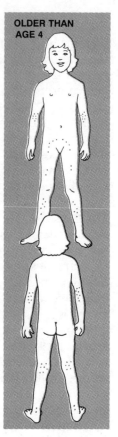

sweating, which transports lipids and water from the skin, leaving it dry and pruritic.

Tell the patient that *contact dermatitis* is an acquired disorder, resulting from prolonged, repeated contact with an allergen. It causes intense pruritus and, depending on the severity, a rash that progresses similarly to that of atopic dermatitis. The rash is typically localized but in severe cases, it may generalize. Warn the patient that subsequent exposures to the allergen may produce a reaction in 24 to 48 hours. Inform him that usually contact dermatitis isn't chronic but can become chronic with repeated exposure.

Complications
Emphasize that strict compliance with the prescribed treatment may help the patient avoid or postpone complications. Without proper treatment, dermatitis can cause permanent skin damage, including lichenification (a thickening and hardening of the skin,

with exaggerated normal markings), altered pigmentation, and scarring.

Warn the patient that uncontrolled *atopic dermatitis* increases his susceptibility to bacterial and fungal infections—and viral infections, such as vaccinia and herpes simplex, which can lead to the potentially fatal Kaposi's varicelliform eruption.

Tell the patient with severe, *chronic contact dermatitis* that the disorder can progress to exfoliative dermatitis—a medical emergency. In this disorder, peeling disrupts the skin's integrity and barrier function, causing thermoregulatory problems, electrolyte imbalances, protein and iron losses, and secondary infection. What's more, if the patient has heart disease, he may experience congestive heart failure. Urge the patient to seek immediate medical attention for localized dermatitis that spreads.

Describe the diagnostic workup
Inform the patient that the doctor diagnoses dermatitis from the patient's and his family's health histories, the lesions' appearance, and blood and allergy test results.

Tests for atopic dermatitis
Describe a simple test for atopic dermatitis: The doctor will firmly stroke the patient's skin with a blunt instrument. Then he'll watch for a white—*not reddened*—dermatographism (hive) to appear. This skin response commonly occurs in patients with atopic dermatitis.

Then explain that the doctor will order blood tests to check for elevated IgE and eosinophil levels, which are indicators of atopic dermatitis. Add that he'll also order tissue cultures to rule out bacterial, fungal, or viral superinfections. (Patients with chronic dermatitis typically have chronic *Staphylococcus aureus* infections.) Finally, he'll order allergy testing if there is any indication of allergic rhinitis or asthma with the clinical skin manifestations.

Tests for contact dermatitis
Tell the patient that the doctor diagnoses contact dermatitis in the same way as atopic dermatitis, but that he'll also examine lesion distribution, which may help to pinpoint allergens. For example, if the lesions appear only on a woman's ear, wrist, and finger, the allergen may be a metal found in jewelry.

Then after treatment to "quiet" the skin during the acute phase, the doctor will probably order patch testing to help identify the allergen. For more information, see *Identifying allergens,* page 582. Also provide the patient with a copy of the teaching aid *Finding the cause of your contact dermatitis,* page 587, to help him identify allergens.

Describe the *patch test* procedure. Explain how the doctor applies allergens to small disks of filter paper attached to aluminum and coated with plastic. Then he tapes these disks to clear, hairless skin on the patient's back or inner forearm to see if the patches cause the skin to react—typically with hives, redness, and

What triggers atopic dermatitis?

If your patient has atopic dermatitis, he'll want to discover what triggers his attacks so that he can take steps to avoid them. Tell him that common triggers include:
• irritants, such as soaps, household cleansers, chemicals, and certain fabrics, for example, wool
• activities that induce sweating
• inhaled or ingested allergens (or both)
• scratching or other skin trauma
• emotional stress
• infections
• environmental temperature changes and heat and humidity.

Identifying allergens

Different allergens produce reactions on different parts of the body. Use this diagram to target contact points and identify possible allergens.

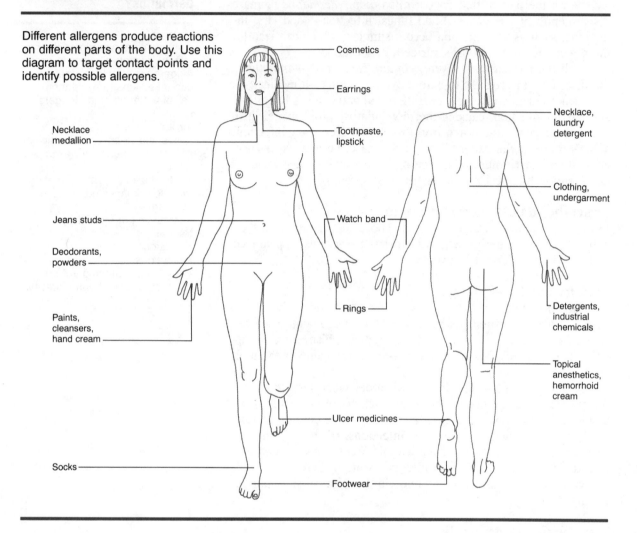

Cosmetics

Earrings

Toothpaste, lipstick

Necklace medallion

Necklace, laundry detergent

Clothing, undergarment

Jeans studs

Watch band

Deodorants, powders

Paints, cleansers, hand cream

Rings

Detergents, industrial chemicals

Topical anesthetics, hemorrhoid cream

Ulcer medicines

Socks

Footwear

pruritus if the patch contains an allergen. Tell the patient not to touch the patches for 48 hours. However, if pain, pruritus, or irritation develops, he should remove them immediately.

Inform the patient that a skin reaction proves contact sensitivity to an allergen, but he should bear in mind that it doesn't necessarily confirm that the specific allergen caused the dermatitis. It is possible that no allergen will be identified.

Teach about treatments

Explain that the best treatment for dermatitis is prevention—avoiding known allergens and other aggravating factors. When this fails, adhering to the prescribed skin care regimen becomes all-important. This regimen includes using medications (topical corticosteroids and bland emollients), taking tepid baths, using nonperfumed soaps, and applying wet wraps or wet-to-dry dressings (depending on whether the skin is erythrodermic or exudative).

Other measures may include activity and diet restrictions and systemic antihistamines to control itching.

Activity
Tell the patient with *atopic dermatitis* that he'll have to curtail his activities temporarily for treatment when his disorder flares up. Otherwise, he can perform his usual activities with the following two exceptions: He should avoid strenuous exercise or any activity that makes him perspire because sweating compounds symptoms. And he should try to avoid activities that cause stress, which can aggravate his symptoms.

Encourage him (especially if he's a child), however, to pursue moderate activity. Then teach him how to cleanse and moisturize his skin after exercise. If he can't avoid stress, refer him to a counselor or encourage him to find a local stress management support group.

Inform the patient with *contact dermatitis* that he needn't restrict activities unless they involve contact with an allergen.

Diet
Explain that diet's value in dermatitis treatment remains controversial. Although patch tests and elimination diets may be used to identify food allergies, test results aren't always reliable. Besides, elimination diets are tedious and difficult to follow, especially for children. Explain that the patient's best bet is to avoid any food that he knows precipitates dermatitis. Common food allergens include eggs, cow's milk, shellfish, and foods containing soybeans, nuts, and wheat.

Medication
Tell the patient that prescribed medications help to reduce inflammation, relieve pruritus, and promote healing. Then describe a typical medication regimen that includes a systemic antihistamine, a topical corticosteroid, and a bland emollient. If severe dermatitis doesn't respond to topical treatment, the doctor may order systemic corticosteroids.

Other possible medications include antibiotics for bacterial infections and antifungals, antivirals, and anti-infectives, as needed. Warn the patient against self-treatment. Explain that some home remedies and well-advertised, over-the-counter "miracle cures" may contain substances (allergens) that do more harm than good.

Antihistamines. Discuss how systemic antihistamines, such as hydroxyzine hydrochloride (Atarax) and diphenhydramine hydrochloride (Benadryl), relieve pruritus. Tell the patient that he may have to take antihistamines around the clock until the scratch-itch-scratch cycle breaks. Suggest that he drink water or use ice chips if the drug causes dry mouth. Warn him that he'll feel drowsy at first, so he should approach physical activity with extra caution. Reassure him that his drowsiness will decrease with continued drug use (see *Questions patients ask about antihistamines,* page 584).

584 Dermatitis

Questions patients ask about antihistamines

Can I become addicted to antihistamines?
No, you can't. Besides being used to relieve itching, antihistamines are sometimes used for their mild, calming effect. However, unlike other drugs used for this same purpose, antihistamines aren't physically addictive.

I get so sleepy at work when I take antihistamines. What can I do to wake up?
First, try taking the drug when you're at home and see how you react. Then take it at work. If drowsiness begins to interfere with your job performance, tell the doctor. He may be able to change the amount you take or switch you to another antihista-mine that won't make you as tired. Sometimes people who take antihistamines for a long time begin to tolerate the medicine and don't feel quite so tired.

Of course, if your job involves driving a car, operating machinery, or performing any other task that requires 100% percent alertness, you'll have to take time off while you're on antihistamines.

Can I drink while I'm taking antihistamines?
No. Alcohol and antihistamines intensify each other's effects. You become drowsier and tipsier faster than if you were either taking an antihistamine or drinking an alcoholic beverage.

Tell the parents of a child taking diphenhydramine hydrochloride that the drug may induce hyperexcitability rather than drowsiness. If this happens, they should contact the doctor who may then order a different antihistamine.

Corticosteroids. Explain that topical corticosteroids reduce pruritus and inflammation and act as skin barriers. They also act as vasoconstrictors to counteract vasodilation and inflammation associated with erythroderma. Mention that corticosteroids are available as cream or ointment, but that ointments are preferred for dermatitis because they're more occlusive. Then explain that corticosteroids come in varying strengths.

Inform the patient that the doctor chooses a corticosteroid based on the severity of dermatitis and the body area affected. Some areas absorb topical drugs more completely than other areas, which increases the risk of toxicity. That's why the doctor rarely prescribes high-potency corticosteroids, such as clobetasol (Temovate) and betamethasone dipropionate (Diprolene), for extensive dermatitis. And that's why such high-potency fluorinated corticosteroids as betamethasone valerate (Celestoderm-V) are never applied to the face, axillae, or groin.

The doctor may recommend midpotency corticosteroids, such as triamcinolone acetonide (Kenalog), for acute dermatitis on all areas except the face, axillae, and groin. These areas respond well to hydrocortisone acetate (Cortef).

Urge the patient to follow application instructions precisely, especially with long-term use. Show him how to apply all topical medications with downward strokes. Explain that stroking in the direction of hair growth minimizes the risk of folliculitis.

Discuss possible adverse reactions. Tell the patient to watch for skin atrophy, easy bruising, and striae. Other possible reactions include slight burning, pruritus, dryness, and skin eruptions.

Explain that percutaneous absorption can increase with long-term use, with occlusion, or with application to broken skin. Inform him that systemic effects occur only after years of use. Instruct him to discontinue the medication and notify his doctor if he develops any adverse reactions or if his dermatitis doesn't seem to be responding.

Bland emollients. Inform the patient that the doctor may recommend using a bland emollient, such as petrolatum, along with a topical corticosteroid. This creates a better skin barrier to maintain homeostasis and skin hydration. Advise him to apply the emollient after the corticosteroid. Explain that with remission the doctor may advise him to discontinue corticosteroid therapy and use emollients only. Tell him to apply emollients after he takes a therapeutic bath.

Procedures

Explain self-care procedures to help dermatitis, including therapeutic baths, wet wraps, wet-to-dry dressings, and for severe dermatitis, occlusive dressings.

Therapeutic baths. Although some doctors restrict bathing because of its drying effect, others suggest soaking in tepid water containing nonperfumed bath oil or colloidal oatmeal. This soothes the skin by helping it retain moisture and, thus, reduce pruritus. Caution the patient to avoid hot baths because heat induces pruritus by increasing vasodilation. Instruct him to use a soft towel to pat excess moisture from his skin (rubbing induces pruritus) and immediately apply the recommended hydrophobic occlusive preparations (such as corticosteroid ointment, petrolatum, or even vegetable shortening). This helps to seal in moisture, enhancing water absorption. To help prevent exacerbations, the patient should continue this regimen even after dermatitis resolves.

For daily cleanliness, advise the patient to use mild, nonperfumed soap with minimal defatting (detergent) activity and a neutral pH—or a prescribed nonsoap cleansing agent.

Wet wraps. For severe or persistent dermatitis in children or adults, the doctor may recommend wet wraps to optimize hydration and topical therapy. To do a total body wrap, tell the patient first to soak a pair of pajamas or long underwear in water and wring out the excess moisture. Then instruct him to apply his medication and step into the wet pajamas or long underwear.

Next, tell him to cover the wet clothes with dry pajamas, dry clothes, or a dry or plastic sweatsuit. He should cover his hands and feet with wet tube socks and then with dry ones. Or he can wrap his hands and feet with wet Kerlix gauze followed by dry elastic bandages.

Instruct him to cover his face with two layers of wet Kerlix gauze, then two layers of dry Kerlix gauze, holding the layers in place with a tubular bandage retainer (such as SurgiNet or Spandage). Naturally, he'll cut holes for his eyes, nose, and mouth. Explain that the gradual water evaporation will reduce inflammation and pruritus. Caution him to keep the room warm so that he doesn't become chilled.

Wet-to-dry dressings. Show the patient with oozing lesions how to apply a wet-to-dry dressing. Then give him a copy of the patient-teaching aid *How to apply wet-to-dry dressings,* page 590, for later review.

Occlusive dressings. In severe dermatitis, show the patient how to use an occlusive dressing. For example, hands with severe contact dermatitis may require a topical corticosteroid and occlusion with gloves to increase drug absorption and skin hydration.

Other care measures

For patients with *atopic dermatitis,* stress the importance of identifying and avoiding aggravating factors and allergens. Remind the patient to wear rubber gloves when cleaning and to rinse his laundry twice to ensure that all detergent washes away. Suggest that he investigate possible irritants associated with his daily life. For example, if he's a house painter, could he be allergic to paint thinner? Do his coveralls make him feel itchy? Do they rub or occlude his skin? Finally, remind him to seek medical attention for such signs of infection as chills, fever, pain, tenderness, warmth, or drainage from sores.

For patients with *contact dermatitis,* discuss the importance of finding the source of the inflammation and then avoiding it. Stress that this involves the cooperation of the patient, nurse, and doctor. Tell the patient to think carefully about substances he comes into contact with regularly, such as cosmetics, drugs, or home remedies. Chances are he's allergic to one or more of them. And don't forget plants—for example, poison ivy, oak, and sumac. They can cause severe contact dermatitis. Offer him a copy of the patient-teaching aid *Recognizing plants that cause dermatitis,* pages 588 and 589.

Sources of information and support

American Dermatologic Society of Allergy and Immunology
Department of Dermatology, Mayo Clinic, Rochester, Minn. 55905
(507) 284-2555

Dermatology Foundation
1563 Maple Avenue, Evanston, Ill. 60201
(312) 328-2256

Further readings

Adams, R.M., et al. "What's New in Occupational Dermatitis?" *Patient Care* 21(12):151-53, 157-58, 160+, July 15, 1987.
Fisher, A.A., et al. "When to Suspect Cosmetic Dermatitis," *Patient Care* 22(11):29-31, 35-38, 43-45+, June 15, 1988.
Grimstone, D. "Occupational Health: Rash Behavior," *Nursing Times* 83(41):47-48, 50-51, October 14-20, 1987.
Nicol, N.H. "Atopic Dermatitis: The (Wet) Wrap-Up," *American Journal of Nursing* 87(12):1560-63, December 1987.
Parker, F. "The Skin and the Elements: Sun, Plants, and Stinging and Biting Organisms," *Emergency Care Quarterly* 4(3):21-31, November 1988.
Sampson, H.A. "Late-phase Response to Food in Atopic Dermatitis," *Hospital Practice* 22(12):111-18, 121, 127-28, December 15, 1987.

PATIENT-TEACHING AID

Finding the cause of your contact dermatitis

Dear Patient:

Once you find what's causing or aggravating your dermatitis, you've won half the battle. But finding it may take some detective work.

First, think of the things you come in contact with daily—at work, at home, and outside. And don't overlook your toiletries and cosmetics. You may develop an allergy to something you've been using for years. Besides, manufacturers commonly change product formulas.

Mark the substances that you suspect from the following list.

Allergic to something at work?

Depending on your occupation, your skin may react to animal bites, anesthetics, arsenic, benzene, carbon paper, cement, chrome, cleaners, dry cleaning fluid, dyes, fabric finishes, or formaldehyde. Also consider glue, grease, ink, jewelers' rouge, lacquers, lead, nickel, oil, paints, plastics, rubber, solvents, or turpentine.

Allergic to something at home?

Your skin may react to animal hairs, antibiotics, antiseptics, bleaches, detergents, disinfectants, feathers, insecticides, jewelry, laundry products, polishes, or raw meats. Consider what you wear: fur, silk, or wool.

Allergic to something outside?

Whether you do yard work or just admire nature, you may find you're allergic to flowers, such as chrysanthemums and geraniums, or to fertilizers, grasses, pesticides, or trees. You may also be allergic to insect bites or stings or to plants, especially poison ivy, oak, and sumac. Consider also extreme weather, fungi, ivy, mites, and molds.

Allergic to cosmetics?

Cosmetics and toiletries are among the worst offenders. They contain many substances that can cause rashes. Read labels. Even some "hypoallergenic" preparations contain ingredients that cause allergic reactions. Look for *formaldehyde, lanolin, PABA, parabens, quaternium-15, 3-diol (Bronopol), 2-bromo-2-nitropropane-1, ureas,* and *wool wax.*

Contact with the following products may cause dermatitis.
- Bath products: astringents, antiperspirants, bubble bath, deodorants, lotions, moisturizers, oils, perfumes, powders, and soaps
- Eye products: false eyelashes and glue, liners, mascara, pencils, and shadows
- Face products: blusher, creams, makeup bases, masks, and powders
- Hair products: colors, rinses, shampoos, sprays, and tonics
- Lip products: glosses, liners, lipsticks, and lotion
- Nail products: conditioners, cuticle removers, false fingernails and glue, hardeners, and polishes
- Shaving products: aftershave lotions, creams, and depilatories
- Other products: douches, sun lotions, sunscreens, and topical anesthetics

Recognizing plants that cause dermatitis

Dear Patient:

Although many plants can cause allergic reactions in sensitive people, three plants cause them in almost everyone. These plants are poison ivy, poison oak, and poison sumac.

All three plants produce *urushiol,* a strong allergy-causing oil. Poison ivy, in fact, produces this oil year-round, even in the winter when the leaves dry up.

If you're sensitive, you can get dermatitis without even touching these plants. For instance, you could get a rash simply from minute, airborne particles of these plants in the smoke of burning brush. Or you could break out from touching pets, sports equipment, or gardening tools that have had contact with urushiol.

By far the most common way to contract dermatitis from these plants is by touching them. Your best defense is to get to know them—and then avoid them.

Poison ivy
Remember the old saying about poison ivy: "Leaves of three, quickly flee." Watch for a small, harmless-looking plant, vine, or low shrub with shiny grean leaflets that grow in groups of three. Waxy, yellow-green flowers and, later, greenish berries, decorate the leaf stems. In the fall, look for the leaves to turn red.

Poison ivy grows everywhere in the United States, except California and parts of adjacent states. It flourishes in the eastern and central states.

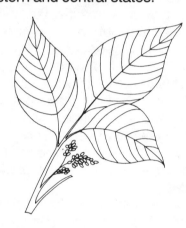

Poison oak
The leaves of poison oak also grow in groups of three. Shaped like oak leaves, they have hairy, light green undersides and darker green surfaces. Poison oak shrubs or vines that bear fruit (not all do) have clustered greenish or creamy white berries. The plant grows on the West Coast from Mexico to British Columbia.

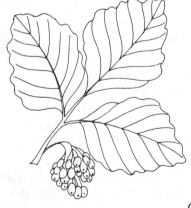

continued

Recognizing plants that cause dermatitis — *continued*

Poison sumac

With 7 to 13 long, smooth, paired leaves, the poison sumac branch is topped with a single velvety leaf. Bright orange in springtime, the plant's leaf surfaces later turn a glossy dark green with a pale green underside — only to change to reddish orange in the fall. Poison sumac has drooping clusters of green berries; nonpoisonous sumac has upright red berries.

If you're in the eastern United States, you can't miss these colorful woody shrubs. They grow from 5 to 25 feet tall and thrive in swampy areas.

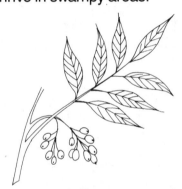

If you're exposed

Even if you've never had a reaction to poison ivy, oak, or sumac, you're not home free. Some people become allergic to them only after years of repeated exposure. Here's how to protect yourself:

- Immediately after contact, wash the affected skin with soap and cold water. (Hot water may make you itch.) Use yellow or brown laundry soap if you have some. Use nonperfumed bath soap if you don't. Lather several times, rinsing the area in running water after each sudsing.
- Use your hands to create the lather. Don't use a brush that could scratch your skin.

- If you're in the woods far from modern plumbing, try to find a brook or stream. Washing your hands and skin in this naturally running water should do the job.
- Wash, rewash, and thoroughly rinse any clothing that touched a plant containing urushiol.
- Wash any pet that touched the plant, too. But first put on rubber gloves so you don't come in contact with your pet's fur. Throw away the gloves when you're finished.

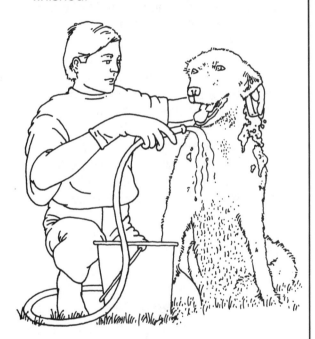

If you get a rash

If preventive measures fail and you notice a mild rash developing, apply cool compresses soaked in water or Burow's solution. Spread calamine lotion or other preparation with calamine in it, such as Caladryl, over the rash to help dry the area while also relieving the itching. If you get a severe rash, don't treat it yourself. Ask your doctor for advice.

How to apply wet-to-dry dressings

Dear Patient:

Wet-to-dry dressings can help relieve flare-ups of dermatitis; soothe inflammation, itching, and burning; remove crusting and scales from dry lesions; and help dry up oozing lesions.

What's more, using these dressings may prevent such complications as bacterial or fungal infections. You can apply the dressings in four steps. Here's how:

For an acute flare-up

1 Moisten a piece of gauze or a soft, clean cloth with warm tap water, normal saline solution, or Burow's solution. Squeeze out the excess moisture. Don't squeeze the gauze or cloth completely dry; it should still make a squishy sound when gently squeezed.

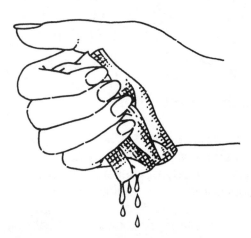

2 Apply the wet dressing to the affected skin area, making sure you cover all of the rash.

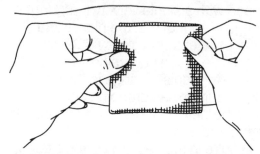

3 Hold the dressing in place with dry roller gauze or pin a towel to hold the dressing in place. Allow the dressing to air dry for about 20 minutes.

Note: Don't hold the dressing in place with tape because the adhesive may irritate your skin.

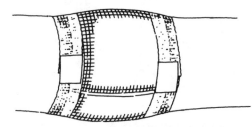

4 Remove the dressing without remoistening it, and apply the topical preparations as prescribed by your doctor.

Repeat the entire procedure every 4 to 6 hours, changing the dressing material every 24 hours.

For a generalized flare-up

Follow the steps above. At step 2, first apply the ointment or cream your doctor prescribed. Then apply the wet dressing as directed. This will make your blood vessels constrict, leaving your skin feeling cool. It also will help your sore, irritated skin absorb the medicine and decrease inflammation and itching.

Alopecia

Because alopecia, or hair loss, has many causes and affects many kinds of patients—from cancer patients to new mothers—you'll thoroughly review your patient's health history to individualize your teaching. Whether hair loss is mild or severe, temporary or permanent, it can exact a high emotional toll, so be prepared to offer plenty of emotional support along with your teaching.

What topics will you cover? Include a review of normal hair growth and of the kinds and causes of alopecia. Explain tests the patient may undergo to determine the cause of hair loss. As you adapt your teaching strategies to the patient's situation, you'll discuss possible treatments, surgery to transplant or graft hair, cosmetic options (wigs or hairpieces), a healthful diet, and daily hair care. With cancer patients, you'll cover ways to minimize hair loss and to care for the hair and scalp during cancer treatment.

Discuss the disorder

Tell the patient that alopecia involves partial or total hair loss usually from the scalp but also from other body areas. Alopecia may progress slowly and irreversibly with changes in hair structures, or it may progress rapidly and temporarily from a disruption in the normal hair-growth cycle (see *Reviewing the normal hair-growth cycle,* page 592, and *What causes alopecia?* page 593).

As you discuss normal hair growth, make sure to cover normal hair loss, noting that a healthy person loses about 100 hairs a day simply from brushing, shampooing, and shedding. Add that the hair grows back at the same rate. Problems arise when hair loss exceeds new growth.

Review the main types of alopecia: scarring and nonscarring. Explain that *scarring alopecia* involves inflammation and destruction of the follicular structure, which may cause irreversible hair loss. Typical signs and symptoms include patchy hair loss, erythema, and excessive scaling that leaves a pale, shiny, smooth scalp. In contrast, *nonscarring alopecia* seldom involves destruction of the follicular structure. This means that the hair follicle can usually reproduce hair. Explain that several types of nonscarring alopecia are potentially reversible. For more information, refer to *Signs and symptoms of nonscarring alopecia,* page 594.

Describe the diagnostic workup

Tell the patient that tests for alopecia are simple and painless. The doctor starts by observing the patient's hair and scalp. He does a "pluck" or "pull" test, firmly and smoothly tugging a group of 8

CHECKLIST

Teaching topics in alopecia

☐ Explanation of normal hair growth
☐ Types of alopecia—scarring and nonscarring
☐ Causes of alopecia
☐ Diagnostic tests, including microscopic examination, trichogram, and scalp biopsy
☐ Importance of a nutritious diet for healthy hair
☐ Medications, including minoxidil, and their use
☐ Ways to minimize alopecia during cancer treatment by using scalp tourniquets and cold caps
☐ Hair transplantation surgery and tunnel grafting
☐ Cosmetic measures, such as wigs and toupees
☐ Hair care tips
☐ Hair and scalp care during cancer treatment
☐ Sources of information and support

Pamela J. Currie, RN, MSN, CRNP, who wrote this chapter, is a nurse practitioner at the University of Pennsylvania Student Health Service, Philadelphia.

Reviewing the normal hair-growth cycle

Inform the patient that disruption in the normal hair-growth cycle can result in unusual hair loss. Sum up the normal hair-growth process by explaining that as hair cells multiply, they are forced upward and become keratinized (converted to keratin, the protein that composes hair). These keratinized cells grow for long periods until they die, shed, and are replaced by new hairs. Then familiarize the patient with the terminology used to describe hair structure and hair-growth stages.

Hair structures
Describe the *shaft* or visible part of the hair and the *root,* which is embedded in the scalp. The root and its inner and outer root sheaths form the bulb-shaped hair *follicle.*

Below the follicle, the *dermal papilla,* which is a loop of capillaries encased in connective tissue, supplies blood and innervation. Over the papilla lie clusters of epithelial cells that reproduce, eventually forming the hair shaft.

Three stages of hair growth
Tell the patient that hair grows through three stages. From 80% to 90% of a healthy person's scalp hair is in the *anagen (growth) stage.* This stage lasts for 3 to 10 years.

The *catagen (transitional) stage* follows the anagen stage and lasts for about 3 weeks. During this stage, the blood supply to the follicle diminishes; thinning and decreased pigmentation occur; and the follicle thickens, forming a short "club" hair that gradually moves closer to the skin surface. This stage progresses as the club hair pushes upward and the follicle below shortens until it's only a small nipple, called a "secondary germ."

In the *telogen stage,* which also lasts for about 3 weeks, the developing anagen hair forces the club hair through the scalp. Between 10% and 20% of scalp hair is in the telogen stage at any time.

Inform the patient that as long as anatomic structures remain intact and alive and as long as the cycle remains uninterrupted, hair will eventually regrow.

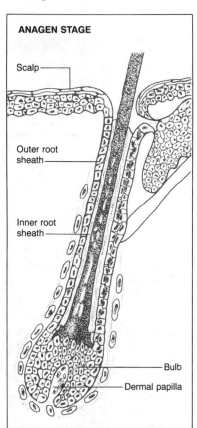

ANAGEN STAGE

Scalp

Outer root sheath

Inner root sheath

Bulb

Dermal papilla

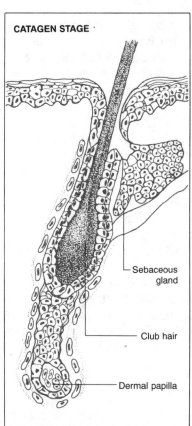

CATAGEN STAGE

Sebaceous gland

Club hair

Dermal papilla

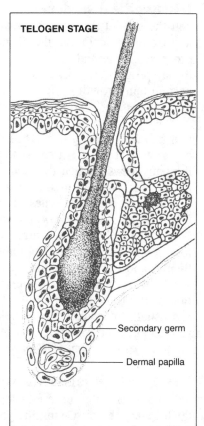

TELOGEN STAGE

Secondary germ

Dermal papilla

to 10 hairs. If more than 4 hairs come out, the patient probably has alopecia. Other tests include microscopic analyses, Wood's lamp examination, trichogram, and biopsy. Mention that the doctor may order other studies—usually blood tests—to rule out a systemic disease (such as syphilis) as a cause of alopecia.

Microscopic analyses
If the results of the "pluck" test are positive, the doctor will probably examine some hairs under a microscope to check for structural abnormalities or signs of infection.

Wood's lamp examination
If the doctor suspects a fungal infection, he'll examine the bald patch under a Wood's fluorescent lamp. He'll watch for the area to glow, or fluoresce (a positive sign). Then he may scrape the scalp lightly and view the scrapings microscopically to identify the fungus.

Trichogram
Once he diagnoses alopecia, the doctor may use a trichogram to determine the ratio of anagen to telogen hairs. This enables him to evaluate the severity and predict the course of the patient's alopecia. Explain that the doctor will grasp about 50 hairs with rubber-tipped forceps and place them on a slide for observation. Later, he may repeat the test to chart progression or improvement.

Biopsy
Explain that a scalp biopsy may help determine alopecia's cause. For this brief test, the doctor numbs the biopsy site with a local anesthetic and then obtains a scalp tissue sample (usually with a punch instrument). Tell the patient that pressure will be applied to control minimal bleeding. Caution him not to shampoo his hair or brush it vigorously for 24 hours after the test.

Teach about treatments
Advise the patient that treatment depends on the amount of hair loss and the type of alopecia. Unfortunately, for some patients no treatment can restore hair. For others, medication (minoxidil, corticosteroids, and other drugs to treat systemic diseases causing alopecia) or surgery (hair transplantation) may help. As appropriate, discuss ways to minimize hair loss from chemotherapy (scalp cooling and scalp tourniquets). Also discuss cosmetic interventions (hairpieces and hair weaving or bonding), a healthful diet, and proper hair care.

Diet
Tell the patient that a well-balanced diet with adequate protein promotes healthy hair. Review the four food groups, emphasizing foods high in protein. Warn against crash diets and fasting, which may cause dry, brittle hair and hair loss. As appropriate, refer the patient to a dietitian or nutritionist for help with meal planning. If alopecia results from excessive vitamin A, advise the patient to avoid vitamin A supplements.

What causes alopecia?

No matter what kind of alopecia your patient has, he'll most want to know why he's losing his hair. Check below for the most common causes:

Scarring alopecia (usually irreversible)
• physical trauma, such as burns
• severe infections, such as folliculitis or herpes simplex
• chronic fungal disorders, such as *Microsporum* infections
• certain systemic diseases, such as lupus erythematosus, scleroderma, destructive skin tumors, granulomas, and follicular lichen planus
• chronic tension on the hair shaft, such as that caused by long-term tight braiding or a ponytail hairstyle

Nonscarring alopecia (may be reversible)
• febrile illness, such as scarlet fever
• endocrine disorders, such as hypothyroidism and hyperthyroidism
• infections of the scalp or hair follicles, such as tinea capitis (ringworm)
• medications, such as cytotoxic drugs used in chemotherapy, heparin, or oral contraceptives
• nutritional insult, such as hypervitaminosis A
• chemical toxicity, such as thallium excess
• trichotillomania (compulsive hair pulling)
• hormonal changes, such as those that accompany childbirth and aging (menopause)
• genetic predisposition, such as male pattern baldness

Signs and symptoms of nonscarring alopecia

Inform the patient that about 90% of all hair loss can be attributed to nonscarring alopecia.

Alopecia areata
Most common in young and middle-aged adults, this sudden hair loss leaves smooth, round, almost bare patches. Causes are unknown.

Anagen effluvium
This sudden diffuse shedding of growing hair typically follows cytotoxic drug or radiation therapy.

Male pattern baldness
Starting at the roots, hair gradually thins—with or without increased shedding. In men, the hairline recedes and the crown becomes bald. In women, the part widens and the front scalp or crown becomes visible. Causes include genetics, aging, and androgen levels.

Telogen effluvium
Sudden diffuse shedding starts at the hair roots after severe illness, surgery, childbirth, drug therapy, nutritional changes, or stopping of oral contraceptives, and usually is irreversible.

Tinea capitis
Patchy hair loss with scaling, redness, and stubble or black dots (which indicate breakage) may result from a fungal infection, such as ringworm.

Trichorrhexis nodosa
Hair breaks, grows unevenly, or doesn't grow beyond a short length. Trichorrhexis nodosa may follow overuse of chemicals or heat.

Trichotillomania
Most common in children and adolescents, patchy hair loss occurs in a random or geometric pattern. The dotlike stubble indicates breakage, but the surrounding scalp usually looks normal.

Medication
Drugs prescribed to help restore hair include minoxidil (Rogaine) and corticosteroids. Other drug therapy may include photochemotherapy with methoxsalen (Oxsoralen) and ultraviolet light, dermatomucosal agents, such as anthralin (Anthra-Derm), antibiotics for bacterial infections, or antifungals for fungal infections.

Minoxidil. Inform the patient that minoxidil may help to restore hair loss from male pattern baldness or, possibly, alopecia areata. Tell him that about 40% of patients report moderate to dense hair growth after a year of regular treatment. Explain that ongoing research will establish the drug's effectiveness and safety in long-term use. If appropriate, give him the patient-teaching aid *Learning about topical minoxidil*, page 596.

Corticosteroids. If your patient has alopecia areata, tell him that corticosteroids such as betamethasone dipropionate (Diprolene), halcinonide (Halciderm), and triamcinolone acetonide (Kenalog), in topical form or by intralesional injection, may help to stimulate hair growth if hair loss is confined to small patches.

Review possible adverse reactions to corticosteroid therapy. Instruct the patient to report signs and symptoms of skin infection, such as pain, redness, or pus-filled blisters. He also should contact the doctor if he has new blistering, burning, itching, or peeling; numbness in his fingers; weight gain; facial puffiness; thinning skin with bruising; and any unusual loss of hair.

Instruct the patient to take the medication exactly as directed. Caution him not to use it on any area other than the treatment area and not to share it. Remind him that applying medication in gel, lotion, or spray form may sting mildly.

Procedures
Because so many patients experience alopecia as a side effect of chemotherapy (see *Which cancer drugs cause alopecia?*), discuss procedures that reduce the blood supply to the scalp and thereby preserve more hair structures. Explain that these procedures—scalp tourniquet or cold cap applications—aren't appropriate for patients with leukemia, lymphoma, or highly metastatic tumors because cancer drugs must be allowed to perfuse the scalp area to eradicate cancer cells. Typically, circulation-reducing devices interfere with perfusion. Explain the process and give your patient the teaching aid *Minimizing hair loss from chemotherapy*, page 597.

Surgery
If the patient with male pattern baldness asks, inform him about hair transplantation and tunnel grafting. Usually these procedures are performed out of the hospital.

Explain that the most common hair transplantation technique is "punch grafting." Plugs, or grafts, of the patient's own hair are punched out of hairy areas and moved to bald areas. Advise the patient that if this expensive procedure is successful, it usually fills in the bald areas but not profusely. His new hair growth will appear thinner than the hair that he lost.

Tell the patient that tunnel grafting involves inserting tubes beneath the scalp skin, then using fibers to attach the tubes permanently to a toupee.

Other care measures
Discuss cosmetic options, such as a wig, hairpiece, or toupee. Hairpieces or toupees may be taped to the scalp or attached by interspersing supplemental hair into the existing hair. This expensive hair-weaving technique must be renewed about as often as a haircut. In another semipermanent technique called hair bonding, the toupee is glued to the scalp or to existing hair. Explain that rarely the patient may have an allergic reaction to scalp adhesives.

If your patient will undergo cancer therapy with drugs that cause alopecia or if he's scheduled for radiation, suggest that he select a hair substitute before treatment starts. In this way he can match his natural hair color without guessing. Explain that human hair wigs appear more natural, but they're usually more expensive than synthetic wigs and require more care. Mention that health insurance may cover the cost. Then discuss ways to conserve remaining hair (see *Hair care tips*).

Whether your patient chooses or refuses a wig, suggest keeping alternatives, such as a scarf, turban, or hat on hand for variety and comfort. And make sure to give him the teaching aid *Caring for your hair and scalp during cancer treatment*, page 598.

Sources of information and support

Medical Information (Rogaine)
The Upjohn Company
7000 Portage Road, Kalamazoo, Mich. 49001
(800) 253-8600

National Alopecia Areata Foundation
714 C Street, Suite 216, San Rafael, Calif. 94901
(415) 456-4644

Further readings
Cohen, E., and Woodyard, C. "The Use of Topical Minoxidil in Alopecia," *Physician Assistant* 12(11):27-33, 36, 114, November 1988.
David, J., and Speechley, V. "Scalp Cooling to Prevent Alopecia," *Nursing Times* 83(32):36-37, August 1987.
Giaccone, G. "Scalp Hypothermia in the Prevention of Doxorubicin-Induced Hair Loss," *Cancer Nursing* 11(3):170-73, June 1988.
Keller, J.F., and Blavsey, L.A. "Nursing Issues and Management in Chemotherapy-Induced Alopecia," *Oncology Nursing Forum* 15(5):603-07, September-October 1988.
Molitor, L. "An Underweight Infant with Localized Alopecia," *Journal of Emergency Nursing* 14(6):392, November-December 1988.
Parker, R. "The Effectiveness of Scalp Hypothermia in Preventing Cyclophosphamide-Induced Alopecia," *Oncology Nursing Forum* 14(6):49-53, November-December 1987.
Price, V.H., et al. "Sorting Out the Clues in Alopecia," *Patient Care* 23(14):70-74, 76, 81, September 15, 1989.
Schindler, A.M. "The Boy Whose Hair Came Back," *Hospital Practice* 22(9):185-86, 88, September 15, 1987.
Schlesselman, S.M. "Helping Your Cancer Patient Cope with Alopecia," *Nursing88* 18(12):43-45, December 1988.

Which cancer drugs cause alopecia?

If your patient's undergoing cancer chemotherapy, explain that certain drugs can cause hair loss, ranging from complete baldness to sporadic thinning. Some drugs damage hair follicles and cause hair roots to atrophy.

Severe alopecia
cyclophosphamide (Cytoxan)
daunorubicin (Cerubidine)
doxorubicin (Adriamycin)
vinblastine (Velban)
vincristine (Oncovin)

Moderate alopecia
busulfan (Myleran)
etoposide (VP-16)
floxuridine (FUDR)
methotrexate (Folex)
mitomycin (Mutamycin)

Mild alopecia
bleomycin (Blenoxane)
carmustine (BiCNU)
fluorouracil (5-FU)
hydroxyurea (Hydrea)
melphalan (Alkeran)

Hair care tips

Remind your patient that regular care and grooming can keep remaining hair and any new growth healthy. Offer these tips:
• Don't use harsh hair chemicals, such as permanent wave solutions, hair bleaches, or dyes. These can damage hair, causing splitting and shedding.
• Avoid burning hair with devices such as curling irons and hair dryers at high settings.
• Try smooth rather than toothed rollers and avoid hot curlers.
• Change hairstyles if hair loss comes from traction caused by tight braids or ponytails.
• Camouflage hair loss by restyling hair to cover thinning spots.

Learning about topical minoxidil

Dear Patient:

Your doctor has prescribed minoxidil (also called Rogaine) to treat your hair loss. When applied to the skin, this drug causes hair to grow back.

Before you start using minoxidil on your skin, review the information below. If you have any questions, ask your doctor, nurse, or pharmacist.

How to use minoxidil

• Apply minoxidil once in the morning and again at bedtime.

• Use only the amount specified on the label. Don't use more of the drug and don't use it more often than ordered. Extra amounts won't speed up hair growth or prompt more to grow. Too much of the drug might even cause unwanted side effects.

• Before applying your morning dose, shampoo your hair and towel dry it thoroughly. Then use the supplied applicator to spread the drug. Begin at the center of the bald area.

• If you apply the drug by hand, wash your hands when you're finished.

• Don't use a hair dryer if you're using minoxidil because this might make the drug less effective.

• Let the drug dry for at least 30 minutes after applying your bedtime dose. That way, more will be absorbed by your scalp, less by your pillowcase.

• If you forget to use minoxidil, apply a missed dose as soon as possible. Then resume your regular schedule. However, if it's almost time for your next

dose, skip the missed one and go back to your regular schedule. Don't apply the drug twice or try to make up for a missed dose some other way.

• Stop using the drug temporarily if your scalp gets irritated or sunburned—but check with the doctor first.

• Don't apply any other medicines to your scalp while using minoxidil. Another medicine could interfere with minoxidil's effect or could cause unwanted side effects.

Be alert for side effects

Minoxidil may cause side effects in some patients. The most common ones—dry, flaking, or reddened skin—should subside as your body adjusts to the drug. Other side effects can occur, however, if your body absorbs too much minoxidil. Report the following side effects to your doctor right away:

• breathing difficulties, chest pain, fast or irregular heartbeat, flushing

• headache, dizziness or faintness, numbness or tingling in your hands, feet, or face

• rapid weight gain and swelling of your feet or lower legs.

Also report burning or itching of your scalp, facial swelling, and rash.

Be patient

You may have to use minoxidil for 4 or more months before you see results, and you must use it every day. If you stop using it, hair growth stops and you can expect to lose any new hair within a few months.

Minimizing hair loss from chemotherapy

Dear Patient:

If you're having chemotherapy, you may lose some or all of your hair. However, a scalp tourniquet or a cold cap can help to minimize the extent of your hair loss. Here's how these devices work.

Scalp tourniquets

A scalp tourniquet decreases the blood supply to your scalp. This limits the amount of cancer drug that penetrates your hair follicles.

The nurse will apply the tourniquet 15 minutes before she starts the drug infusion. Either she'll inflate a blood pressure cuff or tie flat latex tubing around your head in sweatband fashion.

SCALP TOURNIQUET

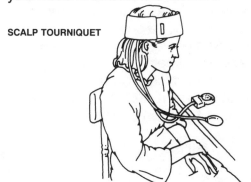

She'll leave this tourniquet in place during the infusion and for at least 10 minutes after the infusion stops.

To keep the tourniquet from loosening, hold your head still and don't talk. However, tell the nurse if you feel dizzy or if the pressure annoys you or gives you a headache.

To avoid these effects, the nurse may offer you acetaminophen (Tylenol) before your treatment.

Cold caps

By using cold to narrow your blood vessels, a cold cap slows the circulation of blood to your scalp. The cooler your scalp becomes, the less drug your scalp tissues will absorb. As a result, your hair will sustain less damage.

The nurse starting the infusion may fashion a cold cap for you. She may use a sturdy plastic bag containing a frozen gel or ice bags filled with crushed ice. She'll mold the bags to your scalp, secure them with gauze, and wrap a towel over them, turban-style.

Or she may give you a commercial chemotherapy cap or a thermocirculator device that pumps a liquid coolant through a nylon cap you'll wear.

CHEMOTHERAPY CAP

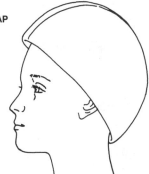

Whichever device you wear, you'll put it on about 15 minutes before your infusion, and you'll wear it for about 30 minutes afterward.

To ward off possible discomfort, the nurse may give you acetaminophen before your treatment. Be sure to report any headache, chills, dizziness, or pressure sensations. Ask for a blanket if you think you'll feel cold.

Caring for your hair and scalp during cancer treatment

Dear Patient:

Some hair loss may be inevitable during chemotherapy or radiation therapy. But *sometimes* you can help minimize hair loss by keeping your hair and scalp clean and treating them gently. Just follow these suggestions.

If you're having chemotherapy
• Keep your hair and scalp clean by shampooing regularly — every 2 to 4 days. (Shampooing every day may be too harsh.)

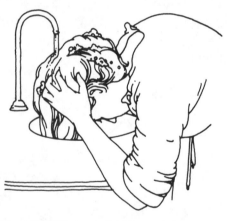

• Use a mild *protein-based* shampoo — for example, Appearance, an apple pectin shampoo. (Baby shampoo isn't necessarily mild.) You may want to talk with a hairdresser to determine which shampoo is best for you.
• Use a creme rinse or conditioner after shampooing.
• Gently pat your hair dry.
• If your scalp is very dry and flaky, try massaging it with mineral oil, castor oil, or vitamin A and D ointment after shampooing and rinsing your hair.

• Brush and comb your hair very gently, using a soft-bristled brush and a wide-toothed, pliable comb.

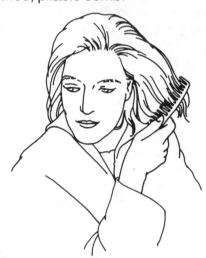

• Avoid harsh chemicals, permanents, and dyes. Also, avoid tight curls or braids. Don't use a curling iron, hot rollers, or a hair dryer. And don't sleep with curlers in your hair.
• To minimize friction on your hair, try sleeping on a satin pillowcase. And to keep your hair from shedding, try using a hair net.
• Wear a hat to protect your scalp from sunburn.

If you're having radiation therapy
• Don't use anything on your scalp except Aquaphor or Eucerin cream. You can buy these products at your local pharmacy without a prescription.
• Once your hair starts to grow back, follow the hair and scalp care instructions listed above.

Index

i refers to an illustration; t refers to a table